Third Edition

ACSM's
Exercise Management for Persons With Chronic Diseases and Disabilities

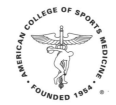

**AMERICAN COLLEGE
of SPORTS MEDICINE**
w w w . a c s m . o r g

J. Larry Durstine, PhD, FACSM
University of South Carolina

Geoffrey E. Moore, MD, FACSM
Cayuga Center for Healthy Living, Ithaca, NY

Patricia L. Painter, PhD, FACSM
University of Minnesota

Scott O. Roberts, PhD, FACSM
California State University

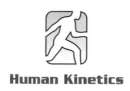

Human Kinetics

Library of Congress Cataloging-in-Publication Data

ACSM's exercise management for persons with chronic diseases and disabilities / American College of Sports Medicine ; editors, J. Larry Durstine ... [et al.]. -- 3rd ed.

p. ; cm.

Rev. ed. of: ACSM's exercise management for persons with chronic diseases and disabilities / American College of Sports Medicine. 2nd ed. c2003.

Includes bibliographical references and index.

ISBN-13: 978-0-7360-7433-9 (hard cover)

ISBN-10: 0-7360-7433-3 (hard cover)

1. Exercise therapy. 2. Exercise tests. 3. Chronic diseases--Exercise therapy. 4. People with disabilities--Rehabilitation. I. Durstine, J. Larry. II. American College of Sports Medicine. III. American College of Sports Medicine. ACSM's exercise management for persons with chronic diseases and disabilities. IV. Title: Exercise management for persons with chronic diseases and disabilities.

[DNLM: 1. Exercise Therapy--standards--Practice Guideline. 2. Chronic Disease--rehabilitation--Practice Guideline. 3. Disabled Persons--rehabilitation--Practice Guideline. 4. Exercise Test--methods--Practice Guideline. WB 541 A187 2009]

RM725.A3 2009

615.8'2--dc22

2009009155

ISBN-10 (print): 0-7360-7433-3

ISBN-13 (print): 978-0-7360-7433-9

ISBN-10 (Adobe PDF): 0-7360-8466-5

ISBN-13 (Adobe PDF): 978-0-7360-8466-6

Copyright © 2009, 2003, 1997 by the American College of Sports Medicine

The Web addresses cited in this text were current as of January 2009, unless otherwise noted.

Acquisitions Editor: Loarn D. Robertson, PhD; **Managing Editor:** Melissa J. Zavala; **Assistant Editor:** Christine Bryant Cohen; **Copyeditor:** Bob Replinger; **Indexer:** Nancy Ball; **Permission Manager:** Dalene Reeder; **Graphic Designer:** Bob Reuther; **Graphic Artists:** Patrick Sandberg and Tara Welsch; **Cover Designer:** Keith Blomberg; **Photographer (interior):** © Human Kinetics, unless otherwise noted; **Photo Asset Manager:** Laura Fitch; **Photo Production Manager:** Jason Allen; **Art Manager:** Kelly Hendren; **Associate Art Manager:** Alan L. Wilborn; **Illustrator:** Alan L. Wilborn; **Printer:** Thomson-Shore, Inc.

ACSM Publications Committee Chair: Jeffrey L. Roitman, EdD, FACSM

ACSM Group Publisher: Kerry O'Rourke

Printed in the United States of America   10   9   8   7   6

The paper in this book is certified under a sustainable forestry program.

Human Kinetics
Web site: www.HumanKinetics.com

United States: Human Kinetics
P.O. Box 5076
Champaign, IL 61825-5076
800-747-4457
e-mail: humank@hkusa.com

Canada: Human Kinetics
475 Devonshire Road, Unit 100
Windsor, ON N8Y 2L5
800-465-7301 (in Canada only)
e-mail: info@hkcanada.com

Europe: Human Kinetics
107 Bradford Road
Stanningley
Leeds LS28 6AT, United Kingdom
+44 (0)113 255 5665
e-mail: hk@hkeurope.com

Australia: Human Kinetics
57A Price Avenue
Lower Mitcham, South Australia 5062
08 8372 0999
e-mail: info@hkaustralia.com

New Zealand: Human Kinetics
P.O. Box 80
Torrens Park, South Australia 5062
0800 222 062
e-mail: info@hknewzealand.com

Contents

Contributors

Senior Editors

J. Larry Durstine, PhD, FACSM
University of South Carolina

Geoffrey E. Moore, MD, FACSM
Syracuse University

Patricia L. Painter, PhD, FACSM
University of Minnesota

Scott O. Roberts, PhD, FACSM
California State University, Chico

Section Editors

Peter H. Brubaker, PhD, FACSM
Wake Forest University

Lorraine E. Colson Bloomquist, EdD, FACSM
University of Rhode Island

Christopher B. Cooper, MD, FACSM
UCLA School of Medicine

Michael J. LaMonte, PhD, FACSM
University of Buffalo

Terry Nicola, MD, MS
University of Illinois, Chicago, IL.

Kenneth H. Pitetti, PhD, FACSM
Wichita State University

Contributors

Ann L. Albright, PhD, RD
Centers for Disease Control and Prevention

Ross Arena, PhD, PT, FACSM
Virginia Commonwealth University

J. Edwin Atwood, MD
Walter Reed Army Hospital

Stephen P. Bailey, PhD, PT, FACSM
Elon University

David L. Balfe, MD
UCLA School of Medicine

Constance Mols Bayles, PhD, FACSM
Center for Healthy Aging, University of
Pittsburgh

Vanina Dal Bello-Haas, PhD, PT
University of Saskatchewan

Thomas J. Birk, PhD, MPT, FACSM
Wayne State University

Susan A. Bloomfield, PhD, FACSM
Texas A&M University

Selena Chan, BS
Center for Healthy Aging, University of
Pittsburgh

Christopher J. Clark, MD
Hairmyers Hospital, University of Glasgow,
Scotland

Lorna M. Cochrane, MD
Hairmyers Hospital, University of Glasgow,
Scotland

Tamar Derghazarian, PT
McGill University

Wesley D. Dudgeon, PhD
The Citadel

M. Kathleen Ellis, PhD
University of Rhode Island

Patricia Fegan, PhD
Special Olympics Maryland, Inc

Stephen F. Figoni, PhD, RKT, FACSM
VA Greater Los Angeles Health Care System

Emma Fletcher, MA
University of South Carolina

Barry A. Franklin, PhD, FACSM
William Beaumont Hospital
Wayne State University

Daniel Friedman, MD, FACSM
New Mexico Presbyterian Heart Group

Andrew W. Gardner, PhD
University of Oklahoma Health Sciences Center

Neil F. Gordon, MD, PhD, MPH, FACSM
Nationwide Better Health

Gregory A. Hand, PhD, FACSM
University of South Carolina

Kimberly B. Harbst, PhD, PT
University of Wisconsin-La Crosse

W. Guyton Hornsby, Jr., PhD, CDE, FACSM
West Virginia University

Connie C.W. Hsia, MD
University of Texas Southwestern Medical Center

Reed Humphrey, PhD, PT, FACSM
University of Montana

Dori S. Hutchinson, ScD
Boston University

Kurt Jackson, PhD, PT, GCS
University of Dayton

Jason R. Jaggers, MS
University of South Carolina

Joseph Jankovic, MD
Baylor College of Medicine

Kirsten L. Johansen, MD
University of California, San Francisco

Tracy Karasinski, MSW
Community College of Rhode Island

Donald R. Kay, MD
University of Missouri Health Sciences Center

Steven J. Keteyian, PhD, FACSM
Henry Ford Hospital

Joanne B. Krasnoff, PhD
University of California, San Francisco

Lisa Stroud Krivickas, MD
Harvard Medical School, Massachusetts General Hospital, Spaulding Rehabilitation Hospital

James J. Laskin, PT, PhD
University of Montana

Kathy Lemley, PT, MS
Concordia University Wisconsin

Larry J. Leverenz, PhD, ATC
Purdue University

Michael Lockard, MA
Willamette University

G. William Lyerly, MS
University of South Carolina

Anthony P. Marsh, PhD
Wake Forest University

Barbara B. Meyer, PhD
University of Wisconsin-Milwaukee

Marian A. Minor, PhD, PT
Missouri Arthritis Rehabilitation Research and Training Center

Janet A. Mulcare, PhD, FACSM
Wright State University

Jonathan N. Myers, PhD, FACSM
Palo Alto VA Medical Center
Stanford University

Raha Nael, MD
University of Oklahoma Health Sciences Center

Karl Otto Nakken, MD, PhD
National Center for Epilepsy, Sandvika, Norway

Patricia A. Nixon, PhD, FACSM
Wake Forest University

Karen Palmer-McLean, PhD, PT
University of Wisconsin-La Crosse

Mark H. Pedrotty, PhD
Carrie Tingley Hospital

J. Brent Peel, MS
University of South Carolina

Donna Polk, MD, MPH
Hartford Hospital

Elizabeth J. Protas, PhD, PT, FACSM
University of Texas Medical Branch

Shahla Ray, PhD
Indiana University

James H. Rimmer, PhD
University of Illinois at Chicago

William F. Riner, PhD, FACSM
John Morrison White Clinic

Joseph Robare, MS, RD, LDN
Center for Healthy Aging, University of Pittsburgh

David J. Ross, MD
UCLA School of Medicine

Richard J. Sabath, EdD, FACSM
Children's Mercy Hospital

Anna L. Schwartz, PhD, ARNP, FAAN
Arizona State University

Maureen J. Simmonds, PhD, PT, MCSP
McGill University

Gary S. Skrinar, PhD, FACSM
Boston University

Donald L. Smith, MS, RCEP
University of Illinois at Chicago

Susan S. Smith, PT, PhD, CCD
Drexel University

Rhonda K. Stanley, PhD, PT
A.T. Still University

Mark A. Tarnopolsky, MD, PhD
McMaster University Medical Center

Janet P. Wallace, PhD, FACSM
Indiana University

Che-Hsiang Elizabeth Wang, PT, MS
Drexel University

Michael West, MD
Loveland Health Systems

Christopher J. Womack, PhD, FACSM
James Madison University

Preface to the Third Edition

J. Larry Durstine, PhD, FACSM
Geoffrey E. Moore, MD, FACSM
Scott O. Roberts, PhD, FACSM
Patricia L. Painter, PhD, FACSM

The first, second, and now third editions of *ACSM's Exercise Management for Persons With Chronic Diseases and Disabilities*, which we informally call CDD, were conceived and written to serve as cursory resources to assist exercise professionals in managing exercise programs for persons with chronic diseases and disabilities. Although other textbooks provide sound reviews of current scientific knowledge of various chronic diseases and disabilities, they tend to be inadequate in providing sufficient recommendations with respect to *what to do* with these persons when considering "real-life" situations. Moreover, there are limited resources that provide exercise guidelines and recommendations for persons with multiple chronic diseases.

Also available in E-BOOK format

We have always worked closely with the contributing authors to craft an integrated approach to each condition based on the author's respective clinical experience, while drafting each chapter in a uniform format to provide practical information throughout the text, as well as tables regarding exercise testing and prescription. Each edition of this book was written with the assumption that the reader 1) has a strong working knowledge of exercise science, and 2) that he or she is using the information to supplement a solid foundation of clinical exercise science for conditions outside his primary expertise. In addition, we have always strived to provide an overview of exercise management that addresses a wider spectrum of chronic diseases and disabilities than any other published textbook.

The third edition of CDD includes updated scientific content and improved guidance to enhance problem solving. We also have added discussions on exercise as medicine and on working with multiple chronic conditions. Another new chapter was added on stress and neuropsychiatric disorders. New information and references for evidence-based medicine, as well as new Web sites, are provided when available with the hope of helping the reader gain greater insight into these conditions. Finally, new case studies have been added for each disease and disability.

All of those involved, including editors and authors, are truly delighted at how well this book has been received. Our goal for the third edition is the same as for the previous two editions: To help the reader translate the *science* of exercise physiology into the *art* of practicing exercise medicine. We hope you find this textbook to be a substantial improvement and a worthy reference for your library.

Preface to the First Edition

J. Larry Durstine, PhD, FACSM
Geoffrey E. Moore, MD, FACSM
Lorraine E. Colson Bloomquist, EdD, FACSM
Stephen F. Figoni, PhD, RKT, FACSM

Patricia L. Painter, PhD, FACSM
Kenneth H. Pitetti, PhD, FACSM
Carol J. Pope, PhD
Scott O. Roberts, PhD, FACSM

The fifth edition of *ACSM's Guidelines for Exercise Testing and Prescription* provides the basic principles of testing and training for normal healthy individuals and for those with cardiovascular disease. There is growing interest in the use of exercise for clients with other chronic diseases and disabilities. The purpose of this book is to provide a framework for determining functional capacity and developing appropriate exercise programming to optimize functional capacity in persons with chronic diseases and/or disabilities. The basic principles for exercise testing and training stated in *ACSM's Guidelines for Exercise Testing and Prescription* provide the foundation for this book. When not otherwise stated, these principles are assumed to apply. However, some special situations created by a disease pathology, disability, or treatment alter these basic principles. For example, exercise testing is an important aspect of the approach used in this book, but some people will not have completed an exercise test before starting an exercise program. Participation in regular physical activity can enhance functional capacity, and a primary goal of this book is to get more individuals physically active. Thus, for many people, exercise testing may not be absolutely necessary before starting a low-level physical activity program.

Exercise management for persons with a chronic disease and/or disability is now provided by a wide variety of health care and exercise professionals. Presently, management techniques depend on the provider's experience and are loosely, if at all, coordinated with other providers. A second goal of this book is to develop an integrated model of care so that everyone can work together in a program in which exercise is coordinated with other aspects of health care.

This is not an all-encompassing book on exercise testing and prescription for the populations of interest. Rather, it is a reference manual to use as a guide for managing people with a condition outside the exercise professional's primary expertise. The editorial board and authors were chosen by virtue of their clinical and research experience in exercise programming for persons with chronic diseases and disabilities. The editors established a format for the book and then worked with the authors in writing the text. During the writing process, each chapter was peer-reviewed and then revised accordingly. Before printing, the entire book was reviewed by individuals with a broad expertise in the use of exercise. The authors have suggested reading materials for more in-depth information; these are listed at the end of each chapter and are strongly recommended. If the reader is unable to solve a clinical problem using this manual and the suggested readings, we recommend contacting the chapter author or section editor for advice.

Many people who have a chronic disease or disability enter a downward spiral toward exercise intolerance, so exercise intervention programs should be designed to resist this spiral and optimize functional capacity. Within any given population, there is a wide range of abilities determined by several factors: progression of the disease, response to treatment, and presence of other concomitant illnesses. Expected outcomes of exercise training are not always known. Realistically, optimal exercise and medical programming may yield improvements or merely prevent further deterioration. This book at times may recommend tests or programs that have not been validated, but that experience has shown to be successful. It is hoped that optimal management will bring the individual greater independence and improved quality of life.

Exercise programming must be regularly updated and adapted to the individual's clinical state. The prescription may change depending on the needs of the person, the progression/stabilization of the condition, or the therapy. As a result of disease progression, exercise programming may need to be discontinued—exercise at all costs is not our intent. Rather, we desire appropriate exercise management, including the astute clinical judgment of the exercise professional, leading to successful exercise programs.

We hope that this book will help improve the quality of life for individuals with chronic diseases or disabilities.

Preface to the Second Edition

J. Larry Durstine, PhD, FACSM
Geoffrey E. Moore, MD, FACSM
Lorraine E. Colson Bloomquist, EdD, FACSM
Peter H. Brubaker, PhD, FACSM
Christopher B. Cooper, MD, FACSM

Stephen F. Figoni, PhD, RKT, FACSM
Patricia L. Painter, PhD, FACSM
Kenneth H. Pitetti, PhD, FACSM
Scott O. Roberts, PhD, FACSM

The first edition of this book, *ACSM's Exercise Management for Persons with Chronic Diseases and Disabilities*, which we informally called CDD, was designed to be a quick reference to assist exercise professionals in managing exercise programs for persons with chronic diseases and disabilities. Existing textbooks were good reviews of scientific knowledge, but they fell short of providing guidance on *what to do*. Moreover, there were almost no sources of guidance for persons with multiple chronic diseases. We sought to provide a rational and consistent approach to helping anyone in need of an exercise program. We developed an integrated approach based on clinical experience and, working closely with the contributing authors, crafted a chapter format containing helpful tables on testing and prescription. CDD provided an overview of exercise management that addressed a wider spectrum of chronic diseases and disabilities than any other textbook on "special populations." CDD assumed that readers (1) had a strong working knowledge of exercise science and (2) sought only simple guidance in areas outside their primary expertise. CDD was about how to solve complex problems with a fairly simple set of clinical guidelines.

The second edition, *ACSM's Exercise Management for Persons with Chronic Diseases and Disabilities*, which we call CDD2, takes the same approach but with updated scientific content and improved guidance in problem solving. The biggest change is the inclusion of example cases in almost every chapter about a disease or disability. Some of these cases are simple, some complex, but all are real cases drawn from the clinical practices of the authors. These case studies strengthen this second edition because they illustrate that our recommendations are based not on academic theory but on knowledge from scientific research tempered by clinical experience. All cases are formatted to a uniform style to improve clarity and ease of use.

The limited scope of what we can achieve within our content constraints may leave some readers disappointed. We empathize with you. We would love to provide an encyclopedic book that addresses virtually all diseases and disabilities—a bona fide all-encompassing textbook—but are unable to do so for reasons of cost and (in some cases) lack of published data. We have, however, added several new diseases and disabilities as well as expanded discussion to this second edition. These include a chapter in section I on growth and development, and a new section containing five chapters on pulmonary diseases: Chronic Obstructive Pulmonary Disease, Chronic Restrictive Pulmonary Disease, Asthma, Cystic Fibrosis, and Lung and Heart-Lung Transplantation. The CDD chapter on organ transplantation has been broken into three chapters in CDD2, including the aforementioned lung and heart-lung transplant chapter as well as the chapters Cardiac Transplant and Abdominal Organ Transplant (Kidney, Liver, Pancreas). We have also added the chapters Atrial Fibrillation and Fibromyalgia. Finally, we have greatly expanded the appendix on medications, adding two appendixes on the effects of drugs on exercise capacity, and have also added a list of Web resources.

Chapter topics were chosen mainly on the basis of prevalence in the United States, although we have included some chapters because they happen to cover a relatively large knowledge base. Lack of peer-reviewed publications continues to be a problem, a fact that underscores the necessity of becoming a skilled practitioner. Historically, exercise scientists studied cardiovascular and pulmonary conditions before moving on to musculoskeletal, neurologic, and metabolic diseases. As a result, there is an uneven depth of knowledge between various diseases and disabilities. Over time, as our knowledge grows, we hope it will be possible to broaden our palette to include a wider spectrum of conditions. For now, the exercise professional must be capable of appropriately improvising to individualize exercise management.

We are truly thrilled at how well CDD has been received. Our goal is to help the reader translate the *science* of exercise physiology into the *art* of practicing exercise medicine. We hope you find CDD2 to be a substantial improvement and a worthy reference for your library.

PART I

Framework

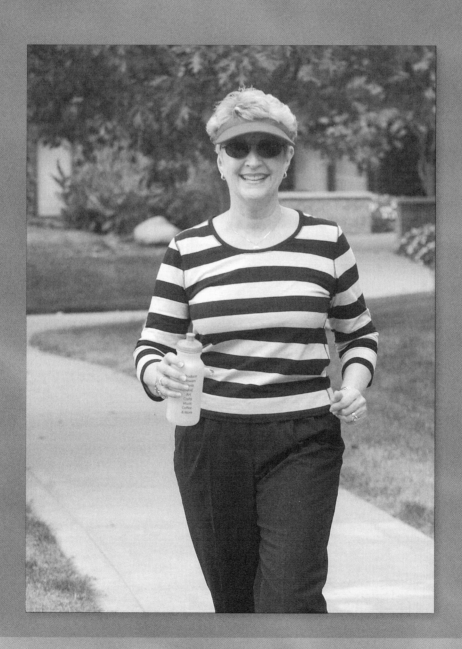

Introduction

Geoffrey E. Moore, MD, FACSM ■ Scott O. Roberts, PhD, FACSM
J. Larry Durstine, PhD, FACSM

In general, our society has a bias toward curative rather than palliative medicine, toward making the disease go away rather than finding ways to cope with disease. An unfortunate consequence of this perspective is that for individuals with chronic disease or disability, the palliative benefits of preserving functionality and well-being are devalued. Recent improvements in social awareness of individuals with disabilities, of the elderly, and of persons with terminal or end-stage disease have brought attention to medical issues surrounding individual rights of autonomy and self-determination. Beginning in the early 1960s, exercise has been promoted as a method of extending life, largely through prevention and moderation of cardiovascular disease. But in the 1980s, research and clinical applications for exercise expanded to populations with a variety of chronic diseases and disabilities, for whom exercise is perhaps more fundamentally related to quality of life than to quantity of life. Perhaps the greatest potential benefit of exercise is its ability to preserve functional capacity, freedom, and independence.

The exercise or health professional looking for guidance in managing exercise programs for people with chronic disease or disability soon discovers that most textbook chapters are grouped by diagnosis, and written by specialists who discuss precautions and caveats for the performance of exercise in the context of a specific disease or disability. Since many diseases and disabilities have yet to be sufficiently studied to yield exact dose–response information,

recommendations are often vague in this regard, originating from empiricism and anecdote instead of controlled trials. While this approach is often valid, it is important to recognize that its origins lie not in physiology but in the structure of academia and the perception that exercise is an adjuvant therapy.

A major shortcoming of diagnosis-oriented management is that many individuals have multiple concomitant problems and do not easily fit into a single group or population. Furthermore, many diseases involve multiple organ systems. Exercise professionals need a useful paradigm, one that is based on the effects of disease or disability, on the acute response to exercise, on the adaptations to training, on the interaction of exercise with medicines, and on the expected dose–response relationship.

Problem-oriented exercise management provides a fundamental framework through which to approach any individual with any combination of diseases or disabilities. Problem-oriented exercise management yields many advantages: It uses exercise testing to reveal physiologic dysfunction; it directs exercise therapy toward problems that might be improved by training; it integrates exercise into medical management; it assigns responsibility to the individual, thereby reinforcing the individual's sense of self-determination and autonomy; and, perhaps most importantly, it transforms problems of overwhelming complexity into components that are more manageable.

CONCEPT OF EXERCISE IS MEDICINE™

The American College of Sports Medicine (ACSM) and the American Medical Association (AMA) have joined forces through the joint initiative titled Exercise is Medicine™ in an effort to educate and encourage all physicians to assess and review every patient's physical activity program at every visit. The editors strongly support of the mission of the ACSM–AMA initiative and believe that the fundamental premise that exercise is medicine has always been one of the primary reasons and guiding forces behind the initial concept and all of the editions of this manual. One of the chapters new to this edition is chapter 3, "Exercise Is Medicine."

EVIDENCE-BASED GUIDELINES

Also new to *Exercise Management for Persons With Chronic Diseases and Disabilities (CDD3)* is the inclusion of specific information within each chapter pertaining to evidence-based medicine (EBM).

Evidence-based medicine is the practice of medicine that is guided by or based on recommendations originating in objective tests of efficacy and published scientific literature, rather than anecdotal observations. The premise of EBM is that one should make every effort to achieve the best outcomes possible for each patient by assessing the quantity and quality of available evidence relevant to the risks and benefits of treatments, or lack of treatments, on a case-by-case basis. The ability to effectively utilize EBM requires clinical expertise, as well as expertise in locating, interpreting, and applying the results of scientific investigations, and then communicating the risks and benefits of various courses of action to patients. Table 1.1 includes selected sources of EBM that readers may find useful. Note that there are far more published EBM guidelines dealing with traditional medical treatments than ones specific to exercise (see Example of Selected Evidence-Based Exercise Guidelines). However, once oriented to EBM guidelines, one may research the literature and assimilate the treatment options, including physical rehabilitation or exercise for a particular medical issue, and develop individual patient treatment plans incorporating EBM.

TABLE 1.1

Select Sources of Evidence-Based Medicine

Source	Description
Agency for Healthcare Research and Quality (AHRQ), formerly known as the Agency for Health Care Policy and Research (AHCPR): Clinical Guidelines and Evidence Reports* www.ahrq.gov/clinic	The AHRQ Web site includes links to the National Guideline Clearinghouse, Evidence Reports from the AHRQ's 12 Evidence-based Practice Centers (EPC), and Preventive Services.
American College of Physicians Journal Club (ACPJC) www.acponline.org/journals/acpjc/jcmenu.htm	ACP Journal Club evaluates evidence in individual articles.
Bandolier* www.jr2.ox.ac.uk/bandolier/	Features short evaluations and discussions of individual articles dealing with evidence-based clinical practice.
Centre for Evidence Based Medicine (CEBM) www.cebm.net/	The CEBM aims to promote evidence-based health care and provide support and resources to anyone who wants to make use of them. The Web site provides links to evidence-based journals and EBM-related teaching materials.

Source	Description
Center for Research Support, TRIP Database www.tripdatabase.com/index.html	The AHRQ began the Translating Research into Practice (TRIP) initiative in 1997 to implement evidence-based tools and information. The TRIP database features hyperlinks to the largest collection of EBM materials on the Internet, including NGC, POEM, DARE, Cochrane Library, CATbank, and individual articles. A good starting place for an EBM literature search.
Clinical Evidence, BMJ Publishing Group* www.clinicalevidence.org	Searches BMJ's Clinical Evidence Compendium for up-to-date evidence regarding effective health care. Lists available topics and describes the supporting body of evidence to date (e.g., number of relevant randomized controlled trials published to date). Concludes with interventions "likely to be beneficial" versus those with "unknown effectiveness." Individuals who have received a free copy of *Clinical Evidence* Issue 5 from the United Health Foundation are also entitled to free access to the full online content.
Cochrane Database of Systematic Reviews* www.cochrane.org/	Systematic evidence reviews that are updated periodically by the Cochrane Group. Reviewers discuss whether adequate data are available for the development of EBM guidelines for diagnosis or management.
Database of Abstracts of Reviews of Effectiveness (DARE)* www.crd.york.ac.uk/crdweb/	Structured abstracts written by University of York CRD reviewers (see NHS CRD). Abstract summaries review articles on diagnostic or treatment interventions and discuss clinical implications.
Effective Health Care* www.york.ac.uk/inst/crd/ehcb.htm	Bimonthly, peer-reviewed bulletin for medical decision makers. Based on systematic reviews and synthesis of research on the clinical effectiveness, cost effectiveness, and acceptability of health service interventions.
Essential Evidence Plus* www.essentialevidenceplus.com	Includes the InfoRetriever search system for the complete POEMs database and six additional evidence-based databases. Subscription is required.
Evidence-Based Medicine* www.evidence-basedmedicine.com	Bimonthly publication launched in 1995 by the BMJ Publishing Group. Article summaries include commentaries by clinical experts. Subscription is required.
Institute for Clinical Systems Improvement (ICSI)* www.ICSI.org	ICSI is an independent, nonprofit collaboration of health care organizations, including the Mayo Clinic (Rochester, MN). Web site includes the ICSI guidelines for preventive services and disease management.

(continued)

TABLE 1.1 *(continued)*

Source	Description
National Guideline Clearinghouse (NGC) www/guideline.gov/	Comprehensive database of evidence-based clinical practice guidelines from government agencies and health care organizations. Describes and compares guideline statements with respect to objectives, methods, outcomes, evidence rating scheme, and major recommendations.
National Health Service (NHS) Centre for Reviews and Dissemination (CRD) www.york.ac.uk/inst/crd/	Searches CRD databases (includes DARE, NHS Economic Evaluation Database, Health Technology Assessment Database) for EBM reviews. More limited than TRIP database.
Primary Care Clinical Practice Guidelines http://medicine.ucsf.edu/resources/guidelines	University of California, San Francisco, Web site that includes links to NGC, CEBM, AHRQ, individual articles, and organizations.
U.S. Preventive Services Task Force (USPSTF)* www.ahrq.gov/clinic/uspstfix.htm	This Web site features updated recommendations for clinical preventive services based on systematic evidence reviews by the U.S. Preventive Services Task Force.

EBM = evidence-based medicine.

*These Web sites are AAFP-approved sources of systematic evidence reviews. When these sources are used to prepare continuing medical education clinical content according to guidelines issued by the AAFP Commission of Continuing Medical Education, the content will qualify for the special designation of evidence-based CME. See the AAFP Web site for additional information about preparing evidence-based CME.

Reprinted with permission from "How to Write an Evidence-Based Clinical Review Article," January 15, 2002, American Family Physician. Copyright © 2002 American Academy of Family Physicians. All Rights Reserved.

Example of Selected Evidence-Based Exercise Guidelines

de Jong ORW, Hopman-Rock M, Tak EC, Klazinga NS. An implementation study of two evidence-based exercise and health education programmes for older adults with osteoarthritis of the knee and hip. Health Educ Res. 2004;19(3):316-325.

Humpel N, Iverson DC. Review and critique of the quality of exercise recommendations for cancer patients and survivors. J Support Care Cancer. 2005;13(7):493-502.

Levy CE, Giuffrida C, Richards L, Wu S, Davis S, Nadeau SE. Botulinum toxin A, evidence-based exercise therapy, and constraint-induced movement therapy for upper-limb hemiparesis attributable to stroke: A preliminary study. Am J Phys Med Rehabil. 2007;86(9):696-706.

Martin Ginis KA, Latimer AE, Buchholz AC, et al. Establishing evidence-based physical activity guidelines: Methods for the Study of Health and Activity in People with Spinal Cord Injury (SHAPE SCI). Spinal Cord. 2008;46(3):216–221.Myslinski MJ. Evidence-based exercise prescription for individuals with spinal cord injury. J Neurol Phys Ther. 2005;29(2):104-106.

Ottawa panel evidence-based clinical practice guidelines for therapeutic exercises and manual therapy in the management of osteoarthritis. Phys Ther. 2005;85(9):907-971.

Pulmonary rehabilitation—joint ACCP/AACVPR evidence-based clinical practice guidelines. Chest. 1997;112(5):1363-1396.

Roddy E, Zhang W, Doherty M, et al. Evidence-based recommendations for the role of exercise in the management of osteoarthritis of the hip or knee—the MOVE consensus. Rheumatology. 2005;44(1):67-73.

Selig SE, Hare DL. Evidence-based approach to exercise prescription in chronic heart failure. Br J Sports Med. 2007;41:407-408.

HOW TO USE THIS BOOK

CDD3 outlines how to effectively manage exercise for someone with chronic disease or disability. To use this manual, the reader should have extensive knowledge about exercise physiology, exercise testing, and exercise training. Successful exercise management should also involve close teamwork among physicians, nurses, and allied health care providers. The editors assume that readers and users of this content information are appropriately skilled in these matters and can adapt to individual circumstances. Readers should consult *ACSM's Resource Manual for Guidelines for Exercise Testing and Prescription, Sixth Edition*, and *ACSM's Guidelines for Exercise Testing and Prescription, Eighth Edition*, for information on a variety of exercise protocols, although some specific protocols or exercise devices are described here. The present manual does not provide detailed instruction on exercise physiology or disease, so supplementary reading may be needed for a full understanding of exercise management. For detailed information on diseases and disabilities, the reader should refer to standard physiology, medical, and adapted physical activity texts.

Each chapter deals with a common chronic disorder or disability that might limit functional capacity. Each chapter briefly outlines the physiologic nature of the disease or disability, its effects on the exercise response and adaptation, the effects of commonly used medicines, and any unique circumstances that should be considered. Recommendations for testing and programming are presented in tables for easy reference. The reader should refer to the chapter(s) relevant for each individual and use the information in those chapters as guidelines in developing an individualized exercise program.

Each chapter begins with an overview of essential pathophysiology relevant to the given topic. The third edition includes updated prevalence data, advances in pathophysiology knowledge, advances in diagnosis and treatment when applicable, and additional information on basic key concepts that are either very complex or quite rare in comparison to other topics covered throughout the manual. Readers with more advanced education and training may find some of this information very familiar, while other less seasoned readers will benefit from assimilating the content more thoroughly. The editors of this manual have strived to ensure that essential and timely information is covered in sufficient detail that readers will be able to identify the most important factors within each chapter related to the safe and effective delivery of exercise programs for individuals with chronic disease and disability.

To develop an integrated model, the editors have aggregated and consolidated old conventions and tried to create a newer, comprehensive system. The first four chapters introduce these new conventions; all remaining chapters follow this model. Some terms and concepts are used interchangeably, such as "exercise prescription" and "exercise programming." Other concepts may be rather new to some readers, such as "model of best practice" or "evidence based."

The authors and editors have strived to use correct and current terminology but have simplified when appropriate. Some of the discussions of concepts in this manual remain complex, since there is simply no easy approach and no substantial benefit to simplifying. For example, aerobic exercise intensity is expressed in a variety of ways: percentage of maximal oxygen consumption ($\dot{V}O_{2max}$), percentage peak heart rate, percentage heart rate reserve, and so on. These choices were largely left to each author's preference. One important convention in this book is the use of the words "clients" or "individuals or persons or people" instead of "patients," where applicable. This convention was chosen because not all exercise managers are health care professionals in a patient–caregiver relationship.

PROBLEM-ORIENTED MANAGEMENT

A method of exercise management that uses problem-oriented techniques is one that is recommended by the editors and is incorporated throughout all of the chapters. This technique uses the SOAP notes commonly employed by health care professionals. For readers unfamiliar with this technique, the problem-oriented system is a common organizational tool used in medicine. SOAP stands for subjective data, objective data, assessment, and plan of action. Notes, to oneself and others, are written in the SOAP outline style to clarify one's own thinking process and the rationale for one's course of evaluation, therapy, or both. Problems and unique needs are identified and the intervention is documented, largely so that follow-up evaluations can be compared to earlier visits and success or failure can be fairly judged.

One of the key benefits of problem-oriented management is that several problems can be independently tracked in their own time frame but within the context of the patient's overall situation. In apparently healthy, able-bodied individuals, there is little need for this system, and there may not be much need even in individuals with a single chronic disease or disability that doesn't alter the physiologic response to activity (e.g., a sensory disorder such as deafness or visual impairment). Problem-oriented management is particularly useful when individuals have multiple chronic disease or disability circumstances that can affect exercise performance. The key to the effective use of problem-oriented management is identifying all problems and needs and then following each problem in its own appropriate time frame. A sample case, in SOAP note format, is provided in each chapter.

HOW TO USE THE TABLES

Each chapter contains tables describing appropriate exercise tests and programs for the chronic disease or disability addressed in that chapter. Columns contain categories of recommendations, and rows contain families of exercise tests as described in chapter 2. Each row contains recommendations regarding the given family of exercise. For testing tables, the recommendation categories are Methods (to use), Measures (to take), Endpoints (and way-points) to specifically note, and general Comments. For programming tables, the categories are Modes (of training), Goals (of the program), Intensity/Frequency/Duration (in the prescription), and Time to Goal. In earlier editions of this book both testing and programming tables had sections that describe appropriate medications and special considerations. This information is now found only in the text.

HOW TO READ THE TABLES

To determine which exercise test to conduct for a particular chronic disease or disability, the reader is encouraged to look at the testing table in the relevant chapter. In the first column, headed "Methods," identify the most appropriate exercise test to use relative to the individual's diagnosis, current medical problems, and desired outcome for the test. Next, read across to the second column, headed "Measures," to determine the physiologic measurement(s) recommended for the specific test selected. The third column, headed "Endpoints," lists relevant indications for terminating the test, although some "endpoints" are relevant way-points, or measurements taken during the test (e.g., ventilatory threshold). The final column, headed "Comments," lists issues relevant to the specific disease or disability. In addition, special attention should be given to the sections in each table on appropriate medications and special considerations, as these provide important safety precautions and recommendations.

Similarly, to develop an individualized exercise program, the reader should look at the exercise programming table. In the first column, headed "Modes," look for the family of exercises desired for the individual in question. Within each exercise family are recommended generic modes of training. Reading across to the second column, headed "Goals," identify the appropriate program objectives for your client. Continuing to read across within the family of exercise, find the appropriate Intensity, Frequency, and Duration recommendations in the third column. The fourth column, headed "Time to Goal," provides an idea of how long it will take to reach an established goal. As with exercise testing, special note should be taken of the medications and special considerations sections now found in the text.

WHAT'S IN THE TABLES

Each table contains material summarized from the chapter as well as recommendations about exercise testing and programming. Protocols and programs are usually listed generically, rather than in specific terms, because detailed listing of all known protocols would be overly cumbersome. We assume that readers know how to conduct exercise tests and design exercise training programs.

WHAT'S NOT IN THE TABLES

Although many tables are complete and comprehensive, many are not. Some tables contain areas that are left blank or omit mention of a particular family of exercises, usually because the author or section editor felt that insufficient data were available to justify a recommendation. Some tables list only a mode or a method because knowledge is insufficient to allow recommendations of specific protocols but the author's experience has been that the suggested modes and methods can be used successfully. Sometimes recommendations for exercise testing and programming for a particular disease or disability don't match; again, the reason is usually that research on exercise testing and training procedures is incomplete. Finally, in the testing and programming tables in chapters 48 through 52, some sections are combined because the disability doesn't alter the normal response to exercise or adaptations to exercise training (e.g., visual impairment).

Suggested Web Site

U.S. Department of Health and Human Services. www.health.gov/PAGuidelines/guidelines/default.aspx

Approach to Exercise and Disease Management

Geoffrey E. Moore, MD, FACSM ■ Anthony P. Marsh, PhD
J. Larry Durstine, PhD, FACSM

This chapter introduces a method of managing exercise in individuals with chronic disease or disability. The first section provides an overview of this model; subsequent sections offer greater detail about specific factors to consider when one is prescribing exercise.

First and foremost, an exercise history should be taken from the individual to obtain subjective data on aerobic ability, anaerobic ability (for athletes), endurance, strength, flexibility, neuromuscular skill, and overall functional performance. The information collected in the exercise history defines the individual's medical problems and conditions, which one can then consider collectively when deciding what exercise tests should be performed to provide objective data. The objective data quantify the individual's limitations in physiologic terms, and this information is used to assess the cause(s) of exercise intolerance. From the objective assessment, an exercise training plan is developed. Formulation of a plan is complex and takes into account (1) medication effects, (2) exercise dose-response (desired goal; type of exercise; intensity, duration, and frequency of training; adaptability to training as well as exhaustion or overtraining limits), (3) risks of training, (4) the cost–benefit ratio, and (5) any necessary coordination among members of the health care team.

PROBLEM-ORIENTED EXERCISE MANAGEMENT

Problem-oriented exercise management (POEM) is the cornerstone to approaching exercise for individuals with chronic disease and disability. POEM was developed in the late 1960s and since that time has been useful to a variety of health care professionals. The major benefit of this approach is that it provides a systematic way of organizing extremely complex problems into simpler parts that make them easier to track and solve. Given the complexity of exercise in chronic disease and disability, one may not be able to successfully manage certain individuals without the use of this technique. POEM consists of five steps, commonly documented in the SOAP format. SOAP is defined as the (1) collection of Subjective data, (2) collection of Objective data, (3) Assessment and generation of a problem list, (4) formulation of a Plan that is diagnostic or therapeutic (or both), and (5) periodic reassessment (follow-up). Because the format provides a quick conceptual reminder of the situation and any progress made, SOAP notes are useful not only to the manager but also to any colleagues who may be assisting in the treatment processes.

Obtaining Subjective Data

Prior to conducting any formalized testing with individuals with chronic disease or disability, identifying and describing the individual's problems in detail is of upmost importance. A medical history should include a comprehensive review of past and current physical activity and exercise habits, as well as related medical problems, including any current complaints or symptoms. With regard to exercise intolerance, symptoms might include shortness of breath, exertional chest pain, overall weakness, ease of fatigability, or back pain. Identifying the reason an individual has been referred for exercise testing or training is important, as is determining what people's past experiences with exercise have been, what physical or emotional limitations they might have, and what types of injuries they have suffered in the past, as well as all of their current medical problems (including heart, lung, circulatory, gastrointestinal, metabolic, and neurological and musculoskeletal problems). Lastly, a complete list of all current medications and results of any recent medical and exercise tests should be obtained.

A thorough review of the information described will help guide decisions that need to be made regarding exercise testing and training. Many of the problems that limit functional capacity can and should be evaluated through exercise testing. For example, if an individual has difficulty going to the store because he or she gets easily winded or fatigued, aerobic and endurance exercise testing may be indicated. If an individual can't go to the store because he or she is too weak to carry the bags home or out to the car, strength testing may be indicated. For someone who is too clumsy to walk to the store, neuromuscular and functional performance testing may be indicated. Recommending a full battery of exercise tests for every individual is neither helpful nor cost effective, nor is it wise to use only certain tests for individuals with a specific disease or disability. In order to provide a complete diagnosis, prescribed tests should be neither too broad nor too narrow. Obtaining and reviewing subjective data helps in the decision-making process when one is deciding which tests to use.

Obtaining Objective Data

Objective data include information collected during a physical examination and from laboratory studies. Once an individual's problem or problems have been identified, the most appropriate exercise tests can be selected—those that will best characterize the exercise capacity of the individual. Appropriate medical and laboratory tests may provide measurements that confirm or rule out possible causes of symptoms. Because of the tremendous number of exercise tests and test protocols available today, they have been grouped into seven categories based on their purpose, or what they are designed to quantify:

1. Aerobic tests: assess the ability to perform exercise using a high rate of oxygen consumption ($\dot{V}O_{2max}$)
2. Anaerobic tests: assess the ability to perform short-term, high-intensity exercise
3. Endurance tests: assess the ability to sustain submaximal aerobic exercise for an extended time
4. Strength tests: assess the ability to sustain low-intensity muscular contractions over time or maximal force produced during high-resistance, short-duration exercise
5. Flexibility tests: assess the ability to move joints through their range of motion
6. Neuromuscular tests: assess the ability to do activities that require coordination and skill
7. Functional performance tests: assess the ability to do specific physical activities of daily living

Exercise testing protocols should be selected to suit each individual and as a result provide the best possible information for developing the management plan. To achieve this task, an estimation of an individual's potential exercise capacity is often necessary. This estimate, along with personal professional knowledge and expertise, as well as information and guidelines presented in this manual, may then be used to attain optimal test and exercise results.

The Assessment

Use of the information obtained from the subjective and objective data-gathering steps should make it possible to generate a list of specific problems. For example, an individual may have (1) low aerobic capacity, (2) low ventilatory threshold, (3) low endurance at 75% of aerobic capacity, and (4) weak hip and knee extensors. This assessment may explain the individual's problems or lead to further assessment of problems that are not evident or have not been elucidated yet. A complete assessment may require a series of testing and reassessment before enough information is available to allow clear identification of all the problems. Organizing the assessment either by family of exercise test or by physiologic problem may be helpful; then one should number the problems in priority of importance. This process of assessment will help track all of the problems in a systematic format.

Formulating a Plan

In medicine as with anything in life, without a plan of action one is less, if at all, likely to achieve a goal. A plan of action begins with the collection of subjective and objective data during the assessment, then proceeds to the diagnosis of an individual's primary and secondary problems and finally to a treatment plan, including exercise therapy. Creating this plan tends to be more difficult for individuals with chronic disease or disability than suggested by the previously outlined steps because in these cases the exercise prescription is often complex, involving numerous confounding variables. The initial plan for some individuals may require performing further assessment or obtaining additional data from another source; but no matter how long it takes, one must formulate a treatment plan including exercise programming. Executing the plan can also be difficult because the plan includes following a single problem or multiple problems for a period of time. This time period can be a few days, a few weeks, or a few months and involves numerous health care providers. When a number of problems are present, involving numerous health care providers, it is easy to lose track of some of the specific treatment objectives over time, making sequential numbering or prioritizing of the problems important.

Steps in Formulating an Exercise-Based Treatment Plan

Firstly, the exercise prescription must include both short- and long-term individualized goals based on the subjective and objective findings of the assessment, among other things. For those not familiar with goal-setting strategies, we encourage using the popular acronym SMART. SMART stands for the following descriptors for goals:

▪ Specific: Goals need to be defined precisely. Saying that an individual should exercise more does not express a goal that will be kept. Saying that the person needs to exercise 20 to 30 min each day, three to four days a week, much more clearly and specifically expresses a goal.

▪ Measurable: Measurability is closely related to specificity but also includes a way to make sure the individual stays on track. A goal that tells an indi-

vidual to increase functional capacity and change body composition isn't measurable. A goal of 15% to 20% improvement in functional capacity and a reduction in body fat from 25% to 20% in six months is far more measurable.

▪ Actionable: The goal should be something that the individual believes in and truly desires. In stating their goals, people might say that they hope all their fears and worries about heart disease will go away once they start the exercise program. A better way for the individual to state the same goal would be to say "I hope this exercise program makes me feel better and helps me reduce my fears about developing angina when I play golf."

▪ Realistic: Goals that are actually achievable are much better and far more motivating than less realistic goals. Individuals will feel better about themselves when they reach a realistic goal than if they constantly shoot for unrealistic goals and fall short. Realistic goals should not be so easy that people easily attain them every single time but should not be so hard that they never reach them at all.

▪ Time oriented: Time orientation is similar to measurability in that a definite time frame for the accomplishment of a goal is provided. Deadlines help people achieve their goals.

Second, consider any unique circumstances an individual might have, such as prosthetics, medications, exercise facilities, and other conditions that may require modification of a more typical program. In addition, it is important to evaluate the risks, benefits, and costs of the program and discuss any concerns the person might have about these aspects. Remember that anyone who exercises will have some activity-dependent risks, including mild to moderate injuries. However, people with a chronic disease or disability have risks related to their disease or disability that are more permanent. The risks of exercise are commonly considered in terms of highest to lowest risk, with heart attacks and sudden deaths representing the highest risk; but even these high risks are really disease-dependent risks for individuals with heart disease. Heart attacks and sudden death are distinctly uncommon in people who don't have heart disease, so other disease-dependent risks may prove more important. The relative risks of any activity are based on the severity of the disease and the inherent danger of the activity engaged in. The most important benefits of exercise will usually be an increase in physical activity levels, quality of life, or both, but may well include a reduction in medications taken or a noticeable reduction in disease severity. The costs of attending an exercise program can be measured in time and energy, particularly for individuals who perform unsupervised exercise, although equipment and facility costs must also be considered.

Third, an exercise program should incorporate each of the considerations discussed to this point. Begin with the individual's current fitness and choose practical levels of intensity, duration, and frequency of exercise sessions. It is wise not to be bound to standard program formats such as 20 to 40 min, three to four times per week. While many standardized exercise programs typically have the goal of improving fitness and in some cases reducing cardiac morbidity and mortality, they may not be the best programs for the goals of individuals with chronic disease or disability. Choose a realistic time frame for achieving the goals, and pay close attention to the necessary rate of improvement. Care should be given to avoid overtraining individuals, since there is no real purpose in overtraining someone with limited reserve who is not a competitive athlete. This is not to say that some individuals with chronic diseases or disabilities can't participate in athletic competition but rather to note that before they do, the risk and benefits of such training and competition need to be carefully analyzed.

Fourth, develop a schedule for follow-up reassessment for each individual client. Occasionally it will seem easy to make an action plan that is logical, readily apparent, and easy to follow. More often, however, the assessment and plan are iterative processes—assessment, data collection, reassessment, more data collection, more reassessment, until the problem is solved or goals are achieved. A therapeutic trial is one way to obtain objective data, allowing observation of how well empiric therapy solves the problem or is working toward achieving the goals of the individual. Once a solution has been settled upon, the appropriate time between reassessments is determined by individual circumstances. Following up too soon is a poor use of time and resources, but following up too late risks letting an old problem get out of control or a new problem go unnoticed. During the follow-up, evaluate the progress and reassess the appropriateness of the prescription for each problem that is not stable and needs more attention. Problems that are not relevant may or may not be skipped.

Organizing problems by category of exercise has many advantages, including maintaining the context of the exercise test and prescription, focusing strategy, and helping track minor problems. Note that the tables for recommended testing and programming found in each chapter of this book are organized by category of exercise.

CATEGORIES OF EXERCISE TEST MEASURES

The exercise tests in this manual are grouped into seven categories of laboratory measurements that characterize the capacity to perform specific activities: (1) aerobic, (2) anaerobic, (3) endurance, (4) strength, (5) flexibility, (6) neuromuscular skill, and (7) functional performance. These generic groupings provide a rationale for selecting an appropriate laboratory test and prescribing a training program. From a physiologic perspective, these groupings overlap to an extent; but in a problem-oriented system these families of exercises are nonetheless useful for organizational purposes. Measures that characterize each family of exercise are as follows:

1. Aerobic exercise tests measure the ability to perform exercise requiring high rates of oxygen consumption. Examples of aerobic test measures are $\dot{V}O_{2max}$, peak oxygen consumption ($\dot{V}O_{2peak}$), maximal steady-state oxygen consumption ($\dot{V}O_{2MSS}$), ventilation (e.g., spirometry), 12-lead electrocardiogram (ECG), heart rate, blood pressure, perceived exertion, metabolic equivalents (METs), time to exhaustion, and lactate threshold.

2. Anaerobic exercise tests measure the ability to exercise at an intensity that exceeds $\dot{V}O_{2max}$ or $\dot{V}O_{2peak}$. Examples of anaerobic tests are capacity for oxygen debt, 30 s peak power output, time trial performance, and peak lactate. These types of tests are useful mostly for athletes.

3. Endurance exercise tests measure the ability to sustain submaximal aerobic exercise for an extended time. Examples of endurance tests are time trial performance, 6 and 12 min walk, 1-mile (1.6K) walk, time to exhaustion or rate of perceived exertion at a constant work rate, and maximal number of repetitions.

4. Strength exercise tests measure the ability to do unsustained work against a high resistance. Examples of strength tests are maximal number of repetitions, isokinetic work and peak torque, maximal voluntary contraction, and peak power output.

5. Flexibility exercise tests measure the ability to move joints through a prescribed range of motion (ROM). Examples of flexibility tests are sit-and-reach distances and goniometry.

6. Neuromuscular exercise tests measure the ability to do activities that require coordination and skill. Examples of neuromuscular tests are gait

analysis, balance times, hand–eye coordination, and reaction time.

7. Functional performance tests measure the ability to do specific physical activities of daily living. Examples of functional performance tests are sit-and-stand scores, lifting, timed walk, and gait.

The redundancy among the categories reflects the integrated nature of physical activity and therefore provides an effective means of characterizing specific aspects of exercise. Note that this manual usually recommends the mode of exercise; for example, in the aerobic category, this would include walking, jogging, cycling, rowing, combined arm and leg cycling, stair climbing, swimming, and aerobic dance.

Daily activities are complex physical activities that require integrated function between many of the organ systems and use all seven categories of exercise. Thus factors such as endurance and neuromuscular skill can determine daily activities and quality of life more than measures of oxygen consumption, strength, flexibility, or combinations of these measures.

Aerobic Exercise Tests

The ability to sustain aerobic exercise is very important for completing activities of daily living, and is commonly tested in the laboratory setting through the use of graded exercise tests. Maximal oxygen consumption is an important physiologic measurement, but many persons with a chronic disease or disability do not achieve a "true" $\dot{V}O_{2max}$. Rather, they reach a point at which they cannot continue. Such individuals are said to reach symptom-limited exhaustion, referred to as $\dot{V}O_{2peak}$. The distinction is important, because $\dot{V}O_{2max}$ is limited by oxygen supply, while $\dot{V}O_{2peak}$ is limited by other factors such as fatigue.

Another critical point that can be revealed during exercise testing is the point at which the person experiences a transition from an exercise intensity that can be sustained more or less indefinitely to an intensity that can be sustained for only a short time. A variety of methods are used to measure this transition, including lactate threshold, onset of blood lactate accumulation, ventilatory threshold, and Conconi heart rate threshold. Several protocols designed to detect this transition are available. For our purposes, the transition from sustainable to unsustainable exercise is the common aspect and will be referred to as $\dot{V}O_{2MSS}$.

Measurement of $\dot{V}O_{2max}$ is important in individuals with chronic disease or disability. Many of these individuals have a very low $\dot{V}O_{2peak}$, usually less than 25 ml · kg^{-1} · min^{-1} and often less than 20 ml · kg^{-1} · min^{-1}. The usual range for $\dot{V}O_{2MSS}$ is 40% to 70% of $\dot{V}O_{2max}$. Most common activities of daily living, usually taken for granted by those who are healthy and able-bodied, require oxygen consumption in the range of 12 to 30 ml · kg^{-1} · min^{-1}. For example, window cleaning, sweeping the floor, and mowing the lawn require approximately 12.6, 11.4, and 17.4 ml · kg^{-1} · min^{-1} respectively. Individuals with a chronic disease or disability have a $\dot{V}O_{2max}$ or $\dot{V}O_{2peak}$ below that required for activities of daily living, employment, and maintenance of individual independence, resulting in a lower quality of life.

In general, constant-increment or continuously increasing (or ramp) work rate protocols are preferred over some standard protocols (e.g., Bruce protocol). Many standard protocols increase work rate in relatively large, often nonlinear increments and are effective in screening for ischemic heart disease. In exercise management, however, we are more interested in characterizing the exercise response in the submaximal range. Ramp protocols are far superior in this regard because they indicate submaximal exercise responses while still detecting coronary artery disease.

A disadvantage of using a standardized ramp protocol is that one cannot individualize exercise tests so that each subject can complete the test in 8 to 10 min. Many unconditioned individuals have a low endurance exercise capacity and will be unable to exercise for this length of time. At the same time, tests lasting for 12 to 15 min or longer can give falsely low results. Therefore, one must know the client's approximate ability, estimate his or her peak exercise capacity, and design a test to yield four to eight changes in work rates during an 8 to 10 min test period. Low-level ramp protocols may require special programming and manual operation, and may be difficult to reproduce on equipment that is imprecise at low exercise levels. For example, some persons can generate only 10 W and will not be able to pedal a standard stationary cycle against any measurable resistance. Therefore, the subject must be tested using freewheel pedaling, in which only the pedaling rate is increased. With careful consideration and planning, successful exercise testing can be accomplished for nearly everyone.

Anaerobic Exercise Tests

Anaerobic tests usually consist of short-term exercise that supplements strength test data or offers data on ability to do brief periods of high-intensity exercise. In several chronic diseases, this type of test correlates closely with a variety of measures of functional capacity, including $\dot{V}O_{2max}$. Anaerobic tests may also be of value for athletes preparing for competition.

Endurance Exercise Tests

Endurance tests are potentially useful because many inactive persons cannot exercise longer than 5 min but can sustain exercise for 1 h or more after training (even without an increase in $\dot{V}O_{2peak}$). Unfortunately, endurance tests have not been well developed and often lack test–retest reliability, well-defined endpoints, and clear physiologic meaning. Claudication tests (e.g., walk distance to onset of pain, maximal walk distance) are useful in arterial insufficiency because they satisfy these criteria.

Strength Exercise Tests

Muscular strength is a critical component of exercise capacity, particularly in individuals with a chronic disease or disability. Resistance testing is essential because skeletal muscle weakness can limit functional capacity. Like aerobic exercise response, skeletal muscle function can be evaluated in myriad ways—for example, maximal repetitions for a given weight (using either free weights or a machine); isokinetic force, work, and power; and isometric force. Each of these forms of testing has its own advantages and disadvantages, and the method chosen should be carefully matched to the problems being addressed and to the person's situation. Resistance testing can reveal several important aspects of strength, including maximal force, the smoothness of contraction and relaxation (lack of spasticity), balance of strength between extensor and flexor muscle groups, symmetry between left and right sides, and resistance to fatigue. Resistance training is also an excellent addition to a rehabilitation program and is often overlooked in cardiovascular rehabilitation programs. Strength training may well belong in virtually every program for persons with a chronic disease or disability.

Flexibility Tests

Flexibility is also a critical aspect of exercise programming. Range of motion is important because muscle force, in order to be useful, must be applied through a full range of movement for the proper performance of physical work. Normal joint and spine movement can maintain symmetry of function and protect muscles, joints, and bones from strain and injury. Like other forms of exercise testing, assessment of flexibility can be performed in a variety of ways; but the easiest, most versatile, and least expensive is the use of a simple goniometer.

For our purposes, goniometry is probably most worthwhile in people with neuromusculoskeletal disability, such as those with extreme scar tissue in joints, contractures, spasticity, and so on. Many exercise programs complete flexibility training (i.e., stretching) during the warm-up and cool-down segments of an exercise training session. Some individuals may require more extensive stretching, perhaps in combination with specific programs, to regain and maintain flexibility.

Neuromuscular Tests

Neuromuscular tests, which assess coordination and skill, are most useful in individuals with a neuromuscular disability or those who are severely debilitated from chronic disease or are frail. As a result, these types of tests are more commonly used by physical, occupational, and kinesiology therapists than by exercise physiologists. Examples include reaction time, hand–eye coordination tests, and gait analysis. These kinds of tests should be used, for the most part, in persons with neuromuscular deficits who need specific assessment and programming.

Functional Performance Tests

A wide range of test batteries have been developed to assess functional performance. These test batteries vary in their total number of tasks, but typically the tasks are timed or ranked using a simple scale. Many functional performance measures have components that relate directly to the mobility and strength of an individual. Independent living and freedom from disability require performance above a threshold level of function, so individuals who barely surpass these functional thresholds of mobility and strength are at risk for future disability.

Functional performance tests should mimic real tasks, should be objective, and should be brief as well as easy to administer. When choosing a test, one should consider its reliability, the availability of normative data, the ability to detect change over time, and clinical applicability. It is recommended that a performance-based measure be a familiar task with a distinct start and endpoint. This enhances the test's reliability and objectivity. The exercise specialist should become adept at administering functional performance tests, and this may require some training so that the tests are administered according to established protocols.

Several tasks are commonly used in performance-based test batteries, including time to walk a given distance (an indicator of cardiovascular endurance; e.g., 6 min walk test); time to rise from a chair and return to a seated position a given number of times (an indicator of lower extremity strength); ability and time to stand in challenging positions (an indicator of postural control; e.g., feet together in a side-by-side, semitandem, or tandem position, or one-leg balance time); a measure of freely chosen gait speed (e.g., over a 20 ft [6.1 m] distance); and the timed "get up and go" test, which is a combination of chair rises and gait.

Physical functioning may also be assessed using a self-report questionnaire. Many such self-report questionnaires measure limitations in activities, modifications in performing activities (e.g., takes longer to perform routine activities, needs assistance in performing activities), and level of difficulty in performing routine activities. As in functional performance tests, any questionnaire you choose should be valid, reliable, and tested in the population of interest. Like functional performance tests, many of these questionnaires are highly predictive of outcomes in diseased populations and can provide insight into the level of limitation and possibly the potential for future disability.

Developing an Exercise Prescription Without an Exercise Test

One predicament that exercise professionals frequently encounter is the need to design a program without having any exercise test data. Although certainly helpful when exercise test data are available, it is not absolutely necessary to have an exercise test in order to begin a program. Developing a safe and effective exercise program is possible with the use of two or more techniques to measure relative intensity (e.g., heart rate and perceived exertion), which then can be compared against each other, as well as with use of prior experience to guide decisions. It is always best to err on the conservative side when developing an exercise prescription for anyone, whether the person is healthy or has a chronic disease. A more pragmatic approach, however, is to improvise an informal submaximal exercise study in the form of an exercise session, or several studies over the course of a week. The simple rules recommended in this chapter and the protocols in the exercise testing table in each chapter provide useful information. For example, you can perform a submaximal cycle ergometer study by using a ramped protocol and recording heart rates and rating of perceived exertion (RPE) up to a level of 17 on a 20-point scale. You would then prescribe a range of exercising heart rates based on perceived exertion.

Behavioral Assessment

Behavioral medicine has made substantial advances in recent years, and there are now many instruments available that assess quality of life, self-efficacy, or readiness to change. It may be tempting to rely on one's own counseling or coaching skills, but using one of these instruments to obtain some objective data is worthwhile. Having such a measurement to gauge progress can be invaluable to a specialist managing an exercise program. Getting a client to exercise regularly at higher doses may well be the best help you can offer. Because this is largely a matter of lifestyle, having an understanding and appreciation of each client's barriers to change is very important for the exercise specialist. You should use instruments that are validated, reliable, well tested, and used for the special population in which you intend to use the instrument. For almost all the chapters in this book, there are quality-of-life instruments that have been designed with the specific population in mind. There are also instruments designed to be used for any population. The proper use of these instruments is beyond the scope of this text, although their application may be mentioned by some chapter authors. Many readers will find it necessary to enlist the aid of a psychologist or behavioral medicine expert.

Summary of Exercise Test Measures

The exercise specialist working with individuals with a chronic disease or disability must be able to employ techniques from each of the seven categories of exercise tests. In the past, much of the emphasis has been on aerobic exercise testing, largely because of the prevalence of cardiovascular disease and the popularity of aerobic exercise. However, many exercise professionals have long used measures of strength, flexibility, neuromuscular skill, and functional performance. Because activities of daily living are integrated functions that require some element from each family of exercise, exercise specialists working with chronically diseased or disabled populations should incorporate the various test results in developing a comprehensive exercise management plan. In addition, many of the new exercise machines are useful tools for obtaining these measurements, but exercise specialists at facilities without these specialized machines can still assess exercise intolerance by using simple tools and a little ingenuity. A thorough knowledge of testing and test devices and an ability to improvise will be required. Some exercise specialists may enhance success by collaborating with other specialists who have complementary expertise and skills.

EXERCISE AND MEDICATIONS

Most people with a chronic disease or disability take prescribed medications to treat their medical problems. Quite often little is known about the side effects of medications as they relate to exercise capacity and quality of life. Some medications improve exercise performance in general; some improve exercise performance when used for specific chronic diseases. Some medications reduce exercise performance and thereby can have an adverse impact on quality of life. The development of an exercise management plan includes consideration of drug-induced changes in exercise performance, as well as optimal dosing of medicines to achieve a desired exercise response. Very little is known about the effects of most medications on adaptations to exercise training, but drug effects on exercise adaptability should be a consideration in exercise management.

Understanding the effects that medications have on exercise performance is easier if one considers exercise itself as a medicine. Exercise, in one sense, is an idealized "intensive care unit" in which neural, hormonal, and local factors alter heart rate and redirect blood flow to deliver oxygen and nutrients. Metabolic control of energy resources is profoundly affected while thermal, acid–base, and electrolyte regulation are altered to support exercise activity. Myriad changes constitute what we call the "exercise response," but these physiologic changes reflect biochemical alterations in the body's control of metabolism. No modern intensive care unit can match the body's extraordinary and sophisticated system for delivery of biochemical compounds during exercise, despite the fact that some natural compounds (including hormones) are often used as prescription drugs. In this way exercise is a medicine.

Part of the difficulty in prescribing exercise as a drug is that exercise doesn't allow independent control over each biochemical process. During exercise, many biochemical reactions take place and we are unable to alter the sophistication of the whole process completely to our liking. However, we can take advantage of the interactions between exercise and medicines. Different kinds of physical activity (e.g., aerobic, strength, flexibility) stimulate biochemical and physiologic processes in slightly different ways. Second, most medicines work by blocking or enhancing specific processes and as a result cause the desired (and undesired) effects. Drug–exercise interactions are determined by the blocked or stimulated processes common to both medicine and exercise. Thus, to understand the effect a medicine has on exercise, one must know both the biochemistry and the physiology of the exercise and the medicine. The challenge is to use these differing effects to the person's advantage.

The study of exercise–medication interactions has generally centered on high blood pressure, angina pectoris (chest pain), congestive heart failure, and ergogenic aids (drugs that improve exercise performance). Most of these studies compare exercise response on and off medication or on different medications. This is the case largely for two reasons: (1) These studies are easier to perform than longitudinal drug–training studies, and (2) these kinds of studies are part of Food and Drug Administration approval and pharmaceutical marketing programs. As a result, the effects of drugs on aerobic exercise response are better known than are the effects of drugs on training adaptations. Most drug–exercise studies have dealt with drugs that alter cardiovascular function: alpha- and beta-adrenergic antagonists (alpha- and beta-blockers), calcium channel antagonists (calcium channel blockers), angiotensin-converting enzyme (ACE) inhibitors, angiotensin II receptor blockers, vasoactive nitrates, and diuretics. Many neuromuscular drugs, such as anti-Parkinsonian drugs, have also been studied in relation to functional performance.

Paradoxical Effects

One paradox of exercise–medication interactions is that disease can alter physiologic action so that a drug can have opposite effects on exercise capacity when used in some combinations or in different disease states. Beta-blockers are the most thoroughly studied drugs with regard to exercise and provide a good example of paradoxical effects. In persons with high blood pressure, beta-blockers typically reduce exercise capacity. In persons with congestive heart failure, however, beta-blockers can increase exercise capacity. The ACE inhibitors provide another example of paradoxical effects. In persons with high blood pressure, ACE inhibitors have no effect on exercise capacity; but in those with congestive heart failure, ACE inhibitors usually increase exercise capacity. The beta-blocker example shows that drug therapy can help the person's disease but reduce exercise capacity. The mechanisms of these effects are complex and will not be discussed here, but these examples show that the effect on exercise capacity is inherent not in the drug but rather in how the drug interacts with the biochemistry of exercise.

Adverse Effects

Sometimes drugs are recommended as preferred therapy even though they reduce exercise capacity. Beta-blockers and diuretics are examples. Recommended as drugs of first choice for high blood pressure, beta-blockers and diuretics have been proven to prevent strokes and heart attacks and to increase longevity. Furthermore, they are inexpensive in comparison to newer medicines such as calcium channel blockers, ACE inhibitors, vasodilators, and alpha-blockers. However, beta-blockers and diuretics often impair exercise response, aerobic capacity, and quality of life. The newer drugs generally do not have these particular side effects. Unfortunately, there are few data on efficacy in preventing strokes or heart attacks and prolonging life for most of these newer drugs. Thus, beta-blockers and diuretics are recommended for high blood pressure even though newer (more expensive) drugs may make it possible to control blood pressure with fewer side effects on exercise capacity and quality of life.

Effects on Muscle

Medicines without cardiovascular action can alter exercise response through effects on skeletal muscle. Corticosteroids, beta-blockers, and ACE inhibitors are examples. Corticosteroids are used for suppression of inflammatory and autoimmune diseases, as well as for immunosuppression in transplant recipients. In the absence of exercise, corticosteroids cause peripheral muscle wasting. In contrast, corticosteroids have no effect on the usual muscle adaptations to exercise training. Beta-blockers also act on skeletal muscle and may attenuate skeletal muscle adaptations to training. On the other hand, long-term ACE inhibitor therapy appears to increase muscle blood flow, although this might be a result of increased physical activity. These examples suggest that the poorly understood effects of medicines on skeletal muscle may be critically important in people who are weak and lacking in endurance.

Drugs That Affect Metabolism

Use of hormones that regulate metabolism can alter functional capacity and response to training. Thyroid hormone and insulin are examples. Hyperthyroidism and hypothyroidism both reduce exercise performance, and over- or underreplacement of thyroid hormone can reduce exercise capacity. However, persons on adequate thyroid replacement have normal exercise performance. In one remarkable example, sprinter Gail Devers suffered from severe hyperthyroidism but recovered after therapy to win gold medals in both the Olympic Games and world championships. Insulin is used to control blood sugar in persons with diabetes, but insulin dosing usually should be reduced (or a snack eaten before exercise) to prevent life-threatening lowering of blood sugar during exercise.

Drugs That Affect Thermoregulation

Drugs with anticholinergic activity block sweat gland excretion, which will lead to decreased heat dissipation and thus increase the risk of heat illness during exercise. Other drugs that interfere with thermoregulation include centrally acting drugs that disrupt hypothalamic thermoregulation and sympathomimetics that cause cutaneous vasoconstriction. In order to prevent heatstroke and further complications relating to heatstroke (e.g., death) individuals who have been prescribed these medications should take precautionary measures to avoid overheating during exercise.

Other Medications

Little is known about the effects of most other drugs on exercise performance. Notable among these are drugs with anti-Parkinsonian activity. Almost nothing is known about the effects of polypharmacy (the use of multiple drugs). Many people take several medications several times a day, and it is well known that under these circumstances people forget to take their medicines. Furthermore, when adherence to or timing of a medication dose varies, the exercise response may be affected. Finally, while the effects of exercise on medicines are generally unexplored, it is worth noting that even less is known about the effects of exercise on the metabolism of medicines (i.e., whether it is increased or decreased).

The examples in this section provide no details about the interactions between medicines and exercise. (See the appendix for the effects of selected medications.) Nonetheless, exercise professionals must know (or learn) about the medications their clients are taking and must be able to assess how the medicine may alter each person's physiology. A pharmacology textbook should be a standard reference for anyone attempting to manage exercise for someone who takes medicines. Exercise professionals should establish a working relationship with the individual's physician so that suggestions about changing medications or dosing schedules can be smoothly integrated into overall medical management.

EXERCISE DOSE-RESPONSE

Prescribing exercise for persons with chronic disease or disability is a complex art. The objective is to decrease physiologic limitations and improve physical capacity through specific therapies. The biggest dilemmas are not in determining which therapies to use but in defining the goals and choosing the appropriate training intensity, duration, and frequency. The key question is, What is the dose–response relationship of exercise training for each disease and disability?

In considering exercise programming for individuals with chronic disease or disability, one often has few data on which to base decisions. Recommendations for preventing death from heart disease are based on large studies; but because these studies generally have not included persons with chronic disease or disability, present data may not be applicable. Furthermore, restoring and maintaining functional capacity and independence are very different goals from preventing cardiovascular disease. Unfortunately, exercise training to optimize functional capacity has not been well studied in the context of most chronic diseases or disabilities. As a result, many exercise professionals have used clinical experience to develop their own methods for prescribing exercise. Many of the recommendations in this manual were derived in this manner.

Experience is an acceptable way to guide exercise management, but a systematic approach would be better. One logical alternative would be to model exercise in the same way that pharmacologists model medications, since exercise and medical prescriptions are similar. Medicines are prescribed by action (type of chemical), bioavailability (which determines the dose), therapeutic level (the goal of therapy), and half-life (metabolism of the medicine). Prescription of exercise is quite similar, in that the family of exercise specifies the action (e.g., aerobic training increases $\dot{V}O_{2max}$; strength training increases muscle strength and mass); exercise dose is a function of intensity and duration (i.e., hard workouts at high intensity or long duration yield a higher number of total MET-minutes); and exercise frequency is determined by the desired fitness level (therapeutic goal) and the length of time for recovery from an exercise session (half-life).

These principles explain some common practices in exercise science and sport. Athletes exercise daily or even twice daily, whereas wellness enthusiasts exercise three or four times a week. People who recover quickly can exercise on the day after a big workout, whereas others may need an intervening day of rest, particularly after a very-high-dose session. Like people who are sensitive to medicines and require lower doses, those with low functional capacity are easily exhausted, and it is common to prescribe short, low-intensity workouts with long rest periods (low-dose exercise). Just as a therapeutic drug level in the blood can be achieved with the use of a lower dose more frequently, conditioning can be achieved through use of lower-intensity exercise two or three times a day. Just as slowly metabolized drugs must be given less often, persons who are slow to recover and adapt need more rest between exercise sessions.

Prescribing the right dose of exercise is important because one can experience an acute "overdose" of exercise. Like marathoners "hitting the wall," persons with chronic disease or disability can suddenly become worn out, often by small amounts of exercise. Common sense suggests that one should probably avoid exhaustion (an exercise overdose), but there are few data to support or refute this notion. In comparison, overtraining is essentially a chronic overdose of exercise, and is associated with psychological and physiological decompensation as well as musculoskeletal injury. Acute exercise overdoses and chronic overtraining must be avoided in persons who have limited reserve because of chronic disease or disability.

One area in which pharmacologists are ahead of exercise specialists is in following the therapeutic effect of medicines. Pharmacologists can do this by measuring drug levels in the blood. This information can then be used to help guide dose frequency. Exercise specialists can try using exercise tests to assess progress, but this information is not as helpful as data on drug level in the blood are to pharmacologists. A systematic way to guide frequency of exercise training has not been developed, largely because we do not fully understand fatigue and adaptation.

The individual's starting level, resistance to fatigue, and adaptability to training are probably what determine the total dose of exercise required to achieve a given fitness level. Perceived fatigue is not like perceived exertion, which is proportional to exercise intensity (e.g., the 20-point Borg scale). Fatigue seems to have a threshold. After this threshold is reached, exhaustion occurs quite rapidly. Adaptability is also poorly understood. It is possible to increase the adaptation rate by training harder (e.g., increasing the intensity or frequency of exercise sessions), but training too hard leads to decompensation or injury. Thus, all we can say at present is that high doses of exercise increase the risk of exhaustion and that high frequency of exercise superimposes more training on incomplete recovery and risks overtraining.

RISK, COST, AND BENEFIT

The most common risks associated with exercise are musculoskeletal injury, heart attack, and sudden death. Individuals who are apparently healthy and able-bodied are at risk largely for musculoskeletal injuries. For example, despite highly publicized cases of sudden death, basketball players are at greater risk for spraining their ankles. Only the basketball players with heart disease are at risk for sudden death. So exercise involves two kinds of risks: disease-dependent and activity-dependent risks. Disease-dependent risks are the adverse effects of exercise that are a consequence of disease. Activity-dependent risks are the adverse effects of exercise that are a consequence of accidents occurring during an activity. Activity- and disease-dependent risks must be considered for each person with a chronic disease or disability.

In general, the most important risks are disease dependent: Arthritic joints can become more inflamed, diabetics can lose control of their blood sugar, people with high blood pressure can have a stroke or heart attack, clients with heart failure can have abnormal heart rhythms, clients with poor balance can fall, prosthetics can cause skin trauma and irritation, and so on. The most common activity-dependent complications are probably musculoskeletal injury and exhaustion, while the most feared risks, of heart attack and sudden death, occur largely in people with heart disease. Accurate estimates of these risks are not available. Although few clinical exercise trials in persons with a chronic disease or disability have reported life-threatening complications, virtually all studies have used small, selected populations that precluded high-risk subjects. Some data suggest a high incidence of musculoskeletal injury with the use of intense exercise in weak and frail individuals, although this has not been a universal finding. Although the data on risk are generally not clear, it is prudent to monitor vigilantly for potential complications.

The costs of exercise training include time, energy, and money put into the program. Fortunately, exercise can be inexpensive compared to other modern medical therapies (particularly so for unsupervised exercise). Even so, exercise is far from cost free. Membership in a YMCA or YWCA, health club, or fitness center can cost hundreds of dollars per year. Some individuals may need to choose a center that caters to persons who have special medical circumstances and need medical supervision. Investment in the appropriate clothing, shoes, and assorted equipment can also be substantial. This can be particularly true for those who must invest in prosthetic equipment or sport or racing wheelchairs. Protective equipment such as pads, gloves, skin protection materials, and helmets must not be overlooked. Since very few people can participate in a lifetime of exercise and be totally free from medical complications (especially activity-dependent problems), it may be reasonable to assume that there will be at least some associated medical costs. Lastly, personal time and energy are major costs of any program, but these are difficult to quantify in monetary terms.

The various investments in an exercise program must be weighed against the probable benefits. Benefits from exercise training are usually related to functional capacity and quality of life, although some populations also benefit from decreased morbidity and mortality. Furthermore, it is sometimes possible to decrease the doses of medications and reap a direct financial return on investment. There has been some success in predicting outcome for cardiac rehabilitation clients, and this technique may be useful for other populations. In the meantime, an exercise trial is probably worthwhile in any person with a chronic disease or disability. In contrast, a person who has several diseases or disabilities may gain little from exercise training or may even be adversely affected by it. Thus, it is difficult to know who is too sick to benefit from exercise. In people who are too sick to improve, it usually becomes apparent that exercise is of little benefit. Unfortunately, it is not currently possible to know how much someone will benefit from a given exercise program, and in many cases it is impossible to compare the benefits to costs in monetary terms. Better methods of predicting adaptation would improve goal setting and improve risk–benefit as well as cost–benefit analyses.

PUTTING IT ALL TOGETHER

Some of the techniques suggested in this manual will be new to exercise specialists, who will need time to learn the techniques and become proficient in their use. Successful exercise management does not require the use of these principles, but thinking about exercise in the contexts presented here can help determine what exercise tests to use, how to accommodate medicines, how to develop goals, how to estimate the dose-response, and how to assess the risk–benefit and cost–benefit relationships. These considerations may be particularly complicated in individuals with a low exhaustion threshold, frequent concurrent illness, multiple chronic diseases, and poor adherence. In someone with only one relatively minor medical problem or disability, these tasks may be simple and straightforward. In someone with a severe chronic disease or disability or multiple chronic diseases or disabilities, these tasks are highly complex. Problem-oriented exercise management using SOAP notes is one mechanism that can be employed to solve these problems. When using this approach, be sure to follow some key steps.

When taking subjective data:

- Uncover the nature of the problem as it relates to exercise.
- Ask about old and new musculoskeletal injuries.
- Look at the person for obvious problems.

When choosing exercise tests (objective data):

- Select the category of exercise tests that provide insight into the problem.
- Use modes and protocols that can be individualized.
- Use tests providing specific measures that either will further define the problem or will determine specific aspects of the exercise program.
- Be aware of medications that may affect the test results, and know the times they are taken.
- Be aware of concomitant conditions and any special circumstances.

When making an assessment:

- Organize the assessment either by family of exercise or by physiologic problem.
- Consider possible need for additional tests.
- Be flexible in assessing multiple problems, and attack each one independently (but watch for interactions).
- Be aware that each problem may follow its own time course.
- If unsure, consider a therapeutic trial.

When developing an exercise program:

- Choose the category and modes of exercise that best treat the problem.
- Choose goals that are realistically attainable to increase the chance of success.
- Adjust exercise doses on the basis of exercise test measures, perceived exercise intensity, and the "fatigue threshold."

- Recommend frequency of training based on the total exercise dose and the person's adaptability.
- Accommodate any need for prosthetic, orthotic, or assistive devices.
- Consider the potential interactions of exercise and medications.
- Consider the disease-dependent and activity-dependent risks.
- Be aware that most of the benefits are probably related to quality of life.

When monitoring:

- Beware of the sudden onset of exhaustion, as well as insufficient recovery and overtraining.
- Monitor stability of the underlying medical problems and changes in medications.
- When in doubt about safety, or if an activity causes pain, don't do it.
- When in doubt about progression, increase in small increments.
- Do not allow clients to push themselves hard unless they are well warmed up.

When following up:

- Report progress in terms meaningful to the individual, not in exercise jargon.
- Estimate dose-response and be willing to consider failure to benefit.
- Always follow up on unresolved problems.
- Use the numbers you assign to the problems to help keep track of everything.
- Most interventions take weeks (if not months) to achieve a benefit, so be patient.

To make the process of writing SOAP notes quick and easy, follow these guidelines:

- Be concise.
- Avoid sentences; use key phrases instead.
- Discuss only currently relevant problems; leave out irrelevant information.
- Organize the problems by exercise family (i.e., aerobic, strength, flexibility, etc.).
- Assign a number to each problem, and always refer to that problem by its number.
- Always follow up unresolved problems.

Exercise Is Medicine

J. Larry Durstine, PhD, FACSM ■ J. Brent Peel, MS
Michael J. LaMonte, PhD, FACSM ■ Steven J. Keteyian, PhD, FACSM
Emma Fletcher, MA ■ Geoffrey E. Moore, MD, FACSM

Exercise has had a natural role in daily human life since preindustrial societies. The conviction that good health is achieved through proper nutrition and physical activity predates the historical writings of classical Greek philosophy and medicine. Greek physicians such as Hippocrates (460-370 B.C.) and Galen (A.D. 129-210) were outspoken and adamant in their belief that disease was not the result of mystical forces, but rather the product of environmental factors, specifically diet and living habits. To enjoy a healthy life required a certain amount of self-discipline in giving proper attention to healthful living habits. Hippocrates has been widely credited with the quote "If we could give every individual the right amount of nourishment and exercise, not too little and not too much, we would have found the safest way to health." Galen, another prominent ancient Greek physician, may have been the first to promote the principle of specificity when he stated, "Those movements which do not alter respiration are not called exercise." Other notable scientists, such as A. Cornelius Celsus (ca. 25 BC-50 AD) and Hieronymus Mercuralis (1530-1606), spoke specifically about the health-related benefits of exercise.

Despite having only a crude understanding surrounding physical activity and regular exercise participation, these notable physicians and healers of the Renaissance and preindustrial eras pushed forward and encouraged the concept that the body is engineered for movement. Physical activity was thought to be a key factor underpinning proper function of human biochemistry and physiology.

It is somewhat ironic, but encouraging, to see that the wisdom about exercise and medicine that our forefathers offered over 2000 years ago has come full circle.

We are also deeply indebted to modern-day physicians such as Joseph B. Wolffe, MD, a founding father of the American College of Sports Medicine (ACSM); Ralph Paffenbarger Jr., MD, DrPH; and Kenneth Cooper, MD, MPH. These influential men have enlightened physicians and laypersons alike through their evidence-based promotion of exercise is medicine. Gratitude is also given to the many contributors from the fields of exercise physiology, epidemiology, psychology, and medicine for their contributions in advancing the use of exercise for the purpose of achieving medical and health benefits. The 20th century was a period of awakening to the clinical merits of regular exercise participation. Knowledge and application related to exercise is medicine have come from diverse and sometimes unexpected sources and experiences. For example, medical services in the military have provided insight into the idea that exercise is rehabilitative in caring for wounded soldiers. Collaborations among physicians, engineers, and biomechanists have led to the development of innovative corrective and therapeutic techniques to treat individuals suffering from chronic musculoskeletal pain as well as from postural and muscular imbalances. Historical wisdom dictated that exercise therapy was of little value to cardiac patients. Seminal reports on the benefits of early chair sitting and on the marked cardiovascular deconditioning following prolonged bed rest provided critical information that segued into modern-day cardiopulmonary exercise rehabilitation programs. More recently, randomized clinical trials have shown that increases in exercise participation, and improvements in other lifestyle behaviors such as dietary intake, are better than standard pharmacotherapy at managing diabetes risk and clinical depression. Indeed, the application of physical activity and exercise training in a medicinal context is far broader than was the case a century past.

Scientists and practitioners are at the forefront of an ever-expanding critical mass of scientific evidence from which to derive the rationale for exercise alone or in combination with other therapeutic regimes as a form of both primary and secondary medical therapy. Modern research techniques are providing exciting new information pertaining to the biochemical, molecular, and genetic mechanisms through which exercise affects health. In the last decade, considerable progress has been made in defining appropriate titration of exercise frequency, intensity, duration, and type for a variety of parameters related to health and physical functioning. Clinical and public health guidelines now call for exercise promotion in conjunction with nutritional and pharmacologic therapies for the prevention and management of disease and disability. Exercise is one of the few therapeutic agents with well-characterized dose–response relationships, associated with a broad spectrum of conditions that does not require approval by the Food and Drug Administration (FDA) or another governmental agency in order to be prescribed. The rigors with which physical activity and exercise training are evaluated and prescribed for medical therapy must accord with existing government standards and polices for all medical treatments and procedures. In his 1993 J.B. Wolffe Memorial Lecture, William Haskell, PhD, provided FDA-type criteria that when properly used provide a means for evaluation of the efficacy, effectiveness, safety, dose-response, and mechanisms of action for exercise that could then be used in developing an appropriate individualized exercise prescription. Continued growth of the scientific evidence will propagate a broader dissemination of the clinical and public health benefits of regular physical activity. Eventually, the medical and lay communities will more uniformly acknowledge a view widely held by exercise scientists and practitioners for over a century—that exercise really is medicine.

TERMINOLOGY

An important distinction to make is that physical activity refers to a behavior, specifically body movement that occurs from skeletal muscle contraction and that results in increased energy expenditure above resting metabolic rate. It now is accepted that the volume of activity-related energy expenditure, or the total dose of physical activity, is more important for health benefits than is the specific type of physical activity (e.g., walking, running, cycling, or occupational activities). Exercise, or "exercise training," is a subcategory of physical activity that is systematically structured toward enhancing one or more components of physical fitness. Physical fitness is a set of physiological attributes (e.g., cardiorespiratory fitness, body composition, muscular strength and endurance, flexibility, agility, and balance) that may be enhanced through exercise training or through regular participation in physical activity, and that may also favorably influence health and quality of life. In most individuals, particularly among those who are sedentary, increases in physical activity through lifestyle activities or through planned exercise training result in increases in physical fitness, whereas fitness declines soon after cessation of exercise. Whether improvements in physical fitness are required to achieve exercise-induced changes in health status remains an area of study. Proper use of the aforementioned terminology is critical to ensure accurate and consistent interpretation of research findings and clinical or public health guidelines. To avoid circumvolution, we use the term "exercise" throughout this writing, noting the various distinctions in terminology just discussed.

EPIDEMIOLOGY

The hypothesis that a sedentary lifestyle leads to premature morbidity and mortality has been extensively tested in numerous scientific studies. An estimated 90 million Americans are currently living with a chronic health condition, and this figure is projected to rise sharply in the years to come as a result of the rapidly expanding older population subgroup. Treating chronic health conditions is very costly, in terms of both direct medical costs and indirect costs such as lost wages and productivity. For example, the direct medical costs of caring for individuals with chronic diseases accounted for more than 75% of the nation's $2 trillion medical care budget in 2005 (table 3.1). Until such time that physicians, practitioners, and employers more readily embrace the idea that physical inactivity is a key antecedent to most chronic diseases and disablements and thus should be a cornerstone of targeted intervention, there will be little impact on controlling or reducing medical costs associated with chronic disease.

In addition to the economics of chronic disease, there are the more humanistic issues related to physical inactivity, such as a lower quality of life, loss of functional independence, depression and mood disorders, and decreased longevity. Cardiovascular disease is currently the primary cause of death within the U.S., and approximately 53% of all cardiovascular disease-related deaths are attributed to coronary artery disease (see figures 3.1 and 3.2). It is disheartening to witness the undue human suffering associated with premature chronic disease given the abundance of scientific literature confirming that individuals who maintain at least moderate levels of functional capacity have lower rates of morbidity and mortality than those with low functional capacity. The Centers of Disease Control and Prevention (CDC) supports the contention that physical inactivity is one of the major underlying causes of premature mortality in the United States. Regular exercise participation throughout the life span is a goal that our society must make a serious commitment to in order to both prevent and treat chronic disease. Clearly an active and fit way of living is a cost-effective, relatively safe, and efficacious approach to reducing premature morbidity and mortality and improve quality of life for all Americans.

Numerous prospective studies, beginning with the pioneering work by epidemiologists Jeremy Morris, MD, and Ralph Paffenbarger Jr., MD, during the 1950s and 1960s have confirmed the role of physical inactivity in chronic disease etiology and premature mortality. For example, in the seminal 1996 *Surgeon General's Report on Physical Activity and Health,* experts evaluated epidemiologic evidence from 12 studies relating physical activity or cardiorespiratory fitness levels to total cardiovascular disease (CVD) risk, 41 studies on coronary heart disease (CHD) risk, and 14 studies on stroke risk. Based on the strength and consistency of evidence, a conclusion for causality was established for total CVD and CHD. The risk of CHD events is at least twofold higher in sedentary persons than in active individuals when the findings are summarized across studies adequately designed to examine this relationship. As is seen with other major CHD risk factors, the prevalence of sedentary lifestyle is relatively high and the distribution worsens across CHD-prone population subgroups such as older adults, groups who are obese or who have diabetes, groups in the lower strata of education and socioeconomic status, and racial or ethnic minority groups. Given the prevalence of sedentary living habits and its strong association with CHD risk, the population burden of CHD is substantial. Assuming that a sedentary lifestyle is causally related with CHD, scientists previously estimated that approximately 35% of CHD deaths could be attributed to being sedentary—a fraction second only to that for hypercholesterolemia (43% of CHD deaths) when compared with other major CHD risk factors.

TABLE 3.1

Selected Chronic Diseases Precipitated by Physical Inactivity and Resulting Health Care Costs in the United States

Chronic disease	Annual cost of condition in United States (U.S. dollars)
Heart disease and stroke	$448 billion (projected 2008)
Diabetes	$174 billion
Obesity	$117 billion
Cancer	$89 billion (direct medical cost)
Arthritis	$81 billion (medical care cost) $128 billion (medical care and loss of productivity)
Cognitive and psychological disorders	Cost not known

Data from Center for Disease Control 2008.

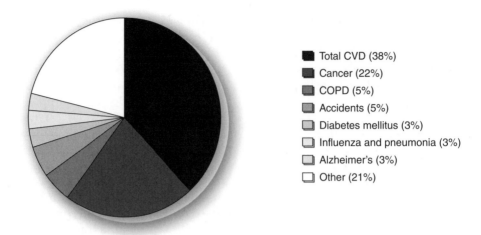

Figure 3.1 Distribution of total deaths by underlying cause.

Data from National Center for Health Statistics 2006.

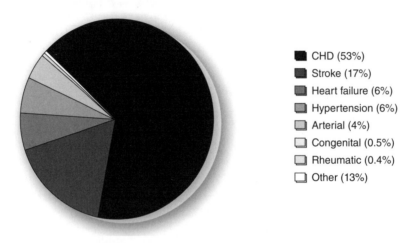

Figure 3.2 Distribution of CVD deaths.

Data from National Center for Health Statistics 2006.

Biological factors are potentially responsible for reduction in the risk of chronic disease and premature death associated with routine exercise participation and daily physical activity. Here is a selected list:

1. Improved body composition
   - Decreased abdominal adiposity
   - Preservation of lean body mass
2. Improved lipid lipoprotein profiles
   - Decreased triglycerides
   - Increased HDL-C levels
   - Decreased LDL-to-HDL ratio
3. Improved glucose homeostasis and insulin sensitivity
4. Reduced blood pressure
5. Improved autonomic tone
6. Enhanced immune system function
7. Reduced systemic inflammation
8. Decreased blood coagulation
9. Improved coronary blood flow
10. Augmented cardiac function
11. Enhanced endothelial function
12. Improved psychological well-being
    - Reduced stress, anxiety, and depression
    - Important in the prevention and management of chronic diseases

A major advancement in the exercise is medicine paradigm has been the growth of a critical evidence base supporting the health benefits of resistance exercise over and above those conferred by aerobic exercise. Higher levels of muscular fitness are associated with significantly better risk factor profiles, lower risk of all-cause mortality and cardiovascular events, improvements in bone density and articular tissue strength, and lower risk of developing functional limitations and nonfatal disease. The positive effect of muscular fitness on health outcomes is reported more often in men than in women and generally is independent of measures of physical activity or cardiorespiratory fitness levels and body size. Muscular fitness may be particularly important in the elderly. In one study, greater muscular strength was associated with significantly lower all-cause mortality risk, even after overall exercise levels and comorbid conditions were accounted for. In fact, controlling for thigh muscle mass has little effect on the association between strength and mortality, which suggests that muscle quality may be more important than muscle quantity as a determinant of health outcomes. Whether the protective effect of muscular fitness derives from maximum muscular strength per se, regular participation in resistance exercise, or both remains to be addressed in future studies.

EXERCISE AND CARDIOVASCULAR DISEASES

The secondary prevention benefits derived from regular exercise are also well documented in individuals with established conditions. For example, several systematic reviews and meta-analyses of clinical trials clearly demonstrate that regular exercise improves CVD risk factors and may arrest, even potentially reverse, CVD progression. Compared with patients receiving usual care, patients in comprehensive cardiac rehabilitation programs report fewer CVD complications, continued utilization of hospital services, and better risk factor profiles; and they experience, on average, a 20% to 25% lower mortality rate. The favorable outcomes and improved health-related benefits recently reported in cardiac rehabilitation patients are likely owing to a more comprehensive and multidisciplinary framework for delivering rehabilitative services that include not only exercise and aggressive pharmacologic risk factor reduction, but also education and training in patient self-monitoring and in risk-reducing lifestyle changes.

Hypertension, defined as a systolic blood pressure of ≥140 mmHg or greater and/or a diastolic pressure of ≥90 mmHg or greater, or the use of antihypertensive medication, is a serious public health problem, particularly among older adults. Hypertension prevalence is estimated to be 29% among all U.S. adults and as high as 65% among adults 60 years and older. Higher levels of exercise are associated with a lower incidence of new-onset hypertension in women and men, younger and older alike. The magnitude of blood pressure lowering in response to exercise is greatest in individuals with higher baseline blood pressure levels, and these exercise reductions are not altered by age, gender, or ethnicity.

Diabetes, principally type 2 diabetes, is the sixth leading cause of death and a major cause of disability in the United States. The risk of all forms of CVD is two- to eightfold greater in adults with diabetes compared to those without diabetes; mortality rates are likewise increased by the presence of diabetes. Epidemiological studies have consistently shown that exercise, alone or in combination with diet therapy, reduces the progression to clinical diabetes in adults with impaired glucose tolerance and promotes better utilization of blood glucose in individuals already diagnosed with type 2 diabetes. Both aerobic and resistance exercise are associated with decreased risk in individuals with type 2 diabetes, primarily as a result of improved blood glucose homeostasis.

Over the past 50 years the role of dyslipidemia has been established in the development of CHD and other chronic disease. An estimated 107 million Americans have clinically elevated blood cholesterol levels defined as fasting total cholesterol >200 mg/dl; approximately 38 million have levels that exceed 240 mg/dl, placing them at high risk for a CHD event. Clinical trials have consistently shown that improving blood lipid and lipoprotein concentrations significantly lowers CHD risk. Exercise training also has been shown to favorably affect blood lipid and lipoprotein profiles. Pharmacological intervention remains primary for dyslipidemic disorders while lifestyle modifications are considered adjunctive therapies. Because exercise and diet work synergistically to enhance blood lipid and lipoprotein profiles, they are the cornerstone lifestyle changes incorporated into a comprehensive blood lipid management plan.

Higher levels of physical activity and cardiorespiratory fitness are associated with lower death rates among individuals with existing diseases such as CHD, hypertension, and diabetes, even after differences in traditional risk factors for each condition have been accounted for. Higher levels of physical activity and cardiorespiratory fitness also confer protection against early mortality among overweight and obese individuals. For example, mortality rates among obese men and women with moderate and higher fitness levels are 50% lower than those experienced by lean men and women with low fitness levels. Furthermore, men with diabetes and low fitness levels are four times more likely to die prematurely than men with diabetes and a high fitness level; this finding was materially unchanged when obesity status and other mortality predictors were considered in analyses.

BIOLOGICAL PLAUSIBILITY

The clinical benefits of exercise are the result of a complex web of interrelated physiologic mechanisms, each having a potentially unique exercise dose–response relationship. Some of these physiologic responses and adaptations to exercise are improved weight control and body composition, lipid and lipoprotein profiles, blood glucose homeostasis and insulin sensitivity, fibrinolysis and thrombolysis capacity, coronary blood flow and arrhythmic threshold, and endothelial function and blood pressure regulation, as well as lower levels of circulating inflammatory and thrombogenic factors. What has yet to be fully elucidated is the dose (e.g., frequency, intensity, and duration of aerobic or resistance exercise) required to improve specific mechanisms, individually or in combination, and their associated clinical sequellae.

Longitudinal studies involving individuals with CHD show that aerobic exercise training, in combination with diet and other risk factor interventions, can prevent the progression and perhaps reduce the severity of atherosclerosis. Numerous studies show that endurance exercise is associated with increased high-density lipoprotein cholesterol (HDL-C), which enhances reverse cholesterol transport and antioxidant activity in the arterial wall, thereby protecting against atherosclerosis. Even a single exercise session can positively alter blood lipid and lipoprotein profiles. A principal mechanism responsible for exercise-induced lipid and lipoprotein changes is through upregulation of lipoprotein lipase activity, which enhances removal of cholesterol and triglyceride from the blood. Another benefit of exercise involves lower levels of circulation inflammatory biomarkers, like C-reactive protein (CRP) and tumor necrosis factor alpha (TNFa), which are strongly associated with

many chronic diseases including CVD, diabetes, and certain types of cancer.

Basic science also has advanced the understanding of how exercise affects type 2 diabetes. Biochemical mechanisms responsible for exercise adaptations in diabetics include enhanced glycolytic enzymes, increased glucose transport proteins (specifically, GLUT-4 protein), greater messenger RNA (mRNA) expression, and activation of an exercise alternative mechanism for skeletal muscle glucose uptake. These new scientific insights provide diabetic exercise practitioners with additional means for promoting regular exercise participation.

Another growing area for new knowledge is the role of exercise in cancer prevention. The literature clearly shows reduced mortality associated with regular exercise. In addition, the exercise-induced mechanisms responsible for these associations are different for each specific cancer. Factors associated with prevention include reduced endogenous reproductive hormone levels, decreased body weight and adiposity, altered circulating levels of insulin and insulin-like growth factors (IGFs), and enhanced immune function that directly affects tumor development and growth.

Exercise has also recently been associated with improved mental health and psychologic well-being, which may in itself be an important consideration in the prevention and management of other non-psychological diseases. Some scientists suggest that exercise-induced changes in neurotransmitters including norepinephrine, dopamine, and serotonin are important mediators of the psychological benefits conferred by regular exercise. The psychosocial aspects of exercise, such as increased opportunity for social interaction, relief from daily stressors, and increased self-efficacy, also have been identified as important aspects of improved mental health.

CURRENT AND FUTURE PRIORITIES

Given that many of the relationships between exercise and chronic diseases likely are causal, large numbers of people will die or become ill each year unnecessarily because of a sedentary lifestyle. It therefore is imperative that continued epidemiologic, basic and applied, and clinical exercise research be funded and completed to further expand the already large evidence base supporting Exercise Is Medicine, as well as more broadly to diffuse Exercise Is Medicine into existing clinical and professional training paradigms. The dose–

response relationship of exercise with most putative risk factors and their associated chronic diseases is not completely defined. Studies also demonstrate that the greatest benefits occur when least active individuals become moderately active. Current recommendations are for a minimum exercise volume of approximately 1000 kcal per week expended in activities of at least moderate intensity. People already achieving this level of activity-related energy expenditure likely will benefit further from higher activity levels.

Amid ubiquitous advertising and marketing of exercise products that require "little effort and time to use and result in rapid improvement in fitness and health," exercise epidemiologists and physiologists face the challenge of better understanding the most efficacious dose of exercise for health benefits, as well as the most effective strategies for affecting population-wide adoption and maintenance of targeted exercise programs. Scientists will continue to consider different perspectives in evaluating and improving the exercise is medicine paradigm. For example, only in recent years have exercise scientists considered delineating the use of exercise in manipulating and understanding the molecular basis for change. In addition, only now have scientists learned to use exercise as we would use pharmacotherapy to manipulate exercise practices to gain optimal exercise adaptations and health outcomes. One area currently gaining much attention is the increasing use of genomic and proteomic techniques to understand the various ways in which exercise influences the entire physiologic system, and in turn how medications are used to optimize physiologic and exercise-developed health outcomes. In this regard, future exercise practitioners will perhaps develop exercise prescriptions that utilize not only target heart rates but also measures of skeletal muscle fatigue. Exercise scientists have known for quite some time that some individuals respond and adapt to exercise training better than others do. Researchers have coined the term "nonresponder" as a way of identifying those individuals who do not respond or adapt to exercise as well as matched controls do. For example, men with the apo E3 genotype have greater plasma HDL-C increases after six months of endurance exercise than men with the apo E2 or E4 genotype. In this case, exercise scientists and practitioners can work together to improve the exercise adaptations in people who are nonresponders, perhaps by coupling an exercise prescription with genotype-targeted pharmacologic therapy designed to maximize the patient's adaptations to exercise.

There is no intensive care unit or pharmacological compound in the world capable of accurately mimicking the exercise response. A very real challenge for exercise scientists and exercise medicine professionals of the 21st century is finding specific ways to overcome the generalities of exercise prescription (frequency, intensity, time, and type) and to develop risk factor– and disease-specific exercise therapies.

EDUCATION FOR EXERCISE PROFESSIONALS

At the end of the day, the hope is that medical doctors and health practitioners will prescribe exercise as therapeutic medicine. The achievement of this goal will require a multidisciplinary effort to institutionalize appropriate educational and practical training experiences at the preprofessional and professional levels to effectively change current health care delivery. Thus, is it not logical that the training of those prescribing exercise as a therapy stand up to a rigorous comparison to other conventional specialties?

The American Medical Association membership (AMA) made public their opinion on this matter. In the November 8, 2007, issue of *AMA eVoice*, a weekly publication of the AMA, then-President Ronald Davis, MD, posed the following question to AMA members: "If you learned that a single prescription could prevent and treat dozens of diseases, such as diabetes, hypertension, and obesity, would you prescribe it to your patients?" The simple act of including Dr. Davis' question in an AMA-affiliated journal is a sign that we already have come a long way in getting physicians to embrace the concept of exercise is medicine. Time will tell as to the extent that physicians respond to Dr. Davis' "call to action."

Since 1975, ACSM has taken a leadership role in training and certifying professionals charged with delivering exercise prescriptions to apparently healthy adults and those with chronic disease or disability. In fact, across a variety of certification offerings, ACSM has now certified well over 35,000 exercise professionals. A list of the current certifications offered by ACSM is shown in table 3.2. Before describing each certification, we offer a brief explanation regarding the rigorous standards and processes that ACSM voluntarily meets in order to offer these examinations.

All of ACSM's certification products are accredited by the National Commission for Certifying

Agencies, whose role is to independently verify that all ACSM examinations offered are developed, evaluated, revised, and scored using methods that meet or exceed best-practice industry standards and reflect well the job duties of professionals working in the field today. Extensive work goes into developing and revising ACSM certification examinations, including the work done by content experts teaching or working in the field who develop or revise the knowledge, skills, and abilities (KSAs) that define and describe the scope of practice for each certification. With use of an electronic survey distributed to currently certified professionals, the KSAs unique to each examination that ACSM offers are evaluated via what is referred to as a Job Task Analysis (JTA). The purpose of the JTA is to gather from practitioners in the field their opinion about how frequently each KSA is performed as part of their routine work duties and about how important or critical each KSA is relative to work conduct. Once survey results are compiled, new examinations are developed or current examinations revised to ensure that they are weighted and partitioned in a manner that best reflects the scope and importance of duties identified in the JTA. Finally, beta or test versions of the new or revised examination are released to consumers to evaluate the quality of each question before the new examination becomes part of an ACSM certification. To ensure that all ACSM examinations remain contemporary and best reflect changes in the field, a new JTA is conducted every three to four years.

Table 3.2 also contains the key characteristics associated with the various ACSM examinations. The ACSM Certified Personal Trainer℠ is ACSM's entry-level certification and is aimed at exercise professionals who primarily work with apparently healthy individuals interested in improving their physical fitness. However, industry trends suggest that more and more personal trainers are helping train select patients with stable, chronic diseases such as hypertension and obesity. The ACSM Certified Health Fitness Specialist℠ (CHFS), formerly ACSM Health/Fitness Instructor® (HFI), represents the next-level exercise professional, who works not only with apparently healthy people but also with many people who have a stable, chronic disease or disability. The CHFS must possess a minimum of an associate's degree (or be in the last semester of the program) in a health-related field. The CHFS is educated and experienced in developing appropriate and safe exercise prescriptions, overseeing fitness testing and training, helping to coordinate or lead the activities of other exercise professionals, and providing general risk factor education and counseling.

Like the CHFS, the ACSM Certified Clinical Exercise Specialist℠, formerly ACSM Exercise Specialist® (ES), must also have completed an academic degree prior to sitting for the exam. The CCES is required to have a bachelor's degree in an allied health field. The focus of the CCES certification is on the advanced testing and training of patients with a cardiac, pulmonary, or metabolic (e.g., diabetes, chronic kidney disease) disorder. Professionals certified as an ACSM CCES℠ may work in a hospital- or university-based setting and represent the "front-line" provider charged with both ensuring safe exercise and facilitating compliance with prescribed therapies. The most advanced or comprehensive clinical certification offered by ACSM is the Registered Clinical Exercise Physiologist® (RCEP). Prior to sitting for this examination the candidate must have completed a master's degree in exercise science or a related field; and, in addition to being educated in clinical exercise programming such as cardiac, pulmonary and metabolic disorders, he or she is tested on KSAs addressing the pathophysiology and exercise-related issues germane to patients with musculoskeletal, neuromuscular, neoplastic, immunologic, and hematologic disorders.

Finally, as previously mentioned, academic credentials are required for several of ACSM's certifications. Since 2004, ACSM, and nearly a dozen other professional organizations that now compose the Committee on the Accreditation of the Exercise Sciences (CoAES), developed, in conjunction with the Committee on Accreditation of Allied Health Education Programs, the academic standards and guidelines for colleges and universities offering exercise science–related degrees. Currently, academic standards and guidelines exist for a one-year certificate in personal training, a bachelor's degree in exercise science, and a graduate degree in exercise physiology, with the latter having two areas of focus: clinical and applied. Additional information and application materials are available for schools interested in undergoing program accreditation; such schools are encouraged to visit the CoAES Web site at www.coaes.org.

As highlighted throughout this book, clinicians now appreciate the important and efficacious role of exercise in medicine. To this end, the ACSM continues to take a leadership role in preparing and certifying the exercise professionals who work with patients having a chronic disease or disability,

TABLE 3.2

Key Characteristics of ACSM's Certification Programs

ACSM certification	Candidate profile	Working environment or setting	Scope of practice (abridged)
ACSM Certified Personal Trainer^SM	College students, professionals new to the field not necessarily with a health-related degree	In-home or community or commercial fitness center	Works with healthy individuals or those with medical clearance to exercise Performs basic fitness assessments and field tests Designs, leads, and progresses one-on-one exercise programs
ACSM Certified Health Fitness Specialist^SM	Graduates of two-year or four-year health-related degree programs	University, community, corporate, or commercial fitness center	Conducts risk factor stratification Works with special populations (elderly, obese, etc.) Works with individuals with controlled disease Has competence in exercise testing and comprehensive exercise prescription Has competence in program administration
ACSM Certified Clinical Exercise Specialist^SM	Undergraduates with a degree in relevant allied health field; 600 h of practical experience in a clinical setting	University, community, or corporate fitness center; public health setting; hospital or clinic for direct patient care	Works with individuals with controlled cardiovascular, pulmonary, or metabolic disease or some combination thereof Has mastery of clinical exercise testing and data interpretation Has competence in conducting and interpreting ECGs at rest and during exercise
Registered Clinical Exercise Physiologist®	Graduates with master's degrees in exercise physiology, exercise science or related field; minimum of 600 h of clinical experience	Hospital or clinic for direct patient care; research-based clinical settings	Works with individuals referred by, or currently under the care of, a physician Works with individuals with cardiovascular, pulmonary, metabolic, orthopedic/musculoskeletal, neuromuscular, or immunological/hematological disease or combinations thereof Has mastery of clinical exercise testing, data interpretation, complex exercise prescription, and counseling

with the purpose of ensuring that the clinical and quality-of-life benefits derived from regular exercise are experienced by an ever-increasing number of people. Additionally, in 2008, ACSM helped establish a new membership affiliate organization called the Clinical Exercise Physiology Association (CEPA). The sole purpose of CEPA is to advance the profession of clinical exercise physiology through advocacy, education, and career development. Further information about CEPA membership and activities can be found at www.cepa-acsm.org.

SUMMARY

The lack of regular exercise is a major contributor to the population burden of chronic disease resulting in an estimated 250,000 premature deaths each year, nearly $1 trillion in annual health care costs, and immense human anguish and pain. Billions of dollars are spent each year on drug development for use in primary, secondary, and tertiary disease prevention, while those scientists studying one of the most potent preventive therapeutics, exercise, struggle to gain funding. These observations may seem dreary, but perspectives may be changing. The use of exercise in disease prevention (primary, secondary, and tertiary alike) is gaining acceptance. We believe that through combined efforts from members of the science, medicine, and public health communities, society will soon formally recognize that Exercise Is Medicine.

Suggested Web Sites

American College of Sports Medicine. www.acsm.org

Centers for Disease Control and Prevention. www.cdc.gov

Exercise is Medicine. www.exerciseismedicine.org

National Cholesterol Education Program. www.nhlbi.nih.gov/about/ncep/index.htm

US Department of Health and Human Services. www.health.gov/PAGuidelines/guidelines/default.aspx

4

Managing Exercise in Persons With Multiple Chronic Conditions

Geoffrey E. Moore, MD, FACSM ■ Patricia L. Painter, PhD, FACSM
G. William Lyerly, MS ■ J. Larry Durstine, PhD, FACSM

OVERVIEW
OF THE PATHOPHYSIOLOGY

The role of exercise for individuals with multiple chronic diseases or disability (or both) is poorly understood. Little published research on this topic is available because of the inherent complexity in the design and methodology involved in completing such research. This complexity entails interactions between pathophysiology of the comorbidities, interactions between medications, alterations in the response to exercise, a perception of the potential for exercise to do harm, diminished biological reserve, and perhaps a reduced ability to adapt to exercise training. Exercise in the context of just a single chronic disease is difficult enough to study; thus, very few scientists have any incentive to take on the complexity of multiple chronic diseases. Even when such studies are attempted by qualified researchers using well-designed protocols, the results often raise additional questions because of all the complex and cofounding variables. When multiple chronic diseases involving a neuromusculoskeletal disability such as polio or a hemiparetic stroke are studied, the problem becomes too difficult to examine scientifically.

Unfortunately, far too many individuals are living today with multiple comorbidities and orthopedic or musculoskeletal conditions; these people desire and deserve help at maintaining the best achievable health for independent living and wish to enjoy the highest quality of life possible. Frequently, medicine or surgery does nothing to help restore an individual's functional capacity; and when this scenario occurs, the person's only hope is the potential benefits achieved from exercise. With a well-designed program, most such individuals respond fairly well, although others do not. Our experience as authors, clinicians, and practitioners reveals that nonresponders are uncommon, and that what may appear to be a nonresponse to exercise is likely overshadowed by responses of other types that are not physiological or clinical (hope, quality of life, desire, etc.). In some cases, the exercise program may not cause an improvement in functional performance or capacity per se, but in fact is preventing or delaying deterioration—a less obvious but nevertheless important benefit of exercise training. In renal failure, for example, life expectancy on hemodialysis is approximately five years, with significant data to support a measurable decline in functional capacity over time. Without interventions to address this functional capacity deterioration, the overall health of a dialysis patient would decline rapidly. Any intervention program that maintains body functioning, despite the possibility of an increased risk for an adverse affect (e.g., a heart attack is considered an overall positive intervention given the natural deterioration in body function due to the disease).

Because the permutations and combinations of multiple chronic conditions are virtually infinite, a discussion of specific pathophysiology within this chapter is not possible. Rather, we provide generic advice on how to approach the problem of working with the individual who has multiple chronic diseases or disabilities. Several very common combinations of multiple chronic diseases are frequently seen in exercise training or rehabilitation programs, so it would be prudent for lifestyle intervention teams to become familiar with the management of persons with these combinations, which include the following:

- Generic "heart disease": hypertension, hypercholesterolemia, myocardial infarction ± heart failure

- Emphysema and "heart disease"

- Obesity, arthritis or back pain or both, and "heart disease"

- Obesity, type 2 diabetes, arthritis or back pain or both, and "heart disease"

- Obesity, type 2 diabetes, stroke, arthritis or back pain or both, and "heart disease"

- Obesity, type 2 diabetes, stroke, arthritis or back pain or both, and renal failure

- Any or all of the above with depression, anxiety, or both

Overall Case Management

In 1904 R. Tait McKenzie, a physician (perhaps even the first physician to specialize in sports medicine), developed a philosophy of care for physical therapists and physical educators. He also became the University of Pennsylvania's first Professor of Physical Education. McKenzie's childhood friend, James Naismith, who some may know as the inventor of the game of basketball, kindled McKenzie's early interest in physical education while both were undergraduate students at McGill University. McKenzie believed that through physical education and other health activities, students could learn how to preserve their health and physical efficiency and learn new muscular and sport-related skills. While giving an opening address in a gymnasium at the University of Pennsylvania, McKenzie presented his argument for combining the "hospital clinic, a great deal of the classroom and laboratory, and a little of the arena." McKenzie's theme was that exercise kept human beings well, serving as a preventive measure

against illness, and thus that physical education and health activities had a beneficial relationship with the academic program in higher education. Exercise professionals are wise to apply McKenzie's views to their interactions and dealings with individuals who have complex multiple chronic diseases.

Because many people with a chronic illness typically receive extensive medical care, the therapist must be familiar and comfortable with all aspects of the physician's medical management plan. Such preparation includes knowledge of the medical management, pathophysiology, and interactions of pharmacologic interventions. When exercise therapists are unfamiliar with a particular medical treatment, dialysis for example, they must take the initiative to study the treatment in order to develop an appropriately designed exercise intervention or program. An understanding of the disease burden or treatment of symptoms (or both) will also assist the therapist in developing effective motivational strategies. Sound knowledge of a specific medical treatment will enhance the credibility of the therapist within the health care team and with the patient and family members. Enlistment of the health care team in encouraging exercise for the patient is critical.

Novice exercise therapists and students often make the assumption that individuals with a chronic disease or disability respond to exercise in the same way as apparently healthy individuals, which of course is not the case. Usually people in these circumstances have disease-specific or treatment-specific exercise capacity limitations or adaptations to exercise training. While considerable data exist regarding the response to a single exercise session in many chronic conditions, less is known about exercise training adaptations for these conditions. The exercise specialist must have knowledge of existing evidence-based guidelines, recommendations, and precautions, and also be keenly aware of all the risks associated with exercise and the ways in which those risks increase due to the nature of a chronic disease. Health care teams often are concerned about exercise-associated risk especially in chronic conditions for which exercise is not among the diagnostic tools (e.g., medical specialties other than cardiology, pulmonary, and orthopedics).

Lastly, because of the vast amount of individual variability inherent with chronic diseases, exercise therapists are likely to encounter certain chronic conditions for which there are no scientific data regarding the role of exercise. One must remember that the majority of volunteer subjects for most clinical exercise research projects are weeded out by inclusion and exclusion criteria. Some research clinics, on the other hand, essentially enroll anyone who comes in asking for help; and by definition, the vast majority of these individuals are not typical of the subjects included in most clinical research studies. Much of the time, exercise therapists have to improvise using their knowledge, experience, and judgment. It is most helpful, but not absolutely required, to have skills in athletic training or adaptive physical education when one faces these difficult situations. Exercise therapists who go "only by the book" and who cannot improvise and adapt to suit the client's individual needs will have poor success rates and can even be a danger to themselves as well as those they work with. The more complex the client, the more flexibility and creativity are required in order for the exercise specialist to effectively implement an exercise program.

Delivery System People with multiple chronic conditions, particularly the common ones mentioned earlier, need more than an exercise program; they require an integrated lifestyle modification program designed to help them solve the multifactorial interactions of stress, diet, exercise, and sometimes smoking cessation. While this manual focuses on the role of exercise in lifestyle change, unequivocally exercise alone is rarely sufficient as a sole intervention for chronic disease or disabilities. One must address factors such as perceived and real barriers to exercise, stress-related factors associated with an individual's exercise program, motivation and goal strategies, and support systems and strategies for relapse in order to ensure that people have the best opportunities for success. Because of the diverse needs of medically complex patients, a team of allied health professionals must be available and involved in the design and periodic review of the exercise prescription.

In the following we describe what a "team" approach might look like for delivering appropriate exercise programming for individuals with multiple chronic conditions.

The Case Manager The case manager's role is to guide clients toward the programs that meet their needs. Very few physicians are sufficiently trained to address and coordinate healthy lifestyle interventions. Therefore most patients benefit from having a case manager to fulfill the role of lifestyle modification program coordinator. A variety of health professionals can assume this role, but they clearly need the proper education and training in all aspects of lifestyle change. Perhaps the most important aspect of the case manager's role is to become a good counselor and advisor, one who provides objectivity and wisdom when helping to guide the client through various lifestyle choices.

Unfortunately, few education programs exist that specifically prepare one to become a "lifestyle" case manager. In most allied health care professions, additional training or experience or both are required to prepare people for this role. Appropriate combinations of education and training for such a role may include exercise science and psychology, exercise science and physical therapy, nutrition and psychology, exercise science and nutrition, physical therapy and nutrition, training as a nurse practitioner, or training as a physician assistant in general medicine with psychiatry experience. Ideally, a clinical exercise physiologist would assume the role of the case manager because these professionals are comprehensively trained for this position. Nonetheless, the use of a midlevel provider (nurse practitioner or physician's assistant) is very helpful in that these services are billable services.

Use of Allied Health Care Specialists In a multifactorial lifestyle modification program designed to help individuals with multiple comorbidities, many allied health specialists have important, varied, and often dual roles. Ideally, these roles will involve expertise in physical therapy; cardiac rehabilitation; medically supervised exercise training; aquatic exercise training; community-based exercise programming; specific education on proper diet, exercise, weight management, diabetes, smoking cessation, advanced stress management skills; and individual and group psychotherapy for depression and anxiety. Given the diversity of needs, the allied health professionals who are part of the team include exercise physiologists, nurses, physical therapists, respiratory therapists, dieticians, psychologists, and health educators. Lastly, some individuals with disabilities might also benefit from having access to a prosthetist to assist with adaptive exercise needs.

Basic Approach

In the management of persons with chronic diseases and disorders, the model of approach includes both a preparticipation exam and problem-oriented exercise management.

Preparticipation Physical Exam Model Case managers for a chronic disease exercise program are often not involved in the evaluation of new or undiagnosed problems; rather, they tend to focus on the evaluation of lifestyle modifications and establish and follow up on referrals.

For exercise programming, the most appropriate model to follow is that of the sport preparticipation physical exam (PPE). The team or family physician, who usually conducts PPEs, is mainly interested in detecting whether an athlete is vulnerable to injury or sudden death. In a lifestyle program PPE, the case manager is more concerned with how the exercise program affects the risk of exacerbation of a chronic condition (e.g., of triggering a complication such as rhabdomyolysis in a patient on a statin for heart disease) or the risk of other complications such as falls, hypoglycemic episodes, hypertensive responses to exercise, and heart attacks or sudden death. Fortunately, in clients with multiple comorbidities, the concern is usually maintaining an active, free-living lifestyle, and the primary emphasis is on lower-level exercise intensities (the level of activities of daily living, ADLs). Thus, even though many of these clients are at high risk for cardiac complications, experience has shown that adverse events are extremely rare. After all, clients who are not safe to perform ADLs probably belong in the hospital.

The lifestyle program PPE is therefore primarily aimed at detecting neuromusculoskeletal and biomechanical problems that could affect the exercise response. These potential problems are typically either existing soft tissue problems like bursitis and tenosynovitis, which are essentially overuse injuries in persons with abnormal biomechanics and poor postural control. These problems may or may not require pharmacological intervention, even local cortisone injections, and usually respond very favorably to physical therapy. The PPE should also identify psychological and motivational issues, most commonly depression and anxiety that may affect initiation of and ability to sustain a program of exercise.

Problem-Oriented Exercise Management The principles of problem-oriented management and use of SOAP notes are well suited to managing the problems of individuals with multiple comorbidities. The medical system generally ignores functional capacity, which is the primary focus of the exercise professional. However, the exercise professional must still be able to work within the traditional medical system while simultaneously serving the exercise needs of the individual. A useful approach to problem-oriented exercise management is to create a problem list consisting of medical diagnoses (those that have an existing ICD-9 diagnosis code), as well as specific exercise-related problems (such as poor endurance, easy fatigability, and weakness). In this way, the "reasons" for the individual's referral to the program by the physician are easily tracked (which also facilitates reimbursement), and

the functional capacity needs of the individual are not lost sight of.

Common situations that deserve special comment are (a) obesity with joint pain in the knees and hips and (b) atypical symptoms during exertion. Many obese individuals have joint pain, making adherence to walking programs difficult, especially when the orthopedist says there is nothing he or she can do for the pain. If bursitis or tenosynovitis is preventing the patient's participation in a walking program, then the weight management program must include therapy and perhaps even cortisone injections. Bursitis or tenosynovitis will usually go away with good conservative care and physical therapy. In addition, people with morbid obesity and joint pain may do well in an aquatic program as the bridge to a more active lifestyle.

Occasionally patients are referred to exercise-based programs who complain of symptoms such as atypical angina pectoris or another symptom of cardiovascular or pulmonary disease; however, dyspnea on exertion is the most common complaint. Additionally, many individuals with type 2 diabetes are at risk for silent ischemia, and the case manager must remain alert for these two coexisting problems. Many physicians are not as thoroughly trained in exertional symptomatology as is the exercise physiologist or physical therapist. Clients with these problems are best served by referral and probably should be sent for diagnostic studies as well as being enrolled in a lifestyle modification program. While the evaluation is being completed, the client may start the lifestyle modification interventions but should refrain from physical activities more intense than common ADLs.

Following the PPE, the individual is referred to the appropriate team members for interventions. The order of these referrals may differ depending on what is determined in the PPE and what are identified as priorities by the case manager and the patient. The case manager makes appropriate referrals, develops a plan for regular follow-up with the patient, reviews the participant's progress, and revises the plan as needed.

Summary Points

- Be very familiar with the common combinations of chronic diseases and disabilities.
- Know the medical management of each of your client's conditions.
- Know the exercise literature for each condition and the limits of applicability.
- Know how to improvise exercise training to suit the individual.

- Develop resources for comprehensive lifestyle modification, with exercise as the centerpiece.
- Case managers should use a PPE approach and refer accordingly.
- Use a team approach that facilitates meeting the multidisciplinary needs of those with multiple conditions.
- Problem-oriented SOAP notes help keep track of all the multifactorial issues to solve.
- Many clients have soft tissue overuse injuries from biomechanical problems.
- Some clients have exertional symptoms that need diagnostic evaluation.
- Musculoskeletal complications of exercise are common; cardiac complications are rare.
- The case manager will make appropriate referrals and schedule follow-ups to review participation and progress and revise the lifestyle management plan.

EFFECTS ON THE EXERCISE RESPONSE

The effects of multiple health conditions on the exercise response are extremely varied. Many individuals with several conditions have profound limitations of functional capacity, while others are surprisingly athletic. In many cases, the role of an exercise evaluation is to determine whether or not there is one particular condition that is most limiting. For example, if a client with New York Heart Association (NYHA) class II heart failure also has osteoarthritis in the knees, knee pain may render him or her functionally equivalent to a NYHA class IV. Such scenarios are very common because of the high prevalence of knee osteoarthritis and back pain. One of the most important points to recognize about the exercise response in multiple comorbidities is that exercise invokes integrated physiology responses and as such can reveal any "weak links" that are preventing individuals from achieving a better functional capacity. The type of evaluation completed depends on symptoms and the goals of the program. Symptomatic individuals with heart disease are referred for an appropriate medical workup, while asymptomatic individuals are evaluated using exercise tests that determine a starting exercise level and are sensitive to changes in functional capacity resulting from regular exercise participation. Thus, for those who have relatively high functioning, a symptom-limited treadmill or cycle ergometry test is appropriate. A submaximal protocol is also appropriate for this type of exercise testing. However, for most patients with multiple comorbidities who are older, more frail, or severely deconditioned, one or more physical performance measures such as a 6 min walk, shuttle walk, gait speed, sit-to-stand test, or "get up and go" are more appropriate for establishing a physical functioning baseline and for assessing exercise adaptations.

ROLE OF EXERCISE TRAINING

Pursuant to the concept of integrated physiology, the following are the main goals of exercise training:

- To mediate the effects of a particular condition limiting functional ability
- To increase overall functional capacity and strength
- To increase lifestyle physical activity and daily energy expenditure
- To enhance metabolism of carbohydrates and lipids
- To promote normalization of cardiovascular function

In many people with multiple conditions, sequential goals should be developed and integrated into a lifestyle modification program. The primary cause of death in individuals who have multiple chronic diseases or disabilities is heart disease. In very few conditions are there compelling data to indicate that an exercise-based lifestyle modification program will prevent death from heart disease, but there is often compelling data indicating that a more active lifestyle improves medical management (e.g., glucose metabolism in type 2 diabetes). Most likely the client is primarily interested in the first two of the goals on the preceding list, and the exercise specialist in conjunction with all the program staff must help the person understand the role of the last three goals.

With regard to normalization of cardiovascular function, there are three main goals.

- To increase peak work (aerobic) capacity
- To improve neural control of vascular function (especially in resistance vessels in skeletal muscle)
- To improve endothelial function (primarily, but not only, in the coronary arteries)

Individuals with a metabolic condition such as type 2 diabetes mellitus, impaired fasting glucose, or hypertriglyceridemia must combine exercise programming with dietary interventions designed to improve overall energy metabolism and normalize blood glucose and lipids. In people with a disability or musculoskeletal comorbidity, the goal of exercise is to minimize the effect of that condition on overall functional capacity, which is usually best addressed initially with a referral to physical therapy.

RECOMMENDATIONS FOR EXERCISE TESTING

Most people with multiple chronic conditions are not eligible for third-party reimbursement for treadmill or cycle ergometer graded exercise testing, because most insurers view an exercise test as a means for diagnosing coronary artery disease and not for developing an exercise program. If one can obtain such a test, however, the information is valuable. The most important information from an exercise test relates to

- cardiac chronotropic response,
- pressor response,
- peak work rate, and
- limiting symptoms.

Use of electrocardiogram (ECG) monitoring is a key clinical judgment made by the exercise specialist, case manager, and physician. In general, ECG monitoring is worthwhile but not strictly essential. However, any individual displaying cardiac symptoms is eligible for a diagnostic exercise test in conjunction with ECG monitoring. Strength testing, goniometry, and neuromuscular skill tests are advantageous depending upon the chronic health condition. These tests are beneficial primarily for individuals with musculoskeletal disorders, but are also frequently used with people who are frail and profoundly deconditioned. Functional testing is generally the most valuable test to perform in these populations. Other tests commonly used include sit to stand, gait speed (3 or 4 m), 6 min walk, and standing balance tests. The shuttle walk test and the get up and go test are also useful. Because these tests are specific to ADLs, the client has a better understanding of how they relate to functional ability, so they are practical as teaching tools.

RECOMMENDATIONS FOR EXERCISE PROGRAMMING

With patients having multiple chronic conditions, it is difficult to provide specific exercise programming advice; however, setting general overarching exercise training goals is entirely possible. While many individuals have specific exercise-related goals, interest in the use of exercise as an integrated lifestyle modification program is becoming common. As stated earlier, in very few conditions do outcome data suggest that an exercise-based lifestyle modification program will prevent death from heart disease, but a plethora of research demonstrates that a more active lifestyle improves medical management and overall health. In frail or older individuals, the goal is to increase the number of active years instead of adding survival time.

The exercise program is the aspect of management in which the exercise specialist is most likely to improvise, because often there are no published data on exercise training in persons with a particular combination of conditions. The following is one approach to designing a program for each individual:

- Review what is known about exercise in each of the conditions.
- Evaluate your client in light of these data.
- Consider what unique characteristics about the client don't fit the knowledge base.
- Determine this client's own goals and objectives.
- Determine what the client is currently able to do.
- Prioritize parts of the program primarily to suit the client's goals, but also aim to achieve health goals.
- Use physical therapy, medically supervised exercise, and so on as a bridge to a home-based long-term plan.
- Integrate the exercise component into the client's overall lifestyle modification plan.

Special Considerations

- When exercise testing, be prepared for the client to stop unexpectedly.
- When exercise testing or training, be prepared for atypical exercise responses.
- See each relevant chapter in this book for disease-specific special considerations.

CASE STUDY

Multiple Chronic Diseases

Renal failure often involves multiple chronic diseases, disability, or both. The most common causes of renal failure are diabetes and hypertension. Renal function also deteriorates with age. When kidney function deteriorates to the point of end-stage disease, the patient is typically hypertensive and often develops hyperparathyroidism secondary to the loss of kidney function in activating vitamin D to its active form. Most patients also develop anemia (because the kidney normally makes two-thirds of the body's erythropoietin), and the most common cause of death is coronary artery disease. Thus, end-stage renal failure is almost by definition a multiple chronic disease.

S: "I am just tired all the time and feel like my muscles just don't work."

O: A 68-year-old female with stage 4 chronic kidney disease, hypertension, and type 2 diabetes was overweight and experiencing muscle weakness, joint stiffness, and overall fatigue. She was having difficulty climbing a flight of stairs (stopping several times to rest and use the handrail) and was unable to walk more than one block without stopping.

Vitals

HR: 92 contractions/min
Temp: Afebrile
Weight: 178 lb (80.9 kg)
BP: 162/88 mmHg
Height: 5 ft 6 in. (1.67 m)
BMI: 28.7 kg/m^2

General observation

Mildly overweight woman, fatigued appearance, in no acute distress

Head and neck

Unremarkable with grossly normal cranial nerves 2-12, without lid lag, proptosis, or thyromegaly

Chest

Respirations unlabored with normal I:E

Cardiovascular

Good color in face and extremities with no clubbing, cyanosis, or edema

Abdomen

Obese without splinting or guarding

Musculoskeletal

Wide-based stance with mildly unstable gait, mild osteoarthritic changes with no tenderness, normal range of motion, mild atrophy in upper and lower extremities, motor 4-5/5 throughout in upper and lower extremities, sensation intact to touch, normal reflexes

Medications

Glipizide: 10 mg BID (twice daily)
Lisinopril: 20 mg QD (once daily)
Carvedilol: 6.25 mg BID
Erythropoietin: 2000 U/month
Ferrous sulfate: 325 mg BID
Calcitriol: 0.25 mg three times weekly with dialysis

Notable Labs

Glucose: 135 mg/dl
Creatinine: 2.5 mg/dl
BUN: 48 mg/dl
Serum Ca: 9.0 mg/dl
Phosphorus: 4.7 mg/dl
EGFR: 20 ml/min/1.73 m^2 (stage 4)
Hemoglobin: 11.6 g/dl
Hematocrit: 34
Total cholesterol: 120 mg/dl
Triglyceride 240: mg/dl

A: 1. Chronic kidney disease, stage 4
   2. Type 2 diabetes mellitus
   3. Hypertension, poor control
   4. Anemia
   5. Sarcopenia secondary to #1 and inactivity
   6. Fatigue, multifactorial (#1, #2, #4, #5, inactivity)

P: 1. Maintain mobility
   2. Improve glucose control
   3. Prevent weight gain
   4. Increase strength

Exercise Testing

1. 4 m walk speed: 0.7 m/s
2. 6 min walk: 1020 ft, no cardiopulmonary symptoms reported
3. Sit to stand: 27 s

Exercise Programming

1. Resistance: 10 reps each, twice daily—sit to stand, step-ups, leg lifts, toe raises, bridging
2. Balance: 30 s each, twice daily—semitandem stand, tandem stand, one-legged stand
3. Flexibility: 30 s each, twice daily—calf stretches, sit and reach
4. Aerobic/endurance: Walk as much as possible to fatigue limit, starting in hallway, progressing to outside/mall

Lifestyle Modification

1. Diabetes education class
2. Discuss motivation/adherence issues
3. Consider senior center group/other support program

5

Physical Activity for Children and Adolescents

William F. Riner, PhD, FACSM ■ Richard J. Sabath, EdD, FACSM

A generation defined by physical inactivity, labor-saving technological advances, and an abundant supply of high-fat, energy-dense foods has in part accelerated the development of adult-related chronic disease conditions in children and adolescents, ensuring an extended period of pain and suffering throughout their lifetime unless something is done soon to reverse this trend. A 2007 report on the state of chronic disease conditions in children and adolescents published in the *Journal of the American Medical Association* paints a daunting picture:

- More than 7% of U.S. children and adolescents were hindered in their daily activities by an illness or chronic health condition that lasted three months or longer in 2004, compared to just 1.8% of children in 1960.

- Chronic conditions affect an estimated 15% to 18% of children and adolescents, and these estimates don't fully account for obesity and mental health problems.

- Some of the most serious and prevalent chronic health conditions facing children and adolescents today include obesity, which rose from 5% in the early 1970s to more than 18% today; asthma, which has nearly doubled in prevalence from the 1980s to 9%; and type 2 diabetes, which has sharply risen from an estimated prevalence of 1% to 4% in the 1990s to anywhere from 8% to 43%.

In perspective, the sudden and dramatic rise in the number of children and adolescents living with at lease one or more chronic health conditions is strongly correlated with the origin and prevalence of childhood and adolescent obesity. Over the past three decades, the prevalence of childhood obesity has more than doubled in children aged 2 to 5 years and adolescents 12 to 19 years of age, and tripled in children aged 6 to 11 years. An estimated 9 million children over 6 years of age are currently considered obese. In concurrence with data on adults, obesity in children and adolescents is associated with significant health risks, including hypercholesterolemia, hypertension, risk for heart disease and cancer, sleep apnea, orthopedic problems, liver disease, and asthma, as well as lower self-esteem and social stigma. In addition to obesity, chronic health conditions in children and adolescents include congenital and acquired conditions of the heart, lungs, kidneys, and neuromuscular and skeletal systems, as well as sensory, cognitive, and central nervous system dysfunction.

As the role of physical activity in the medical management of chronic disease and disability in adults becomes increasingly more defined and employed, it is important to consider that children and adolescents obtain benefits from exercise training that are similar to, if not the same as, those for adults. Although preventive and therapeutic exercise training programs for children and adolescents are less widespread than those for adults, child and adolescent referrals to clinically based exercise programs are becoming increasingly common. Because of the higher risk associated with exercise training in any individual with a known or suspected chronic disease or disability, care should be taken by the physician or other health professional to screen all children and adolescents prior to any physical activity, especially when any organic disease is present. Both physical activity and exercise can be effective therapies in reducing the signs and symptoms of chronic disease as well as improving quality of life and health outcomes in the future. As in adults, illness and disability can influence the exercise responses in children and adolescents, in addition to age-specific differences in the response to exercise.

EFFECTS OF HEALTH STATUS AND PHYSICAL ACTIVITY ON GROWTH AND DEVELOPMENT

The regulation of growth and development in children is affected by environmental influences, such as social, cultural, economic, geographic, and nutritional factors, as well as biological factors like genetics and hormonal factors. These same factors play a role in determining health status, including the presence and consequences of many chronic diseases and disabilities. Genetic abnormalities in biological mechanisms can affect metabolic function and body composition as well as neuromuscular and cardiorespiratory function. The environment in which a child lives can also be responsible for an illness or disability, whether congenital or acquired. The environment additionally affects the way in which those conditions are handled by children, their families, and the health care providers who treat them.

Growth charts are an important way to monitor the overall health and wellness of children and adolescents. Growth charts provide important information about the rate of maturation and height and weight status, all of which can be influenced by factors such as sleep and rest, proper nutrition, and physical activity. The nutritional status of a child may also be affected by illness or its treatment, as in the case of cancer. Resulting deterioration or retarded development of bone and muscle tissue may cause a child to measure low on the growth charts, perhaps never achieving normal height and weight for his or her age. Low levels of physical activity, imposed by restriction during the acute stages of illness or treatment, may also impede growth. Although the impact may be less dramatic, otherwise healthy children may also experience impaired skeletal, muscular, and functional development as well as obesity if they are not physically active. The impact of health status and physical activity on normal growth and development is well established and should be given appropriate consideration by all who treat children affected by chronic ailments.

NORMAL RESPONSES TO PHYSICAL ACTIVITY IN CHILDREN AND ADOLESCENTS

Although children and adolescents respond and adapt to exercise and physical activity in much the same way that adults do, physiological differences between children and adults do exist and must be considered when one is exercise testing and evaluating physiological function of children.

Aerobic Exercise Response

The aerobic capacity of children is measured most frequently in a laboratory setting using a treadmill or cycle ergometer. The mode of evaluation is often determined by exercise professionals, the child's preference, size of the child, space available for testing, and the physiological parameters to be evaluated. Maximal oxygen consumption ($\dot{V}O_{2max}$) is generally considered the best indicator of aerobic fitness; however, peak oxygen consumption ($\dot{V}O_{2peak}$) is perhaps more appropriate for describing fitness levels in children, as many of them have difficulty achieving a true plateau in $\dot{V}O_{2max}$ during exercise testing. During childhood there is relatively little difference in absolute $\dot{V}O_{2max}$ between the sexes; but by the onset of puberty, gender differences in absolute $\dot{V}O_2$ begin to increase such that male $\dot{V}O_{2max}$ values are approximately 20% greater by the late teen years. These differences persist even when oxygen consumption is expressed in relative terms. Significant improvements also occur in measures of cardiovascular endurance in both males and females throughout the maturation process.

The maximal heart rate of children and adolescents is generally considerably higher than in adults. Children also have higher submaximal heart rates than adults at a standard exercise intensity.

Maximal heart rate remains essentially unchanged in both males and females throughout childhood (approximately 200-205 contractions per minute), while resting heart rate declines. Frequently, as a sequela of correction for congenital heart defects, children will experience chronotropic deficits of approximately 20 contractions per minute. This deficit requires the practitioner to modify the exercise prescription with regard to target heart rate expectations. As with adults, maximal heart rates achieved during exercise testing are dependent on both the mode and type of exercise, with treadmill running producing higher values than walking or cycle ergometer exercise.

Pulmonary parameters are important variables for health care professionals to monitor during spirometry and evaluation of maximal oxygen uptake. Children and adults differ in resting respiratory rate (i.e., breaths per minute). Resting breathing rate decreases progressively during childhood, resulting in lower relative minute ventilation as children age. However, absolute minute ventilation increases throughout the pediatric years. Maximal breathing frequency also declines as the child ages.

Children have immature thermoregulatory systems and tend to sweat less than adults during exercise in hot or humid weather, resulting in a decrease in evaporative cooling. Children also take longer to acclimatize to exercise in hot or humid conditions and at high altitude. Furthermore, children experience a greater rise in core temperature during hot weather exercise due to voluntary hypohydration. Inadequate fluid intake may lead to blood volume depletion and an increased susceptibility to heat injuries, as well as a decreased ability to exercise efficiently in the heat. From an exercise management perspective, children should be exposed to warm weather exercise gradually and given frequent opportunities (e.g., every 15-20 min) for fluid replacement. Younger children usually need to be encouraged to drink because the need for fluids is often greater than the desire to ingest them.

The blood pressure response of children and adolescents follows the same general pattern as that of adults during aerobic exercise, although the magnitude of change observed in systolic blood pressure is not as great. Normal adults usually increase their systolic blood pressure 6 to 8 mmHg for each metabolic equivalent (MET) increase in work rate. Young children normally experience a 2 to 3 mmHg rise, while adolescents show increases in systolic blood pressure of 4 to 6 mmHg per MET increase in exercise intensity.

Regulating exercise intensity in children may be somewhat more difficult than in adults. Younger children are frequently unable or find it difficult to count heart rate accurately. Rating of perceived exertion (RPE) appears to work reasonably well in children over the age of 8 years, but young children are cognitively unable to use the RPE scale accurately and consistently. Use of the simple walk–talk principle seems to work satisfactorily in most children.

Anaerobic Exercise

The anaerobic capacities of children and adolescent males and females are lower than those of adults, whether expressed per unit of lean body mass or in absolute units; children rank lower than adolescents and adults, and females rank lower than males. Anaerobic power increases throughout childhood and adolescence, with peak values achieved in early adulthood.

Neuromuscular Function

Muscle strength increases during childhood primarily as the result of normal growth and development. Males demonstrate significant increases in muscle size and strength that are temporally related to the time of their peak height velocity. This maturation-driven change produces significant disparities in muscular strength between adolescent males and females and is most noticeable in terms of upper body strength. While maturation and serum testosterone levels play a major role in increasing muscular size and strength after puberty, studies have shown that strength may be improved by resistance training in both sexes prior to the onset of puberty, primarily as a result of neural adaptation versus muscle hypertrophy. Maturation-enhanced local muscle endurance also occurs and leads to improved performance in endurance activities.

Psychological-Social Function

Engaging in physical activity and exercise has been shown to have a positive effect on children's and adolescents' self-concept, self-efficacy, and self-esteem. However, the data are more limited and less conclusive with respect to the effect of physical activity on body image. While physical activity seems to have a positive effect on the symptoms of depression and in reducing stress in children, its effect on anxiety is inconclusive. Physical activity has also been found to be positively associated with several measures of psychological well-being.

EXERCISE TESTING OF CHILDREN AND ADOLESCENTS

To achieve optimal results during exercise evaluations of children, the proper testing environment is critical. The laboratory should be physically attractive to children, containing age-appropriate pictures of interest. The lab should be a minimum of 400 to 600 ft^2 (37-56 m^2) and have good lighting and ventilation. Room temperature should be maintained between 20° and 22° C (~72° and 76° F) with a relative humidity of less than 60%. Enthusiastic, compassionate, and encouraging staff members who enjoy working with children are essential in successful pediatric exercise testing. With younger children, it is necessary to proceed much more slowly than with adults. Age-appropriate language should be used to describe each piece of equipment and the desired objectives during the test. Pictures of children performing various aspects of the exercise test are also useful in helping younger children to understand what is expected and to feel more at ease. Using this approach, treadmill evaluations have been routinely performed on children as young as 4 years of age.

The use of appropriately sized equipment and protocols is critical. Since children achieve steady state faster than adults, treadmill protocols using 2 or 3 min stages are appropriate. The mode of exercise is also important in determining the results. In children and adolescents, treadmill testing will produce $\dot{V}O_{2max}$ values 7% to 10% greater than cycle ergometers, and treadmill running has been found to elicit $\dot{V}O_{2max}$ values 6% to 10% higher than treadmill walking. Test protocols should be designed to last between 8 and 12 min.

From a test administration perspective, children consistently rate submaximal exercise lower on RPE charts than do adolescents and adults. Younger children are often intimidated about communicating with unfamiliar adults in new situations. The test administrator must continuously monitor the child by asking frequent questions to assess his or her status as the test progresses. To avoid false positive answers and early test termination, refrain from asking leading questions or describing specific symptoms (e.g., chest or leg pain, dizziness, shortness of breath). Younger, unfit adolescent clients may require strong verbal encouragement to achieve satisfactory intensity levels during exercise evaluation.

Exercise prescriptions for children should take into consideration the attention span of the child as well as the extent to which the parent(s) provide appropriate role models. Prescribed activities should be enjoyable and relatively nonspecific, with increased movement as the initial goal, especially if the child has a long history of physically inactivity.

Benefits of Exercise Testing

The potential benefits of conducting exercise tests in children with various diseases or disabilities include the following:

- Documenting any impairment in cardiac or pulmonary functional capacity
- Detecting and managing exercise-induced asthma
- Detecting myocardial ischemia
- Assessing physical work capacity
- Assessing the results of rehabilitation programs
- Documenting functional changes during the course of a progressive disease
- Providing indications for surgery, therapy, or additional tests
- Assessing cardiac rate and rhythm as well as blood pressure response
- Assessing exercise-related symptoms
- Evaluating the effects of therapy
- Increasing confidence, in the child and parents, in the ability of the child to exercise safely

Risks of Exercise Testing

Although less validated than in adults, exercise testing in children is considered relatively safe and is generally thought to carry a much lower risk than testing in adult clients. The use of side rails and handrails can help reduce the potential risk of falling. Detailed guidelines for conducting pediatric exercise tests are available from the American Heart Association and the American College of Sports Medicine (ACSM).

GENERAL PHYSICAL ACTIVITY CONCERNS FOR CHILDREN WITH A CHRONIC HEALTH CONDITION OR DISABILITY

Special care is taken in working with children, as any child constantly changes during growth and development and each child does so at different rates. When children or adolescents present with a disease or disability, these growth and development concerns may be even more significant due to the effect of the health status on the maturation process. Although physical activity should be expected to provide many of the same benefits to all children, the individual's health status may impose limitations. A condition or its treatment may retard growth and affect the development of functional systems integral to physical performance, thereby limiting the individual's ability to participate in activity. Parental apprehension about the child's involvement in activity must be considered and adequate measures taken to address those concerns. This will require reassurance by the physician, program professionals, and activity leaders. Parents should be allowed to observe (unobtrusively) all sessions and must be fully informed of all details of the child's participation.

Fitness and health assessments for children and adolescents with chronic diseases or disabilities are essentially the same as for normal children, with the addition of precautions appropriate to the condition. Besides condition-specific clinical evaluations to facilitate appropriate exercise prescription and intervention, assessments of body composition, neuromuscular function, and aerobic and anaerobic fitness should be performed in children with chronic diseases and disabilities. Methodologies and protocols suitable for these children are discussed in detail in numerous sources.

The benefits, risks, and precautions that apply to healthy children are generally the same for those affected by disease or disability. The primary benefit of participation in physical activity for all children is improved quality of life with respect to social, psychological, and physical well-being. For the child affected by disease or disability, the therapeutic consequences of exercise can be significant. Self-esteem, self-efficacy, and self-concept, especially as the child ages, can be greatly enhanced if he or she can have a nearly normal lifestyle of activity. Furthermore, for these children, regular exercise should have the same primary preventive benefits with respect to other diseases, such as coronary artery disease, osteoporosis, hypertension, diabetes, and obesity.

Depending on the particular characteristics of a disease or disability, special consideration must be given to the intensity of an activity, the environmental conditions, and the risk for contact injury. Very-high-intensity efforts can lead to injuries in any child, but those with chronic lung disease such as cystic fibrosis, congenital heart defects, or sickle cell disease have an increased risk of injury and

must be considered accordingly. Children are less able than adults to accommodate very high or very low environmental temperatures, and those with a compromised health status may be even less able to adapt to such environmentally stressful conditions. Activities like climbing and diving may not be appropriate for children with certain conditions. Each case should be evaluated on its own merits.

SELECTED DISEASES AND DISORDERS OF CHILDREN AND YOUTH

As already discussed, all children respond and adapt to exercise somewhat differently than do older youth and adults. Those who are affected by disease or disability may display even greater variation. This section addresses response issues within selected conditions, as well as how the role of physical activity in the growth and development of normal children might be altered by the child's health status.

Congenital and Acquired Heart Defects

In every 1,000 live births, approximately eight infants have some type of heart defect ranging from mild to very severe. Most children with congenital heart defects (CHD) do not require activity restrictions and can participate in normal physical activity. However, some children with severe or very complex CHD may need to avoid strenuous activity or competitive sport. Common forms of CHD include atrial and ventricular septal defects, patent ductus arteriosus, and atrioventricular canal. These conditions can range from mild to severe. Some, as in the case of small septal defects, may repair themselves spontaneously; others may require significant surgical intervention. Usually no special modifications in exercise testing modes are necessary for children with CHD. Many individuals with these defects can participate in a wide range of physical activities without modification. Those with pulmonary hypertension, arrhythmia, or evidence of myocardial dysfunction, however, may need to restrict their exercise to low-intensity activities as indicated by the 2005 Bethesda conference guidelines.

Cyanotic defects result in decreased oxygen delivery to the body with a subsequent alteration in skin coloration. This coloration is dark blue or purplish when the condition is severe. Numerous defects constitute this class of CHD (e.g., tetralogy of Fallot, tricuspid atresia, and pulmonary atresia; transposition of the great arteries; truncus arteriosus; and total anomalous pulmonary venous connection). A detailed description of the complex anatomy and physiology associated with each of these defects is beyond the scope of this chapter. Children with cyanotic defects often have mild to moderate decreases in their aerobic capacity. Those with significant residual problems following surgical repair may be more limited. Limitation in competitive sport increases as the degree of residual problems increases after surgery. Children with good surgical repair of these defects and those with no (or minimal) residual effects can often participate in various types of competitive sports (refer to the Bethesda conference guidelines for full recommendations). Postsurgery clients who experience oxygen desaturation during exercise require individualized exercise prescriptions.

Obstructive CHD occurs when one of the heart valves or blood vessels returning to or carrying blood from the heart becomes stenotic or atretic. The most common obstructive conditions are coarctation of the aorta and pulmonary and aortic stenosis. Defects of this type are classified from trivial to severe. As the severity of the defect increases, the potential for functional impairment also increases. Physical activity and competitive athletic competition restrictions are likely at the most severe levels of obstructive CHD. Children with mild to moderate obstructive CHD can normally participate in unrestricted or low-intensity levels of physical activity if the Bethesda conference guidelines are followed. Valvular stenoses may worsen as the child with CHD grows. Thus, regular assessment via echocardiography, exercise testing, and perhaps cardiac catheterization is usually necessary. Most children with obstructive CHD can perform modified Balke protocols as well as cycle ergometer protocols without significant alteration. Exercise evaluation of children with severe obstructive CHD may be contraindicated.

Any of these conditions or their treatments can have either a temporarily or permanently deleterious effect on growth and development. This should be addressed as appropriate with the child and his or her parents. Physical activity may be among the most effective means by which those effects can be offset.

Obesity

The increased incidence of childhood obesity is well documented The Centers for Disease Control and Prevention (CDC) has compiled a normative table based on body mass index (BMI) for age and gender. Although some variation in the interpretation of the values exists, many consider children with a BMI between the 85th percentile and the 94th percentile to be overweight. Children at the 95th percentile and above are considered obese. Regardless of the interpretation or the definitions used, there is concern about the effects of obesity on health, both acutely and long term. The most serious acute risk in children, type 2 diabetes, is discussed next. The long-term chronic health conditions include cardiovascular disease, some types of cancer, and arthritis. Contributing factors to overweight and obesity include excessive energy intake and lack of caloric expenditure. Thus, poor eating habits, sedentary lifestyles, and lack of physical activity are the most frequently investigated issues concerning childhood overweight and obesity. Recommendations regarding overweight and obesity are presented in chapter 25.

Diabetes Mellitus

Although treatment for diabetes mellitus (DM) has greatly advanced in recent years, the disease can make life difficult for children and their families. The freedom and spontaneity of childhood can be severely affected. Insulin-dependent diabetes mellitus (IDDM), the type previously associated with early onset and affecting only 5% to 10% of the population, is no longer the only concern for children. Increases in sedentary behavior and the resulting obesity markedly increases the incidence of childhood non-insulin-dependent diabetes mellitus (NIDDM), which was previously expected to occur in middle-aged persons. Thus, an increasing number of young people will be exposed to the consequences of DM for much longer time periods.

There is evidence regarding the benefits of exercise in the management of NIDDM, and to a lesser extent IDDM, through several mechanisms. The primary mechanisms include an increase in sensitivity to insulin, increases in glucose transport protein (GLUT-4), and glycogen synthase activity. Intestinal absorption of glucose may also be affected by exercise. A physically active lifestyle may aid in preventing or delaying the onset of NIDDM, primarily through the control of obesity, in all age groups. Additional benefits of regular activity include serum lipid reduction, increased aerobic fitness, and overall improvement in quality of life. The negative impact on social and psychological well-being can be mitigated for the child through involvement in a normally active lifestyle.

Precautions that should be considered for the diabetic (IDDM) child involved in physical activity include careful attention to preventing hypoglycemia by monitoring and regulating insulin levels and glucose intake. Special attention must be given to both the intensity and duration of the activity. High-intensity activity and physical exhaustion in young people with IDDM may cause an abnormal reaction, resulting in sustained hyperglycemia. Also, careful management of wounds and other injuries must be maintained. The stabilization of glucose levels is much more difficult in cases of IDDM than in those of NIDDM. Glucose control is much more structured, resulting in an even more severe intrusion into the life of the child. Nevertheless, the benefits are worth the effort. The more knowledgeable the child is about his or her daily care and the more involved, the more successful the management. If the diabetic child can get through the adolescent years in otherwise good condition, without excessive weight gain or other chronic conditions, the prognosis for health in the future is likely better. Exercise recommendations for individuals with diabetes are discussed in chapter 24.

Neuromuscular Disorders

A limited amount of research has been done on the implications of exercise testing and therapy for children affected by various progressive neuromuscular disorders (both congenital and acquired). Because the focus of this type of problem is on the muscular system, including muscular strength, endurance, power, and the metabolic cost of movement, all testing and therapeutic procedures should address these areas. Another area of concern relates to children with gait and coordination disorders that are often subclinical, thereby frequently receiving little or no attention.

Exercise testing can be effective in assessing and tracking delayed development or progressive deterioration in coordination as well as the efficacy of interventions. Although there are relatively few controlled studies, some evidence indicates that therapeutic modalities involving exercise training (aerobic, anaerobic, and resistance) may be beneficial in slowing the progression of some conditions and in maintaining or improving functional abilities. The difficulties involved in designing and carrying out the type of studies necessary to provide conclusive clinical data are significant. However, it seems reasonable that having affected children involved in appropriate physical activity would do no harm. Indeed, this would most likely yield some benefits related to normalizing growth and development.

Pulmonary Disorders

Bronchial asthma (which includes exercise-induced asthma), and cystic fibrosis (CF), are the most commonly occurring chronic pulmonary diseases among children. Both of these conditions result in limitations on exercise tolerance and in cardiorespiratory responses that vary from those normally expected in children. Although chronic asthma attacks may be initiated by a number of environmental factors, such as allergens and pollution, exercise-induced asthma has been attributed to several mechanisms. These vary from the rather simple cooling, drying, and rewarming of the airways with increased ventilation to more complex effects involving chemical inflammation mediators. CF is an inherited condition of genetically defective sodium and chloride ion transport, which results in extracellular dehydration. Multiple organs and functions are affected by the thick mucus, which blocks ducts, tubules, and small airways. The function of affected organs, especially the lungs, is impaired to the point of causing early death. Although both asthma and CF can be life threatening, long-term survival and a relatively normal life can be expected with well-managed asthma. CF has a poor prognosis, however. Nevertheless, the benefits of regular exercise in persons with these disorders have been demonstrated. These relate mostly to improvement in aerobic fitness for both persons with asthma and those with CF and to increased ventilatory muscle endurance and strength in the individual with CF. The possibility of increased mucus clearance has also been reported, although benefits in pulmonary function are limited, if present at all. Caution is necessary when individuals with CF are exposed to heat and altitude. They are usually capable of normal thermoregulation, but special attention must be paid to fluid and electrolyte replacement. There is a risk of oxygen desaturation if oxygen tension in the environment is low.

The usefulness of exercise testing in diagnosis and prognosis determination for both conditions has been well documented. Determination of exercise tolerance and aerobic fitness not only is beneficial for the health care provider, but also instills confidence in both clients and parents.

SUMMARY

Children, like adults, are frequently affected by chronic disease and disability. Childhood afflictions can be even more tragic than adulthood onsets, simply because the onset of a limiting condition in childhood means that the individual will have to cope with the problem for a much longer period of time. Thus, an underlying goal for the practitioner is to be sensitive to these concerns and always be alert for ways to help chronically ill children deal with their problems. Further complicating effective management, many children may present with multiple problems. The practitioner must be creative and resourceful in using exercise testing and prescription to evaluate current status and progression, as well as to facilitate as active a lifestyle as possible for the affected child. The desired outcome will be an improved quality of life and possible mitigation of the long-term consequences of disease or dis-ability. Being physically active is in the nature of a child. This nature should be foremost in the minds of everyone working with children, whether sick or well.

Evidence-Based Guidelines

The pediatric evidence-based care guidelines developed at Cincinnati Children's Medical Center. www.cincinnatichildrens.org/svc/alpha/h/health-policy/ev-based/default.htm

Suggested Web Site

American Academy of Pediatrics. www.aap.org

PART II

Cardiovascular Diseases

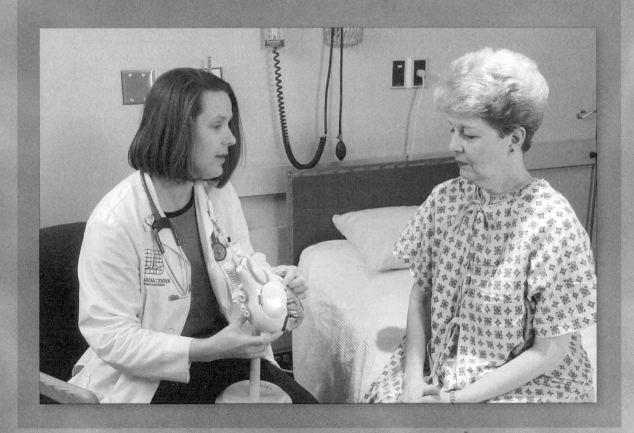

Myocardial Infarction

Barry A. Franklin, PhD, FACSM

OVERVIEW OF THE PATHOPHYSIOLOGY

Coronary atherosclerosis or disease (CAD) is a progressive, chronic disease associated with endothelial dysfunction; vascular inflammation; and the accumulation of lipids, macrophages, blood-clotting elements, calcium, and fibrous connective tissue within the inner lining of coronary arteries. Atherosclerotic changes over time result in the formation of atheromatous plaques or lesions, vascular remodeling, and luminal stenosis, culminating in the impairment or obstruction of normal blood flow. Any transient impairment or obstruction of blood flow to the myocardium secondary to CAD is referred to as myocardial ischemia, whereas the complete obstruction of blood flow is termed myocardial infarction (MI). Atherosclerotic lesions that reduce the normal diameter of a major coronary artery (i.e., the left anterior descending, the left circumflex, or the right coronary artery) by at least 50% are considered clinically significant and an indication for possible revascularization surgery, medical therapy, or other intervention. Lesions with 50% or greater stenosis are responsible for the majority of MI's; however, lesions that have much less stenosis (~30%) but are unstable can also cause an MI. Lesions with 70% or greater stenosis are most commonly associated with myocardial ischemia and angina. Judgment of whether a lesion is clinically significant or not based solely on diameter is imprecise, since diameter alone does not take into account the length of the lesion or the effect of blood flow when entering and exiting the lesion, all of which can affect blood flow dynamics.

Clinically significant lesions that produce myocardial ischemia and left ventricular dysfunction most often develop in the proximal, epicardial segments of coronary arteries at sites of abrupt curvature or branching. The effects of atherosclerotic lesions are further complicated by hemorrhage, ulceration, calcification, or thrombosis. Plaque, which is composed of fibrous tissue and to a lesser extent lipid, can be either active and unstable or quiet and stable. Unstable plaques, even mild- to moderate-sized plaques (~50% stenosis), can fissure, rupture, swell, or undergo a combination of these processes. The occurrence of these events at vulnerable regions within coronary arteries can result in a sudden and complete obstruction of a coronary artery, leading to an acute myocardial infarction (AMI). Nearly 90% of AMIs involve lesions with <70% obstruction in the months to years prior to an MI. Rupture of a vulnerable atherosclerotic plaque with resultant thrombus formation is believed to be the most important mechanism underlying rapid progression of less severe lesions to severe stenosis or total coronary artery occlusion.

The clinical outcomes associated with plaque instability and AMIs can be dramatically decreased following reductions in total and low-density lipoprotein cholesterol (LDL-cholesterol). Recent research has shown that inflammation plays a key role in the atherosclerotic process and coronary artery disease (CAD), as well as the triggering of an AMI. Immune cells govern the early stages of atherosclerotic plaque formation, while immune cell effector molecules accelerate progression of the lesions. Selected blood markers of active inflammation, including C-reactive protein (CRP) and lipoprotein-associated phospholipase A2 (PLAC), are significantly correlated with CAD risk and possible future MIs. CRP has been shown to reflect inflammation and strongly predicts coronary risk in middle-aged men and women, whereas PLAC has been shown to help predict cardiovascular events in patients who have relatively low levels of LDL-cholesterol, that is, <130 mg/dl. Prolonged ischemia (>60 min) causes irreversible cellular damage and necrosis, leading to acute MI. More than 1.5 million Americans have an MI each year, including a similar number of men and women; of these, approximately 500,000, or one-third, will die.

MI's are classically characterized by a diagnostic triad of signs and symptoms, including the following:

- Severe, prolonged chest pain or pressure, which may radiate to the arms, back, or neck, frequently associated with sweating, nausea, or vomiting
- Increased serum levels of cardiac enzymes released by the necrotic myocardial cells (e.g., CK-MB >5% of total CK; CPK or CK: women >70 U/L, men >90 U/L; troponin I ≥0.5 ng/ml)
- Electrocardiographic changes in the leads overlying the area of infarction, manifested as ST-segment elevation and T-wave inversion, resulting from ischemic injury and disappearing over timePronounced Q-waves, which represent myocardial necrosis and irreversible damage to the myocardium

MI's, which usually affect the left ventricle, are associated with permanent cessation of contractile function in the necrotic area of the myocardium and impaired contractility in the surrounding ischemic muscle. Two types of infarctions are generally described, depending upon the amount of myocardial tissue involved:

- Transmural infarction (i.e., Q-wave MI), which involves the full thickness of the ventricular wall
- Subendocardial infarction (i.e., non-Q-wave MI), which is limited to the inner half of the myocardium

Infarctions are further described according to the involvement of the coronary circulation and location on the ventricular wall. For example, anterior infarctions result from lesions in the left anterior descending coronary artery and involve the anterior wall of the left ventricle, whereas inferior wall infarctions are generally the result of right coronary artery

lesions. Other commonly designated infarct sites are lateral, posterior, and septal or (with extensive infarctions involving large portions of the ventricle) combinations of these locations (e.g., anteroseptal, inferolateral).

The risk of future cardiovascular morbidity and mortality after acute MI is largely determined by three variables:

- The extent of left ventricular damage or dysfunction, using ejection fraction as the reference criterion (mean normal [±SD] left ventricular ejection fraction at rest is 62.3 ± 6.1%).
- The degree of residual myocardial ischemia (suggesting additional myocardium in jeopardy), manifested by exertional angina pectoris, ST-segment depression, technetium (Tc)-99m Sestamibi (Cardiolite) or thallous (thallium) chloride-201 transient perfusion abnormalities, or combinations thereof.
- The level of cardiorespiratory fitness, expressed as metabolic equivalents (METs; 1 MET = 3.5 ml $O_2 \cdot kg^{-1} \cdot min^{-1}$), as measured or estimated during peak or symptom-limited exercise testing. In fact, recent studies suggest that a reduced exercise capacity (<4 METs) more accurately predicts five-year mortality than does left ventricular ejection fraction in patients with ST-elevation MI treated with percutaneous coronary intervention.

EFFECTS ON THE EXERCISE RESPONSE

AMI's can alter an individual's cardiorespiratory and hemodynamic responses to both submaximal and maximal exercise. Individuals who have suffered a previous MI often have a reduced level of cardiorespiratory fitness (50-70% of age and gender predicted). The reduced oxygen transport capacity is primarily due to diminished cardiac output (stroke volume, heart rate, or both) rather than a reduction in peripheral extraction of oxygen. In some individuals, a primary limitation appears to be the decreased contractile force of the left ventricle due to residual ischemia or necrosis, causing a progressive decrease in ejection fraction and stroke volume, which often manifests itself as a blunted or decreasing systolic blood pressure response during progressive exercise (exertional hypotension). In others, cardiac output may be limited by the restriction in the rise of the heart rate due to intrinsic disease of the sinoartial

(SA) or atrioventricular (AV) node (chronotropic impairment), or by the appearance of anginal symptoms, with or without ischemic ST-segment depression, which precludes exercising to a higher level. Potential life-threatening exercise-induced ventricular arrhythmias occur more commonly in individuals with a history of a previous MI than in individuals without heart disease, especially in the presence of ischemic ST-segment depression, angina pectoris, left ventricular dysfunction, or combinations thereof. In addition, clients with a history of a previous MI are often taking medications to decrease heart rate and blood pressure (and myocardial oxygen demands); the type and dose of these medications should be noted before the client undergoes exercise testing or training.

EFFECTS OF EXERCISE TRAINING

Potential benefits of exercise training in individuals with a history of a previous MI include the following:

- Increased maximal oxygen consumption ($\dot{V}O_{2max}$) (mean ~20%), which generally varies inversely with the pretraining $\dot{V}O_{2max}$
- Improvement in the ventilatory response to exercise
- Improvement in the anaerobic or ventilatory threshold
- Relief of anginal symptoms secondary to reductions in heart rate or blood pressure (or both) and myocardial oxygen demand at any given somatic oxygen uptake or submaximal work rate
- Increased heart rate variability
- Modest decreases in body weight, fat stores, blood pressure (particularly in hypertensives), total blood cholesterol, serum triglycerides, and LDL-cholesterol
- Increases in the "antiatherogenic" high-density lipoprotein (HDL)-cholesterol subfraction
- Improved psychosocial well-being and self-efficacy
- Protection against the triggering of MI by vigorous physical exertion (i.e., ≥6 METs)
- Decreased coronary inflammatory markers (e.g., CRP, PLAC)
- Increased numbers of endothelial progenitor cells and circulating angiogenic cells—cell populations that promote angiogenesis and vascular regeneration
- Decreased blood platelet adhesiveness, fibrinogen, and blood viscosity and increased fibrinolysis
- Increased vagal tone and decreased adrenergic activity

An important note is that conventional exercise training as an isolated intervention generally has little effect on increasing left ventricular ejection fraction and myocardial perfusion. Numerous training studies have demonstrated improved exercise tolerance in individuals with impaired left ventricular function, despite the lack of improvement in resting hemodynamics or ejection fraction. However, those who have both left ventricular dysfunction and exercise-induced myocardial ischemia show little or no increase in $\dot{V}O_{2max}$ after early outpatient cardiac rehabilitation.

Meta-analyses of randomized controlled clinical trials of rehabilitation with exercise after MI have now shown a 20% to 25% reduction in total and cardiovascular-related mortality, with no difference in the rate of nonfatal recurrent events. Although it has been suggested that current thrombolytic and revascularization procedures may diminish the impact of adjunctive contemporary cardiac rehabilitation programs on survival, at least one meta-analysis has demonstrated that the benefits of cardiac rehabilitation persist in modern cardiology.

Recommending vigorous exercise training for individuals with the following characteristics has previously been questioned:

- Individuals with exertional ST-segment depression without symptoms (silent ischemia)
- Those recovering from an MI involving a large portion of the anterior wall

And while at least one isolated report has suggested that vigorous exercise training in these individuals may actually worsen cardiac function, other studies suggest that increased fibrosis, infarct expansion, and deterioration in left ventricular function are unlikely outcomes of exercise training.

MANAGEMENT AND MEDICATIONS

The medical management of individuals with CAD and those recovering from an MI is essentially palliative, undertaken to minimize the severity of clinical sequelae and to potentially slow, halt, or even reverse the progression of disease. Individuals at moderate to high risk may likely experience a reduction in mortality from successful percutaneous transluminal coronary angioplasty or coronary artery bypass graft surgery. Risk factor interventions aimed at smoking cessation, lipid and lipoprotein modification, hypertension control, increasing physical activity, weight reduction (if appropriate), and efficacious drugs (including beta-blockers, angiotensin-converting enzyme [ACE] inhibitors, HMG-CoA reductase inhibitors [e.g., statins], clopidogrel [Plavix], and aspirin) have produced remarkably consistent reductions (approximately 20-25%) in cardiovascular-related morbidity and mortality. When risk factor interventions are selectively combined, even greater reductions in subsequent cardiovascular events are likely to be achieved. Although vitamin supplementation (vitamin E; folic acid, with or without vitamin B6 and/or vitamin B12) has not been shown to promote added cardioprotective benefits in patients with cardiovascular disease, food sources that provide omega-3 fatty acids—especially the longer-chain fatty acids from marine sources—are now widely recommended to decrease cardiovascular risk.

Appropriate pharmacotherapy decreases mortality after an AMI, attenuates the manifestations of acute ischemic syndromes, improves symptoms in stable angina and heart failure, suppresses atrial and ventricular arrhythmias, and inhibits platelet function and fibrin formation. Accordingly, many people take one or more medications following an AMI, including anti-ischemic drugs (e.g., beta-blockers, calcium channel blocking agents, nitroglycerin, and longer-acting nitrate drugs), platelet inhibitors, anticoagulants, medications for the treatment of heart failure (e.g., digitalis, diuretics, ACE inhibitors), vasodilators, antiarrhythmic drugs, and lipid-altering drugs (see chapter 22).

SPECIAL PRECAUTIONS

Several cardiovascular medications can potentially influence the responses to exercise testing and training, as follows:

- Diuretics do not alter chronotropic reserve or aerobic capacity (except possibly in individuals with congestive heart failure). Thus, the prescribed exercise heart rate can be determined in the standard fashion. However, diuretics may precipitate ventricular ectopy if hypokalemia or hypomagnesemia occurs, resulting in a "false positive" test result.

- Beta-blockers decrease submaximal and maximal heart rate and sometimes exercise capacity, especially with nonselective agents. These drugs may also prevent or delay signs or symptoms of myocardial ischemia and increase exercise tolerance in clients with exertional angina. Nevertheless, exercise trainability appears to be unaffected, despite therapeutic doses and a reduced training heart rate. Because beta-blockers do not alter the remarkably consistent relationship between $\%\dot{V}O_{2max}$ and $\%HR_{max}$, the generally prescribed metabolic load for training (60-80% $\dot{V}O_{2max}$) may be achieved at the conventional relative heart rate recommendation for training (70-85% HR_{max}).

- Vasodilators, ACE inhibitors, and angiotensin receptor blockers do not generally affect the heart rate response to exercise. Consequently, exercise training intensity can be prescribed in the usual manner. Individuals on these medications may be subject to hypotensive episodes during the postexercise period unless an adequate cool-down period is allowed.

- Calcium channel blockers do not generally impair functional capacity or exercise trainability and may increase exercise tolerance in individuals with angina. However, certain calcium channel blockers (e.g., bepridil, diltiazem, verapamil) may decrease the heart rate response at rest and during exercise, and prevent or delay manifestations of myocardial ischemia. Consequently, the prescribed training heart rate should be based on the medicated client's response to an exercise test.

- Central nervous system–active drugs, including clonidine, guanfacine, and guanabenz, can have attenuating effects on heart rate and blood pressure during exercise. Thus, the potential for hypotension, dizziness, and syncope necessitates careful monitoring.

- Alpha receptor blockers significantly lower systolic and diastolic blood pressure but appear to have minimal effects on heart rate and metabolic responses to exercise. Therefore, training heart rates may be prescribed in the usual manner.

- Antiarrhythmic agents can cause false negative (quinidine) or false positive (procainamide) test results; however, they do not substantially alter the heart rate response or aerobic capacity in persons with or without heart disease. In contrast, a decrease of 20 contractions per minute in exercise HR_{max} has been reported in clients taking amiodarone.

■ Digitalis appears to have little effect on the hemodynamic and metabolic responses to exercise. ST-segment depression can be induced or accentuated during exercise in persons with or without heart disease who are taking digitalis. In individuals who are taking digitalis, marked ST-segment depression may indicate myocardial ischemia, particularly when it is accompanied by a prolonged QT interval. Nevertheless, exercise-induced ST-segment depression should be interpreted with caution in the presence of digitalis therapy.

RECOMMENDATIONS FOR EXERCISE TESTING

Low-level exercise testing (generally ≤5 METs) is utilized with individuals recovering from uncomplicated MIs to assess functional status, as well as to provide diagnostic, prognostic, and therapeutic guidance. Exercise testing also serves to promote client confidence, providing reassurance that routine activities can be undertaken safely. Abnormal findings (e.g., angina, ischemic ST-segment depression) suggest that additional areas of myocardium are served by stenosed coronary vessels and remain in jeopardy.

The test protocol for peak or symptom-limited testing should focus on accommodating the individual's ability to perform lower-extremity exercise (see table 6.1). People who are unable to perform treadmill or cycle ergometer exercise may be alternatively evaluated with arm crank ergometry or pharmacologic stress testing (e.g., dobutamine, dipyridamole, Persantine, and adenosine) at rest.

The exercise test should begin at an intensity level considerably below the anticipated peak or symptom-limited capacity and increase gradually in 2 or 3 min stages, with hemodynamic measures made at each progressive stage. If possible, exercise capacity should be directly measured using gas exchange techniques rather than predicted from work rate (e.g., treadmill speed and grade or duration), which tends to overestimate aerobic fitness. Increments in work rate should be chosen so that the total test

time to volitional fatigue approximates 10 ± 2 min. Contraindications to testing and indications for terminating exercise should be closely observed.

The primary objectives of exercise testing for individuals recovering from or having a history of an MI are to evaluate quantitatively and accurately the following functions:

■ Chronotropic capacity and heart rate recovery
■ Aerobic capacity ($\dot{V}O_{2max}$)
■ Myocardial aerobic capacity, estimated by the peak rate–pressure product
■ Exertional symptoms (e.g., increasing chest pain or light-headedness)
■ Associated changes in electrical functions of the heart (e.g., arrhythmias, ST–T-wave changes)

The data collected during an exercise test are critical to categorize risk status (e.g., low, moderate, high) and establish a safe and effective metabolic load for aerobic exercise training. Indicators of an adverse prognosis in the post-MI client include the following:

■ Ischemic ST-segment depression at a low level of exercise
■ Functional capacity <4 METs
■ Low peak rate–pressure product (i.e., ≥21,700 mmHg × contractions per minute)
■ Hypotensive blood pressure response to exercise

Exercise testing for individuals on "long-acting" beta-blockers should be conducted at approximately the same time of day the subject will be exercising, because the significant reduction in exercise heart rate may dissipate over time. Because ST-segment abnormalities that develop during exercise are not interpretable in the presence of digitalis, substantial ST-segment depression at rest, left ventricular hypertrophy, left bundle branch block, or pacemaker rhythms, exercise testing with myocardial perfusion imaging is often recommended to screen for myocardial ischemia in individuals with these conditions.

RECOMMENDATIONS FOR EXERCISE PROGRAMMING

Simple exposure to orthostatic or gravitational stress, including intermittent sitting or standing, during the bed rest stage of hospital convalescence

TABLE 6.1

Myocardial Infarction: Exercise Testing

Methods	Measures	Endpoints*	Comments
Aerobic			
Cycle (ramp protocol 17 W/min; staged protocol 25-50 W/3 min stage) Treadmill (1-2 METs/3 min stage)	■ 12-lead ECG, HR	■ Serious dysrhythmias ■ >2 mm ST-segment depression or elevation ■ Ischemic threshold ■ T-wave inversion with significant ST change	■ Use low-level treadmill protocol for acute MI clients. ■ Important in establishing a safe training intensity. ■ Chronotropic impairment results in poor prognosis.** ■ Minimal treadmill speed should be ≤1.0 mph.
	■ BP, rate–pressure product	■ SBP >250 mmHg or DBP >115 mmHg	■ Exertional hypotension (drop of ≥20 mmHg or failure to rise) suggests poor prognosis.
	■ RPE (6/20) ■ Angina scale	■ +3 or earlier on +1 to +4 scale	
	■ Gas analysis ($\dot{V}O_{2peak}$ or $\dot{V}O_{2max}$) ■ Radionuclide testing		■ Only if exact measures are indicated, ventilatory threshold is often useful. ■ Is more sensitive and specific than exercise ECG in assessing ischemic heart disease.
Strength			
Isokinetic or isotonic	90% maximal voluntary contraction (MVC), greatest load lifted 2 or 3 times	3 consecutive reps	Use 1RM (estimated from 90% MVC) to establish training work rate.

*Measurements of particular significance; do not always indicate test termination.

** A delayed decrease in the heart rate (< 12 contractions/min) during the first min of recovery is also a powerful predictor of overall mortality.

(often referred to as Phase I cardiac rehabilitation) can prevent much of the deterioration in exercise performance that normally follows an AMI. Rhythmic exercise involving large muscle groups such as walking, cycle ergometry, rowing, or stair climbing is appropriate for outpatient (Phases II-IV cardiac rehabilitation) physical conditioning. People should be encouraged to perform whole-body exercises, involving both sets of limbs, to achieve maximal benefits from exercise. Mild to moderate resistance training can be a safe and effective method for improving cardiovascular function, body composition, coronary risk factors, flexibility, and muscular strength and endurance in clinically stable cardiac clients. Individuals should also be counseled to integrate multiple short bouts of physical activity into their daily lives. Pedometers can be helpful in this regard, as can programs that use them (e.g.,

America on the Move), to enhance awareness of physical activity through progressive increases in daily step totals.

Mode, intensity, frequency, and duration recommendations for structured or formal exercise training or physical activity can be found in table 6.2. They are summarized as follows:

- Intensity generally corresponds to 40% to 80% of $\dot{V}O_2R$ or maximal heart rate reserve, using rating of perceived exertion (RPE; 11 to 16 [on the Borg scale of 6-20]) as an adjunct to heart rate as an intensity guide. A recent analysis of 23 training studies in coronary patients concluded that ~45% of the oxygen uptake reserve (~69% of HR_{max}) should be considered the minimal effective intensity for improving cardiorespiratory fitness in this population.

- Frequency of exercise should be at least four to seven (nonconsecutive) days per week.

- Duration of training involves 20 to 60 min of continuous or accumulated (interval) exercise, preceded and followed by warm-up and cool-down periods of 5 to 10 min.

- Mode of exercise should include, in addition to a formal or structured program, increasing the adoption and maintenance of physical activity in daily living; maximum benefit requires 5 to 6 h per week of physical activity.

TABLE 6.2

Myocardial Infarction: Exercise

Modes	Goals	Intensity/Frequency/Duration	Time to goal
Aerobic Large muscle activities Arm/leg ergometry	■ Increase aerobic capacity ■ Decrease BP and HR response to submaximal exercise ■ Decrease submaximal myocardial $\dot{V}O_2$ demand ■ Decrease CAD risk factors ■ Increase ADLs	■ RPE 11-16/20 ■ 40-80% $\dot{V}O_{2max}$ or HR reserve ■ ≥3 days/week ■ 20-60 min/session ■ 5-10 min of warm-up and cool-down activities	4-6 months
Strength* Circuit training	■ Increase ability to perform leisure and occupational activities and ADLs ■ Increase muscle strength and endurance	■ 30-40% 1RM (upper body), 50-60% 1RM (lower body) (avoid Valsalva) ■ 2-3 days/week ■ 2-4 sets of 12-15 reps ■ 8-10 different exercises ■ Resistance gradually increased over time	4-6 months
Flexibility** Upper and lower body ROM activities	Decrease risk of injury	■ Static stretches: hold for 10-30 s ■ 2-3 days/week	4-6 months

*A single set of exercises to volitional fatigue is highly effective, at least over the initial months of training.

**Strength and flexibility training are often used, but not well researched. Typical programs are recommended here.

CASE STUDY

Myocardial Infarction

A 59-year-old college professor presented to the emergency department about 4 h after experiencing symptoms, including a rapid heart rate and mild throat tightness and discomfort. His coronary risk factors were generally unremarkable; however, his history included a slightly elevated LDL-cholesterol (range: 140-190 mg/dl) and a slightly reduced HDL-cholesterol (range: 32-36 mg/dl). He walked on a regular basis, was normotensive, did not smoke cigarettes, was not diabetic, and was slightly overweight: 5 ft 9 in. (1.8 m), 183 lb (83 kg). At the time of his cardiac event, he was working 70 to 80 h per week, attempting to meet several "deadlines."

S: *"I've developed a heart rhythm irregularity that feels extremely rapid—like a fluttering in my chest. What a strange sensation."*

O: Vitals

BMI = 27 kg/m^2
HR: Atrial fibrillation; ventricular rate ranged from 150-180 bpm
BP: 146/86 mmHg
Middle-aged male in distress; symptomatic
ECG: Atrial fibrillation, poorly controlled concomitant inferolateral ST-segment depression (~1.0-1.5 mm); patient reverted to NSR with drug therapy
Cardiac enzymes: On the first blood draw these were normal; however, on the subsequent blood draw the levels of CK-MB and troponin I had risen considerably, >5% of total CK and >0.5 ng/ml, suggesting the early evolution of acute myocardial infarction.

Cardiac Catheterization

Total occlusion of the proximal RCA; otherwise, unremarkable
Ejection fraction: 50%
Percutaneous emergent transluminal coronary angioplasty successful

Graded Exercise Test (Post-PTCA, Day 3, Low Level)

Peak exercise: 4-5 METs
Peak HR: 112 contractions/min
No ECG changes, threatening arrhythmias, or symptoms of myocardial ischemia
Medications: Metoprolol, ASA, clopidogrel, statin

A: 1. Atrial fibrillation with acute inferior wall MI
   2. CAD with successful emergent PTCA
   3. Overweight
   4. History of lipid/lipoprotein abnormalities
   5. High stress; type A personality; workaholic

P: 1. Refer to home-based cardiac rehabilitation program: comprehensive lifestyle modification.
   2. Reduce body weight/fat stores (goal weight = 160-165 lb [73-75 kg]).
   3. Lipid/lipoprotein modification (patient was prescribed Lipitor, once per day; niacin 500 mg, twice daily; and omega-3 fish oil, 1200 mg capsules, twice daily) in addition to his other cardiac medications.
   4. Patient was counseled to refrain from work for 4-6 weeks and to resume and maintain a reduced workload/schedule.
   5. Initiate a program of weight reduction, dietary modification, stress reduction.
   6. Target HR: 84-96 contractions/min
   7. RPE: 11-13 (fairly light to somewhat hard)
   8. Distance walking training: ≥30 min/session, 3-5 days/week

Exercise Program Goals

1. Peak exercise tolerance; 8.9-10.9 METs (corresponding to a moderate level of cardiorespiratory fitness)
2. Increase functional capacity

Aerobic	3 days/week	20 min/session	THR (90-102 contractions/min) RPE 11-13/20	Increase to 40 min @ 60-70% THR after 8 weeks
Strength (all major muscle groups)	3 days/week	1 set ≤10 reps	50-70% 1RM	Increase to 2 sets of 10-12 reps after 12 weeks
Flexibility (anterior chest, hip flexors, plantarflexors)	3 days/week	20 s/stretch	Maintain stretch below discomfort point	Discomfort point should be at higher ROM
Warm-up and cool-down	Before and after each session	10-15 min	RPE <10/20	Maintain

3. Reduce body weight/fat stores
4. Improve lipid/lipoprotein profile
5. Stress reduction; reduce work-related activities
6. Reinforce lifestyle changes/adhere to prescribed medications/regular exercise/medical management

Follow-Up

Approximately 14 weeks after his MI, the client completed 11 min on a Bruce protocol (4.2 mph, 16% grade, 10-11 METs). Peak heart rate was 132 contractions/min. The test was terminated due to volitional fatigue, without significant ST-segment depression or anginal symptoms. Isolated PVCs were noted during and after exercise. The exercise prescription was updated, and he continued his home-based rehabilitation program.

Evidence-Based Guidelines

Canadian Cardiovascular Society, American Academy of Family Physicians, American College of Cardiology, American Heart Association, Antman EM, Hand M, et al. ACC/AHA guidelines for the management of patients with ST-elevation myocardial infarction. J Am Coll Cardiol. 2004;44:671-719.

Minhas R, Cooper A, Walsh JD, Williams H, Nherera L, Guideline Development Group of the NICE guideline for secondary prevention after MI. Evidence based secondary prevention following a myocardial infarction (MI): The new NICE guideline. Int J Clin Pract. 2007;61(10):1604-1607.

Suggested Web Sites

American Heart Association. www.americanheart.org

American Association of Cardiovascular and Pulmonary Rehabilitation. www.aacvpr.org

American College of Cardiology. www.acc.org

American College of Sports Medicine. www.acsm.org

7

Revascularization
CABGS and PTCA or PCI

Barry A. Franklin, PhD, FACSM

OVERVIEW OF THE PATHOPHYSIOLOGY

Coronary artery atherosclerosis or disease (CAD) involves a localized accumulation of lipids, macrophages, platelets, calcium, and fibrous connective tissue within coronary arteries, resulting in the formation of atheromatous plaques and progressive narrowing of the lumen, eventually causing impairment or obstruction of normal blood flow. Atherosclerotic lesions that result in 50% or greater stenosis in a major coronary artery should be considered clinically significant and an indication for possible revascularization intervention. The following are the aims of revascularization:

- To increase blood flow and oxygen delivery to ischemic myocardium beyond an obstructive arterial lesion
- To decrease or eliminate the potential consequences or manifestations of myocardial ischemia, including significant ST-segment depression, angina pectoris, threatening ventricular arrhythmias, or combinations thereof
- To potentially reduce cardiovascular-related morbidity and mortality

The two most common revascularization techniques are coronary artery bypass graft surgery (CABGS) and percutaneous transluminal coronary angioplasty (PTCA) or percutaneous coronary intervention (PCI). The surgical technique involves passing the critically obstructed coronary artery with a saphenous vein, removed from the client's leg(s), or an internal mammary artery, one of the major arteries carrying blood to the chest wall, or both. Recent variations of the technique include minimally invasive direct CABGS, wherein the surgeon operates with fiberoptical scopes through small incisions between the ribs to work directly on a contracting heart, and off-pump coronary artery bypass, wherein surgeons operate on the contracting heart without the use of the heart–lung machine. With PTCA, a balloon or double-lumen dilation catheter is directed to the site of a coronary lesion until it lies within the vascular stenosis. Inflation of the balloon produces

- plaque compression and redistribution, and
- stretching of the vessel wall with an increase in the overall vessel diameter.

Today, the majority of individuals diagnosed with ischemic heart disease who are referred for revascularization intervention undergo PTCA (>700,000 patients a year).

CABGS

Current indications for CABGS, after coronary anatomy and left ventricular function have been defined by cardiac catheterization, are as follows:

- Relieve anginal symptoms that are refractory to pharmacologic therapy or when PTCA is contraindicated
- Prolong life in clients with left main coronary artery disease, triple-vessel disease, double-vessel disease, left ventricular dysfunction, proximal left anterior descending coronary artery disease, or some combination of these diseases
- Preserve left ventricular function in clients with diffuse or left main coronary artery disease and significant additional myocardium in jeopardy, particularly when previous myocardial infarction has already compromised left ventricular function

Among patients with three-vessel or two-vessel disease, those treated with CABGS have significantly lower adjusted rates of death and of death from myocardial infarction than those treated with drug-eluting stents. Individuals who undergo CABGS today are characteristically older, are more likely to have three-vessel disease, and have intrinsically poorer pump function. The left ventricular ejection fraction in clients who undergo CABGS averages 38%; the value for those undergoing PTCA is 55%.

Complications of CABGS, including perioperative infarction in 5% to 12% of all cases, occur more frequently in older clients, diabetics, women, obese clients, clients with left ventricular dysfunction (ejection fraction <30%), and clients undergoing emergency bypass surgery. Current patency rates for saphenous vein grafts are 90%, 80%, and 60% after 1, 5, and 11 years, respectively. The greatest incidence of graft occlusion occurs between five and eight years after surgery, often heralded by recurrent angina pectoris, diminished physical work capacity, or both. In contrast, internal mammary grafts have a 93% 10-year graft patency and appear to be resistant to atherosclerosis. This fact may partially explain the impressive 10-year actuarial survival advantage in clients undergoing CABGS who received internal mammary grafts as compared with those who received saphenous vein bypass grafting. Total relief of angina pectoris typically occurs in 70% of clients undergoing CABGS at five years; approximately 50% are asymptomatic at 10 years.

PTCA or PCI

Although the use of PTCA was initially restricted to elective cases of low-risk individuals who had discrete, proximal, single-vessel lesions, indications for the procedure have since broadened to include individuals with two-vessel or three-vessel disease, impaired left ventricular function, and acute occlusion during myocardial infarction. Individuals electing to undergo PTCA must also consent to undergo emergency CABGS should dilation fail or complications occur. Compared with CABGS, which generally requires a hospital stay of five to seven days, the recovery period following elective PTCA is much shorter (one or two days), and the cost is considerably less. However, arterial injuries, blood clotting–related complications, and restenosis remain the major limitations of PTCA. Approximately 30% of clients undergoing PTCA will develop restenosis of the treated vessel within six months of the procedure. Also important to note is that the restenosis rate is 5% to 8% for those undergoing PTCA with a drug-eluting stent.

In 1994, the U.S. Food and Drug Administration approved the use of the Palmaz-Schatz stent, a tiny, flexible metal cylinder inserted into the restored coronary artery to maintain patency. More recently, clinicians have employed stents coated with sirolimus, a drug-eluting stent that attenuates the potential for inflammation of the inner walls of blood vessels, to further reduce the likelihood of subsequent restenosis.

Although PTCA is known to improve survival when done to restore blood flow during an acute myocardial infarction, until recently few data have been available regarding the time frame for coronary intervention for subacute infarct-related coronary artery occlusion to achieve long-term patency and improve ventricular function. Two major clinical trials (Occluded Artery Trial [OAT] and the Total Occlusion Study of Canada [TOSCA-2]) have confirmed that patients who had angioplasty to restore blood flow in a coronary artery 3 to 28 days following their acute myocardial infarction fared no better than those who were medically treated to prevent a recurrent cardiac event.

In 2004, more than 1 million coronary stent procedures were performed in the United States, and approximately 85% of these procedures were undertaken electively in patients with stable coronary artery disease (CAD). Nevertheless, few studies have examined the ability of PTCA to improve outcomes over and above modern, optimal medical therapy in patients with stable CAD. In 2005, investigators performed a meta-analysis of 11 randomized trials comparing PTCA with conservative treatment in patients with stable CAD. They concluded that there was no significant difference between the two treatment strategies for any of the outcome variables tested; if anything, there was a trend for more cardiac deaths or acute myocardial infarctions, particularly nonfatal events, in patients who underwent PTCA. More recently, the COURAGE Trial randomized low-risk symptomatic patients with CAD to PTCA with optimal medical therapy versus optimal medical therapy alone, and again, lack of mortality benefit from PTCA was observed.

Risks and possible complications associated with PTCA or stent (or both) include, but are not limited to, the following:

- Bleeding at the catheter insertion site (usually the groin, but the arm may be used in certain circumstances)
- Blood clot or damage to the blood vessel at the insertion site
- Blood clot within the vessel treated by PTCA/ with or without the use of a stent
- Infection at the catheter insertion site
- Cardiac dysrhythmias and arrhythmias (abnormal heart rhythms)
- Myocardial infarction
- Chest pain or discomfort
- Rupture of the coronary artery, requiring open heart surgery

EFFECTS ON THE EXERCISE RESPONSE

Successful revascularization may favorably alter the exercise response to a single exercise session in several ways. By increasing the blood flow and oxygen supply to myocardial regions beyond an obstructive coronary arterial lesion, CABGS or PTCA may reduce or eliminate electrocardiographic changes resulting from ischemia, such as T-wave inversion and ST-segment depression, as well as anginal symptoms on exertion. The relief of exertional angina may serve to increase physical work capacity in individuals who are symptomatic at low levels of exercise. Correcting the imbalance between myocardial oxygen supply and demand may also improve ventricular contractility and wall motion,

favorably altering the hemodynamic response to exercise. Chronotropic impairment, a delayed heart rate recovery immediately after exercise, or exertional hypotension (or a combination of these irregularities) may normalize after revascularization. Ischemia-related ventricular arrhythmias may also be diminished or eliminated altogether following successful CABGS or PTCA.

EFFECTS OF EXERCISE TRAINING

The benefits and limitations of exercise training for individuals undergoing successful CABGS or PTCA are similar to those for survivors of an acute myocardial infarction (see chapter 6). Surveillance for the development of threatening ventricular arrhythmias during exercise-based cardiac rehabilitation following CABGS may improve medical management and prognosis by facilitating the early detection and treatment of electrical instability in selected high-risk individuals. The average improvement in physical work capacity and maximal oxygen consumption ($\dot{V}O_{2max}$) in this population is approximately 20%. Moreover, training-induced reductions in heart rate and blood pressure serve to decrease myocardial demands at rest and at any given submaximal work rate. Research has suggested that post-CABGS patients should increase their level of additional physical activity beyond that of the cardiac rehabilitation program in order to improve their cardiac autonomic control (e.g., heart rate recovery). Even short-term endurance training in clients rehabilitated after CABGS promotes favorable modification of glucose metabolism, presumably by a decrease in insulin resistance.

Although results from several meta-analyses have demonstrated a 20% to 25% reduction in fatal cardiovascular events and total mortality after myocardial infarction, the contribution of exercise training to the survival of individuals following CABGS and PTCA has, until now, received less attention. At least one study has shown that in patients with stable CAD and an angiographically documented stenosis amenable to PTCA, who undertook a 12-month exercise training program resulted in a higher event-free survival rate and exercise capacity at lower costs when compared with PTCA. Each 1 MET (metabolic equivalent) increase in exercise capacity appears to confer an 8% to 17% reduction in mortality.

MANAGEMENT AND MEDICATIONS

Treatment of individuals following revascularization procedures has progressed from the use of nitrate drugs and beta-blocking agents to an aggressive multimodality approach using coronary risk factor modification, pharmacologic therapy (e.g., aspirin, clopidogrel, calcium channel blocking drugs, antiarrhythmic and lipid-lowering drugs), thrombolytic enzymes, PTCA, surgical interventions, and, when necessary, the automatic implantable cardioverter defibrillator. Nevertheless, lifestyle interventions designed to slow, halt, or even reverse the underlying atherosclerotic disease process remain the mainstay of treatment, including

- regular aerobic exercise,
- blood pressure control,
- smoking cessation,
- cholesterol lowering,
- diabetes management, and
- reduction of body weight and fat stores.

Smoking cessation, for example, is associated with a higher prevalence of disease-free bypass grafts over time and increased survival. Cessation of smoking at age 60, 50, 40, or 30 gains, respectively, about 3, 6, 9, or 10 years of life expectancy.

Empiric experience has shown that close observation and monitoring of revascularization clients during exercise-based cardiac rehabilitation can often detect deterioration in clinical status. Exercise-related signs or symptoms that may indicate restenosis of a treated vessel, occlusion of vein grafts, or progression of atherosclerotic disease include the following:

- Recurring anginal pain (e.g., chest pain or pressure, an ache in the jaw or neck, pain across the shoulders or back)
- Dizziness or light-headedness
- Threatening forms of ventricular ectopy (e.g., frequent paired or multiform ventricular premature contractions, couplets, or ventricular tachycardia)

Cardiac and lipid-lowering medications commonly used to treat revascularization clients are summarized elsewhere (see chapters 6 and 22), with specific reference to their hemodynamic and electrocardiographic effects. With the exception of drug-eluting stents, interventions to prevent restenosis have been largely ineffective. Repeat PTCA is the usual treatment for restenosis, and most clients experience sustained improvement in signs and symptoms after the procedure.

RECOMMENDATIONS FOR EXERCISE TESTING

Exercise testing can follow general protocols and procedures outlined for postmyocardial infarction (post-MI) clients (see table 7.1). Treadmill or cycle ergometer testing three to five weeks after CABGS has proved valuable in assessing exercise tolerance and in prescribing levels of physical activity; in contrast, arm ergometer testing at this time may be inappropriate because of midsternal incisional pain. Follow-up testing procedures are similar to those after acute MI (e.g., following an additional three to six months of exercise training and yearly thereafter). For the purpose of risk stratification, symptomatic individuals five years or less and all individuals more than five years after CABGS may benefit from exercise testing with concomitant myocardial perfusion imaging. An exercise capacity of 4 METs or less indicates a higher-mortality group, whereas an exercise capacity of 9 METs or more identifies a cohort with an excellent long-term prognosis, regardless of the underlying extent of CAD or its ischemic manifestations. Submaximal effort tolerance upon intake and completion of a 12-week cardiac rehabilitation program is also a strong and age-independent predictor of mortality in patients who have had recent CABGS.

Exercise testing following PTCA may be performed sooner and more frequently than is typically recommended after an MI or CABGS. A rather new procedure using supine cycle ergometer and echocardiography has been shown to be a safe and reliable tool for detecting exercise-induced wall motion abnormalities following PTCA and providing prognostic information in the risk assessment of clinical restenosis. Among asymptomatic individuals with single-vessel disease, the detection of restenosis following PTCA via conventional exercise testing remains unreliable, especially when quantitative coronary angiography is used as a reference. However, the presence of 75% or more cross-sectional narrowing shown by intravascular ultrasound is well correlated with 1 mm or more ST-segment depression at follow-up treadmill testing

TABLE 7.1

CABGS and PCTA: Exercise Testing

Methods	Measures	Endpoints*	Comments
Aerobic			
Cycle (ramp protocol 17 W/min; staged protocol 25-50 W/3 min stage)	▪ 12-lead ECG, HR	▪ Serious dysrhythmias ▪ >2 mm ST-segment depression or elevation ▪ Ischemic threshold	▪ ST-segment displacement can occur with restenosis or partial occlusion. ▪ Important in establishing a safe training intensity.
Treadmill (1-2 METs/3 min stage)		▪ T-wave inversion with significant ST change	▪ Chronotropic impairment suggests poor prognosis. ▪ Minimal treadmill speed should be ≤1.0 mph.
	▪ BP, rate–pressure product	▪ SBP >250 mmHg or DBP >115 mmHg	
	▪ RPE (6-20) ▪ Gas analysis ($\dot{V}O_{2peak}$ or $\dot{V}O_{2max}$)		
Strength			
Isokinetic or isotonic	▪ 90% MVC ▪ Greatest load lifted 2 or 3 times	3 consecutive reps	▪ Use 1RM (estimated from 90% MVC) to establish training work rate. ▪ Should not be performed until sternum has healed.

*Measurements of particular significance; do not always indicate test termination.

after PTCA. The addition of QT dispersion (QTd) ($QTd = QT_{max} - QT_{min}$) to ST-segment depression during exercise testing also improves the diagnostic value and can be used as a noninvasive tool in the diagnosis of restenosis after PTCA. Preliminary signs or symptoms of restenosis, manifested as significant ST-segment depression, the provocation of angina pectoris, or both, may be apparent with exercise testing as early as two or three days after PTCA. A more accepted time period for initial evaluation of PTCA clients is two to five weeks, followed by another exercise test at six months. Thereafter, exercise testing once a year is generally considered adequate.

RECOMMENDATIONS FOR EXERCISE PROGRAMMING

Simple exposure to orthostatic or gravitational stress during the abbreviated bed rest stage of hospital convalescence and soon thereafter may prevent much of the deterioration in cardiorespiratory fitness that normally follows CABGS and, to a lesser extent, PTCA. A significant increase in aerobic capacity generally occurs in the weeks following coronary revascularization, even in individuals who undergo no formal exercise training. Research indicates that self-care and other out-of-hospital activities performed by cardiac clients soon after hospital discharge frequently lead to sustained increases in heart rate and oxygen uptake that exceed the minimal effective intensity (i.e., 40% to 50% heart rate or $\dot{V}O_{2max}$) commonly prescribed for training. Transient fluxes in cardiorespiratory activity may promote a training effect and account, at least in part, for the spontaneous improvement in aerobic capacity during the early weeks after coronary revascularization.

Walking is highly recommended as a primary mode of exercise soon after CABGS or PTCA. Numerous studies have shown that brisk walking is of a sufficient intensity to elicit a training heart rate (defined as ≥70% of measured maximal heart rate) in all but the most highly fit clients with coronary disease. Walking distance, in men who underwent an exercise-based rehabilitation program, was found to be a strong independent predictor, and a greater guide to prognosis, than gains in $\dot{V}O_{2max}$. General recommendations for exercise training are found in table 7.2. Compared with MI clients, clients after CABGS typically

- begin inpatient exercise rehabilitation sooner,
- progress at a more accelerated rate, and
- devote more attention to upper extremity range of motion (ROM) exercises.

Persons who undergo CABGS may experience significant soft tissue injury and bone damage of the chest wall. If these areas do not receive ROM exercise in the early postsurgical period, the musculature can become weaker and foreshorten, resulting in more discomfort for the client during convalescence and a prolonged recovery period. ROM exercises used in the inpatient program for the CABGS client typically include shoulder flexion, abduction, and internal and external rotation; elbow flexion; hip flexion, abduction, and internal and external rotation; plantarflexion and dorsiflexion; and ankle inversion and eversion.

TABLE 7.2

CABGS and PCTA: Exercise Programming

Modes	Goals	Intensity/Frequency/Duration	Time to goal
Aerobic - Large muscle activities - Arm/leg ergometry	- Increase aerobic capacity - Decrease BP and HR response to submaximal exercise - Decrease submaximal O_2 demand - Decrease CAD risk factors - Increase ADLs	- RPE 11-16/20 - 40-80% $\dot{V}O_{2max}$ or HR reserve - Intensity must be kept below ischemic threshold - 4-7 days/week - 20-60 min/session	4-6 months
Resistance Circuit training	- Increase ability to perform leisure and occupation activities and ADLs - Increase muscle strength and endurance - Decrease rate–pressure product during lifting or carrying objects	- 40-50% MVC (avoid Vasalva) - 2-3 days/week - 2-4* sets of 12-15 reps - 8-10 different exercises - 1-2 lb (0.5-0.9 kg) to start (wait 12 weeks post-CABGS before using heavier weights) - Resistance gradually increased over time	4-6 months
Flexibility - Upper and lower body - ROM activities	- Decrease risk of injury - Maintain ROM	- 2-3 days/week - Static stretches held for 10-30 s	4-6 months

*A single set to volitional fatigue is highly effective, at least during the initial months of training.

However, CABGS clients who experience sternal movement or have postsurgical sternal wound complications would not perform these exercises unless medically cleared. Upper body ergometry or traditional resistance training exercises that may cause pulling on the sternum should be minimized until healing is complete (generally 12 weeks after CABGS and sternotomy). Often, however, patients receive advice after surgery involving sternotomy that is vague or overly restrictive (or both), not taking into account which muscle groups patients could safely use without risking damage to the surgical site. The sternum should be checked for stability by an experienced health care professional before a resistance training regimen is initiated or at any time symptoms of chest discomfort or clicking develop.

Middle-aged and older individuals may begin to resume normal activities, including light- to moderate-intensity exercise such as brisk walking, within 24 to 48 h following PTCA. Appropriately selected PTCA clients who wish to initiate a resistance training program may benefit by first participating in an aerobic exercise regimen for two weeks or more, whether in a home-based or a medically supervised program. Exercise-based cardiac rehabilitation (Phase II) provides close monitoring and supervision in which failures (restenosis) are detected early.

CASE STUDY

Coronary Artery Bypass Surgery

A 60-year-old automobile executive had recently experienced substernal chest discomfort while shoveling snow, and again while climbing a flight of stairs. These symptoms were generally precipitated by physical exertion and sometimes occurred after heavy meals or stressful situations. Six years earlier, the client had experienced an inferolateral MI. Additional coronary risk factors included a history of hypertension, hypercholesterolemia (total cholesterol consistently >240 mg/dl, LDL-cholesterol >150 mg/dl), obesity, and a family history of premature CAD. He had a positive exercise stress test, and cardiac catheterization revealed triple-vessel disease (total right coronary obstruction from his previous MI, 90% proximal left anterior descending obstruction, 60-70% obstruction of the mid circumflex coronary artery) with inferolateral wall hypokinesis and an ejection fraction of 40%. Coronary artery bypass surgery was performed, and he was referred to cardiac rehabilitation.

S: "I had bypass surgery a couple of months ago."

O:Vitals

HR: 80 contractions/min
BP: 146/90 mmHg
BMI: 32.6 kg/m²
Male, no acute distress; no jugular venous distension
Lungs: Clear
Heart: Regular rate, irregular rhythm; no gallops or murmurs; distal pulses 2+ and nondelayed; no peripheral edema
ECG: Sinus rhythm with infrequent PVCs; nonspecific ST–T-wave abnormalities with Q-waves in leads III and aVF

Graded Exercise Test (Treadmill, Modified Bruce Protocol)

Rest HR: 88 contractions/min
BP: 146/90 mmHg

Peak HR: 124 contractions/min
Peak BP: 160/84 mmHg
Peak exercise: 2.5 mph, 12% grade (1 min); test terminated due to fatigue (RPE 17/20) at an estimated aerobic capacity of 5.6 METs
No significant ST-segment depression symptoms; isolated PVCs
Isotope imaging showed a fixed defect in the inferior wall and no evidence of ischemia-induced perfusion abnormalities
Medications: Metoprolol, Lipitor, aspirin

A: 1. Recent bypass surgery and prior MI
2. Deconditioning

P: Initiate a 12-week cardiac rehabilitation program.

Exercise Program Goals

1. Peak exercise tolerance >7.5 METs (moderate fitness for age/gender)
2. Increase low functional capacity
3. Adjunct to diabetes/weight management
4. Reinforce lifestyle changes/medical management

Follow-Up

Approximately six months after bypass surgery, the client completed 7 min of the conventional Bruce treadmill protocol (1 min at 3.4 mph, 14% grade, ~7.6 METs) to volitional fatigue, without significant ST-segment depression or angina. Isolated PVCs were noted during and after exercise, and the client achieved a peak heart rate of 130 contractions per minute. He chose to continue cardiac rehabilitation in a medically supervised Phase III program.

Mode	Frequency	Duration	Intensity	Progression
Aerobic	3 days/week	20 min sessions as tolerated	THR (96-108 contractions/min) RPE 12-15/20	Increase to 40 min/session at 60-80% THR after 8 weeks.
Strength (lower extremity, upper extremity delayed until sternum well healed)	3 days/week	1 set ≤10 reps	40-50% of 1RM	increase to 2 sets of 10-12 reps after 12 weeks.
Flexibility (shoulders, elbows, wrists, hips, knees, ankles)	3 days/week	20 s/stretch	Maintain stretch below discomfort point	Discomfort point should occur at higher ROM.
Warm-up and cool-down	Before and after each session	10-15 min	RPE <10/20	Maintain.

Evidence-Based Guidelines

ACC/AHA guidelines for percutaneous coronary intervention (revision of the 1993 PTCA guidelines). Circulation. 2001;103:3019.

Suggested Web Sites

American Association of Cardiovascular and Pulmonary Rehabilitation. www.aacvpr.org

American College of Cardiology. www.acc.org

American College of Sports Medicine. www.acsm.org

American Heart Association. www.americanheart.org

8

Angina and Silent Ischemia

Daniel Friedman, MD, FACSM ■ Scott O. Roberts, PhD, FACSM

OVERVIEW OF THE PATHOPHYSIOLOGY

The heart relies almost exclusively on aerobic energy metabolism; consequently, it requires a constant, reliable supply of oxygen to survive. Under normal conditions, the heart closely regulates coronary blood flow (CBF) in response to variations in myocardial oxygen ($M\dot{V}O_2$) demand. This tight coupling of CBF with $M\dot{V}O_2$ demand is essential, given that resting myocardium extracts nearly 80% of the available oxygen from surrounding blood. During exercise, CBF increases in response to elevated myocardial tension, contractility, and heart rate (HR), which together account for the heart's higher oxygen demand during exercise. When the oxygen supply/demand ratio is reduced either by a decrease in oxygen delivery relative to demand as with vascular stenosis due to coronary artery disease (CAD), or by an increase in demand relative to supply, tissue hypoxia occurs.

Myocardial ischemia is usually the result of an obstruction in the coronary arteries caused by atherosclerosis. Less common causes of myocardial ischemia include focal spasms in the coronary arteries that reduce flow independent of atherosclerosis and, in rare occurrences, a very high demand in the absence of flow restriction. When myocardial ischemia causes pain or discomfort in the chest it is referred to as symptomatic ischemia, or angina.

Angina is typically categorized as a heavy, squeezing, or constricting feeling that typically originates behind the sternum and can radiate to the shoulders, arms, neck, or jaw. Some people experience shortness of breath, nausea, or diaphoresis as well. Atypical features, described as sharp, stabbing or knife-like pain, may also be present. Symptoms generally last from 2 to 10 min, depending on the severity of the disease. Chest pain is a nonspecific symptom that can have cardiac or noncardiac causes. Noncardiac causes include spasm of the esophagus; reflux of acid from the stomach; hiatal hernia; inflammation of the bones or cartilage of the chest wall or sternum; or muscular pain from muscles of the chest wall, back, shoulder, or arms.

Stable angina is usually associated with a specific amount of physical exertion, emotional stress, or exposure to cold and is predictably relieved promptly with rest or sublingual nitroglycerin. Stable angina is usually the result of a fixed stenosis in a particular segment of a coronary artery. When a coronary artery lumen diameter is narrowed by more than 70%, the reduced blood flow may be sufficient to serve the cardiac oxygen needs at rest but be insufficient for increases in demand during exercise when myocardial oxygen requirements may go up as much as 10-fold. As CAD progresses

Acknowledgment

The editors wish to acknowledge the previous authors of this chapter, Adam Gitkin, MS; Martha Canulette, MSN, RN; and Daniel Friedman, MD, FACSM.

over time, the frequency and intensity of angina episodes often increase.

Unstable angina (UA) poses significantly greater risk than stable angina because the onset of symptoms is far less predictable, often occurring at rest or following markedly lower than normal levels of physical exertion than in the past. The traditional definition of UA, an intermediate state between stable angina and a myocardial infarction, may be too limiting today, given that UA often indicates at least a transient complete blockage of an artery. Contemporary opinion is to include UA within the continuum of the acute coronary syndromes (myocardial infarction, non-Q-wave myocardial infarction, and UA). The following are the three principal presentations of UA:

- Angina that occurs at rest or upon awakening from sleep, lasting more than 20 min
- New onset, or first experience, of anginal chest pain
- Increasing severity, frequency, duration, or threshold pattern (level of activity that reproduces the pain) of previously diagnosed angina

The latter two, however, may occur in stable angina when the degree of obstruction becomes sufficient to result in symptoms.

The pathogenesis of UA is multifactorial and includes one or more of the following:

- Rupture and hemorrhage into an atherosclerotic plaque
- Platelet aggregation or thrombosis (clot) at a site of coronary artery narrowing
- Transient periods of vasospasm at the atherosclerotic plaque

UA can be a precursor to a myocardial infarction, and must be treated immediately with anticlotting (anticoagulant) drugs or emergency balloon angioplasty.

Variant, vasospastic, or Prinzmetal's angina occurs when the coronary arteries spasm, or contract suddenly. Angiograms of this type of angina show no obstruction or stenoses and very little evidence of atheroma. However, most spasm does seem to occur in the setting of some degree of atherosclerosis. Intense vasospasm (i.e., a form of cramp of the vessel wall muscles) can cause a transient narrowing capable of independently reducing coronary oxygen supply, resulting in angina. Medications such as calcium channel antagonists and nitrates that reduce coronary spasms are an effective treatment for this

type of angina. In general, the prognosis is thought to be good.

Some individuals with CAD do not have symptoms consistent with myocardial ischemia. Angina in the absence of typical symptoms is called silent ischemia. Laboratory techniques, such as cardiac stress testing and continuous ambulatory electrocardiography, are used to diagnose silent ischemia. As in symptomatic ischemia, ST-segment and T-wave changes are commonly seen, as well as horizontal or downward sloping ST-segment depressions and T-wave flattening or inversions. Silent ischemia is particularly common among diabetics, possibly related to impaired pain sensation due to peripheral neuropathy. Treatment for persons with silent ischemia is similar to that for people with angina.

EFFECTS ON THE EXERCISE RESPONSE

Given the relatively high oxygen requirements of myocardium at rest relative to blood flow, when myocardial demand increases during the transition from rest to exercise, an increase in CBF is the primary, if not only, way in which the myocardium receives increased oxygen supply. During periods of vigorous exercise, CBF can increase four to six times above resting levels in an effort to keep pace with the high metabolic demand. Rarely is CBF a limiting factor in exercise tolerance in healthy individuals. However, when $\dot{M}VO_2$ demand increases in the presence of diseased arteries, supply may not be able to keep up.

The degree to which myocardial ischemia limits exercise tolerance is largely dependent on the severity of coronary artery obstruction and the extent to which collateral blood flow supports affected areas of the heart. Other limiting factors in diseased arteries include reduced production of the dilating compound nitric oxide (also known as endothelial-derived relaxing factor) and an increase in platelet aggregation caused by release of thromboxane A2, a chemical that strongly constricts blood vessels, increasing the likelihood of clotting.

Since the heart relies almost exclusively on aerobic energy metabolism, hypoxic conditions, as with myocardial ischemia, result in functional, metabolic, and morphological alterations to the myocardium, including arrhythmias, poor contractility, and electrophysiological abnormalities. Further consequences of a hypoxic myocardium include reduced stroke volume, left ventricular ejection fraction, and cardiac output and a drop in perfusion pressure, which collectively limit skeletal muscle perfusion and overall exercise tolerance. A decreased stroke volume may also lead to a compensatory increase in HR, putting a further strain on the heart. For these reasons, a longer warm-up is recommended for anyone with diagnosed angina.

EFFECTS OF EXERCISE TRAINING

Exercise training is generally beneficial for individuals with stable angina. Exercise alone, or in combination with other lifestyle behavior changes, helps to reduce overall cardiac risk and can slow, prevent, or even reverse atherosclerotic plaques. The overall goal for people with angina is to raise their ischemic threshold, or the point during physical stress at which angina symptoms occur. Optimal pharmacological therapy will also help enhance exercise performance. Following exercise training, most people are able to perform greater leisure- and exercise-related physical activity without signs and symptoms of angina. Improved exercise tolerance and decreased severity and extent of exercise-related myocardial ischemia are usually due to a reduction in $M\dot{V}O_2$ demand, as well as increased efficiency of the exercising skeletal muscle.

The majority of individuals with stable angina achieve many, if not all, of the same benefits of exercise as apparently healthy people. One of the most important benefits of exercise for those with angina is a reduced HR and blood pressure (BP) at any given level of submaximal work. A lower HR and BP at the same relative workload prior to exercise corresponds to a lower $M\dot{V}O_2$ demand. Heart rate and systolic blood pressure (HR × SBP), often referred to as the double product or rate–pressure product (RPP), is a useful indirect measure of myocardial oxygen consumption during exercise. The RPP index can be used to document specific workloads at which signs and symptoms of angina occur and improvements in functional capacity relative to the onset of symptomatic ischemia.

Exercise training can also improve the supply of oxygenated blood to the heart at rest and during exercise. Two of the possible mechanisms for improved CBF following exercise are greater nitric oxide production and improved coronary arterial smooth muscle function. Studies have shown that long-term exercise training (e.g., four to seven times a week for 12 weeks or more) stimulates the production of nitric oxide, which improves the control and degree of vasodilation of the coronary arter-

ies. Training-induced changes in coronary arterial smooth muscle function due to either a decrease in coronary tone (vasoconstriction) or an increase in vasodilation (relaxation), or both, can lead to improved blood flow in coronary arteries.

MANAGEMENT AND MEDICATIONS

The primary goals for treatment of myocardial ischemia include increasing $M\dot{V}O_2$ supply and decreasing demand through a combination of medications, exercise, and other lifestyle modifications. Accepted strategies used to increase $M\dot{V}O_2$ supply include controlling multiple CAD risk factors (e.g., smoking cessation, hypertension control, weight loss, stress management), direct revascularization of ischemic myocardium (e.g., balloon angioplasty with or without stenting), and coronary artery bypass graft surgery (CABG). Primary drug categories used to treat angina include antiplatelet drugs, beta-blockers, calcium channel antagonists, nitrates (nitroglycerin), and a newer agent called ranolazine.

Antiplatelet drugs (e.g., aspirin) decrease the adherence of platelets to the walls of blood vessels and decrease the aggregation of platelets. Antiplatelet drugs inhibit thromboxane A2, a potent platelet aggregator and blood vessel constrictor, which ultimately helps inhibit the clotting process and thus assists in preventing myocardial ischemia.

Beta-blockers (e.g., atenolol) decrease $M\dot{V}O_2$ demand by exerting a negative chronotropic (i.e., HR) and inotropic (i.e., force of contraction) effect on the heart. Beta-blockers block the effects of adrenaline on beta receptors in the heart, which slows down the nerve impulses traveling through the heart.

Calcium channel blockers (e.g., verapamil) reduce $M\dot{V}O_2$ demand, myocardial contractility, and systemic BP by blocking calcium entry into cardiac muscle and blood vessels. The lower levels of intracellular calcium reduce contractility of the heart and vascular smooth muscle contractility, which enhances arterial vasodilation.

Nitrates (both short- and long-acting nitroglycerin) decrease $M\dot{V}O_2$ demand and peripheral resistance. Nitrates dilate peripheral blood vessels, thereby reducing venous return and cardiac preload (myocardial wall tension to achieve contraction). At the same time, nitrates increase oxygen supply through an increase in coronary perfusion and a decrease in coronary vasospasm.

The recently approved anti-ischemic or anti-anginal drug ranolazine (brand name Ranexa) is a new treatment for chronic angina in patients who have failed to respond to prior angina therapy. Ranolazine reduces angina and myocardial ischemia without reducing HR or BP or increasing the RPP at maximal exercise levels. Recent clinical trials have shown that ranolazine significantly decreases the frequency of angina attacks and need for nitroglycerin and improves exercise tolerance compared to other standard cardiac medications.

RECOMMENDATIONS FOR EXERCISE TESTING

Exercise testing is a valuable diagnostic tool for diagnosing CAD, evaluating and guiding medical therapy, and stratifying overall risk as well as prognosis (see table 8.1). However, when the risk of performing an exercise test outweighs the benefits, other tests should be considered. Current evidence-based guidelines for the evaluation and treatment of UA/non-ST-segment elevation MI (NSTEMI) state that exercise testing is contraindicated in patients with acute ischemia but can be performed in patients with nondiagnostic electrocardiograms (ECGs), negative cardiac biomarkers, and no resting angina within the past 6 h. In addition to standard clinical measures obtained during exercise testing (HR, ECG, BP, signs and symptoms, etc.) anginal symptoms, rating of anginal pain, and the exact onset and duration of angina (if they occur) should be documented when testing patients with a history of angina. In addition to commonly accepted indications for terminating an exercise test, as outlined by the American College of Sports Medicine Guidelines, the following indications are highlighted because they relate specifically to myocardial ischemia, angina, and UA.

Absolute Indications

- Drop in SBP >10 mmHg from baseline despite an increase in work rate, accompanied by other evidence of ischemia
- Moderately severe angina (defined as 3 on standard 1-4 angina scale)
- ST elevation (+1.0 mm) in leads without diagnostic Q-waves (other than V1 or aVR)

Relative Indications

- Drop in SBP >10 mmHg from baseline despite an increase in work rate, in the absence of other evidence of ischemia
- ST or QRS changes such as excessive ST depression (>2 mm horizontal or downsloping ST-segment depression) or marked axis shift

The presence of ST-segment changes alone does not confirm the presence or absence of CAD unless

TABLE 8.1

Angina and Silent Ischemia: Exercise Testing

Methods	Measures	Endpoints*	Comments
Aerobic			
Cycle (ramp protocol 17 W/min; staged protocol 10-25 W/3 min stage)	■ 12-lead ECG, HR	■ Serious arrythmias ■ >2 mm ST-segment depression or elevation ■ Ischemic threshold ■ T-wave inversion with significant ST change	
Treadmill (1-2 METs/3 min stage)	■ Angina scale, rate–pressure product	■ +3 or greater (1-4 scale)	■ Onset of angina at low work rates is predictive of ischemic heart disease.
	■ BP	■ Plateau or drop in SBP with increased work rate ■ SBP >250 mmHg or DBP > 115 mmHg	■ Drop in BP with exercise is associated with increased prognosis of ischemic heart disease.
	■ RPP		

*Measurements of particular significance; do not always indicate test termination.

these changes are correlated with other pertinent data such as treadmill time, HR and BP responses, signs and symptoms of angina, presence of supra- or ventricular arrhythmias. Sensitivity of exercise testing increases when clinical exercise test guidelines are adhered to and multivariate scoring is used to enhance diagnostic and prognostic confidence.

RECOMMENDATIONS FOR EXERCISE PROGRAMMING

Lifestyle changes, medications, and revascularization all play important roles in reducing or eliminating symptoms of angina and slowing the progression, and in some cases even stimulating the regression, of coronary atherosclerosis. Increased physical activity helps prevent as well reduce CAD risk factors. Evidence-based physical activity guidelines for secondary prevention of CAD have recently been published and are similar to general public health guidelines for apparently healthy persons (see table 8.2).

- The general goal is 30 min, seven days per week (minimum five days per week).
- All CAD patients are encouraged to get 30 to 60 min of moderate-intensity aerobic activity, such as brisk walking, on most, preferably all, days of the week, supplemented by an increase in daily lifestyle activities (e.g., walking breaks at work, gardening, and household work).
- Resistance training two days per week is encouraged.
- Medically supervised exercise programs are advised for high-risk patients (e.g., those with recent acute coronary syndrome or revascularization, heart failure).

More formalized exercise training generally can begin within one or two weeks after revascularized UA/NSTEMI. The initial exercise intensity level should be conservative and well within the functional and disease limitations of the individual. The initial exercise intensity level for stable angina patients starting a formalized exercise program

TABLE 8.2

Angina and Silent Ischemia: Exercise Programming

Modes	Goals	Intensity/Frequency/Duration	Time to goal
Aerobic Large muscle activities	▪ Improve functional capacity ▪ Decrease CAD risk factors ▪ Decrease BP response to submaximal exercise ▪ Decrease $M\dot{V}O_2$ demand	▪ HR 10-15 contractions/min below ischemic threshold ▪ 3-7 days/week ▪ 20-60 min/session ▪ 5-10 min of warm-up and cool-down	4-6 months
Strength Circuit training*	Improve functional capacity	▪ Light resistance; 40-50% of maximal voluntary contraction (avoid Valsalva) ▪ 2-3 days/week ▪ 15-20 min/session	4-6 months
Flexibility Upper and lower body ROM activities	Decrease risk of injury	2-3 days/week	4-6 months

*Avoid isometric exercises.

is conservative and takes into consideration the individual's medical history and current functional status. Unless a recent ET has been performed, a sensible approach is to use inpatient exercise guidelines to start, then modify the intensity based on subjective and objective evaluation of several sessions of exercise. Inpatient exercise guidelines for intensity include the following:

- RPE <13 (6-20 scale)
- Post-MI: HR <120 contractions per minute or HR_{rest} + 20 contractions per minute (arbitrary upper limit)
- Postrevascularization: HR_{rest} + 30 contractions per minute (arbitrary upper limit)
- To tolerance if asymptomatic

Special Considerations

- Prior to exercise training, anyone with a diagnosis of angina must be able to define angina, describe his or her unique symptoms, identify provoking factors, describe the immediate treatment of angina (including the necessity and protocol for taking nitroglycerin), and understand his or her upper limits of exercise (including HR, ratings of perceived exertion, and angina scales).

- The exercise prescription must take into account the effects of all medications on HR, BP, ECG, and exercise capacity.

- If there is a change in frequency, type, or severity of anginal symptoms before, during, or after an exercise session, the patient's physician should be notified.

- If a client develops angina during an exercise session, exercise should be terminated and sublingual nitroglycerin administered according to national EMS or individual facility guidelines.

- Warm-up and cool-down: A prolonged warm-up and cool-down (10 min or more), including range of motion, stretching, and low-intensity aerobic activities, has been shown to have an antianginal effect.

- Intensity: The upper training heart rate (THR) should be set at 10 to 15 contractions per minute below the ischemic threshold (the RPP at which angina symptoms developed during ET or monitored exercise). In addition to the ischemic threshold, the upper limit may be based on other thresholds at which symptoms of cardiovascular insufficiency occur, such as ventricular arrhythmias or plateau or decrease in SBP during exercise. Over time, the THR will need to be modified as training adaptations occur.

- Duration: Initially exercise should consist of short-duration (e.g., 5-10 min each) sessions, two or three per day, separated by short rest periods; sessions can be gradually increased and even combined over time.

- Frequency: The frequency of exercise sessions may start out high (e.g., several short sessions five to seven days per week) and gradually progress to longer-duration, less frequent sessions per week depending on how individuals tolerate and adapt to exercise.

Evidence-Based Guidelines

A Report of the American College of Cardiology/ American Heart Association Task Force on Practice Guidelines. ACC/AHA 2007 guidelines for the management of patients with unstable angina/non–ST-elevation myocardial infarction. J Am Coll Cardiol. 2007;50:652-726.

A report of the American College of Cardiology/ American Heart Association Task Force on Practice Guidelines Writing Group. 2007 chronic angina focused update of the ACC/AHA 2002 guidelines for the management of patients with chronic stable angina. J Am Coll Cardiol. 2007;50:2264-2274.

Suggested Web Sites

American College of Cardiology. www.acc.org

American Heart Association. www.americanheart.org

CASE STUDY

Angina and Silent Ischemia

A 54-year-old man had been having substernal chest pressure for several months. At first it occurred only when he was doing very vigorous activities, but later it was brought on by climbing a flight of stairs. The discomfort occasionally radiated to his left shoulder and was associated with some shortness of breath and nausea. Heart catheterization revealed a 75% mid-right coronary artery stenosis, which was opened to less than 10% stenosis by balloon angioplasty. He was referred to cardiac rehabilitation.

S: "I had one of those balloon jobs."

O: Vitals

BP: 142/75 mmHg
HR: 73 contractions/min
Respiration: 14 breaths/min
Lungs: Clear
Heart sounds: Soft fourth heart sound
Normal peripheral pulses; no edema

Labs

ECG: Normal
Graded Exercise Test (Stress Test; Bruce Protocol): 1.5 mm of flat ST-segment depression in the inferolateral leads at 6 min
Medications: None

A: Exertional angina caused by CAD

P: 1. Refer to Phase II cardiac rehabilitation.
   2. Check fasting lipids; initiate lipid-lowering therapy.
   3. Prescribe aspirin.

Exercise Program Goals

1. Evaluate/improve anginal threshold
2. Increase functional capacity
3. Educate about managing angina symptoms
4. Reinforce lifestyle changes/medical management

Mode	Frequency	Duration	Intensity	Progression
Aerobic	2 days/week	20 min/session	THR 10-15 contractions/min below ischemic threshold	Increase to maintain 10-15 contractions/min below ischemic threshold.
Strength	3 days/week	1 set of ≤10 reps	40-50% of 1RM	Increase to 2 sets of 10-12 reps after 12 weeks.
Flexibility	3 days/week	20 s/stretch	Maintain stretch below discomfort point	Discomfort point should occur at higher ROM.
Warm-up and cool-down	Before and after each session	10-15 min	RPE<10/20	Maintain.

Atrial Fibrillation

J. Edwin Atwood, MD ■ Jonathan N. Myers, PhD, FACSM

OVERVIEW OF THE PATHOPHYSIOLOGY

Chronic atrial fibrillation (AF) is characterized by disorganized atrial activity that results in rapid and irregular ventricular depolarizations. AF is one of the most common arrhythmias encountered clinically, and occurs more frequently with advancing age. Although the pathophysiology of AF is not completely understood, it is believed to be caused by multiple reentrant circuits within the atria. The chaotic and rapid atrial contractions cause an irregular ventricular response, which can impair cardiac pump function and lead to a variety of symptoms attributable to hemodynamic variance. Although AF can often be asymptomatic, its assorted problems are generally thought to include the following:

- Increased risk of thromboembolic events
- Rapid ventricular rates when the atrioventricular (AV) node is inadequately suppressed
- Incomplete ventricular filling causing reduced cardiac output
- Decreased exercise capacity
- Fatigue

AF is also associated with chronic heart failure, cardiomyopathy, significant valvular disease, coronary artery disease, hypertension, and hyperthyroidism. Some of these disorders may be underlying causes of AF, and in some cases they may be manifestations of AF.

EFFECTS ON THE EXERCISE RESPONSE

The most notable hemodynamic feature of exercise in clients with AF is a rapid, irregular ventricular response. Heart rate in individuals with AF is comparatively high at any level of exercise, in part to compensate for the diminished stroke volume and thus cardiac output in AF. Maximal heart rate tends to be considerably higher in clients with AF than in subjects in normal sinus rhythm. There is, however, a marked variability in the maximal heart rate response, as evidenced by standard deviations of 30 contractions per minute, even among subjects of a similar age. The heart rate response is also affected by comorbid conditions commonly associated with AF (e.g., coronary artery disease, chronic heart failure) and the use of AV nodal suppressant drugs such as beta-blockers, calcium channel blockers, and digoxin.

Exercise tolerance is generally reduced in AF relative to that in age-matched normal subjects. The degree of this reduction is typically on the order of 20% but is highly dependent on the presence and extent of underlying heart disease. Individuals with AF alone (no other underlying coronary artery disease) achieve peak oxygen consumption values typical of age-matched subjects in normal sinus rhythm.

Because of the variability in the diastolic filling period, the determination of systolic blood pressure can be difficult and is poorly reproducible.

This is particularly true at rest when, after long RR intervals, Korotkoff sounds may be heard more distinctly.

EFFECTS OF EXERCISE TRAINING

Insufficient scientific literature is available concerning the effects of exercise training specifically in patients with AF. However, because the prevalence of AF is comparatively high in men older than 60 years, individuals with AF have been included in many rehabilitation studies by default. Individuals with AF would not be expected to have a training response significantly different from that of individuals in normal sinus rhythm. The major concern in terms of exercise training in clients with AF is the underlying heart disease, particularly valvular disease, chronic heart failure, and coronary artery disease. The presence of these underlying diseases should be the foremost consideration in exercise programming for individuals with AF.

MANAGEMENT AND MEDICATIONS

Management of AF primarily involves converting the individual to normal sinus rhythm, pharmacologic intervention to maintain sinus rhythm, and, when AF is chronic, strategies to control the ventricular rate response and reduce the incidence of stroke. In many clients initially diagnosed with AF, an effort will be made to convert the client back to sinus rhythm electrically, pharmacologically, or in both ways. This procedure has been shown to improve exercise capacity on the order of 15% to 20%, although functional gains probably do not occur until at least one month after successful cardioversion. While the initial success rate of electrical cardioversion is high, many clients will return to AF within four to six weeks. Conversion and maintenance of normal sinus rhythm is particularly difficult when the duration of AF has been long. Twenty-four hour ambulatory monitoring can be helpful for examining heart rate control. There is currently some controversy regarding whether efforts to restore normal sinus rhythm (through electrical cardioversion, radiofrequency ablation, or a surgical method termed the maze procedure), commonly known as a rhythm control strategy, are preferable in terms of long-term outcomes to simply "accepting" the presence of AF and managing the ventricular rate pharmacologically (commonly

known as a rate control strategy). Because the latter strategy is now common, an increasing number of patients with chronic AF will be referred to rehabilitation programs.

The following are medications used to control the ventricular rate in AF:

- Digoxin
- Beta-blockers (e.g., propranolol, sotalol, metoprolol, atenolol)
- Calcium channel blockers (e.g., diltiazem, verapamil)

Other agents used to convert AF to sinus rhythm, or maintain sinus rhythm once cardioversion is successful, include the following:

- Amiodarone
- Propaferone
- Dofetilide
- Disopyramide
- Procainamide

Also of note, digoxin may help to control the ventricular response during exercise, as digoxin can cause diffuse effects on the ST-segment response and "false positive" electrocardiogram (ECG) changes. Other AV nodal suppressants, including calcium channel blockers and beta-blockers, can mask ischemic changes, and beta-blockers are likely to reduce exercise capacity.

In terms of stroke prevention, several major trials have demonstrated that antithrombotic therapy in clients with AF reduces the risk of stroke. Treatment with warfarin has consistently demonstrated a reduction in stroke risk, on the order of 64% to 84%. This risk reduction is independent of the duration of AF. Aspirin has also been demonstrated to be effective in reducing stroke risk, but clinical trials have shown that aspirin is less effective than warfarin. Lastly, successful anticoagulation therapy is dependent upon regular (e.g., at least monthly) measurements of the international normalized ratio (INR), with careful adjustment to maintain a level between 2.0 and 3.0.

RECOMMENDATIONS FOR EXERCISE TESTING

Maximal exercise testing can be safely performed to objectively characterize the functional capabilities of individuals with AF (see table 9.1). Exercise testing is also helpful in determining the effectiveness of rate control therapy. The reduction in exercise capacity associated with AF is a direct function of the underlying heart disease. Because underlying heart disease is common, moderately incremented protocols such as the Naughton or ramp are recommended.

Contraindications to exercise testing related to comorbidities and other underlying conditions, such as stability of chronic heart failure, valvular disease, or complex ventricular arrhythmias, should take precedence over AF itself. In the absence of other clinical indications for stopping, clients with AF may be safely taken to fatigue or shortness of breath endpoints. The fact that many clients with AF are taking digoxin, beta-blockers, or other antiarrhythmic agents, along with the fact that left bundle branch block and left ventricular hypertrophy are common in AF, complicates the interpretation of ST-segment changes on the exercise ECG. Age-predicted maximal heart rate targets are particularly useless in AF because of the rapid and highly variable ventricular response. Because of the irregular ventricular response, it has been demonstrated that heart rate is most accurately measured using calipers over at least a 6 s rhythm strip during exercise.

Several medications and precautions should be considered during exercise testing:

- Digoxin, digitalis: May control ventricular response; diffuse ST effects.
- Calcium channel blockers: May mask ischemia and decrease exercise heart rate (HR) response (e.g., verapamil).
- Diltiazem, verapamil: Help control ventricular response; may improve exercise capacity.
- Beta-blockers: Help control ventricular response; may reduce exercise capacity. Decrease submaximal and maximal HR and blood pressure (BP) response; sometimes exercise capacity, especially with nonselective medications.
- Age-predicted maximal HR targets are not valid.
- Irregular ventricular response may make BP determination less precise or more difficult.

TABLE 9.1

Atrial Fibrillation: Exercise Testing

Methods	Measures	Endpoints*	Comments
Aerobic			
Cycle (ramp protocol 10-15W/min; staged protocol 20-30 W/min stage)	▪ 12-lead ECG, HR	▪ Serious dysrhythmias ▪ >2 mm ST-segment depression or elevation ▪ Ischemic threshold	
Treadmill (individualized ramp protocol, 8 to 12 min target)		▪ T-wave inversion with significant ST change	
Moderately incremented protocol <1 MET/2-3 min (e.g., Naughton, Balke)	▪ BP, rate–pressure product ▪ RPE (6-20) ▪ Angina scale ▪ Gas analysis ($\dot{V}O_{2peak}$) ▪ Radionuclide testing	▪ SBP >250 mmHg or DBP >115 mmHg ▪ +3 or greater on +1 to +4 angina scale	Better estimate of exercise capacity
Endurance			
6 min walk	Distance walked	Rest stops allowed; note stops in record	
Flexibility			
Goniometry	Angle of flexion/ extension		If lowered ROM

*Measurements of particular significance; do not always indicate test termination.

RECOMMENDATIONS FOR EXERCISE PROGRAMMING

As the population ages, the number of individuals with AF referred for exercise rehabilitation will increase. There are two major factors to consider in exercise programming for clients with AF:

- Concomitant or underlying heart disease
- Inherent unreliability of the pulse rate for prescribing exercise intensity

Because AF is frequently accompanied by ischemic heart disease, chronic heart failure, or valvular heart disease, exercise programming considerations for these conditions should take precedence over AF. In addition, some clients with AF referred to a rehabilitation program will have experienced a stroke, in which case the goals of the rehabilitation program change accordingly (see chapter 38). Regardless of the concomitant disease, all individuals with AF will require frequent monitoring of the INR. Because of the chronically irregular ventricular rate, exercise intensity should be prescribed based on work rate and perceived exertion levels. Frequency, duration, intensity, and progression of exercise are similar to those for clients in normal sinus rhythm referred to a rehabilitation program.

AF can be intermittent (e.g., the client may be in AF one day and in normal sinus rhythm the next);

this will influence not only the client's HR response to exercise but also exercise tolerance and level of fatigue. The rhythm should therefore be determined on a daily basis. When the individual is in AF, a longer sampling of the pulse is often needed to reliably determine HR. Furthermore, AF has varied effects; some patients will experience fatigue while others will not. Finally, many clients will be elderly, and comorbid conditions such as osteoporosis, coronary disease, diabetes, and obesity must be considered in development of the exercise program. Available data, while limited, have demonstrated that individuals with AF can achieve significant functional gains from exercise rehabilitation (see table 9.2).

Several medications and precautions should be considered during exercise programming:

- See the appendix for a list of medications that may influence cardiovascular response to exercise training.
- Longer sampling of pulse may be needed for reliable HR.
- AF has varied effects; some patients will experience fatigue, while others will not.
- Ascertain rhythm on a daily basis.
- AF is frequently intermittent.
- Many clients will be elderly; consider comorbid conditions such as osteoporosis, coronary artery disease, and hypertension.

TABLE 9.2

Atrial Fibrillation: Exercise Programming

Modes	Goals	Intensity/Frequency/Duration	Time to goal
Aerobic ■ Large muscle activities ■ Arm/leg ergometry	■ Increase $\dot{V}O_{2peak}$ ■ Increase ADLs	■ RPE 11-16/20 ■ 50-80% $\dot{V}O_{2peak}$ or HR reserve ■ 3-7 days/week ■ 30-45 min/session	3 months
Resistance Weight machines	Increase strength	■ High reps, low resistance (12-15 reps) ■ 2-3 nonconsecutive days/week	2-3 months
Flexibility Upper and lower body ROM activities	■ Increase flexibility ■ Reduce risk of injury	3-5 days/week	2-4 months

CASE STUDY

Atrial Fibrillation

A 68-year-old male had a five-year history of intermittent AF before it became chronic. After several failed attempts at electrical cardioversion, a decision was made to accept the fact that he had AF and to control the rate pharmacologically and to anticoagulate. He had no history of other cardiovascular disorders but had been taking medication for hypertension for approximately 20 years. He had a 20 pack a year history of smoking, but had stopped smoking approximately 25 years before. He reported an inability to perform daily physical activities at the level he had been able to previously.

S: "I'd like to be able to get through each day without feeling so fatigued."

O: Vitals

Height: 5 ft 9 in. (1.75 m)
Weight: 171.3 lb (77.8 kg)
BMI: 25.3 kg/m^2
HR: 88 contractions/min, irregular
BP: 136/90 mmHg, irregular
Middle-aged male in no distress
Cardiovascular: Irregular rhythm; no rubs, gallops, or murmurs
Medications: Warfarin, Sotalol
INR: 2.12
ECG: Atrial fibrillation with a ventricular response of 88 contractions/min, but otherwise normal; cardiac exam unremarkable

Echocardiogram: Mildly enlarged left and right atria, normal left ventricle, normal wall thicknesses, and normal ejection fraction (55%); aortic and mitral valves show mild thickening; mild mitral and tricuspid regurgitation; findings are similar to an echocardiogram performed one year earlier.

Graded exercise test (Naughton protocol)

Peak exercise: 5.5 METs (70.5% of predicted)
Peak RPE: 18/20
Termination from leg fatigue
Chronotropic response to exercise: Normal
Peak HR: 166 contractions/min
Peak BP: 178/94 mmHg
No significant ST changes during exercise or recovery
No report of chest discomfort

A: 1. Chronic AF
    2. Low exercise tolerance for age
    3. No evidence of significant underlying heart disease

P: 1. Improve resting and exercise ventricular rate pharmacologically.
    2. Begin cardiac rehabilitation program.

Exercise Program Goals

1. Improve cardiovascular endurance
2. Monitor ventricular response to exercise
3. Monitor pressor response to exercise
4. Refer to cardiologist for changes in goals 2 and 3

Mode	Frequency	Duration	Intensity	Progression
Aerobic	3 days/week	20 min/session	THR (50-75% $\dot{V}O_{2peak}$) RPE 11-16/20	Gradually increase to 40 min at 60-80% THR after 4 weeks.
Resistance (all major muscle groups)	3 days/week	1 set of 10-12 reps	50-70% of 1RM	Increase to 2 sets of 10-12 reps after 8 weeks.
Flexibility (all major muscle groups)	3 days/week	20 s/stretch	Maintain stretch below discomfort point	Discomfort point should occur at higher ROM.
Warm-up and cool-down	Before and after each session	10-15 min	RPE <10/20	Maintain.

Evidence-Based Guidelines

Fuster V, Ryden LE, Cannon DS, et al. ACC/AHA/ESC guidelines for the management of patients with atrial fibrillation: A report of the ACC/AHA Task Force on Practice Guidelines and the European Society of Cardiology Committee for Practice Guidelines developed in collaboration with the European Heart Rhythm Association and the Heart Rhythm Society. Circulation. 2006;114:e257-e354.

Management of newly detected atrial fibrillation: A clinical practice guideline from the American Academy of Family Physicians and the American College of Physicians. Ann Intern Med. 2003;139:1009-1017.

Suggested Web Sites

American College of Cardiology. www.acc.org

American Heart Association. www.americanheart.org

10

Pacemakers and Implantable Cardioverter Defibrillators

Scott O. Roberts, PhD, FACSM ▪ Michael West, MD

OVERVIEW OF THE PATHOPHYSIOLOGY

A variety of factors contribute to optimal cardiac functioning, including atrioventricular synchronization and the responsiveness of heart rate (HR) and contractility to neurohormonal control. Any loss of the normal sequence of atrial and ventricular filling and contraction can result in deterioration of hemodynamics and significant symptoms at rest and during exercise. Pacing techniques help improve symptoms, enhance exercise performance, and improve quality of life and are considered largely based on the presence or absence of symptoms attributable to bradycardia. Individuals who cannot increase their HR in response to increased metabolic demand usually have sinus node dysfunction and may require cardiac pacing. Individuals with a history of life-threatening ventricular arrhythmias are sometimes candidates for an implantable cardioverter defibrillator (ICD) or a combined pacemaker and ICD device.

Pacing Terminology

- Chronotropic incompetence: The inability to increase HR during exercise. Chronotropic incompetence is confirmed by a peak exercise HR <85% of age-predicted maximum or failure to reach at least 80% of HR reserve during any stage of an exercise test.

- Symptomatic bradycardia: A pathologic condition caused by a slow HR (often <50 contractions per minute), resulting in symptoms that can include light-headedness, fatigue or weakness, complete or near loss of consciousness (syncope), shortness of breath, and a weak pulse.

- Rate-adaptive pacemakers: Pacemakers equipped with sensors that regulate the pacemaker's rate according to increases in demand (i.e., exercise). These units utilize various types of sensors, including those that respond to physiological, mechanical, or electrical signals.

- Pacemaker syndrome: A constellation of symptoms, including lethargy, fatigue, light-headedness, hypotension, shortness of breath, syncope, neck pulsations, and impaired exercise capacity, that occur in the setting of a pacemaker and from the loss of physiologic timing of atrial and ventricular contractions.

- ICD: A small battery-powered electrical impulse generator implanted in patients who are at risk of sudden cardiac death due to sustained ventricular tachycardia or fibrillation.

■ Tiered therapy: ICDs that utilize antitachycardia pacing, shock therapies, and bradycardia safety pacing in a step-wise approach to the treatment of life-threatening ventricular arrhythmias.

■ Sudden cardiac death syndrome: A life-threatening cardiac emergency, usually caused by ventricular tachycardia (VT), ventricular fibrillation (VF), severe bradycardia or asystole, that requires the immediate use of an automatic external defibrillator (AED) or an ICD to restore normal rhythm.

Pacemakers

The use of a permanent cardiac pacemaker increases survival, decreases symptoms, and improves quality of life in those receiving the pacemaker. The following are some commonly accepted indications for pacemaker implantation:

■ Sick sinus syndrome with symptomatic bradycardia

■ Acquired atrioventricular (AV) block

■ Persistent advanced AV block after myocardial infarction

Other less common indications for use of a pacemaker include the following:

■ Neurally mediated syncope

■ Carotid sinus hypersensitivity

■ AV block intentionally created by ablative procedures

A typical pacemaker system consists of two basic components, a pulse generator and either one or two pacing wires. The pacing wires are insulated and are implanted transvenously into the right atrium, right ventricle, or both. The leads are connected to the pulse generator, which is typically implanted subcutaneously just below the clavicle. The two main functions of the leads are sensing and pacing. Sensing involves receiving electrical signals (i.e., P-waves and R-waves) from the heart. In the absence of such sensed signals, the pacemaker generator will fire, causing the atria or ventricles to contract. Optimally, the pacing system utilizes an atrial and ventricular lead to maintain AV synchrony, which facilitates cardiac output at rest and during exercise.

Pacemakers are categorized by a standardized code. The first letter represents the chamber paced; the second is the chamber sensed; and the third denotes the response to a sensed event. The fourth position is utilized to indicate that the pacemaker has rate-response capabilities. For example, VVIR is the abbreviation used when the ventricle (V) is the chamber being paced and sensed. When the pacemaker senses a normal ventricular contraction, the pacemaker is inhibited (I). The R indicates that the pulse generator is rate responsive during exercise.

Another common pacemaker system is dual chamber paced, dual chamber sensed, dual chamber inhibited response (DDDR), which paces and senses both the atrium and ventricle; the response is to either "trigger" or inhibit a pacing stimulus depending on the presence or absence of atrial or ventricular rhythm (or both) above the programmed rate cutoff. The DDDR pacemaker is widely regarded as the optimal pacing mode in individuals who have normal sinoatrial (SA) node function because it provides AV synchrony and utilizes the client's own sinus rhythm as the sensor-driven HR.

Implantable Cardioverter Defibrillators

ICDs are utilized to electrically terminate life-threatening ventricular tachyarrhythmias. They consist of two basic parts: the lead system and the cardioverter defibrillator. ICDs have lead systems that are placed transvenously, typically by way of the subclavian vein. The ICD leads track the cardiac rhythm and transmit the information to the pulse generator, which is usually implanted subcutaneously in the pectoral region. When a tachyarrhythmia is detected, preprogrammed therapies are sent back to terminate the arrhythmia. The units can pace-terminate an arrhythmia or deliver electric cardioversion or defibrillation shocks, or both. In order to terminate an arrhythmia, the pulse generator is programmed to recognize specific HRs. Ventricular tachycardia and fibrillation are typically recognized by their rapid rates; and if either is sensed, the pulse generator will deliver the appropriate preprogrammed therapy to the heart through the lead system. The modern generation of ICDs can detect both atrial and ventricular arrhythmias, deliver antitachycardia pacing and shocks, are multiprogrammable, have intracardiac electrocardiogram storage, and provide all functions of antibradycardia dual-chamber pacing including rate responsiveness and mode switching.

EFFECTS ON THE EXERCISE RESPONSE

In the absence of normal sinus node function, cardiac conduction, or neurohormonal regulation, rate-adaptive pacemakers generally improve exercise tolerance. Rate-adaptive pacemakers utilize a variety of physiological sensors to initiate to the pacing rate during periods of increased metabolic activity. Following exercise or other physically demanding activity, the pacing rate returns to the previously programmed setting. Individuals with ICDs are at risk of receiving an inappropriate shock during exercise if training HR exceeds the ICD's programmed threshold rate for therapy or if they develop an exercise-induced supraventricular tachycardia. For this reason, individuals with ICDs should be closely monitored during exercise to ensure that their HR does not approach the activation rate for the device.

EFFECTS OF EXERCISE TRAINING

Recipients of new pacemakers or ICDs should be encouraged to resume normal activities of daily living, including daily physical activity, as soon as they receive clearance from their cardiologist. Research has confirmed that exercise is safe and effective and that underlying heart or other medical or health condition has more influence on the ability to exercise than the presence of a pacemaker or ICD. Recent technologic advances have dramatically furthered pacemaker function to the point where pacemakers can nearly mimic normal cardiac function, both at rest and during exercise. It is important that the exercise training upper HR limit in DDDR and VVIR pacemakers be set below the person's ischemic threshold. At least a 10% safety margin between exercise HR and rate cutoff for the device is advised. An inappropriately delivered shock can be proarrhythmic and itself induce a life-threatening ventricular dysrhythmia. Despite a high level of caution, however, inappropriate shocks are common and have many causes. Therefore, full knowledge of individuals' ICD programming is essential before exercise, and close consultation with the client's electrophysiologist is advised.

MANAGEMENT AND MEDICATIONS

Commonly prescribed medications for individuals with pacemakers and ICD patients include angiotensin-converting enzyme (ACE) inhibitors, beta-blockers and channel blockers to control abnormal heart rhythms, and vasodilators in the presence of left ventricular dysfunction. In addition to the precautions associated with a pacemaker or ICD, possible side effects during exercise or exercise

training should be followed on the basis of the type of medications currently being taken.

RECOMMENDATIONS FOR EXERCISE TESTING

Exercise testing can be useful as a diagnostic tool as well as a therapeutic tool in the adjustment of rate-responsive pacemakers (see table 10.1). Once a permanent pacemaker with rate-responsive pacing capabilities has been implanted, exercise testing is useful in the evaluation of pacemaker behavior as well as for optimization of the pacemaker activity response. The exercise protocol selected should be suited to an individual's age, health and medical status, and present functional capacity. Low-level treadmill protocols such the modified Bruce or Naughton or bike ergometer protocols that utilize small watt increases per stage are very useful with this population. Because exercise-induced ST-segment changes may not reflect ischemic changes in individuals with pacemakers, other diagnostic tests such as stress imaging with echocardiography or thallium may produce higher test sensitivity and specificity results. Medications and special considerations for exercise testing and training include the following:

- A risk of receiving inappropriate shocks exists.
- One should ensure that the exercise HR stays below the activation rate of the ICD.
- Radionuclide testing or stress echocardiography may result in greater test sensitivity.
- Peak systolic blood pressure may be blunted, or may decrease or not increase, with left ventricular dysfunction.

RECOMMENDATIONS FOR EXERCISE PROGRAMMING

Once an upper training HR is established and documented, low- to moderate-intensity training can be initiated (see table 10.2). In addition to improving functional capacity, exercise training can help to reduce cardiac risk factors (e.g., through cholesterol modification, hypertension reduction) and improve psychosocial outcomes. Activities should be selected so that the intensity can be carefully regulated during exercise. Because some upper body movement may dislodge implanted leads, upper body exercises are not advised initially for individuals with pacemakers. Current guidelines

TABLE 10.1

Pacemakers and ICDs: Exercise Testing

Methods	Measures	Endpoints	Comments
Aerobic Cycle (ramp protocol 17 W/min; staged protocol 10-25 W/3 min stage) Treadmill (1-2 METs/3 min stage)	■ 12-lead ECG, HR	■ Peak HR must be below activation rate for ICD ■ Serious arrythmias ■ >2 mm ST-segment depression or elevation ■ Ischemic threshold ■ T-wave inversion with significant ST change	■ Peak HR may be blunted. ■ ECG sensitivity is low for detecting ischemia. ■ Know HR activation rate for ICD before testing.
	■ BP, rate–pressure product ■ RPE (6-20) ■ Radionuclide testing or stress echocardiogram	■ SBP >250 mmHg or DBP >115 mmHg ■ Watch for drop or no increase in SBP with increased work rate	■ Peak SBP may be blunted. SBP may decrease or not increase with left ventricular dysfunction. ■ Better guide of intensity because of possible HR inability to increase with exercise. ■ May be more useful in assessing ischemic heart disease.

TABLE 10.2

Pacemakers and ICDs: Exercise Programming

Modes	Goals	Intensity/Frequency/Duration	Time to goal
Aerobic Large muscle activities	■ Increase functional capacity and ability to perform ADLs ■ Circuit training ■ Increase self-efficacy	■ 40-80% $\dot{V}O_{2peak}$ ■ Target HR should be kept below ischemic threshold and ICD activation threshold ■ 4-7 days/week ■ 20-60 min/session	4-6 months
Strength Circuit training	Increase ability to perform leisure and occupational activities and ADLs	■ Low to moderate intensity ■ 2 days/week ■ 15-20 min/session ■ Should be avoided initially after implantation	
Flexibility Upper and lower body ROM activities	Maintain ROM	2-3 days/week	

suggest that traditional resistance training (i.e., 50% of 1-repetition maximum) should not be initiated until four to six weeks postimplantation. Before exercise training, full knowledge of the individual's ICD programming is essential, and close consultation with the client's electrophysiologist is advised. Specific ICD information, including the following, should be well documented and communicated among all personnel:

- The ICD detection threshold setting in beats per minute
- Whether the device is set for VT or VF
- How quickly the HR is allowed to increase before therapy is delivered
- What the sustained VT setting is (how long each episode should last before therapy is delivered)
- What the ICD mode of therapy is (e.g., antitachycardia pacing [ATP] or shocks)

The upper exercise training intensity must be set below the person's ischemic threshold and must not approach a HR causing activation of the ICD. The following are special considerations for exercise testing and training:

- A risk of receiving inappropriate shocks exists in individuals with ICDs.
- One should ensure that the training HR does not approach the activation rate of the ICD (a safe margin is the ICD detection rate minus 20 contractions per minute).
- Upper extremity range of motion may be restricted due to pacemaker and ICD incision.
- Rating of perceived exertion should be used in conjunction with HR to monitor intensity.

Some individuals with pacemakers and ICDs have moderate to severe left ventricular dysfunction, and appropriate precautions for this population should be followed.

Evidence-Based Guidelines

Platonov MA, Gillis AM, Kavanagh KM. Pacemakers, implantable cardioverter/defibrillators, and extracorporeal shockwave lithotripsy: Evidence-based guidelines for the modern era. J Endourol. 2008;22(2):243-247.

Suggested Web Sites

American College of Cardiology. www.acc.org

American Heart Association. www.americanheart.org

CASE STUDY

Pacemaker

A 63-year-old female rancher was referred for a two- to three-week history of palpitations, which she described as forceful, "squishy" heartbeats. An electrocardiogram revealed 2:1 AV block with a right bundle branch block. Carotid sinus massage improved conduction to 1:1, proving that the 2:1 block was distal and likely in need of permanent pacing. The client denied the typical symptoms of "symptomatic bradycardia," such as activity intolerance, dyspnea, light-headedness, or syncope. To better assess for limited aerobic capacity, she was given a regular treadmill test. Her maximal HR was 82 contractions per minute with persistent 2:1 block throughout the exercise period. Remarkably, she completed more than 8 min of a Bruce protocol. After a dual-chamber pacemaker was implanted, she had a follow-up exercise test in which she exercised for over 14 min. The "squishy" heartbeats resolved with pacing.

S: "My heart's been fluttering."

O: Vitals

Height: 5 ft 6 in. (1.7 m)
Weight: 140 lb (63.5 kg)

BMI: 21.97 kg/m^2
RHR: 50 contractions/min
BP: 116/70 mmHg
Medications: Estrogen replacement

Graded Exercise Test (Treadmill, Bruce Protocol)

Duration: 8 min 30 s (3.4 mph at 14% grade)
Max HR: 82 contractions/min with persistent 2:1 block throughout exercise

A: 1. 2:1 AV block
   2. Very active rancher, tolerating AV block well

P: 1. Undergo dual-chamber permanent pacemaker implantation.
   2. Refer to cardiac rehabilitation.

Exercise Program Goals

1. Improve functional capacity
2. Educate about managing angina symptoms
3. Reinforce lifestyle changes/medical management

(continued)

Mode	Frequency	Duration	Intensity	Progression
Aerobic	3 days/week	20 min/session	THR (55-70% $\dot{V}O_{2max}$) RPE 11-14/20	Increase to 40 min at 60-70% THR after 12 weeks.
Strength (all major muscle groups)	3 days/week	1 set of ≤10 reps	50-70% of 1RM	Increase to 2 sets of 10-12 reps after 12 weeks.
Flexibility	3 days/week	30-60 s/stretch	Below discomfort point	
Warm-up and cool-down	Before and after each session	10-15 min	RPE <10/20	

Valvular Heart Disease

Daniel Friedman, MD, FACSM ▪ Scott O. Roberts, PhD, FACSM

OVERVIEW OF THE PATHOPHYSIOLOGY

The human heart is nearly flawless and efficient at forcefully pumping blood forward throughout a closed network of blood vessels. The direction and quantity of blood flow through the heart and between the systemic and pulmonary circuits are regulated by one-way heart valves positioned at the exit of each chamber. Heart valves, which are named after their shape and structure, consist of fibrous flaps called leaflets or cusps that open passively during systole and snap close during diastole when ventricular pressure drops and blood begins to flow backward across them. When heart valves become damaged or diseased, blood flow through the heart can become obstructed or reduced, eventually causing mild to severe symptoms of valvular heart disease (VHD).

Rheumatic fever (RF) is an inflammatory condition resulting from infection associated with strep throat. RF was the leading cause of VHD and death among children in the United States through the mid-20th century. Although rare today due to the introduction of widespread use of antibiotics in the late 1940s, it continues to be a major public health problem among developing countries worldwide. Rheumatic fever can affect any tissue in the body, but its greatest threat is to heart muscle, especially heart valves. Damage to heart valves resulting from RF is caused by an autoimmune response that destroys heart tissue along with the bacteria themselves. Valvular heart disease caused by RF is referred to as rheumatic heart disease (RHD).

The two primary causes of all heart disease are congenital heart defects (present at birth) and acquired disorders (lifestyle, infection, aging, etc.). The leading causes of VHD include RF, congenital defects, infection, and aging. An estimated 5 million U.S. adults have moderate to severe VHD as a result of aging alone, and this number is expected to double as a result of the dramatic changes in aging occurring in the U.S. adult population. Valvular heart disease (RHD and congenital defects) accounts for less than 1% of all cardiovascular disease mortality.

The symptoms and limitations of VHD depend on the following:

- Heart valve(s) involved (i.e., mitral, aortic, tricuspid, pulmonary, or some combination of these)
- Condition of the valve (e.g., narrowing, or stenosis; or failure to close properly, regurgitation or insufficient)
- Severity of the valve lesions
- Presence of coronary artery disease, myocardial dysfunction (congestive heart failure), or other organ system disease

In the early stages of VHD, few if any symptoms may be present, or symptoms may be mistaken for other conditions. Mild symptoms of VHD include fatigue, heart palpitations, chest pain (angina pectoris), and changes in blood pressure. With time, especially with poorly diagnosed and treated VHD or with more serious forms of VHD (aortic stenosis), more serious symptoms, including heart failure, can develop. These include excessive, extreme fatigue;

unexplained coughing; shortness of breath; and swollen legs or feet.

Mitral Valve Prolapse

Mitral valve prolapse (MVP) is the most prevalent form of VHD, affecting an estimated 5% to 10% of the U.S. population. MVP is characterized by bowing of the mitral valve leaflets into the left atrium during systole. Because symptoms are usually nonspecific or absent altogether, the diagnosis of MVP is usually made on physical examination and confirmed by echocardiography. Some individuals, however, may present with chest pain or palpitation-associated arrhythmias, most of which are benign. Auscultation can identify MVP by the presence of a midsystolic "click" or murmur (or both). The click represents the sudden tensing of the involved mitral leaflet or chordae tendineae as the leaflet is forced back toward the left atrium, whereas the murmur represents the regurgitant flow through the incompetent valve. M-mode echocardiography defines MVP as 2 mm or more of posterior displacement of one or both leaflets.

Mitral Stenosis

Mitral stenosis (MS) is a form of VHD characterized by the narrowing of the orifice of the mitral valve, which increases the resistance across the mitral valve and impedes ventricular filling and left ventricular stroke volume and cardiac output (CO). As the pressure gradient across the valve steadily increases, the left atrial pressure is elevated, increasing the risk of pulmonary hypertension. As the condition worsens, the chronic overload to the left atrium stretches the atrial conduction fibers, leading to atrial fibrillation and increased risk of atrial thrombus formation. The causes of MS include RF (60% of cases), a congenital etiology, lupus, carcinoid and amyloid disease. Pathologic features of rheumatic MS include thickening and shortening of the chordae tendineae, calcification of the valve leaflets, and fusion of the commissures (the borders where the leaflets meet).

Dyspnea is usually the presenting symptom, in addition to hemoptysis, chest pain, thromboembolism, infective endocarditis, and hoarseness. Symptoms increase with heart rate, which may limit exercise capacity. On auscultation, a loud S1, an opening snap, and a low-pitched diastolic murmur are present. Echocardiography is helpful in evaluating the left atrial size to assess the presence and severity of MS, degree of mitral regurgitation, and presence of pulmonary hypertension. A reduction of the valve orifice to 2 to 2.5 cm^2 or less (normal is 4 to 6 cm^2) confirms MS, and 1.0 cm^2 as severe MS. Transesophageal echocardiography (TEE) is often used to assess MS when balloon valvuloplasty is feasible.

Mitral Regurgitation

Mitral regurgitation (MR) occurs when the leaflets of the mitral valve do not close properly. Annular dilation is the major cause of MR, most often in the setting of congestive heart failure (CHF). Other factors involved include congenital abnormalities, myxomatous degeneration, MVP, chordae tendineae rupture, bacterial destruction (endocarditis), and annular disease. Symptoms of MR depend on the severity and the rate of development of the MR. Mild MR produces no symptoms. Moderately severe MR can lead to increased left atrial and left ventricular volumes, which can lead in turn to pulmonary venous congestion, elevation of pulmonary artery pressures, and dyspnea. A holosystolic murmur is the most prominent feature during the physical exam. Echocardiography can confirm the etiology and severity of MR as well as help establish long-term therapy. TEE and angiography can also be useful in determining the severity of MR. Patients with significant regurgitation need to be closely monitored for symptoms of ventricular dysfunction, dilation, or pulmonary hypertension.

Aortic Stenosis

Aortic stenosis (AS) is a narrowing of the aortic valve leaflets. A common cause of AS is gradual fibrosis and calcification of the aortic valve, which results in failure of the valve to either open or close normally. Other causes include congenital AS, a bicuspid valve, and RHD. Symptoms of AS include dyspnea (congestive heart failure), angina, syncope, or a combination of these symptoms. Mild degrees of AS are usually well tolerated, but as the stenosis progresses, compensatory ventricular hypertrophy proportional to the degree of obstruction leads to left ventricular (LV) dysfunction, myocardial ischemia, reduced CO and coronary perfusion, and increased myocardial oxygen consumption (MV̇O$_2$). On physical examination, carotid upstrokes are diminished; the second heart sound is single and may be soft; and a harsh systolic murmur at the upper left sternal border (often radiating to the neck) is present. Echocardiography is recommended to diagnose and determine the severity of AS. Except with asymptomatic mild AS, physical activity is generally not recommended until exertional hemodynamics and clinical status are assessed, preferably with exercise testing.

Aortic Regurgitation

Aortic regurgitation (AR) is the result of widening of the aortic root or valve leaflets. AR can develop in the setting of rheumatic disease, infective endocarditis, trauma, congenital lesions, or connective tissue–related diseases; the latter would include Marfan's and Ehlers-Danlos syndrome and other rheumatic conditions. Mild to moderate AR can be tolerated for years, with the only common symptom being exertional dyspnea. As AR worsens, more noticeable symptoms will begin to appear, including fatigue (especially during times of increased activity), shortness of breath, edema, arrhythmias, and angina. Exaggerated arterial pulses, a systolic ejection murmur, and an early diastolic murmur are also often noted. Echocardiography can both diagnose AR and help in determining the appropriate treatment. When the heart begins to dilate or lose contractile strength, surgery is generally considered.

Tricuspid Stenosis

Tricuspid stenosis (TS) is a rare condition resulting from narrowing of the tricuspid valve. It is almost always secondary to RHD and mitral valve disease. Other causes include infection, dilated right ventricle, pulmonary hypertension, tumors, and trauma. A universal symptom of TS is fatigue and swelling in the lower extremity and abdominal regions. Physical examination reveals distended neck veins, significant edema, and normal breath sounds, with the murmur being difficult to auscultate. Echocardiography is the preferred method to determine the presence, cause, and severity of TS.

Tricuspid Regurgitation

Tricuspid regurgitation (TR) is often caused by dilation of the right ventricle and tricuspid annulus, resulting in mild regurgitation. Other causes include Ebstein's anomaly, carcinoid syndrome, RHD, and infections. In the absence of pulmonary hypertension (PPH), TR may not produce any symptoms. The following symptoms are common in the presence of PPH: distended neck veins, generalized swelling, fatigue, and weakness. A holosystolic murmur, increasing with inspiration, is heard at the lower left sternal border. Doppler echocardiography can determine the presence and severity of the lesion as well as estimate right ventricular function (including right ventricular pressure).

Pulmonic Stenosis

Pulmonic stenosis (PS) is a narrowing or tightening of the pulmonary valve resulting in reduced blood flow to the lungs. The causes of PS are congenital heart disease, RHD, and malignant carcinoid tumors. Mild PS generally produces few if any symptoms. Significant PS, however, can produce symptoms of heart failure, exertional dyspnea, syncope, or chest pain and reduced PaO_2. Diagnosis and treatment options are guided by echocardiography.

Pulmonic Regurgitation

Pulmonic regurgitation (PR) is rare and almost always caused by PPH. The major symptoms of PR usually relate to the underlying cause. PR causes a harsh, rapidly louder, then softer, systolic murmur at the upper left sternal border. In significant PR, an early diastolic murmur in the same region can be heard. Echocardiography is used to determine the presence and possible cause of PR. PR itself does not usually cause symptoms, but PPH does; these can include fatigue, dizziness, dyspnea, and signs of poor perfusion. Rarely does this lesion require any intervention.

EFFECTS ON THE EXERCISE RESPONSE

The extent to which VHD affects the exercise response depends in part on the type and severity of lesion and valve involved. With asymptomatic milder forms of VHD there are usually few if any restrictions to physical activity or exercise. As the disease progresses or in the case of severe acute forms of VHD, exercise is contraindicated and physical activity restricted due to the increased risk of abnormal hemodynamics during exercise.

- Mitral stenosis: In severe cases, tachycardia and atrial fibrillation are common. Cardiac output can be blunted during exercise, leading to exercise-induced hypotension. Abnormal exertional hemodynamics, especially in the presence of PPH, cause increased $M\dot{V}O_2$ demand, chest pain, and ST-segment depression.

- Mitral regurgitation: Expect normal hemodynamic responses to exercise with mild to moderate MR. With severe MR, exercise capacity is limited as a result of reduced CO and hypotension.

- Aortic stenosis: With mild asymptomatic AS, the exercise response may be quite normal. Exercise is generally contraindicated in severe, symptomatic

AS because of the following factors: compensatory concentric left ventricular hypertrophy (LVH); diastolic dysfunction; CHF; inadequate $M\dot{V}O_2$ supply; and exertional syncope, dyspnea, and angina.

- Aortic regurgitation: Asymptomatic patients with low to mild AR and good LV function should have normal responses to exercise. As the disease progresses, systolic dysfunction may severely limit exercise tolerance.

EFFECTS OF EXERCISE TRAINING

Despite the fact that the mechanical function of a valve does not improve with exercise, physical activity and exercise is widely accepted and recommended for this population. Exercise can help improve overall quality of life and ability to perform activities of daily living, as well as the ability to tolerate specific medical conditions and therapies better. Only when VHD progresses to the point of causing resting or exertional symptoms or compromised hemodynamics is exercise contraindicated or severely restricted. Physical activity and exercise recommendations should always be guided by good clinical examination and judgment.

MANAGEMENT AND MEDICATIONS

Medications used to manage VHD depend on the valve involved and symptoms. In severe VHD, control of the heart failure is often the goal. Common medications used to treat VHD include the following:

- Angiotensin-converting enzyme (ACE) inhibitors: Widen blood vessels, lower blood pressure, and decrease the work rate of the heart (in the case of valvular regurgitation).
- Antiarrhythmics: Maintain a regular heartbeat and slow rapid heart rhythms; improve overall pump function especially in mitral valve disease.
- Antibiotics: Help prevent or treat infection.
- Beta-blockers: Lower heart rate, blood pressure, and myocardial oxygen demand.
- Anticoagulants: Help prevent the formation of blood clots in the setting of atrial fibrillation and MS.

- Diuretics: Lower excess fluid levels in the body.
- Inotropes: Increase the force of the heart's contractions.

SURGICAL CONSIDERATIONS

Although some heart valves can be repaired, most require replacement. Valve replacement surgery is generally necessary with symptomatic AS. Although balloon valvuloplasty can increase the cross-sectional area of the valve opening, it has not been highly effective in treating this condition. Medical management is generally recommended for mild symptomatic AR with minimally increased or normal cardiac size. Surgery is indicated, however, when the heart dilates significantly. Surgery is considered with MS when symptoms cannot be controlled medically, particularly when the mitral valve area is less than 1.0 cm². Surgery is also an option in MR when the heart dilates or weakens or when a person has symptoms despite medical therapy. Surgical repair is generally considered with tricuspid disease and is usually done at the time of mitral valve surgery. Severe pulmonic valve stenosis can usually be repaired with a balloon valvuloplasty or surgery. With isolated TR, there is usually no intervention.

RECOMMENDATIONS FOR EXERCISE TESTING

Exercise testing can be useful as a diagnostic tool in asymptomatic AS adults to qualify and quantify exertional symptoms and for patients with echocardiographic evidence of moderate AS who report atypical symptoms (see table 11.1). However, the decision to perform exercise testing in this population must take into consideration that it has poor overall diagnostic accuracy for the evaluation of concurrent coronary artery disease (CAD). The high prevalence of LVH and exercise-induced ST-segment depression in asymptomatic AS patients limits the prognostic ability of the test. Exercise testing is clearly contraindicated in symptomatic stenotic patients. Under certain circumstances, exercise testing can be performed to assess exercise capacity, HR, and blood pressure (BP) responses and exercise-induced symptoms provided that a clinical examination has been performed first. Exercise

TABLE 11.1

Valvular Heart Disease: Exercise Testing

Methods	Measures	Endpoints*	Comments
Aerobic			
Cycle (ramp protocol 17 W/min; staged protocol 10-25 W/3 min stage)	▪ 12-lead ECG, HR	▪ Serious arrhythmias ▪ >2 mm ST-segment depression or elevation ▪ T-wave inversion with significant ST change ▪ Ischemic threshold	
Treadmill (1-2 METs/3 min stage)	▪ BP, rate–pressure product	▪ Plateau or drop in SBP with increased work rate ▪ SBP >250 mmHg or DBP >115 mmHg	
	▪ Resting stress echocardiogram		▪ Useful in determining degrees of stenosis, regurgitation, LV function. ▪ Helpful in determining timing of surgery. ▪ ST changes may lose specificity with mitral valve and aortic valve prolapse in terms of diagnosis of CAD.
	▪ RPE (6-20)		▪ May be useful for setting exercise prescription.

*Measurements of particular significance; do not always indicate test termination.

testing can be utilized to quantify the extent of hemodynamic impairment (chest pain, dyspnea, arrhythmias, and other symptoms) consequent to VHD. The results can be used for continued follow-up and to determine appropriate time for interventions.

RECOMMENDATIONS FOR EXERCISE PROGRAMMING

Dynamic, low- to moderate-intensity physical activity is recommended in asymptomatic patients with all forms of mild VHD, including AS (see table 11.2).

▪ Mitral stenosis: Physical activity and exercise are recommended in asymptomatic mild MS. The decision to start, modify, or stop exercise should be guided by signs and symptoms of exertional intolerance.

▪ Mitral regurgitation: Asymptomatic patients with MR of any severity who have normal sinus rhythm and LV function and pulmonary artery pressure can exercise without any restrictions.

▪ Aortic stenosis: With mild asymptomatic AS, the exercise response may be quite normal. Exercise is generally contraindicated in severe, symptomatic AS because of the following factors: compensatory concentric LVH; diastolic dysfunction; CHF; inadequate MVO$_2$ supply; and exertional syncope, dyspnea, and angina.

▪ Aortic regurgitation: Asymptomatic patients with low to mild AR and good LV function should have normal responses to exercise. As the disease progresses, systolic dysfunction may severely limit exercise tolerance.

TABLE 11.2

Valvular Heart Disease: Exercise Programming

Modes	Goals	Intensity/Frequency/Duration	Time to goal
Aerobic Large muscle activities	■ Improve functional capacity ■ Improve muscle function ■ Improve ADLs with decreases in symptoms	■ 4-7 days/week ■ 20-60 min/session ■ After surgery: resting HR + 20-30 contractions/min ■ THR: 40-80% $\dot{V}O_{2max}$ ■ RPE: 11-16/20 ■ 10-15 min warm-up and cool-down	4-6 months
Strength Isotonic or isokinetic	■ Improve muscle function ■ Increase strength for vocational and avocational activities	■ 30-50% MVC (avoid Valsalva) ■ 2-3 days/week ■ 4-8 exercises (major groups) ■ 12-15 reps (increasing 5-10 lb) ■ 2-4 sets ■ <1 h	4-6 months
Flexibility Upper and lower body ROM activities	■ Increase ROM ■ Increase functioning for vocational and avocational activities	■ ≥3 days/week, to a position of mild discomfort ■ 10-30 s/stretch ■ Static (slow, controlled)	4-6 months

SPECIAL CONSIDERATIONS

Refer to appropriate sources for the effects of medications used in this population on HR, BP, electrocardiogram, and exercise capacity. Symptomatic AS is an absolute contraindication to exercise testing. Clarify symptoms prior to testing. Be aware of the low prognostic power when assessing VHD and concurrent CAD. Avoid strength training with significant AS and PS. Exercise is contraindicated in symptomatic AS and PS.

Evidence-Based Guidelines

ACC/AHA. 2006 guideline for the management of patients with valvular heart disease. Circulation. 2006;114:e84-e231.

Vahanian A, Baumgartner H, Bax J, et al. Guidelines on the management of valvular heart disease: The Task Force on the Management of Valvular Heart Disease of the European Society of Cardiology. Eur Heart J. 2007;28(2):230-268.

Suggested Web Sites

American College of Cardiology. www.acc.org

American Heart Association. www.americanheart.org

CASE STUDY

Valvular Heart Disease

A 55-year-old Hispanic male had been told years earlier that one of his heart valves was narrowed. His primary care provider saw him and sent him for an echocardiogram. This revealed normal left ventricular function and severe aortic stenosis with a valve area of 0.5 cm². As a result he was evaluated by a cardiologist.

S: He admitted some shortness of breath on exertion, although he did little exercise. He had not had chest pain, syncope, or presyncope. He smoked one pack of cigarettes daily.

O: Vitals

HR: 80 contractions/min
BP: 120/76 mmHg
RR: 14 breaths/min
Weight: 134 lb (61 kg)
Height: 5 ft 3 in. (1.6 m)
Obese male in no distress

Lungs: Clear to A and P
Heart: III/VI systolic murmur along the left sternal border and a loud S4
Extremities: Trace edema; pulses slightly reduced
ECG: Left ventricular hypertrophy

A: Severe aortic stenosis

P: 1. Left heart catheterization: 99% proximal LAD, 50% proximal and 90% mid RCA lesions
   2. Aortic valve replacement and two-vessel coronary artery bypass
   3. Smoking cessation
   4. Modification of other risk factors
      • Lipid lowering
      • Weight loss
   5. Cardiac rehabilitation with exercise training

Mode	Frequency	Duration	Intensity	Progression
Aerobic	3 days/week	20 min Rest for symptoms	THR (<60% $\dot{V}O_{2max}$) RPE <14/20	Very slow, ≤60 min over several months
Strength	Contraindicated			
Flexibility	3 days/week	20-60 s/stretch	Maintain below discomfort point	
Warm-up and cool-down	Before and after each session	10-15 min	RPE<10/20	

12

Chronic Heart Failure

Jonathan N. Myers, PhD, FACSM   ■   Peter H. Brubaker, PhD, FACSM

OVERVIEW OF THE PATHOPHYSIOLOGY

Chronic heart failure (CHF) is characterized by the inability of the heart to adequately deliver oxygen to the metabolizing tissues. The underlying pathophysiology of CHF is defined by systolic dysfunction, diastolic dysfunction, or both. Systolic dysfunction refers to impaired ventricular contraction due to the loss of myocardium secondary to myocardial infarction (MI) or loss of contractility. Diastolic dysfunction is characterized by an increased resistance to the filling of one or both ventricles, elevated diastolic pressure in the ventricles, and reduced ventricular compliance. Diastolic dysfunction is estimated to be the principal etiology in 40% or more of the estimated 500,000 new cases of CHF each year.

Central hemodynamic changes associated with CHF include the following:

- Decreased cardiac output during exercise, or in severe cases at rest
- Elevated left ventricular filling pressures
- Compensatory ventricular volume overload
- Elevated pulmonary and central venous pressures

In addition to central hemodynamic characteristics, CHF is associated with secondary organ changes, including major disturbances in skeletal muscle metabolism, impaired vasodilation, and renal insufficiency leading to sodium and water retention. Collectively, these changes underlie the hallmark signs and symptoms of CHF, namely, fatigue, dyspnea, and reduced exercise tolerance.

CHF is a serious, debilitating, and costly public health problem that affects an estimated 5 million Americans. Despite continued advances in medical therapy, the prognosis for CHF is poor, confirmed by five-year survival rates of 25% for men and 38% for women. The impact of CHF on the U.S. health care system is staggering, from both an economic and a utilization standpoint. CHF is the most common reason for emergency room visits as well as hospitalizations among the elderly. The estimated cost to treat CHF in the United States in 1998 was over $20 billion, making CHF the single most costly form of cardiovascular disease to treat. Poor self-management of the disease may be a significant contributing factor to the poor overall prognosis seen in individuals with CHF. The prognosis for persons with CHF is generally better for those that take their prescribed medications, follow a very-low-sodium diet, and strive to be physically active.

EFFECTS ON THE EXERCISE RESPONSE

The basis for traditionally recommending bed rest over exercise for individuals with CHF has changed dramatically especially within the last decade, in light of the growing body of evidence demonstrating that exercise in combination with mainstay medical therapy improves functional capacity, quality of life, and morbidity and mortality in individuals with CHF. A number of central, peripheral, and ventilatory abnormalities influence exercise responses among persons with CHF:

- Central factors, including systolic function, pulmonary hemodynamics, diastolic dysfunction, and neurohumoral mechanisms
- Peripheral factors, including blood flow abnormalities, vasodilatory capacity, and skeletal muscle biochemistry
- Ventilatory factors, including pulmonary pressure, physiologic dead space, ventilation–perfusion mismatch, respiratory control, and breathing patterns

Irrespective of etiology (systolic vs. diastolic dysfunction), the primary concern regarding exercise for this population is that CHF causes a reduction in cardiac output relative to the demands of work. This resultant compensatory response leads to the "syndrome" of CHF as well as a number of other characteristic responses to exercise. Poor cardiac output underlies a mismatching of ventilation to perfusion in the lung, causing an elevation in physiologic dead space and leading to shortness of breath. Although dyspnea on exertion is a hallmark sign of CHF, the majority of individuals with CHF are limited by leg fatigue during exercise testing versus dyspnea. The hyperventilation response and early onset of fatigue with exercise in individuals with CHF is largely the result of inadequate blood flow to the working skeletal muscles as well as early accumulation of lactate in the blood at relatively low work rates.

Abnormal neurohumoral mechanisms also contribute to reduced cardiac performance during exercise in individuals with CHF. Elevated catecholamine levels and beta-adrenergic receptors that are less sensitive to endogenous and exogenous beta-agonist stimulation, which together alter normal inotropic regulation of the heart, are the likely cause of reduced contractile function during exercise in individuals with CHF. Altered baroreceptor reflexes have also been observed in humans and animals with heart failure and may contribute to diminished chronotropic responses or to reduced systolic pressure during exercise in this population, with the latter contributing to peripheral perfusion abnormalities as well.

Significant peripheral abnormalities also influence the response to exercise in individuals with CHF. These include not only reductions in blood flow but also abnormal redistribution of blood, reduced vasodilatory capacity, endothelial dysfunction, and abnormal skeletal muscle biochemistry. Abnormalities in skeletal muscle metabolism, including reduced mitochondrial enzyme activities and histological changes (reduced type I aerobic fibers and increased type II fibers), reduce exercise tolerance as a result of greater glycolysis, reduced oxidative phosphorylation, and greater metabolic acidosis.

EFFECTS OF EXERCISE TRAINING

Prior to the mid-1980s, individuals with CHF were generally discouraged from participating in formal exercise training due to concerns over safety and questions about whether or not exercise training caused greater harm to an already weakened heart. In the past two decades, however, numerous studies have documented the safety and benefits of endurance exercise training in individuals with heart failure. Studies suggest that improvements in exercise capacity following training result more from peripheral adaptations (e.g., improvements in skeletal muscle metabolism, endothelial function, vasodilatory capacity, and distribution of cardiac output) than from cardiac changes (e.g., central hemodynamics including volumes, ejection fraction, and pulmonary pressures at rest and during exercise). More recent studies have included resistance training, alone or in combination with aerobic exercise, in the exercise program of stable CHF patients, and favorable outcomes have been reported (increased function, increased strength) without any adverse effects.

There has been some controversy regarding the possibility that endurance or resistance exercise training (or both) in individuals with heart failure could lead to abnormal ventricular remodeling and infarct expansion, particularly when exercise is performed early after an MI. This concern arose primarily because a group of individuals who had ventricular asynergy were initially found to have worsening asynergy, myocardial expansion, and decreased ejection fraction after training. More recent reports, however, including studies using high-intensity training and assessment of the myocardium using Doppler 2-D echocardiography and magnetic resonance imaging (MRI), have dispelled these concerns. Some individuals with reduced ventricular function following an MI will continue to deteriorate despite intensive intervention, but studies continue to demonstrate that exercise training does not lead to further myocardial damage. The majority of studies have shown that exercise training neither harms nor results in significant benefit to the heart muscle in individuals with

CHF. Recent exercise training studies in older individuals with isolated diastolic dysfunction have demonstrated improvements in functional capacity, similar to benefits observed in those with systolic dysfunction. The benefits of such training studies appear to be the result of peripheral adaptations, because no changes in left ventricular function or volumes have been observed.

One of the studies examining the effects of endurance exercise training on the substantial morbidity and mortality associated with CHF demonstrated that endurance exercise training for 14 weeks resulted in a 71% decrease in hospitalizations and a 63% reduction in death. A meta-analysis (ExTraMATCH) determined that individuals with CHF caused by systolic dysfunction who participated in an endurance exercise program experienced fewer deaths and hospital admissions over a two-year period than similar patients who did not exercise. More definitive information on the effects of endurance exercise on morbidity and mortality, as well as many other outcomes, in individuals with CHF will likely emerge as the results of the large multicenter HF-ACTION (Heart Failure and A Controlled Trial Investigating Outcomes of Exercise TraiNing) trial involving more than 2000 patients become available.

MANAGEMENT AND MEDICATIONS

Initial management of CHF involves identifying the underlying cause. For example, a stenotic valve may need to be replaced, hypertension or myocardial ischemia controlled, or alcohol use discontinued. In some individuals, these measures alone may restore cardiac function to normal. A major manifestation of CHF in individuals with systolic dysfunction is increased ventricular volume and pressure; therefore, the second goal is to reduce the overload pharmacologically. Therapy generally reduces symptoms; however, a specific period of time of therapy is required before exercise capacity improves. Since excessive salt and water retention is a hallmark of CHF, most individuals will require the use of diuretics to improve symptoms. Afterload reduction through the use of angiotensin-converting enzyme (ACE) inhibition, ACE-II receptor blockers, or other arterial vasodilators tends to reduce left ventricular end-diastolic pressures and improve stroke volume and cardiac output, as well as overall symptoms of CHF. Angiotensin-converting enzyme inhibition may lower mortality, while digoxin or other inotropic agents tend to increase myocardial contractility.

In recent years, beta-blocking agents have gained acceptance as an effective treatment option for clients with CHF, and studies have demonstrated that these agents improve symptoms and reduce mortality as well. Beta-blockers act by inhibiting sympathetic activation, and their beneficial effects are related to the prevention of the deleterious effects of chronically increased adrenergic stimulation on the failing heart. In terms of pharmacologic management, the primary difference between clients with systolic and diastolic dysfunction is that the latter do not require positive inotropes. In addition, the use of calcium channel blockers has been shown to improve ventricular relaxation, increase end-diastolic volume, and increase functional capacity in clients with diastolic dysfunction.

Biventricular pacemakers for cardiac resynchronization therapy (CRT) and implanted cardiodefibrillators (ICDs) are another form of therapy that is becoming more established in the management of heart failure patients. The synchronization of the right and left ventricles appears to improve cardiac output and exercise performance in many CHF patients, particularly those with a widened QRS (>0.12 s) on the electrocardiogram. Implanted ICDs have also been shown to decrease mortality in individuals with CHF.

RECOMMENDATIONS FOR EXERCISE TESTING

Exercise testing can be a valuable tool to objectively characterize the severity of CHF and to evaluate the efficacy of therapeutic interventions. In general, the standard exercise electrocardiogram offers little insight into the nature of symptoms associated with CHF. It is frequently more appropriate to characterize the cardiopulmonary (ventilatory gas exchange) response to exercise, quantify exercise tolerance, and identify the pathophysiological abnormalities responsible for the limitation in exercise capacity. Exercise capacity measured by gas exchange techniques accurately quantifies functional limitations, identifies ventilatory abnormalities, and helps to optimize risk stratification in persons with CHF. The normal central and peripheral responses to the exercise test may not be present in these individuals. For example, relative to what is seen in apparently healthy individuals, cardiac output is reduced, blood is redistributed abnormally, and peripheral vascular resistance is high. Heightened ventilation is a characteristic feature of the exercise response in CHF. Exercise can cause a drop in ejection fraction, stroke volume, or both, as well as exertional hypotension. Although exercise testing in these individuals has the potential for a higher rate of complications, limited data on the safety of exercise testing in CHF suggest that it is similar to that observed among persons with coronary artery disease (see table 12.1).

The following considerations relate to exercise testing with this population:

- Symptoms are frequently observed under 5 METs (metabolic equivalents), so lower-level, moderately incremented, individualized protocols are recommended (Naughton or ramp).
- Symptoms indicative of unstable or decompensated CHF are a contraindication.

- Respiratory gas exchange measurements (including $\dot{V}O_{2peak}$, VT, $\dot{V}_E/\dot{V}CO_2$ slope) increase precision, optimize risk stratification, and permit assessment of breathing efficiency and patterns; these are particularly useful in clients with CHF.
- 6 min walk tests are an effective supplement to the graded exercise test.
- Exertional hypotension, clinically significant dysrhythmias, and chronotropic incompetence may occur in CHF.
- Test endpoints should focus on symptoms, hemodynamic responses, and standard clinical indications for stopping (and not target heart rate).

TABLE 12.1

Chronic Heart Failure: Exercise Testing

Methods	Measures	Endpoints	Comments
Aerobic Cycle (ramp protocol 10-15 W/min; staged protocol 10-15 W/3 min stage)	▪ 12-lead ECG, HR ▪ BP, rate–pressure product ▪ RPE, dyspnea scales ▪ Respired gas analysis ($\dot{V}O_2$, VT, $\dot{V}_E/\dot{V}CO_2$ slope)	▪ Serious dysrhythmias ▪ T-wave inversion with significant ST change ▪ Hypotensive response ▪ Perceived shortness of breath and fatigue ▪ $\dot{V}O_{2peak}$ and ventilatory threshold	
Treadmill (Naughton or individualized ramp)			Peak performance is often <5 METs, so a low-level ramp or Naughton protocol is preferred.
Endurance 6 min walk	Distance	If breaks for rest are required, be sure to note the duration of the break, the distance walked, and the perceived exertion (note time distance, or both, and perceived exertion)	Useful throughout training program.
Functional Lifestyle-specific tests	Performance related to ADLs		

RECOMMENDATIONS FOR EXERCISE PROGRAMMING

Because of improvements in therapeutic and surgical techniques, individuals with CHF represent one of the fastest-growing segments of cardiac rehabilitation populations, despite limited third-party reimbursement. Formal exercise training programs are effective in reducing symptoms and improving exercise capacity. An improvement in the ability to sustain low-level activities can result in a person's being able to live independently and continue to work instead of being disabled. For these and other reasons, exercise programs may significantly enhance the quality of life in individuals with CHF (see table 12.2). The impact of endurance exercise training will be more clearly understood with the completion of the HF-ACTION trial.

However, the potential complications and outcomes for individuals with CHF differ significantly from those for the standard cardiac rehabilitation population. For example, many with CHF will deteriorate irrespective of exercise or medical therapy; in such cases, the exercise regimen needs to be continually reassessed. People with CHF are at higher risk of sudden death, as well as more frequent episodes of psychosocial and vocational problems brought on by their disease. Some individuals with CHF may be so weak that they experience prolonged fatigue after only a single exercise session. Careful consideration should be given to absolute contraindications, particularly left ventricular outflow obstruction, decompensated CHF, and unstable dysrhythmias. Relative contraindications to exercise are the same for individuals with CHF as for those with normal left ventricular function. Collectively, these considerations necessitate that programs be designed carefully and that the staff be trained to recognize specific needs of this population as well as specific precautions that should be taken.

- Status can change quickly, and clients should be reevaluated frequently for signs of decom-

TABLE 12.2

Chronic Heart Failure: Exercise Programming

Modes	Goals	Intensity/Frequency/ Duration	Time to goal
Aerobic Large muscle activities	■ Increase $\dot{V}O_{2peak}$ and ventilatory threshold ■ Increase peak work rate and endurance capacity	■ RPE 11-14/20 ■ 40-70% $\dot{V}O_{2peak}$ or HR reserve ■ 4-7 days/week ■ 20-60 min/session or 2-3 sessions/day of 10-20 min	3 months
Resistance Circuit training	Reduce atrophy	High reps, low resistance	3 months
Flexibility Upper and lower body ROM activities	Maintain ROM	2-3 days/week	4-6 months
Functional Activity-specific exercise	■ Increase ADLs ■ Return to work ■ Improve quality of life and maintain independence	2-3 days/week	3 months

pensation, rapid changes in weight or blood pressure, worse than usual dyspnea or angina on exertion, or increases in dysrhythmias.

- Warm-up and cool-down sessions should be prolonged.
- Some clients may tolerate only limited work rates and need lower-intensity, longer-duration exercise sessions.

- Duration of activity may need to be adjusted to allow clients more opportunity rest and to progress at their own pace. Some clients may better tolerate discontinuous training involving shorter sessions of exercise interspersed with periods of rest.
- Perceived exertion and dyspnea scales should take precedence over heart rate and work rate targets.

CASE STUDY

Chronic Heart Failure

A 70-year-old male complained of increasing difficulty sustaining recreational activities and household chores. The client had a 10-year history of reduced left ventricular function from ischemic heart disease and had had bypass surgery performed five years before. He was not smoking, but had a 40 pack a year history of smoking. Other risk factors included a sedentary lifestyle, history of high blood pressure (controlled pharmacologically), and slightly excessive weight. He carried nitroglycerin for chest pain and an albuterol inhaler for bronchitis, but he rarely used either one.

S: "I get fatigued when I'm doing things."

O: Vitals

HR: 55 contractions/min
BP: 130/65 mmHg
Elderly male, normal appearance
ECG: Sinus bradycardia
Medications: Lisinopril, Hydrochlorothiazide, Carvedilol, Naproxen
Echocardiogram
LVEF: 30%, mild ventricular hypertrophy, posterior wall dyskinesis, inferior wall akinesis, mild mitral valve thickening and moderate regurgitation, mild tricuspid valve regurgitation

Spirometry

FVC: 2.84 L (60.6% of expected)
FEV1: 70.4% of normal (low)

Graded Exercise Test

Peak exercise: 4.6 METs (estimated)
$\dot{V}O_{2peak}$: 15.3 ml · kg^{-1} · min^{-1} (measured, 62% of age-predicted)
Terminated due to shortness of breath at RPE 17/20
No chest discomfort
Peak HR: 95 contractions/min
Peak BP: 160/70 mmHg
ECG: No significant ST changes during exercise or recovery; occasional PVCs

A: 1. CHF, NYHA class III
2. Coronary artery disease, s/p CABG
3. Mild COPD

P: 1. Introduce home-based exercise.
2. Increase physical activity level.
3. Reevaluate in 6 months.

Exercise Program Goals

1. Improve functional capacity.
2. Monitor for symptoms of worsening CHF.
3. Assist with lifestyle changes to decrease cardiovascular risk.

Mode	Frequency	Duration	Intensity	Progression
Aerobic	Daily	20 min/session as tolerated	THR (40-70% $\dot{V}O_{2max}$) RPE 10-16/20	Increase to 30 min/session as tolerated
Strength	2-3 days/week	1 set of 8-10 reps	50-70% of 1RM	Limit to 2 sets of 10-12 reps
Flexibility	2-3 days/week	20-60 s/stretch	Maintain stretch below discomfort point	
Warm-up and cool-down	Before and after each session	10-15 min	RPE <11/20	

- Isometric exercise should be avoided.
- Electrocardiogram monitoring is required for persons with a history of ventricular tachycardia, cardiac arrest (sudden death), or exertional hypotension.
- Consider ancillary study data (e.g., exercise echocardiogram, radionuclide studies, hemodynamic studies, ventilatory gas analysis) when developing the exercise program. In general, do not exceed a work rate that produces wall motion abnormalities, a drop in ejection fraction, a pulmonary wedge pressure greater than 20 mmHg, or the ventilatory threshold.

Evidence-Based Guidelines

Uddin N, Patterson JH. Current guidelines for treatment of heart failure: 2006 update. Pharmacotherapy. 2007;27(4):12S-17S.

Suggested Web Sites

American College of Cardiology. www.acc.org

American Heart Association. www.americanheart.org

Cardiac Transplant

Ross Arena, PhD, PT, FACSM ■ Reed Humphrey, PhD, PT, FACSM

OVERVIEW OF THE PATHOPHYSIOLOGY

Cardiac transplantation is a life-saving surgery performed on individuals with advanced, irreversible heart failure that involves replacing the patient's damaged or diseased heart with a healthy donor heart. The prognosis for cardiac transplant patients undergoing the orthotopic procedure (the complete removal of the recipient's heart) has improved dramatically in the past two decades, with present average one- and three-year survival rates greater than 80% and 70%, respectively. Of the estimated 5000 cardiac transplant procedures performed worldwide each year, nearly half are performed in the United states (2,192 in 2006). Despite receiving a healthy heart, most patients following orthotopic heart transplantation via bicaval anastamosis often continue to experience exercise intolerance. Causes of postsurgical exercise intolerance include the following:

- Inactivity before surgery
- Reduced aerobic characteristics of skeletal muscle
- Decreased skeletal muscle mass and force production
- Pulmonary diffusion abnormalities
- Left ventricular dysfunction
- Chronotropic incompetence

One of the ways to counteract the expected exercise intolerance following cardiac transplantation is to recommend that stable patients participate in a supervised exercise program prior to cardiac transplantation.

Cardiac transplant recipients are unique in that their hearts undergo autonomic denervation during the surgical procedure. Partial sympathetic reinnervation has been demonstrated in some individuals undergoing cardiac transplant, although, if occurring, it is likely to be a late phenomenon years after transplantation. Younger donor and recipient age as well as a faster, uncomplicated surgical procedure may increase the likelihood of sympathetic reinnervation. Of note, individuals experiencing partial sympathetic reinnervation present with an enhanced cardiac response to exercise and higher aerobic capacity compared to cardiac transplant recipients who have persistent sympathetic denervation. Irrespective of the presence or absence of partial sympathetic reinnervation, skeletal muscle abnormalities and depressed left ventricular function remain in individuals undergoing cardiac transplant surgery. Therefore, while the spontaneous recovery of aerobic capacity following cardiac transplant is significant, values typically remain substantially lower than predicted values, particularly in the absence of an exercise training program.

Acknowledgment
The editors wish to acknowledge the previous authors of this chapter, Steven J. Keteyian, PhD, FACSM; and Clinton Brawner, BS, FACSM.

EFFECTS ON THE EXERCISE RESPONSE

As a consequence of the surgical procedure and medical management, heart rate and hemodynamic response evident at rest and during exercise are different from those of apparently healthy individuals. The following are some of these differences:

- Increased resting heart rate (~20 contractions per minute above that of age- and sex-matched controls)
- Diminished chronotropic response to exercise
- Elevated resting blood pressure, likely due to (a) elevations in catecholamines, (b) the side effects of immunosuppressive medications (cyclosporine and prednisone), and (c) altered baroreceptor function
- Decreased systolic pressure at peak exercise

During exercise, cardiac transplant recipients have a diminished cardiac output response. During light exercise, cardiac output is augmented secondary to an increase in stroke volume (increased venous return and preload) rather than heart rate. Increases in cardiac output during moderate- to high-intensity exercise are attributable to catecholamine- and potentially sympathetic reinnervation-related increases in heart rate and further increases in stroke volume. Despite remarkable adaptations following cardiac transplantation, cardiac output at peak exercise is still only 60% to 70% that of age-matched healthy controls secondary to a combined lower heart rate and stroke volume. The lower than normal stroke volume during maximal exercise is a consequence of persistent left ventricular dysfunction following cardiac transplant. Mechanisms for left ventricular dysfunction may include

- diastolic dysfunction (mismatching of donor–recipient body type, hypertension),
- cardiac allograft vasculopathy,
- oxidative stress, and
- compromised recipient autoimmune response.

During recovery from an acute bout of exercise, heart rate initially remains elevated for a prolonged period, or may actually rise above values observed at maximal exercise, secondary to the absence of parasympathetic innervation to the sinoatrial node and the increase in circulating catecholamines during exercise.

EFFECTS OF EXERCISE TRAINING

Participation in a formal exercise training program has consistently proven to be beneficial to cardiac transplant recipients. Positive physiologic and clinical adaptations have been safely demonstrated for both aerobic and resistance exercise programs. Reported benefits of exercise training in cardiac transplant recipients include the following:

- Decreased blood lactate concentrations at a given work rate
- Improved aerobic characteristics of skeletal muscle
- Improved endothelial function
- Decreased resting heart rate and blood pressure
- Increased $\dot{V}O_{2peak}$ and $\dot{V}O_2$ at ventilatory threshold
- Improved ventilatory efficiency ($\dot{V}_E/\dot{V}CO_2$ slope)
- Increased muscle force production
- Increased bone mineral density
- Counteraction of the deleterious effects of immunosuppressive therapy

MANAGEMENT AND MEDICATIONS

Controlling immune system rejection of the donor heart and avoiding the adverse side effects of immunosuppressive therapy (infections, hyperlipidemia, hypertension, obesity, osteoporosis, renal dysfunction, and diabetes) are primary concerns following cardiac transplantation. Acute graft rejection is common among all transplant recipients, especially within the first year, and is characterized by perivascular infiltration of killer T-lymphocytes into the myocardium, including possible cellular necrosis. Episodes of graft rejection are classified as follows:

- Minimal rejection (1A)
- Small amount of rejection (1B)
- Moderate rejection (2)
- One serious area of rejection (3A)
- Multiple serious areas of rejection (3B)
- Severe rejection (4)

Treatment for acute graft rejection includes aggressive medical management and in rare cases retransplantation.

Two approaches are used to lessen the occurrence of acute rejection. First, since rejection is silent, endomyocardial biopsy (by catheters) is performed both to detect preclinical cellular involvement and to assess the efficacy of therapy. Second, immuno-suppressive agents (e.g., prednisone, cyclosporine, azathioprine, mycophenolate, tacrolimus) are used to prophylactically suppress killer T-lymphocyte function. Doing so, however, renders individuals more susceptible to certain infections and cancers. Presently, tacrolimus (54%) and cyclosporine (40%) are the two most commonly utilized calcineurin inhibitors. While prednisone use is decreasing, 63% of cardiac transplant recipients are still prescribed this agent at one year postsurgery. Depending on the severity of acute rejection episodes, decreasing the volume or intensity or complete discontinuation of the exercise program may be necessary and is at the discretion of the physician responsible for the patient's care.

One year after surgery, the likelihood for acute rejection lessens, but there is increased probability of developing accelerated atherosclerosis (i.e., cardiac allograft vasculopathy) of the donor heart. By five years after transplantation, repeat cardiac transplant, cardiac allograft vasculopathy within the first year, and drug-treated rejection prior to postsurgical hospital discharge are all significant predictors of mortality in these patients.

RECOMMENDATIONS FOR EXERCISE TESTING

Exercise testing for cardiac transplant recipients should follow accepted American College of Sports Medicine standards (see table 13.1). A progressive exercise test using a treadmill or stationary cycle ergometer is recommended. The mode of exercise used for testing should ideally be the same as the primary mode used for training. A conservative exercise testing protocol, with lower increases in work rate per stage (e.g., 0.5-1.0 METs [metabolic equivalents]), should be employed. A number of different conservative incremental or ramping pro-tocols exist for both the treadmill and cycle ergom-eter. Given the altered heart rate response, ratings of perceived exertion as well as oxygen consump-tion, via ventilatory expired gas analysis, should be

TABLE 13.1

Cardiac Transplant: Exercise Testing

Methods	Measures	Endpoints	Comments
Aerobic			
Cycle: 　– Ramp protocol: 10-15 W/min 　– Incremental protocol: 25-30 W/2 to 3 min stage 　– Treadmill: 　– Ramp protocol: ≤1 MET/30 s to 1 min 　– ncremental protocol: ~1-2 METs/3 min stage	■ Heart rate ■ Blood pressure ■ Perceived exertion ■ Dyspnea ■ Angina ■ Peak METs ■ Exercise time ■ Ventilatory expired gas (if available) 　– $\dot{V}O_{2peak}$ 　– $\dot{V}O_2$ at VT 　– Peak RER 　– $\dot{V}_E/\dot{V}CO_2$ slope	■ Subject request ■ Dizziness or signs of poor perfusion ■ Moderate-severe dyspnea or ischemia ■ Peak RER ≥1.1 ■ Drop or abnormal rise in blood pressure ■ ECG evidence of ischemia ■ Arrhythmias (particularly ventricular)	■ Blunted heart rate response to exercise and delayed recovery postexercise secondary to autonomic denervation. ■ Aerobic capacity is typically below age- and sex-predicted norms. ■ Subject may not experience chest pain during ischemic event secondary to autonomic denervation. ■ Consider nuclear or echocardiography assessments in conjunction with exercise test when cardiac ischemia is suspected.

(continued)

TABLE 13.1 *(continued)*

Methods	Measures	Endpoints	Comments
Muscle force production Free weights or machine (loaded weight plates, pneumatic, etc.) – Assess 1RM of large muscle groups Examples of exercises: Chest press Leg press Lat pulldown	▪ Blood pressure ▪ Perceived exertion ▪ Dyspnea ▪ Angina ▪ Maximal resistance achieved for each movement (pounds or kilograms)	▪ Dizziness or signs of poor perfusion ▪ Moderate-severe dyspnea or ischemia ▪ Drop or abnormal rise in blood pressure ▪ Inability to move a given load throughout full range of motion	▪ Closely monitor individual for proper body mechanics and breathing cycle during movements. ▪ Prolonged corticosteroid use can decrease bone mineral density and increase fracture risk. ▪ Consider imaging assessment of bone mineral density when osteoporosis is a significant concern. ▪ Calcium supplementation may increase bone mineral density.
Flexibility Assess active range of motion in major joints Examples of motions: ▪ Spine: flexion/extension ▪ Shoulder: flexion/extension/abduction ▪ Hip: flexion/extension/abduction ▪ Knee: flexion/extension ▪ Ankle: dorsiflexion and plantarflexion ▪ Sit-and-reach test	▪ Range of motion ▪ Pain with motion	Pain-free end range of active motion for a given muscle group	Assess for mechanism when pain with motion or limitation in muscle group range (or both) is detected.
Aerobic Cycle: – Ramp protocol: 10-15 W/min – Incremental protocol: 25-30 W/2 to 3 min stage Treadmill: – Ramp protocol: ≤1 MET/30 s to 1 min – Incremental protocol: ~1-2 METs/3 min stage	▪ Heart rate ▪ Blood pressure ▪ Perceived exertion ▪ Dyspnea ▪ Angina ▪ Peak METs ▪ Exercise time ▪ Ventilatory expired gas (if available) – $\dot{V}O_{2peak}$ – $\dot{V}O_2$ at VT – Peak RER – $\dot{V}_E/\dot{V}CO_2$ slope	▪ Subject request ▪ Dizziness or signs of poor perfusion ▪ Moderate-severe dyspnea or ischemia ▪ Peak RER ≥1.1 ▪ Drop or abnormal rise in blood pressure ▪ ECG evidence of ischemia ▪ Arrhythmias (particularly ventricular)	▪ Blunted heart rate response to exercise and delayed recovery postexercise secondary to autonomic denervation. ▪ Aerobic capacity is typically below age- and sex-predicted norms. ▪ Subject may not experience chest pain during ischemic event secondary to autonomic denervation. ▪ Consider nuclear or echocardiography assessments in conjunction with exercise test when cardiac ischemia is suspected.

assessed. These assessments allow for accurately quantifying functional capacity, developing an appropriate exercise prescription, and determining subject effort. For the latter, assessment of peak respiratory exchange ratio ($\dot{V}CO_2/\dot{V}O_2$) provides a highly objective measure.

Determination of $\dot{V}O_2$ at the ventilatory threshold can help set initial work rates for exercise training. Ventilatory threshold automatically derived from a computerized metabolic system should be confirmed by at least one individual trained in cardiopulmonary exercise testing procedures. $\dot{V}O_{2peak}$ in untrained cardiac transplant recipients is generally ≤20 to 25 ml · kg^{-1} · min^{-1}. If measured before and after a training regimen, $\dot{V}O_2$ at ventilatory threshold can also serve as a marker for change in submaximal cardiorespiratory endurance. Both $\dot{V}O_{2peak}$ and $\dot{V}O_2$ at ventilatory threshold have been shown to significantly improve following training. To assess recovery following maximal or submaximal exercise, combined assessment of systolic blood pressure and heart rate is a better indicator than either one alone.

Although isolated cases of chest pain associated with accelerated graft atherosclerosis have been observed, autonomic denervation reduces the likelihood of anginal symptoms, especially in the initial months or years following surgery when partial reinnervation is less likely. Exercise electrocardiography is also inadequate with respect to assessing ischemia, as evidenced by its low sensitivity (i.e., <25%) for detecting true disease in these individuals. Thus, radionuclide testing may be more useful for assessing suspected ischemic heart disease. For these reasons, professionals experienced in exercise testing in high-risk populations should perform the assessment.

Following an adequate warm-up, assessment of muscle force production can be accomplished using a 1-repetition maximum (1RM) method. In most individuals, 1RM is reached within three to five trials. Be sure to allow at least 3 min recovery between trials.

Although the restoration or maintenance (or both) of range of motion is important for all adults, among people with cardiac transplant there are no unique joint or muscle issues limiting range of motion. A flexibility assessment used in the general population is therefore adequate.

Sternal precautions should be strictly adhered to in the acute phase following cardiac transplantation. These precautions will likely affect the ability to perform strength and flexibility assessments in the initial weeks and months following surgery. The patient's physician or cardiac surgeon (or both)

should be consulted with respect to timing of all fitness assessments. Certain immunosuppressive agents (e.g., cyclosporine) may negatively affect the aerobic capacity of skeletal muscle. Prednisone may cause fluid retention, muscle atrophy, decreased leg strength, and myopathy. The side effect profile of standard pharmacologic agents may therefore contribute to the observed limitation in exercise capacity and performance.

The following are important medication precautions to consider during exercise:

- Prednisone may cause fluid retention, muscle atrophy, and decreased leg strength and may cause myopathy.
- Cyclosporine may cause increases in resting and submaximal blood pressure.
- Calf muscle cramps can occur in ~15% of patients.
- Leg strength deficits are common and result in decreased exercise time.
- Use caution with high-resistance exercise in persons receiving long-term, high-dose corticosteroids, which can decrease bone mineral content and increase risk for fracture.
- Longer periods of warm-up and cool-down are indicated because the physiologic responses to exercise recovery may take longer.

RECOMMENDATIONS FOR EXERCISE PROGRAMMING

As with virtually all individuals with chronic disease, progressive exercise training in people with cardiac transplant is an effective means to (see table 13.2)

- improve cardiorespiratory fitness,
- improve muscle endurance and force production,
- reestablish self-efficacy, and
- improve quality of life.

Less established, however, is whether the modification of cardiovascular risk factors through exercise alters the progression of accelerated graft atherosclerosis, which is the major factor limiting long-term survival in transplant recipients.

The current recommended methods to guide exercise intensity in cardiac transplant recipients include ratings of perceived exertion, fixed distance, percentage of $\dot{V}O_{2peak}$, and work rate achieved at ventilatory threshold. When incorporated into

TABLE 13.2

Cardiac Transplant: Exercise Programming

Modes	Goals	Intensity/Frequency/Duration	Time to goal
Aerobic Large muscle activities	■ Increase self-efficacy ■ Increase cardiovascular fitness ■ Improve risk factors (e.g., body mass, insulin sensitivity, BP)	■ RPE 11-14/20 ■ 40-80% $\dot{V}O_{2peak}$ ■ 4-7 days/week ■ 15-60 min/session or accumulated throughout the day	>6 months
Strength All major muscle groups	■ Increase ability to perform leisure and occupational activities and ADLs ■ Increase muscle strength and endurance ■ Delay or reverse harmful effects of long-term corticosteroid therapy	■ Low to moderate intensity ■ 1-2 sets of 10-15 reps ■ 2-4 days/week	>2 months
Flexibility Upper and lower body ROM activities	Improve upper body ROM following sternotomy	2-3 days/week	>1 month

training studies involving cardiac transplant recipients, these methods have resulted in increases in $\dot{V}O_{2peak}$ ranging between 15% and 40%. The minimal threshold intensity (i.e., 40%, 50%, or 60% of $\dot{V}O_{2peak}$) needed to significantly improve $\dot{V}O_{2peak}$ is not known. However, general principles of exercise training (i.e., overload, specificity, and reversibility), as well as factors to consider for an individualized exercise prescription (mode, intensity, frequency and duration), also apply to the cardiac transplant population.

The use of heart rate alone to guide exercise intensity is not appropriate in this population. In fact, it is not uncommon to find cardiac transplant recipients achieving an exercise heart rate that not only exceeds 85% of measured peak heart rate but is equal to or greater than peak heart rate. Instead, a rating of perceived exertion (commonly between 11 and 14) or a percentage of $\dot{V}O_{2peak}$ or work rate achieved during exercise testing (most commonly 50-85%) should be used to guide training intensity. Also, these persons should perform an aerobic activity most if not all days of the week while pro-

gressively increasing the duration from 15 to 60 min (see table 13.2).

Because muscle endurance and force production deficits exist in cardiac transplant recipients, a progressive resistance training program is vital. Such a program will help negate or reverse the glucocorticoid-induced myopathy and bone loss that occur in these clients after surgery. One or two sets of 10 to 15 repetitions is generally sufficient to accomplish these goals.

These are important medication precautions to consider during exercise programming:

■ Corticosteroids may cause bone- or joint-related disorders because of demineralization effects.

■ Cyclosporine may cause increases in resting and submaximal blood pressure.

■ Start slow. Severe deconditioning is common, especially if prolonged bed rest was required prior to surgery. Intermittent exercise or short periods throughout the day may be needed until longer, continuous exercise can be tolerated.

CASE STUDY

Cardiac Transplant

A 50-year-old African American male underwent heart transplantation because of nonischemic heart failure secondary to idiopathic cardiomyopathy. He underwent left ventricular assist device implantation six months prior to transplantation. Two months following left ventricular assist device implantation, the patient began participation in a cardiac rehabilitation program (three times per week) and maintained that program until transplantation. His past medical history included non-insulin-dependent diabetes, dyslipidemia, and hypertension. One month following successful transplantation he was referred to outpatient cardiac rehabilitation for a reconditioning program and cardiovascular risk reduction.

S: "I had a heart transplant about one month ago. I am having difficulty walking long distances, going up and down stairs, and getting in and out of a chair. My family is very supportive of my rehabilitation."

O: Vitals

HR: 95 contractions/min
BP: 146/88 mmHg
Weight: 185 lb (84.1 kg)
Height: 5 ft 9 in. (1.75 m)
BMI: 27.5 kg/m2
Overweight male post heart transplant
Baseline echocardiogram: Normal left ventricular ejection fraction (60%), mild mitral and tricuspid regurgitation
Estimated PA pressure: 30 mmHg
Total cholesterol: 215 mg/dl
  - HDL: 40 mg/dl
  - LDL: 149 mg/dl
  - Trig: 130 mg/dl
Fasting blood glucose: 110 mg/dl
Subjective measures: Minnesota Living With Heart Failure Questionnaire, 45 out of 105 (scale 0-105; higher value is less favorable); Duke Activity Status Index, 6 METs
Graded exercise test performed on a treadmill with conservative ramping protocol (~0.5 METs/30 s):
Peak exercise: 4.0 METs
$\dot{V}O_{2peak}$: 14.0 ml · kg^{-1} · min^{-1}
Peak RER: 1.14
$\dot{V}_E/\dot{V}CO_2$ slope: 35.0
VO_2 at ventilatory threshold: 9.8 ml · kg^{-1} · min^{-1}
Peak HR: 140 contractions/min
Peak BP: 189/90 mmHg
No ECG changes or ischemia indications
Test terminated by patient primarily due to lower extremity fatigue (RPE = 17/20). Dyspnea also reported (2/4).

HR in recovery at: 1 min = HR decreased by 7 contractions/min; at 3 min = HR decreased by 18 contractions/min
Note: Improved from one month pretransplant exercise test: $\dot{V}O_{2peak}$ = 9.8 ml · kg^{-1} · min^{-1}; peak RER= 1.19; $\dot{V}_E/\dot{V}CO_2$ = 49.0
Medications: Tacrolimus, prednisone, isosorbide dinitrate, pravastatin, furosemide, enalapril, glyburide, aspirin, magnesium

A: 1. Status post cardiac transplant
   2. Reduced exercise tolerance although improved from pretransplant level. Appropriate hemodynamic response, as expected post cardiac transplant (decreased HR, cardiac output); ECG response to exercise within normal limits.
   3. Hypertension persists although pharmacologically managed
   4. Dyslipidemia persists although pharmacologically managed
   5. Type 2 diabetes, fasting blood glucose above desired threshold (<100 mg/dl)

P: 1. Reinstitute supervised aerobic conditioning initiated in the pretransplant stage and progress as tolerated.
   2. Assess muscle force production and initiate resistance exercise training program after one month of aerobic exercise training is completed.
   3. Introduce diabetic, dyslipidemia, hypertension, and dietary education.
   4. Closely monitor resting and exercise HR, BP, and ECG.
   5. Progress patient to unsupervised home exercise program over the next three months.

Goals (12 weeks)

1. Increase functional capacity to 5 METs
2. Increase muscle force production by 10%
3. Decrease BMI to 25 kg/m^2
4. Improve glucose and lipid values
5. Decrease SBP and DBP by 10%
6. Improve perceived quality of life as measured by MLWHF instrument
7. Ability to independently perform activities of daily living
8. Independent management of exercise program, dietary monitoring, and risk factor control
9. Attenuate skeletal muscle atrophy and increase bone density

(continued)

CASE STUDY Cardiac Transplant *(continued)*

Mode	Frequency	Duration	Intensity	Progression
Aerobic Walking, running Ergometry Swimming Stair stepper	Eventual goal: most if not all days of the week	Eventual goal: 30-60 min of continuous activity	• 50-75% of peak METs or $\dot{V}O_{2peak}$ • Work rate approximating $\dot{V}O_2$ at ventilatory threshold • 11-14/20 on RPE scale • Avoid using HR as an index of exercise intensity in cardiac transplant patients	• Begin frequency (2-3 days per week) and duration (10-15 min continuously) conservatively and progress to eventual goal levels over the initial weeks or months following cardiac transplant. • Consider several daily shorter intermittent sessions during the initial phases of the exercise program for significantly debilitated patients or those with a complicated postoperative recovery.
Resistance All major muscle groups for upper and lower extremity: 8-10 exercises Free weights (dumbbell, barbell, or both) Machine Tubing	2-3 nonconsecutive days per week	20-30 min (multijoint exercises more time efficient)	1-2 sets of 10-15 repetitions at ~40-60% of 1RM	• Begin program at or below low end of 1RM percentage (≤40%). • Progress to higher intensity when subject can perform given resistance for 15 repetitions with appropriate body mechanics and breathing technique.
Flexibility All major muscle groups for upper and lower extremity Subject actively moves and statically holds joint at end range of pain-free motion	2-3 nonconsecutive days per week	~15-20 min	• 3-5 repetitions for each muscle group • Each stretch to be held for 20-30 s	No progression required.

- Range of motion and stretching exercises are important for the upper body due to sternotomy; however, these exercises should be limited for up to six to eight weeks after surgery.
- Ratings of perceived exertion should be primary method of monitoring exercise intensity.
- Longer periods of warm-up and cool-down are indicated because the physiologic responses to exercise recovery may take longer than in other people.

Evidence-Based Guidelines

Mehra MR, Jessup M, Gronda E, Costanzo MR. Rationale and process: International Society for Heart and Lung Transplantation guidelines for the care of cardiac transplant candidates—2006. J Heart Lung Transpl. 2006. 25(9):1001-1002.

Suggested Web Sites

American Heart Association. www.americanheart.org

International Society for Heart and Lung Transplantation. www.ishlt.org

14

Hypertension

Neil F. Gordon, MD, PhD, MPH, FACSM

OVERVIEW OF THE PATHOPHYSIOLOGY

Elevated blood pressure (BP) is a major public health problem in most Western industrialized countries. An estimated 37% of U.S. adults have prehypertension (i.e., systolic BP of 120 to 139 mmHg, or diastolic BP of 80 to 89 mmHg, or both), and nearly one in three adults has hypertension (i.e., systolic BP >140 mmHg and/or diastolic BP >90 mmHg and/or use of antihypertensive medication). Recent public health surveillance data indicate that the prevalence of hypertension may be increasing and that control rates among those with hypertension remain low. The risk for nonfatal and fatal cardiovascular disease, especially coronary artery disease and stroke, renal disease, and all-cause mortality increases progressively with higher levels of both systolic and diastolic BP. At any level of high BP, risks of cardiovascular disease are increased severalfold for persons with target organ disease. Cardiovascular risks are also related to the presence of other risk factors.

Table 14.1 depicts how BP in adults is classified according to the 2003 report of the Joint National Committee on Prevention, Detection, Evaluation, and Treatment of High Blood Pressure. In more than 95% of cases, the etiology of hypertension is unknown and is called primary, essential, or idiopathic hypertension, whereas secondary hypertension refers to hypertension with a known etiology. Identifiable causes of hypertension include sleep apnea, drug-induced or drug-related causes, chronic kidney disease, primary aldosteronism, renovascular disease, chronic steroid therapy and Cushing syndrome, pheochromocytoma, coarctation of the aorta, and thyroid or parathyroid disease.

EFFECTS ON THE EXERCISE RESPONSE

A single session of dynamic exercise usually evokes a normal rise in systolic BP from baseline levels in unmedicated individuals with hypertension, although the response may be exaggerated or diminished in certain individuals. However, because of an elevated baseline level, the absolute level of systolic BP attained during dynamic exercise is usually higher in persons with hypertension. In addition, their diastolic BP may not change, or may even slightly rise, during dynamic exercise, probably as a result of an impaired vasodilatory response.

Studies have documented a consistent 10 to 20 mmHg reduction in systolic BP during the initial 1 to 3 h following 30 to 45 min of moderate-intensity dynamic exercise in individuals with hypertension. This training-induced reduction in BP may persist for up to 9 h and appears to be mediated by a transient decrease in stroke volume rather than peripheral vasodilation. Untreated hypertension, as well as the use of certain antihypertensive drugs, may impair exercise tolerance, performance, or both. However, exercise tolerance is typically enhanced through control of hypertension with lifestyle modifications and, if warranted, well-tolerated antihypertensive medications.

TABLE 14.1

Classification and Management of Blood Pressure for Adults*

BP classification	SBP mmHg*	DPB mmHg*	Lifestyle modification	Initial drug therapy	
				Without compelling indication	With compelling indications[†]
Normal	<120	and <80	Encourage		
Prehypertension	120-139	or 80-89	Yes	No antihypertensive drug indicated.	Drug(s) for compelling indications.[‡]
Stage 1 hypertension	140-159	or 90-99	Yes	Antihypertensive drug(s) indicated.	Drug(s) for compelling indications.[‡] Other antihypertensive drugs, as needed.
Stage 2 hypertension	≥160	or ≥100	Yes	Antihypertensive drug(s) indicated. Two-drug combination for most.[†]	

DBP, diastolic blood pressure; SBP, systolic blood pressure.

*Treatment determined by highest BP category.

[†] Initial combined therapy should be used cautiously in those at risk for orthostatic hypotension.

[‡] Compelling indications include heart failure, postmyocardial infarction, high coronary artery disease risk, diabetes, chronic kidney disease, and recurrent stroke prevention. Treat patients with chronic kidney disease or diabetes to BP goal of <130/80 mmHg.

EFFECTS OF EXERCISE TRAINING

Existing evidence indicates that endurance exercise training reduces the magnitude of rise in BP that can be expected over time in individuals at increased risk for developing hypertension. Longitudinal studies further show that endurance training may elicit an average reduction of about 5 to 7 mmHg in both systolic and diastolic BP in persons with stage I or II hypertension. Both the Joint National Committee and the American College of Sports Medicine (ACSM) advocate regular aerobic exercise as a preventive strategy to reduce the incidence of high BP, and indicate that exercise training can be effectively used as definitive or adjunctive therapy for hypertension.

The mechanisms by which exercise training lowers BP have still to be fully elucidated. Possibilities include the following:

- Decrease in plasma norepinephrine levels
- Increase in circulating vasodilator substances
- Amelioration of hyperinsulinemia
- Alteration in renal function

Physically active individuals with hypertension and those with higher levels of cardiorespiratory fitness have been shown to have markedly lower mortality rates than sedentary and less fit persons.

There are several fundamental differences in cardiovascular responses to a single session of resistance exercise compared to endurance exercise. In particular, heavy-resistance exercise elicits a pressor response that involves only moderate increases in heart rate and cardiac output, relative to those seen with dynamic exercise, but a greater elevation in systolic and diastolic BP. Randomized controlled trials examining the effects of concentric and eccentric resistance training on resting BP have yielded conflicting findings. Although resistance training performed according to ACSM's guidelines generally does reduce resting BP in hypertensive adults, the magnitude of reduction is less than that observed with endurance exercise training.

MANAGEMENT AND MEDICATIONS

The goals of antihypertensive therapy are to control BP and to reduce cardiovascular and renal morbidity and mortality by the least intrusive means possible. These aims may be achieved through lifestyle modification alone or in combination with pharmacologic treatment. Individuals with a systolic BP of 120 to 139 mmHg or a diastolic BP of 80 to 89 mmHg (or both) should be considered "prehypertensive" and also require lifestyle intervention.

According to recent evidence-based recommendations from the American Heart Association (table 14.2), the BP goal is <140/90 mmHg for general coronary artery disease prevention; <130/80 mmHg in patients with diabetes mellitus, chronic kidney disease, known coronary artery disease or a coronary artery disease equivalent (i.e., carotid artery disease, peripheral arterial disease, or abdominal aortic aneurysm), or a 10-year Framingham risk score >10%; and <120/80 mmHg in patients with left ventricular dysfunction. Because most individuals with hypertension, especially those older than 50 years, will reach the diastolic BP goal once systolic BP is at the goal level, the Joint National Committee recommends that the primary focus be on achieving the systolic BP goal.

For hypertension control or overall cardiovascular risk reduction, or both, it is recommended

TABLE 14.2

Summary of Main Evidence-Based Recommendations of the American Heart Association

Area of concern	BP target, mmHg	Lifestyle modification†	Specific drug indications	Comments
General CAD prevention	<140/90	Yes	Any effective antihypertensive drug or combination‡	If SBP ≥160 mmHg or DBP ≥100 mmHg, then start with two drugs.
High CAD risk*	<130/80	Yes	ACEI or ARB *or* CCB *or* thiazide diuretic *or* combination	If SBP ≥160 mmHg or DBP ≥100 mmHg, then start with two drugs.
Stable angina	<130/80	Yes	Beta-blocker *and* ACEI or ARB	If beta-blocker contraindicated, or if side effects occur, can substitute diltiazem or verapamil (but not if bradycardia or LVD is present). Can add dihydropyridine CCB (not diltiazem or verapamil) to beta-blocker. A thiazide diuretic can be added for BP control.
LVD	<120/80	Yes	ACEI or ARB *and* beta-blocker *and* aldosterone antagonist *and* thiazide or loop diuretic *and* hydralazine/isosorbide dinitrate (blacks)	Contraindicated: verapamil, diltiazem, clonidine, moxonidine, alpha-blockers

CAD, coronary artery disease; SBP, systolic blood pressure; DBP, diastolic blood pressure; ACEI, angiotensin-converting enzyme inhibitor; ARB, angiotensin receptor blocker; CCB, calcium channel blocker; LVD, LV dysfunction.

Before making any management decisions, clinicians are strongly urged to read the full text of the relevant section of the scientific statement.

*Diabetes mellitus, chronic kidney disease, known CAD or CAD equivalent (carotid artery disease, peripheral arterial disease, or abdominal aortic aneurysm), or 10-year Framingham risk score ≥10%.

†Weight loss if appropriate, healthy diet (including sodium restriction), exercise, smoking cessation, and alcohol moderation.

‡Evidence supports ACEI (or ARB), CCB, or thiazide diuretic as first-line therapy.

that individuals make the following lifestyle modifications:

- Lose weight, if overweight.
- Limit alcohol intake to no more than two drinks a day in most men and one drink a day in women and lighter-weight individuals.
- Perform aerobic physical activity, such as brisk walking, for at least 30 min a day on most days of the week.
- Reduce salt intake as much as possible, ideally to 65 mmol/day (corresponding to 1.5 g/day of sodium or 3.8 g/day of salt).
- Eat a diet rich in fruits, vegetables, and low-fat dairy products and reduced in saturated fat and cholesterol; potassium intake should be increased to 120 mmol/day (4.7 g/day).
- Stop smoking.

The decision to initiate drug therapy requires consideration of several factors, including

- severity of BP elevation,
- presence or absence of clinical cardiovascular disease or target organ disease, and
- presence or absence of other medical conditions and cardiovascular disease risk factors.

Most people with hypertension who require drug therapy in addition to lifestyle modification will need two or more antihypertensive medications to achieve goal BP. If BP is >20/10 mmHg above the goal, consideration should be given to initiating antihypertensive therapy with two agents, one of which should usually be a thiazide-type diuretic.

Thiazide-type diuretics should be used in drug treatment for most patients with uncomplicated hypertension, either alone or combined with drugs from other classes. Certain high-risk conditions are compelling indications for the initial use of other antihypertensive drug classes. Compelling indications include heart failure (diuretics, beta-blockers, angiotensin-converting enzyme [ACE] inhibitors or angiotensin receptor blockers [ARBs], and aldosterone antagonists), postmyocardial infarction (beta-blockers, ACE inhibitors/ARBs, and aldosterone antagonists), high risk for coronary artery disease (diuretics, beta-blockers, ACE inhibitors/ARBs, and calcium channel blockers), diabetes (diuretics, beta-blockers, ACE inhibitors/ARBs, and calcium channel blockers), chronic kidney disease (ACE inhibitors/ARBs), and recurrent stroke prevention (diuretics and ACE inhibitors/ARBs).

After initiation of drug therapy, most patients should return for follow-up and adjustment of medications at approximately monthly intervals until the BP goal is reached. More frequent follow-up may be needed for patients with stage 2 hypertension or with complicating comorbid conditions. Serum potassium and creatinine should be monitored at least one to two times per year. Follow-up visits can usually be at three- to six-month intervals once BP is at goal and stable.

Other cardiovascular risk factors (such as serum lipids and lipoproteins and diabetes) should be treated to their respective goals. Other evidence-based cardioprotective drugs should be initiated if clinically indicated. Low-dose aspirin therapy for cardiovascular risk reduction should be considered only when BP is controlled, because the risk of hemorrhagic stroke is increased in patients with uncontrolled hypertension.

Beta-blockers and, to a lesser degree, the calcium antagonists diltiazem and verapamil reduce the heart rate response to submaximal and maximal exercise. In contrast, dihydropyridine-derivative calcium antagonists and direct vasodilators may increase the heart rate response to submaximal exercise.

With the exception of beta-blockers, most antihypertensive agents do not substantially alter the systolic BP response to a single session of dynamic exercise. However, they do lower the resting BP and therefore the absolute level attained. Beta-blockers have been shown to attenuate the magnitude of rise in systolic BP from the baseline level as well as to reduce the resting BP. Unfortunately, the usefulness of beta-blockers, especially nonselective agents, is often considerably limited by a concomitant impairment of exercise tolerance in persons without myocardial ischemia or heart failure and by a possible blunting of exercise training-induced lowering of BP and triglycerides and increase in high-density lipoprotein cholesterol.

Antihypertensive agents that reduce total peripheral resistance by vasodilation may predispose to postexercise hypotension. This potential adverse effect can usually be prevented by avoidance of abrupt cessation of exercise and use of a longer cool-down period. Diuretics may result in serum potassium derangements and thereby accentuate the risk for exercise-induced dysrhythmias.

RECOMMENDATIONS FOR EXERCISE TESTING

Standard exercise testing methods and protocols may be used for individuals with hypertension. People with an additional coronary risk factor, and those who are male and older than 45 years or female and older than 55 years, should perform an exercise test with electrocardiogram (ECG) monitoring before starting a vigorous exercise program (i.e., >60% of maximum oxygen consumption reserve [$\dot{V}O_2R$]). Irrespective of the intensity of exercise training, persons with symptoms of cardiovascular disease or with known cardiovascular disease should perform an exercise test with ECG monitoring before commencing an exercise program. When exercise testing is performed for the purpose of exercise prescription, the individual should be taking his or her usual antihypertensive medications. A resting systolic BP over 200 mmHg or diastolic BP over 110 mmHg is considered a relative contraindication to exercise testing. Attainment of a systolic BP over 250 mmHg or diastolic BP over 115 mmHg is an indication for exercise test termination (see table 14.3).

RECOMMENDATIONS FOR EXERCISE PROGRAMMING

Individuals with marked elevations in BP (>180/110 mmHg) are encouraged to add endurance training to their treatment regimen only after initiating drug therapy.

Mode: Large muscle, aerobic activities

Frequency: Most, preferably all, days of the week

Duration: >30 min of continuous or accumulated physical activity per day

Intensity: 40% to <60% $\dot{V}O_2R$ recommended for individuals with hypertension as well as apparently healthy adults (see table 14.4)

Interestingly, exercise training at somewhat lower intensities appears to lower BP as much as, if not more than, exercise at higher intensities. This is especially important in certain specific populations of persons with hypertension, such as those who are elderly or who have chronic diseases in addition to hypertension. When exercising, it appears prudent to maintain systolic BP <220 mmHg and diastolic BP <105 mmHg.

Strength or resistive training is not recommended as the only form of exercise training for persons with hypertension because, with the exception of circuit weight training, it has not consistently been shown to significantly lower BP. Thus, resistive exercise training is recommended when done as one component of a well-rounded exercise program. Resistive training using lower resistances and higher repetitions should be prescribed (e.g., one set of 8-12 reps at 60-80% of 1RM).

TABLE 14.3

Hypertension: Exercise Testing

Methods	Measures	Endpoints*	Comments
Aerobic			
Cycle (ramp protocol 17 W/ min; staged protocol 25-50 W/3 min stage) Treadmill (1-2 METs/3 min stage)	■ 12-lead ECG, HR	■ Serious dysrhythmias ■ >2 mm ST-segment depression or elevation ■ Ischemic threshold ■ T-wave inversion with significant ST change	Medications should be taken at usual time relative to exercise session
	■ BP, rate–pressure product	■ SBP >250 mmHg or DBP >115 mmHg ■ Headache or other significant symptoms	
	■ RPE (6-20) ■ Respired gas analysis	■ Volitional fatigue ■ $\dot{V}O_{2max}$	
Strength			
Free weights, machines	1RM or maximal voluntary contraction		Observe for exaggerated pressor response (SBP >250 mmHg or DBP >115 mmHg).

*Measurements of particular significance; do not always indicate test termination.

TABLE 14.4

Hypertension: Exercise Programming

Modes	Goals	Intensity/Frequency/Duration	Time to goal
Aerobic Large muscle activities	■ Control BP at rest and during exercise ■ Improve coronary artery disease risk factors ■ Increase $\dot{V}O_{2max}$ and ventilatory threshold ■ Increase peak work and endurance ■ Increase caloric expenditure	■ 40-80% peak HR ■ 40-60% $\dot{V}O_2R$ or maximal HR reserve ■ RPE 11-13/20 ■ 4-7 days/week (if not all days of the week) ■ 30-60 min/session ■ 700-2000 kcal/week	4-6 months
Strength Circuit training	Increase strength	■ 1 set of 8-12 reps ■ 60%-80% 1RM	4-6 months

Important medications and precautions to consider during exercise programming include the following:

- Beta-blockers: Attenuate HR by ~30 contractions per minute.
- Alpha$_1$ blockers, alpha$_2$ blockers, calcium channel blockers, and vasodilators: May cause postexertional hypotension.
- People should not exercise with resting systolic BP >200 mmHg or diastolic BP >115 mmHg.
- Exercise is allowable when pressor response is well controlled by medications.
- Exercise at 40% to 70% $\dot{V}O_{2max}$ appears to lower resting BP as much as, if not more than, exercise at higher intensities.

- 700 kcal/week should be the initial goal; 2000 kcal/week should be the long-term goal.

Evidence-Based Guidelines

American Heart Association. AHA scientific statement: Evidence-based guidelines for cardiovascular disease prevention in women. Circulation. 2004;109:672-693.

Whitworth JA, World Health Organization, International Society of Hypertension Writing Group. 2003 World Health Organization (WHO)/International Society of Hypertension (ISH) statement on management of hypertension. J Hypertens. 2003 Nov;21(11):1983-1992.

Suggested Web Sites

American College of Cardiology. www.acc.org

American Heart Association. www.americanheart.org

CASE STUDY

Hypertension

A 56-year-old male was interested in starting an exercise program. He had no health complaints but did have hypertension and hyperlipidemia. He was also obese and met the criteria for the diagnosis of the metabolic syndrome. He had been sedentary for many years, did not smoke cigarettes, and had a family history of premature atherosclerosis.

S: "I think I should start an exercise program."

O: Vitals

Height: 5 ft 10 in. (1.78 m)
Weight: 210 lb (95.5 kg)
BMI: 30.2 kg/m^2 HR: 56 contractions/min
BP: 146/94 mmHg
Moderately obese male; no distress
No vascular changes on funduscopic exam; peripheral pulses nondelayed; no bruits
Normal heart sounds, nondisplaced ventricular apical impulse
Medications: Metoprolol SR 50 mg daily, Rosuvastatin 10 mg daily

Graded Exercise Test (Bruce Protocol)

Terminated at 6 min because of leg fatigue
Peak RPE: 18/20
Peak HR: 134 contractions/min
Peak BP: 192/96 mmHg
ECG: No significant ST changes; occasional PVCs
No chest discomfort reported

A: 1. Hypertension
    2. Hyperlipidemia
    3. Obesity
    4. Metabolic syndrome
    4. Sedentary lifestyle/deconditioning

P: Initiate an aerobic exercise program.

Exercise Program Goals

1. Improved blood pressure and pressor response to exercise
2. Weight management
3. Cholesterol control
4. Management of metabolic syndrome

Mode	Frequency	Duration	Intensity	Progression
Aerobic (treadmill, stationary cycling)	Start at 3 days/week	Start at 15 min/session Add ~5 min/week until 30-60 min session	40-59% of HRR (87-102 contractions/min) RPE 11-13/20	Build to 5-7 days/week.
Strength (all major muscle groups)	2-3 days/week	1 set of 10-15 repetitions of 8-10 different exercises	RPE 11-13/20	
Flexibility (anterior chest, hip flexors, plantarflexors)	3 days/week	15-30 s/stretch (all major muscle groups)	Maintain stretch below discomfort point	Progress as tolerated to at least 4 repetitions per muscle group.
Warm-up and cool-down	Before and after each session	2-3 min	RPE <11/20	

Peripheral Arterial Disease

Christopher J. Womack, PhD, FACSM ■ Andrew W. Gardner, PhD
Raha Nael, MD

OVERVIEW OF THE PATHOPHYSIOLOGY

Peripheral arterial disease (PAD) affects an estimated 8 million Americans and is associated with a high rate of morbidity and mortality. PAD is caused by atherosclerotic lesions in the arteries of the lower extremities that restrict blood flow distally. PAD can progress to critical limb ischemia and is associated with a two- to sixfold increased risk of coronary artery disease and a four- to five fold increased risk of cerebrovascular events. Primary modifiable risk factors associated with PAD include cigarette smoking, dyslipidemia, and diabetes; nonmodifiable risk factors include race and age. The prevalence of PAD is significantly higher in blacks than all other races, and with advancing age, especially in those 65 years of age or older.

A common symptom of PAD is intermittent claudication, which is characterized as an aching, cramping pain in the calves, thighs, and buttocks resulting from exercise (especially walking or running) that subsides with rest. However, only a small percentage (≈10%) of individuals with PAD develop the classic symptoms of intermittent claudication (exercise-induced aching, cramping pain in the lower extremities relieved by rest); ≈40% won't develop any signs or symptoms of intermittent claudication and the remaining 50% will experience atypical signs or symptoms. The symptoms associated with intermittent claudication are caused by inadequate blood supply to the muscles as a result of atherosclerosis. The severity of PAD may be classified into the following categories:

- Grade 0 = asymptomatic
- Grade 1 = intermittent claudication
- Grade 2 = ischemic rest pain
- Grade 3 = minor or major tissue loss from the foot

Primary care physicians should be diligent in screening patients who are considered at risk for PAD, because the majority of people with PAD are asymptomatic (Grade 0). Techniques used to diagnose PAD include a medical history, physical exam, ultrasound, X-ray angiography, and magnetic resonance imaging angiography (MRA). Another useful diagnostic assessment for PAD is the ankle-brachial index (ABI). The ABI uses Doppler or pulse volume waveform analysis along with a standard sphygmomanometer to record resting systolic pulse pressures of the posterior tibial and dorsalis pedis arteries and the brachial artery. A normal ABI score is >1.0, whereas a score of <1.0 is abnormal. Diagnostic ABI scoring criteria are as follows:

- Less than 0.95: Significant narrowing of one or more blood vessels in the legs is indicated.
- Less than 0.8: Pain in the foot, leg, or buttock may occur during exercise (intermittent claudication).
- Less than 0.4: Symptoms may occur during rest.
- 0.25 or below: Severe limb-threatening PAD is probably present.

EFFECTS ON THE EXERCISE RESPONSE

The primary effect of PAD during a single exercise session is the development of claudication pain due to insufficient blood flow to meet the metabolic demands of the leg musculature. Time or distance, or both time and distance, to onset and to maximal claudication pain during walking are used as criteria for assessing the functional severity of disease. Ankle systolic pressure and ABI are reduced following exercise because blood flow is shunted into the proximal leg musculature at the expense of the periphery and distal areas of the leg.

EFFECTS OF EXERCISE TRAINING

The role of exercise training in the prevention and treatment of PAD is well established. Individuals with PAD who attain high levels of physical activity have one-third the risk of mortality that their inactive counterparts have. Following a period of supervised exercise training, the majority of individuals with PAD report less severe claudication at any given level of work prior to initiating exercise training. Proposed mechanisms for an increase in exercise tolerance include the following adaptations:

- Increase in leg blood flow
- More favorable redistribution of blood flow
- Improved hemorheological and fibrinolytic properties of blood (e.g., reduced viscosity)
- Greater reliance upon aerobic metabolism because of a higher concentration of oxidative enzymes
- Less reliance upon anaerobic metabolism
- Improvement in the efficiency of walking economy and oxygen uptake kinetics
- Increased free-living daily energy expenditure

MANAGEMENT AND MEDICATIONS

Common medications for intermittent claudication include the following:

- Cilostazol (Pletal)
- Pentoxifylline (Trental)
- Hydroxymethyl glutaryl coenzyme A (HMG CoA) reductase inhibitors (statins)

- Plavix
- Aspirin

Cilostazol improves walking distance by 40% to 60% after 12 to 24 weeks. Cilostazol also improves ABI, walking ability, and quality of life. Pentoxifylline marginally improves pain-free and maximal walking distance but has no effect on ABI. HMG-Co-A reductase inhibitors (statins) are recommended to decrease low-density lipoprotein-cholesterol in patients with PAD to less than 100 mg/dl, and to less than 70 mg/dl in individuals at high risk for cardiovascular disease. Antiplatelet agents, including aspirin and Plavix, are recommended in those with PAD to lower risk of cardiovascular and cerebrovascular events and mortality. Aspirin lowers risk of cardiovascular death by 19% to 32% depending on the dosage. Plavix reduces risk of a cardiovascular event by 23% compared with aspirin.

The interaction of exercise training and medication therapy for treatment of intermittent claudication is not well understood. Cilostazol and pentoxifylline can affect exercise testing by improving time to onset of claudication symptoms. Individuals who have been taking these medications for longer than three months can undergo exercise testing while on their normal regimen. However, people who start these medications less than three months are recommended to refrain from taking them until after exercise testing.

Individuals with PAD also take medications for related forms of cardiovascular disease or related risk factors (e.g., hypertension, hyperlipidemia, diabetes), which can affect exercise testing. For example, persons taking beta-blockers may experience a decrease in time to onset of claudication and a decrease in maximal heart rate response to exercise. However, patients should continue their normal regimen on these medications prior to exercise testing to better ensure consistency in test data and to enhance safety.

RECOMMENDATIONS FOR EXERCISE TESTING

The primary objectives of graded exercise testing for individuals with PAD are as follows:

- To obtain reliable measures of claudication pain times
- To obtain reliable measures of ankle pressure following exercise
- To assess whether coronary artery disease is present

- To obtain information that can be used to set exercise prescription (see table 15.1)

The preferred mode for exercise testing for this population is the treadmill. The following are the procedures for treadmill testing individuals with PAD:

- Ankle and brachial systolic blood pressures are measured and ABI is calculated after the client has been in a supine position for 15 min.
- Blood pressure is measured in both arms and in the posterior tibial and dorsalis pedis arteries of both legs (via Doppler). The artery yielding the higher systolic pressure in each leg is used for the measurement of ankle systolic pressure, and the higher pressure between the two arms is used to calculate ABI.

- An exercise test with gradual increments in percent grade is then performed. Small increments in grade allow claudication times of clients to be stratified according to disease severity. A highly reliable protocol uses a constant speed of 2 mph (3.2 km/h) and an increase in grade of 2% every 2 min beginning at 0% grade.
- A validated pain scale ranging from 0 to 4 (0 = no pain, 1 = onset of pain, 2 = moderate pain, 3 = intense pain, and 4 = maximal pain) is used to assist clients in identifying progression of claudication pain during the test to maximal pain (a score of 4). The time elapsed from the start of exercise to each pain score is recorded. Holding on to the handrails is discouraged, except for brief moments to maintain balance, because this alters metabolic demands, resulting in changes

TABLE 15.1

Peripheral Arterial Disease: Exercise Testing

Methods	Measures	Endpoints*	Comments
Aerobic Treadmill (1-2 METs/stage; preferred)	▪ Time to pain onset ▪ Time to maximal pain ▪ BP, HR, ankle systolic BP after test ▪ 12-lead ECG	▪ Serious dysrhythmias ▪ >2 mm ST-segment elevation or depression ▪ Ischemic threshold ▪ T-wave inversion with significant ST-segment change	▪ Use 4-point claudication scale. ▪ Cycle protocol can underestimate the severity of PAD.
Functional and endurance 6 min walk (majority of patients)	▪ Time of pain onset ▪ Total walking distance	SBP >250 mmHg or DBP >115 mmHg	Use 4-point claudication scale.
Neuromuscular Short Physical Performance Battery Score	Time to walk 4 m; time to complete 5 sequential sit-to-stand transfers; time to hold side-by-side, semitandem, and full-tandem standing positions	Inability to stand from a chair	Quartile scores obtained on the following tasks: 4 m walk, repeated chair rise, standing balance.

*Measurements of particular significance; do not always indicate test termination.

in physiological responses that cause variability in claudication times. Heart rate and brachial blood pressure are recorded during the last minute of each 2 min exercise stage.

- The client recovers in a supine position for 15 min. The time elapsed from the start of recovery to the relief of claudication pain (a score of 0) is recorded. Ankle and brachial blood pressures are recorded throughout the recovery period.

- Use of indirect calorimetry during treadmill testing can alter the client's perception of claudication pain. Repeated tests should be consistent with regard to whether indirect calorimetry is used.

If treadmill testing equipment is not available, the 6 min walk is an excellent alternative for measuring improvements in onset to claudication and maximal distance walked.

The following are special considerations for exercise testing:

- Patients have a high risk for CAD.
- This patient group has a high prevalence of smoking.
- Diabetic neuropathy can mimic claudication.
- Skin ulcers are common in individuals with resting leg pain (Grade 2).

RECOMMENDATIONS FOR EXERCISE PROGRAMMING

Exercise programs for persons with PAD should be designed with a goal of improving claudication pain symptoms and reducing cardiovascular risk factors (see table 15.2). The type of exercise training recommended to improve the signs or symptoms of claudication in individuals with PAD is unique in relation to any other chronic health condition, since exertion to the point of leg pain is required for maximum benefits. Most individuals with PAD should engage in interval walking, pole striding, or

TABLE 15.2

Peripheral Arterial Disease: Exercise Programming

Modes	Goals	Intensity/Frequency/ Duration	Time to goal
Aerobic Large muscle activities (walking highly preferred)	■ Improve pain response, increase walking time and grade achieved on graded exercise test ■ Decrease cardiac risk factors ■ Increase duration before intensity	■ 40-60% $\dot{V}O_{2peak}$, HR reserve ■ Intermittent walk to 3 (out of 4) on claudication scale ■ 3-5 days/week ■ Begin at ≥15 min/session and progress by 5 min every 4 weeks to achieve 30-60 min/session	3-6 months
Functional and endurance Home-based walking	Improve time to onset of pain and 6 min walk distances; improve ADLs and quality of life	Accumulation of ≥30 min of walking daily	3-6 months
Neuromuscular	Improve Short Physical Performance Battery Score	Resistance training: at least 2 days/week 1-2 sets (10-12 reps) of lower and upper body exercise	3-6 months

stair climbing three times a week, at an intensity that causes pain with a score of 3 on a 4-point scale. The onset of claudication should occur in approximately 5 min; full recovery is allowed between intervals. This type of program may start with 20 min of exercise per session at 40% of heart rate reserve and gradually progress to 40 min at 70% of heart rate reserve over a period of about six months. Non-weight-bearing tasks (e.g., cycling) may be used for warming up and cooling down.

There are circumstances in which it is inappropriate for clients with PAD to exercise:

- Exercise training should not be performed until medical clearance, based on a physical exam, blood screening, and graded exercise test, has been completed.

- Exercise should not be performed when there are concomitant comorbidities that may limit exercise tolerance.

Special considerations for exercise programming include the following:

- Improvement in functional capacity may unmask coronary ischemia.

- Changes in comorbidities should be monitored.

- Cold weather may worsen symptoms, necessitating a longer warm-up.

Evidence-Based Guidelines

Hirsch AT, Haskal ZJ, Hertzer NR, et al. ACC/AHA 2005 guidelines for the management of patients with peripheral arterial disease. Circulation. 2006;113(11):e463-654.

Suggested Web Sites

American College of Cardiology. www.acc.org

American Diabetes Association. www.diabetes.org

American Heart Association. www.americanheart.org

National Heart, Lung, and Blood Institute. www.nhlbi.nih.gov

Peripheral Arterial Disease Coalition. www.padcoalition.org/wp

Society for Vascular Medicine. www.svmb.org

Vascular Disease Foundation. www.vdf.org

Vascular Web: Provided by the Society for Vascular Surgery. www.vascularweb.org

CASE STUDY

Peripheral Arterial Disease

A 65-year-old man with history of hypertension, hyperlipidemia, and tobacco use presented with the complaint of cramping and fatigue of his left calf and buttocks with ambulation, which interfered with his ability to work as a mail carrier. The patient noted a significant decrease in his walking ability over the previous year and frequently stopped to relieve the pain. The patient denied pain at rest. He had also developed erectile dysfunction. He was sent to the exercise laboratory for evaluation of intermittent claudication. After the evaluation, he wished to enroll in an exercise program.

S: "The cramps in my left calf and buttocks interfere with my ability to work."

O: Vital signs

Height: 5 ft 10 in. (178 cm)
Weight: 220 lb (100 kg)
BMI: 31.6 kg/m²
RHR: 72 contractions/min
BP: 150/90 mmHg (no blood pressure difference between the two arms)
Medications: Lisinopril 20 mg once daily, Simvastatin 40 mg once daily

Vascular Examination

Neck: Evidence of carotid bruits bilaterally
Cardiac: Regular rate and rhythm
Abdomen: No abdominal bruits, no pulsatile mass
Extremity: 1+ dorsalis pedis (DP)/posterior tibialis (PT) pulses on the left, 2+ DP/PT pulses on the right, evidence of hair loss over the left lower extremity, no evidence of ulcerations
Left ankle/brachial index: 0.70
Right ankle/brachial index: 0.89

Graded Exercise Test

Continuous treadmill at 2.0 mph, 0.0% grade increasing 2% every 2 min
Time to onset of claudication pain: 510 s
Time to maximal claudication pain: 956 s
Free-living daily energy expenditure as measured by accelerometer: 300 kcal/day
6 min walk distance: 1250 ft (231.6 m)

Laboratory

Blood lipids: Total cholesterol, 213 mg/dl; high-density lipoprotein cholesterol, 31 mg/dl; triglycerides, 165 mg/dl; low-density lipoprotein cholesterol, 149 mg/dl

A: 1. Peripheral arterial disease with intermittent claudication
2. Decreased functional capacity caused by early-onset claudication

P: 1. Initiate a treadmill exercise program.
2. Consider starting Cilostazol and antiplatelet medications.
3. Smoking cessation.

Exercise Program Goals

1. Increased time to claudication onset and maximal pain
2. Increased free-living energy expenditure
3. Increased functional capacity

Follow-Up

The six-month rehabilitation program increased the time to onset of claudication pain by 5 min, and the patient no longer terminated the test due to maximal claudication pain. His free-living daily activity increased from 300 kcal/day to 550 kcal/day. One year after completing the formal rehabilitation program, he maintained a 4 min improvement in time to onset of claudication and still did not terminate the test due to maximal claudication pain. Patient was able to resume his job as a mail carrier.

Mode	Frequency	Duration	Intensity	Progression
Aerobic Walking on indoor track lightly touching rail, treadmill	3-7 days/week	15 min/session	60% of $\dot{V}O_{2peak}$ Elicit 3 (of 4) claudication pain	Increase duration by 5 min every 4 weeks to achieve 45 min/session.
Functional and endurance	Daily walking	≥30 min	Elicit 3 (of 4) claudication pain	Progress as tolerated.
Strength	3 days/week	1-2 sets of lower and upper body exercise	10-12 reps/set	Progress as tolerated.
Warm-up and cool-down	Before and after each session	5-10 min	RPE <11/20	

16

Aneurysms

Jonathan N. Myers, PhD, FACSM

OVERVIEW OF THE PATHOPHYSIOLOGY

An aneurysm is a localized dilation or bulge of a blood vessel caused by disease or weakening of an arterial vessel wall, particularly at branching points. Aneurysms typically occur in arteries at the base of the brain and in the aortoiliac region. The cause of most aneurysms is largely unknown; however, congenital defects, acquired diseases, and postinfection or trauma may be contributing factors. The majority of aneurysms have no associated symptoms and frequently are not discovered until they rupture or cause symptoms due to localized pressure on an adjacent tissue. Aneurysms are considered a disease of aging, with a peak incidence rate between 40 and 60 years. Aneurysms are most threatening when they progressively enlarge, develop a tear in the arterial wall (dissection), or suddenly rupture. The possibility of these events applies to any aneurysm, regardless of location in the body.

Aneurysms are most prominent and significant in the aorta. The enlargement usually occurs in a well-defined location, although some regions of this long artery are more susceptible than others. The aortic root (the point where the vessel leaves the heart) is one such region. The abdominal aorta (where the artery branches off to supply the kidneys) is the most common site for developing an aneurysm, affecting between 4% and 8% of men and 0.5% to 1.5% of women over the age of 60; this condition is commonly known as abdominal aortic aneurysm disease. Other regions of the aorta can enlarge at different ages depending on the disease process.

Another common site for aneurysms is within the brain; an aneurysm at this site is known as a cerebral or intracranial aneurysm. Cerebral aneurysms occur in approximately 2% to 5% of the population. Most cerebral aneurysms cause no symptoms or illness during the person's entire life. However, neurologic problems can occur if the aneurysm enlarges, causing increased pressure on a particular area of the brain. A rupture of the aneurysm (cerebral hemorrhage) can cause severe disability or death; or it may cause mild, reversible damage, treatable by medication, surgery, or both. The rupture of an artery in the brain (known as a hemorrhagic stroke) is associated with a 32% to 67% fatality rate and 10% to 20% long-term dependence in survivors due to brain damage.

Although aneurysm enlargement is usually without symptoms, common risk factors associated with cardiovascular disease greatly increase the risk of aneurysm occurrence, enlargement, and rupture. Most aneurysms are acquired; examples are abdominal aortic aneurysms associated with hypertension, atherosclerosis, and other chronic diseases. Cigarette smoking and high blood pressure are the most common risk factors for abdominal aortic aneurysms in older adults. In particular, smoking is associated with a fivefold increase in abdominal aortic aneurysm risk in men. Other causes of aneurysms include inflammation, infection, and injury

Acknowledgment
The editors wish to acknowledge the previous authors of this chapter, Geoffrey Moore, MD, FACSM; and Peter H. Brubaker, PhD, FACSM.

to the aorta (especially deceleration injuries as in automobile accidents). Aneurysms can be acquired from iatrogenic causes, mainly as a complication of surgical attempts to dilate a vessel with atherosclerosis. The most common site for this complication is the coronary arteries, since these vessels commonly undergo angioplasty procedures.

The main congenital cause of aortic aneurysms is Marfan's syndrome. Individuals with Marfan's syndrome often are tall and lanky and have deformities such as scoliosis (curvature of the spine), pectus excavatum (inward-shaped or funnel chest), overly flexible joints, and dislocation of the eye lens. Marfan's syndrome is caused by a genetic defect in the microfibrils forming the elastic fibers of large arteries, as well as in similar microfibrils that give strength and structure to some connective tissues. Marfan's syndrome causes the aortic root to dilate immediately above the aortic valve. As dilatation progresses, the aortic valve may begin to leak (aortic regurgitation), and the risk of dissection increases.

EFFECTS ON THE EXERCISE RESPONSE

Early in the course of aneurysmal disease when dilation is minimal, there is usually no effect on the exercise response. Even in individuals with existing aneurysms, there is likely to be little change in the exercise response other than a delay and blunting in pulse pressure. Indeed, it is more likely that exercise will affect an aneurysm than that the aneurysm will alter the exercise response.

Biomechanical modeling of flow through an aortic aneurysm suggests that exercise training may have detrimental effects on the progression of the disease. Pulsatile flow through an aneurysm creates vortices and turbulence within the aneurysm that markedly increase wall stress. In theory, this may contribute to endothelial damage and stimulation of the inflammatory phase of atherogenesis. However, regular exercise training is known to favorably modify the systemic inflammatory state, and the vascular shear stress caused by moderate exercise training has been demonstrated to improve endothelial function in radial, femoral, and coronary arteries. While regular exercise training may improve hemodynamic conditions and potentially regress aneurysm size, this has not been tested in a scientifically rigorous fashion.

Exercise training has, in rare circumstances, been associated with aneurysm dissection or rupture. This complication has been reported for cerebral,

aortic, renal, and coronary arteries; and any artery is theoretically at risk. In most case reports of such incidents, it was not known whether the aneurysm was present prior to the onset of symptoms. The authors of a study of patients with abdominal aortic aneurysms undergoing maximal exercise testing reported one rupture 12 h after the test (an event rate of 0.4%). Because this was a retrospective survey of a selected population, however, the true risk is not known. Therefore in certain cases, pharmacologic stress testing may be more appropriate for patients with aneurysms than exercise stress testing. Dobutamine stress has not been shown to be associated with aneurysm instability or rupture among subjects with intracranial or abdominal aortic aneurysms.

Athletes with Marfan's syndrome have died while playing sports, including the volleyball Olympic gold medalist Flo Hyman. Such high-profile events have increased the awareness of Marfan's syndrome among team physicians; but, more importantly, they underscore the need for caution when one is managing the exercise training program of a client with aneurysmal disease.

EFFECTS OF EXERCISE TRAINING

Little is known regarding the risks of exercise training in individuals with an aneurysm. In theory, because acute exercise increases blood pressure, the tension on the aneurysm wall increases and thus the risk of dissection or rupture for an already weakened aneurysm is subsequently increased. However, intermittent periods of increased wall stress through regular exercise training have been shown to improve vascular function and possibly even diminish aneurysm expansion rates. Exercise training also has favorable effects on the major risk factors for aneurysm disease (e.g., blood pressure, inflammatory markers, and lipids). In addition, studies have shown that patients in chronic sedentary states (those with spinal cord injury, amputation) are at higher risk for abdominal aortic aneurysm disease. Thus, there is justification for recommending moderate exercise training in these patients. Furthermore, asymptomatic (and undiagnosed) aneurysms are common in the elderly, who in many cases have undoubtedly participated in rehabilitation exercise training programs safely for many years without knowledge of the condition. In light of the paucity of data on the effects of training on aneurysm disease, a conservative approach to exercise training is appropriate, and frequent follow-up with the patient's physician to monitor aneurysm progression is warranted.

MANAGEMENT AND MEDICATIONS

Because aneurysms often go undiagnosed until a serious event such as a rupture occurs, many efforts have been made to assess the mortality benefits and cost effectiveness of screening for abdominal aortic aneurysms. A recent U.S. Preventive Services Task Force recommended that all men between the ages of 65 and 75 with a history of smoking be screened for the disease with ultrasonography. The prevalence of aneurysm is lower in women, and thus a disagreement exists regarding the appropriateness of screening for this disease, although some data suggest that women >65 years with a history of smoking or heart disease should be screened.

For individuals diagnosed with an aneurysm, the key step in medical management is to follow the progress of the enlarged area. This might involve echocardiography, abdominal ultrasound, magnetic resonance imaging, or (less commonly) angiography. The next most important step in managing these patients is to aggressively treat the risk factors that underlie the disease. This includes smoking cessation; lowering blood pressure; and lipid, diabetes, and obesity management. Medications for individuals with aneurysms primarily involve those needed to control cardiovascular risk.

- A beta-adrenergic blocking drug, such as atenolol or propranolol, is ideally suited to blood pressure management because the drug also reduces the strength of arterial pulses. Even those with a low-normal baseline blood pressure should be treated with a beta-blocker if there is not a contraindication to this medicine.
- Statins are commonly prescribed because of their moderating influence on lipids and inflammatory markers.

Aneurysm diameter is progressive in many patients, and the decision regarding surgery for aneurysm repair should be made by a vascular surgeon when appropriate. Given that aneurysms most commonly occur among elderly individuals, there are likely to be other medications used for the various comorbidities prevalent in this population (e.g., other cardiovascular conditions such as coronary artery disease or peripheral vascular disease, hypertension, diabetes).

RECOMMENDATIONS FOR EXERCISE TESTING

Almost all patients about to undergo abdominal aortic aneurysm surgery require preoperative risk assessment (cardiac clearance) prior to the procedure. Limited retrospective data suggest that the risk of complication is low for diagnostic exercise testing prior to surgery. Although maximal exercise testing for individuals with an abdominal aortic aneurysm <5.0 cm is likely to be quite safe, those with known intracranial aneurysms of any type should not undergo maximal exercise testing. Dobutamine stress echocardiography or adenosine nuclear myocardial profusion SPECT (single-photon emission computed topography) testing is often used in place of exercise testing to assist in gaining clearance for surgery. Submaximal exercise tests can be used to optimize therapeutic control of heart rate and blood pressure. In particular, avoiding a substantial increase in the rate–pressure product (HR × systolic blood pressure) is important, as this is a measure of stress on the arteries. Exercise testing can help in adjusting medications so that pulse rate does not rise above 100 contractions per minute (in adults). Virtually no data are available regarding the likelihood that an increase in rate–pressure product will cause an aneurysm to rupture; but in theory, the larger the aneurysm, the more vulnerable it may be to such an occurrence. Thus, testing endpoints should be conservative. Maximal strength testing is contraindicated due to the increased pressure imposed on the body during this type of exercise (thereby raising heart rate and blood pressure to dangerous levels).

RECOMMENDATIONS FOR EXERCISE PROGRAMMING

The recommended modes of exercise training for individuals with aneurysmal disease are limited. In general, contact sports and competition should be avoided. Sports that have low cardiovascular demand, such as bowling, are recommended by the American College of Cardiology for clients with aneurysmal disease. The larger the diameter of the aneurysm relative to the normal diameter of the vessel, the more exercise training should be restricted. In any case, any aerobic activity should be performed at a moderate to low intensity. For individuals taking beta-adrenergic blocking drugs, heart rate is not a good guide of intensity unless the peak heart rate has been ascertained by way of a graded exercise test. If peak heart rate is unknown, perceived exertion scales should be used. Moderate resistance exercise (low resistance) is appropriate for abdominal aortic aneurysms, but resistance training should be avoided for cerebral aneurysms since this type of exercise can markedly increase blood pressure (see table 16.1).

Persons with Marfan's syndrome who have joint involvement should not perform flexibility training (e.g., some yoga positions) because this may risk joint dislocation. Some yoga activities may be useful, however, for blood pressure control (see table 16.2). Those with Marfan's syndrome are also likely to have orthopedic concerns such as joint contractures, hypermobility, scoliosis, hyperlordosis, and kyphosis.

SPECIAL CONSIDERATIONS

One management difficulty with aneurysmal disease is in advising individuals who want to exercise at higher levels, in particular those who wish to engage in competitive sport. Indeed, some people with Marfan's syndrome may be particularly suited to competitive sports because of their stature and flexibility. Unfortunately, the very sports for which these individuals have a predisposition (e.g., basketball) involve body contact and extreme elevation of the rate–pressure product. Furthermore, high doses of beta-blocking medications are likely to decrease aerobic performance, needed for intense competitive sports. The psychological characteristics that lead to athletic success may present problems with adherence to recommendations for limiting these

TABLE 16.1

Aneurysm: Exercise Testing

Methods	Measures	Endpoints	Comments
Aerobic Cycle (ramp protocol 10-15 W/min or 20-30 W/2 min stage) Treadmill (ramp or Naughton protocol)	▪ 12-lead ECG ▪ HR ▪ BP ▪ RPE ▪ Chest pain and dyspnea scales	Endpoint should be conservative; use submaximal testing if appropriate.	Conservative protocols are most suitable.
Endurance Time trial (e.g., 6 min walk)	Distance	Time	Assess low-level exercise endurance.
Strength Not recommended			Increases HR and BP to dangerous levels.
Flexibility Goniometry Sit and reach	ROM		
Functional capacity Balance		Assess need for occupational or physical therapy.	

TABLE 16.2

Aneurysm: Exercise Programming

Modes	Goals	Intensity/Frequency/ Duration	Time to goal
Aerobic Large muscle activities (walking, swimming, cycling)	Increase peak work, endurance, and time to exhaustion	■ 30-40 min ■ 3-4 days/week ■ Emphasize duration over intensity	4-6 months
Strength Not recommended for individuals with cerebral aneurysms Moderate resistance exercise appropriate for abdominal aortic aneurysms		Low resistance should be utilized if resistance training is incorporated	Increases HR and BP to dangerous levels.
Flexibility Stretching	Increase or maintain ROM		
Neuromuscular Gait or balance training	Improve gait (for joint disorders)		
Functional performance Activity specific	Maintain ADLs		

activities and may warrant the involvement of an expert in sport psychology. While individuals with an abdominal aortic aneurysm can safely tolerate typical exercise intensities (50% to 70% of heart rate reserve), those with a cerebral aneurysm generally should avoid heart rates above 100 contractions per minute.

Evidence-Based Guidelines

Hirsch AT, Haskal ZJ, Hertzer NR, et al. ACC/ AHA 2005 guidelines for the management of patients with peripheral arterial disease. Circulation. 2006;113(11):e463-654.

Johnston SC, Higashida RT, Barrow DL, et al., Committee on Cerebrovascular Imaging of the American Heart Association Council on Cardiovascular Radiology. Recommendations for the endovascular treatment of intracranial aneurysms: A statement for healthcare professionals from the Committee on Cerebrovascular Imaging of the American Heart Association Council on Cardiovascular Radiology. Stroke. 2002;33(10):2536-2544.

Suggested Web Sites

American College of Cardiology. www.acc.org

American Heart Association. www.americanheart.org

CASE STUDY

Abdominal Aortic Aneurysm

A 75-year-old male with a history of heavy smoking, hypertension, hyperlipidemia, renal insufficiency, obesity, and abdominal aortic aneurysm was referred for an exercise test as part of a study on the effects of exercise therapy on abdominal aortic aneurysm expansion rates. A sonogram revealed a distal aortic aneurysm of 4.2 cm diameter. He was asymptomatic but reported doing very little activity.

S: "I feel OK, but I know I have a lot of health problems and I'd like to try and become healthier."

O: Vitals

HR: 69 contractions/min
BP: 136/86 mmHg Weight: 215 lb (97.7 kg)
Height: 5 ft 10 in. (1.77 m)
BMI: 30.8 kg/m^2
Abdominal bruit; femoral pulses intact and nondelayed
Medications: Atenolol, amlodipine, atorvastatin, ASA

Graded Exercise Test: Individualized Ramp Treadmill Protocol

2.7 METs (40% of age predicted)
Peak HR: 138 contractions/min

Peak BP: 182/100 mmHg
Terminated due to shortness of breath
No significant ST change during exercise or recovery; occasional PVCs

A: 1. Low exercise tolerance secondary to:
- History of smoking
- Vascular disease
- Deconditioning
2. Abdominal aortic aneurysm (no vascular compromise)

P: 1. Initiate an exercise training program.
2. Refer to smoking cessation program.
3. Reassess aneurysm size in 6 months.

Exercise Program Goals

1. Improve exercise capacity.
2. Monitor risk factors including smoking, lipids, body weight, and hypertension.
3. Special considerations: Monitor changes in aneurysm size.

Mode	Frequency	Duration	Intensity	Progression
Aerobic	3-7 days/week	5 to 10 min intervals	THR (50-65% $\dot{V}O_{2max}$) RPE 10-12/20	Advance to 15-20 min sessions in 3-4 weeks. Progress to goal of 30-45 min total.
Strength				Begin light strength training after 1 month.
Flexibility	3-5 days/week	20 s/stretch		
Neuromuscular				
Functional				
Warm-up and cool-down	Before and after each session	5-10 min	RPE <10	

PART III

Pulmonary Diseases

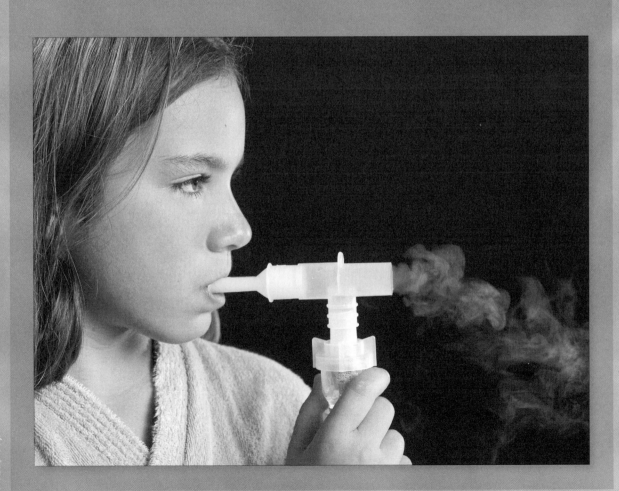

Chronic Obstructive Pulmonary Disease

Christopher B. Cooper, MD, FACSM

OVERVIEW OF THE PATHOPHYSIOLOGY

Chronic obstructive pulmonary disease (COPD) is a progressive lung disease resulting in persistent airway obstruction due to chronic bronchitis, emphysema, or both. COPD is characterized by small-airway inflammation and peribronchiolar fibrosis, eventual irreversible airway obstruction, marked difficulty in breathing, wheezing, and a chronic cough. The primary cause of COPD is cigarette smoking. In fact, an estimated 80% of individuals with COPD are current or former smokers. Other risk factors include occupational and environmental pollutants, alpha$_1$ antitrypsin deficiency, allergies and asthma, poor nutrition, periodontal disease, and low birth weight; COPD is also most commonly found in white men over 60 years of age. COPD is currently the most common lung disease, affecting an estimated 24 million Americans, and is the fourth leading cause of death in the United States. By the year 2020, COPD is projected to be the third leading cause of death for both males and females and the fifth leading cause of disability worldwide.

Besides the obvious impairment of ventilation and gas exchange and accompanying shortness of breath (dyspnea), the systemic effects of COPD are largely the result of compensatory responses to a damaged respiratory system. Pathophysiological consequences of COPD include the following:

Ventilatory Impairments

- Increased airway resistance causing air flow obstruction, mainly during expiration due to a decrease in airway size as lung volume decreases. The air flow obstruction in smoking-related chronic bronchitis slowly progresses over several decades.

- Reduced lung elastic recoil and thus increased compliance in the presence of emphysema, contributing to air flow limitation, air trapping, and hyperinflation.

- Increased work of breathing necessary to overcome the increased airway resistance.

- Ventilatory muscle weakness due to hyperinflation, which places the inspiratory muscles at a mechanical disadvantage.

- Ventilatory inefficiency due to increased dead space (wasted) ventilation. This is reflected in an increase in the ratio between physiological dead space and tidal volume (VD/VT).

- Ventilatory muscle fatigue resulting from increased work of breathing, ventilatory muscle weakness, ventilatory inefficiency, or a combination of these factors.

- Ventilatory failure with inadequate alveolar ventilation, hypoxemia, and hypercapnia. This condition arises in the later stages of very severe COPD.

Abnormalities of Gas Exchange

- Chronic bronchitis causes ventilation–perfusion ($\dot{V}/\dot{Q}$) inequality, whereas emphysema causes destruction of the alveolar-capillary membrane with increased alveolar dead space and loss of diffusing capacity. Each of these abnormalities impairs pulmonary gas exchange.

- High $\dot{V}/\dot{Q}$ abnormalities amount to increased alveolar dead space (wasted ventilation) with increased ventilatory requirement and increased work of breathing that can contribute to ventilatory limitation in some cases.

- Low $\dot{V}/\dot{Q}$ abnormalities amount to venous admixture (wasted perfusion), which causes hypoxemia. The hypoxemia usually worsens during exercise.

Cardiovascular Impairments

- Reduced physical activity often leads to cardiovascular deconditioning, to which individuals with COPD are particularly susceptible.

- Reduced pulmonary vascular conductance occurs due to reflex pulmonary vasoconstriction in response to chronic hypoxemia as well as to destruction of pulmonary capillary bed by emphysema. As a result of the increased pulmonary vascular resistance, the right ventricle is unable to respond adequately to the demand for increased cardiac output during exercise.

Muscular Impairments

- Peripheral muscle deconditioning, which is an inevitable consequence of reduced physical activity in COPD.

- Muscle wasting and weakness are also present due to inactivity and malnutrition. In some individuals with COPD, these problems are made worse by systemic corticosteroid therapy.

Symptomatic Limitations

- Breathlessness (dyspnea) is a frightening symptom with a complex etiology. Dyspnea results from a summation of neurological inputs from chemoreceptors and from mechanoreceptors in the lungs, chest wall, and limbs. Some people have dyspnea that is disproportional to their mechanical limitations or gas exchange failure.

Psychological Disturbances

- Chronic anxiety afflicts many individuals with COPD because of the frightening nature of their symptoms.

- Depression sometimes follows from limited ability to pursue normal daily activities with resulting social isolation, feelings of helplessness, and despair.

EFFECTS ON THE EXERCISE RESPONSE

One crucial aspect of COPD related to the exercise response is hyperinflation that results from impeded exhalation, incomplete lung emptying, and air trapping. Hyperinflation can be static (i.e., measured at rest) due to both reduced lung elastic recoil and increased airway resistance. However, during exercise, additional dynamic hyperinflation is superimposed on static hyperinflation, with further reduction in inspiratory capacity, smaller tidal volume, and higher operational lung volumes with increased elastic and threshold work of breathing. Dynamic hyperinflation has been shown to relate to increases in breathing frequency and occurs even in mild and moderate COPD (FEV_1 >50%). More importantly, dynamic hyperinflation affects the mechanical efficiency of ventilation and is directly linked to the development of breathlessness. Marked changes occur in the pattern of daily physical activity in individuals with COPD compared with age-matched controls. Furthermore, reductions in daily walking time occur early in the course of the disease and constitute an important component of disease progression.

Some individuals with COPD have true ventilatory limitation whereby the ventilatory requirement at maximum exercise equals the ventilatory capacity that can be measured over 12 or 15 s (maximal voluntary ventilation) or calculated from spirometry. This phenomenon might simply result from reduced ventilatory capacity due to mechanical factors, but it is important to assess whether ventilatory limitation is in part due to increased ventilatory requirement through increased VD/VT (wasted ventilation), deconditioning, or both.

In the absence of true ventilatory limitation, exercise can be limited by cardiovascular factors including deconditioning, impaired left ventricular function due to hypoxemia, or reduced pulmonary blood flow secondary to chronic hypoxemia. Peripheral muscle deconditioning can lead to lactic acid accumulation at low work rates, increased CO_2 output from bicarbonate buffering, and consequently an increased ventilatory requirement (which compounds the situation). Impairment of gas exchange occurs in emphysema because of destruction of the alveolar-capillary membrane.

This worsens breathing efficiency by increasing VD/VT and also may cause hypoxemia during exercise, particularly when increases in pulmonary blood flow increase shunting through areas of incomplete gas exchange. Chronic hypoxemia also causes erythrocytosis, and the resulting increase in blood viscosity can further compromise the circulation during exercise. In smokers, increases in carboxyhemoglobin, which does not carry oxygen, impairs blood oxygen transport. Finally, in some people, symptoms (predominantly dyspnea) and psychological factors might limit exercise capacity independently.

EFFECTS OF EXERCISE TRAINING

Almost any level of physical activity including exercise can result in favorable improvements in oxygen utilization, work capacity, and anxiety in individuals with COPD. The following are some of the benefits of exercise for this population:

- Cardiovascular reconditioning
- Reduced ventilatory requirement at a given work rate
- Improved ventilatory efficiency
- Reduced hyperinflation
- Desensitization to dyspnea
- Increased muscle strength
- Improved flexibility
- Improved body composition
- Better balance
- Enhanced body image

The accomplishment of these changes requires careful attention to medications to obtain optimal respiratory mechanics, and may require use of oxygen therapy to maintain adequate oxygenation during exercise.

MANAGEMENT AND MEDICATIONS

The primary objectives of medical management for individuals with COPD are to reduce breathlessness, increase exercise capacity, and improve quality of life. Important secondary objectives are to prevent and treat exacerbations, slow disease progression, and prolong survival. Because individuals with COPD have some degree of physical deconditioning, exercise training is a crucial aspect of clinical management and rehabilitation. The specific goals of management are the following:

- Optimization of respiratory system mechanics by careful attention to bronchodilator therapy, inhaler dosage, and technique
- Correction of hypoxemia whether it occurs at rest, during exercise, or during sleep
- Exercise training to correct physical deconditioning, reduce lactic acidosis, and reduce ventilatory requirement during exercise
- Desensitization to dyspnea, fear, and other potentially limiting symptoms
- Breathing retraining to improve ventilatory efficiency
- Energy conservation through improved coordination, balance, and mechanical efficiency during activities of daily living

All but the last goal are directed toward enabling an individual to perform exercise at higher intensity, thus increasing the potential for obtaining a reconditioning effect from exercise training.

Persons with COPD are often taking several medications that could have implications for exercise testing and training. Furthermore, COPD often coexists with cardiovascular diseases such as coronary artery disease, hypertension, and peripheral arterial disease. The potential effects of medications for these conditions are described in the chapters on the particular condition.

- Selective beta$_2$-adrenoceptor (sympathomimetic) agonists relax bronchial smooth muscle and produce bronchodilation by increasing cyclic adenosine monophosphate (cAMP) and can be considered short acting (SABA: e.g., albuterol, terbutaline, and metaproterenol) or longer acting (LABA: e.g., salmeterol and formoterol). However, they also reduce peripheral vascular resistance and tend to cause tachycardia, palpitations, and tremulousness. Nonselective sympathomimetic drugs (e.g., epinephrine and isoprenaline) should not be used because of unwanted effects on the cardiovascular system.
- Methylxanthines (e.g., theophylline and aminophylline) have potent bronchodilator action but also cause tachycardia, cardiac dysrhythmias, and central nervous system stimulation with increased respiratory drive and the risk of seizures.
- Thiazide diuretics (e.g., hydrochlorothiazide) and loop diuretics (e.g., furosemide) are prescribed to control fluid retention in cor pulmonale. Intravascular volume depletion might cause hypotension during exercise. Hypokalemia might predispose

clients to cardiac dysrhythmias and muscle weakness.

- Glucocorticoids (e.g., prednisone) are prescribed for COPD with the hopes of reducing inflammation and improving pulmonary function. Many individuals with COPD end up on long-term glucocorticoid therapy. Important side effects that influence exercise include skin atrophy and fragility, osteoporosis, muscle atrophy, and myopathy (including the ventilatory muscles).

- Antidepressants (e.g., tricyclics), like many psychotropic drugs, cause resting and exercise tachycardia.

RECOMMENDATIONS FOR EXERCISE TESTING

Exercise testing is extremely valuable in individuals with COPD to distinguish among the possible causes of limited exercise capacity. It is also essential to identify coexistent exercise-induced hypoxemia, hypertension, cardiac dysrhythmias, or myocardial ischemia. Maximal exercise testing is safe with appropriate monitoring and gives the best definition of the limitations, including psychological problems and symptoms. The cycle ergometer offers the best means of controlling external work rate, measuring gas exchange, and blood sampling. A typical protocol might include 3 min of unloaded pedaling followed by a ramp increase in work rate of 5, 10, 15, or 20 W/min, depending on the degree of impairment. Treadmill testing might be more readily accepted by patients and relate better to everyday activities. A near-linear increase in work rate should be attempted with use of incremental adjustments of speed and grade. With either mode of exercise testing, the aim should be to obtain between 8 and 12 min of exercise data.

A constant work rate protocol on a cycle or treadmill ergometer can be used repetitively to compare physiological responses to an identical exercise stimulus. A submaximal constant work rate test of high enough intensity to cause lactic acid accumulation and fatigue offers the best means of showing improvements after therapeutic interventions including exercise training. Valid measures would include exercise endurance time and physiological measures after a standard time interval (iso-time). Treadmill exercise testing is also helpful for the oxygen-dependent person and can be repeated with different oxygen systems and flows to determine the best means of correcting hypoxemia (see table 17.1).

Several functional exercise tests have been utilized in COPD, the most popular of which is the 6 min walking test. Although these tests are difficult to standardize and are strongly influenced by patient motivation, they are quick and easy to perform with few resources.

RECOMMENDATIONS FOR EXERCISE PROGRAMMING

Exercise should be encouraged for all individuals with COPD. The exercise prescription should be individualized and flexible to account for fluctuations in clinical status. Any significant change in the medical condition of the person requires reassessment of the goals and risks of the exercise program.

Exercise rehabilitation should involve several different professionals. Respiratory therapists evaluate, teach, and ensure effective use of bronchodilator medications and oxygen therapy. Physical therapists and exercise professionals evaluate exercise endurance, muscle strength, flexibility, and body composition in addition to determining and adjusting the exercise prescription and demonstrating and supervising techniques for improving flexibility, balance, and muscle strength. Occupational therapists evaluate activities of daily living and quality of life and teach energy conservation and improved body mechanics aimed at reducing the oxygen requirement for specific activities. All therapists teach improved breathing efficiency using methods such as pursed lips and diaphragm breathing, which slow the respiratory rate.

The recommended mode of exercise training can be walking, cycling, swimming, or conditioning exercises based on energy centering and balance, such as tai chi (see table 17.2). The mode of exercise selected should be one that is enjoyable and that directly improves ability to perform usual daily activities. In addition to the accepted specificity of training effect in terms of muscle performance, there is some evidence that desensitization to dyspnea is task specific.

Oxygen should be administered during exercise to individuals who have a documented reduction in arterial oxygen tension to less than 55 mmHg or in oxyhemoglobin desaturation to less than 88%. Prevention of exercise-induced hypoxemia is likely to improve exercise capacity as well as enhance the effects of exercise training. The goal of oxygen therapy during exercise is to maintain oxyhemoglobin saturation above 90%.

TABLE 17.1

Chronic Obstructive Pulmonary Disease: Exercise Testing

Methods	Measures	Endpoints*	Comments
Aerobic Cycle (preferred) (ramp protocol 10, 15, or 20 W/min; staged protocol 25-50 W/3 min stage) Treadmill (1-2 METs/stage)	▪ 12-lead ECG, HR ▪ BP ▪ RPE (6-20), dyspnea scale (0-10) ▪ Pulse oximetry/arterial PaO_2 ▪ Respired gas analysis ▪ Blood lactate	▪ Serious dysrhythmias ▪ >2 mm ST-segment depression or elevation ▪ T-wave inversion with significant ST change ▪ SBP >250 mmHg or DBP >115 mmHg ▪ Maximum ventilations ▪ $\dot{V}O_{2peak}$ ▪ Lactate orventilatory threshold	▪ Clients with COPD often have coexistent CAD. ▪ Breathing pattern analysis may also be helpful. ▪ Lactic acidosis may contribute to exercise limitation in some patients.
Endurance 6 min walk	Distance	Note rest stop distance/time, dyspnea index, vitals	Useful for measurement of improvement throughout program.
Strength Isokinetic or isotonic	▪ Peak torque ▪ Maximum number of reps ▪ 1RM		5 or 10 RMs are acceptable for those unable to perform the 1RM.
Flexibility Sit and reach	Hip, hamstring, and lower back flexibility		
Neuromuscular Gait analysis Balance	▪ Gait speed, distance ▪ Berg Balance Scale ▪ Ashworth Scale ▪ Modified Fatigue Impact Scale		Body mechanics, coordination, and work efficiency are often impaired.
Functional Sit to stand Stair climbing Lifting	Time to 10 reps		

*Measurements of particular significance; do not always indicate test termination.

TABLE 17.2

Chronic Obstructive Pulmonary Disease: Exercise Programming

Modes	Goals	Intensity/Frequency/Duration	Time to goal
Aerobic Large muscle activities (walking, cycling, swimming)	■ Increase $\dot{V}O_{2peak}$ ■ Increase lactate threshold and ventilatory threshold ■ Become less sensitive to dyspnea ■ Develop more efficient breathing patterns ■ Facilitate improvement in ADLs	■ RPE 11-13/20 (comfortable, pace and endurance) ■ Monitor dyspnea ■ 1-2 sessions, 3-5 days/week ■ 30 min/session (shorter intermittent exercise sessions may be necessary initially) ■ Emphasize progression of duration more than intensity	2-3 months to ensure completion
Strength Free weights Isokinetic/isotonic machines	■ Increase maximal number of reps ■ Increase isokinetic torque/work ■ Increase lean body mass	■ Low resistance, high reps 2-3 days/week	2-3 months
Flexibility Stretching Tai chi	Increase ROM	3 days/week	Ongoing
Neuromuscular Walking, balance exercises Breathing exercises	Improve gait, balance Improve breathing efficiency		

Modifications to the duration and frequency of exercise might be necessary. Commonly the person with chronic respiratory disease is unable to sustain 20 or 30 min of exercise, and interval exercise consisting of 5 or 10 min sessions might be necessary until adaptations have occurred that allow reduction of rest intervals and gradual increases in work intervals.

An intensive six-week exercise program with group interaction is helpful to begin the process of physical reconditioning. However, the importance of maintaining a higher level of physical activity cannot be overemphasized. The individual with COPD is at particular risk of relapsing into a state of inactivity and physical deconditioning. Rehabilitative exercise should therefore be lifelong, and membership in a health and fitness facility is worth considering.

Evidence-Based Guidelines

Ries AL, Bauldoff GS, Carlin BW, et al. Pulmonary rehabilitation: Joint ACCP/AACVPR evidence-based clinical practice guidelines. Chest. 2007;131(5):4S-42S.

Suggested Web Sites

American Association of Cardiovascular and Pulmonary Rehabilitation. www.aacvpr.org

American Lung Association. www.lungusa.org

CASE STUDY

Chronic Obstructive Pulmonary Disease

A 52-year-old male presented to his primary care physician for a routine history and physical examination. He had no known prior medical history and took no regular medications. He complained, however, of feeling more breathless on exertion that he had been accustomed to in the past. He also had an occasional cough in the morning productive of mucoid sputum. He smoked about 15 cigarettes per day from age 18 until 30 but then quit and worked all his life as a furnace maintenance man in a steel factory.

S: "I think I am becoming out of shape."

O: Vitals

HR: 80 contractions/min
BP: 140/90 mmHg
Weight: 176 lb (80 kg)
Height: 5 ft 11 in. (1.80 m)
BMI: 24.7 kg/m^2
Exam: Male, well nourished and apparently healthy in appearance
Chest configuration normal, percussion normally resonant; breath sounds diminished with prolonged exhalation phase
Heart sounds regular without murmur; no increased jugular venous pressure or peripheral edema
Truncal obesity; mild degree of muscle wasting affecting all limbs
Chest X ray: Mildly hyperinflated
Medications: No regular medications

Pulmonary Function Tests

FVC: 95% of predicted
FEV$_1$: 65% of predicted with 16% improvement after bronchodilator

FEV$_1$/FVC: 68%
DL$_{CO}$: 72% of predicted

Arterial Blood Gas

pH: 7.43
PCO$_2$: 41 mmHg
Po$_2$: 78 mmHg (breathing room air)

Graded Exercise Test (Treadmill)

Starting settings: 1.0 mph, 1% grade
Maximum settings: 9.0 mph, 8% grade
Duration: 10 min (equal speed increments of 0.9 mph)
$\dot{V}O_{2peak}$: 1.76 L/min (74%); $\dot{V}O_2\theta$ 0.95 L/min (LLN 1.00 L/min).
HR$_{max}$: 165 contractions/min; $\dot{V}_{Emax}$: 120 L/min (75%)
Arterial PO2 decreased to 65 mmHg
RPE: 16/20; breathlessness: 92/100 (visual analog scale)

A: 1. Moderate COPD secondary to tobacco smoking and occupational dust exposure
   2. Deconditioning with marked symptomatic limitation during exercise
   3. Excess fat weight with loss of lean body mass

P: 1. Introduce Combivent MDI 2 puffs as needed up to four times daily.
   2. Substitute tiotropium DPI 18 μg once daily if patient is using Combivent every day.
   3. Recommend a personal exercise program with aerobic and resistance exercise prescriptions.

Exercise Program Goal

Improve functional capacity to increase activities of daily living and restore more normal lifestyle.

Mode	Frequency	Duration	Intensity	Progression
Aerobic	3 days/week	30 min/session	THR (110 contractions/min) RPE 11/20	Progress as tolerated over 6-week program to 13/20 RPE
Strength (upper and lower extremities)	2 days/week	2 sets of 12 reps	To fatigue	Add resistance until 12 reps achieves fatigue
Flexibility	3 days/week	Hold 20-60 s/stretch	Below discomfort point	Progress as ROM allows
Neuromuscular (walk drills, balance drills, breathing exercises)	Daily	5 min each	As tolerated	Maintain skill level
Functional (O.T.)	If needed for ADL tasks	Match to ADL tasks as needed	As tolerated	As tolerated
Warm-up and cool-down	Before and after each session	10 min	RPE <10/20	Maintain

18

Chronic Restrictive Pulmonary Disease

Connie C.W. Hsia, MD

OVERVIEW OF THE PATHOPHYSIOLOGY

Chronic restrictive pulmonary disease (CRPD), also known as interstitial lung disease (ILD), comprises a group of chronic lung disorders that cause inflammation and scarring (fibrosis) of the lungs. CRPD is characterized by reduced lung volume, loss of lung compliance, incomplete lung expansion, and increased lung stiffness. A variety of disorders cause reduction or restriction of lung volumes; however, a common characteristic of CRPD regardless of exact etiology is reduced lung volume. The different disorders of CRPD are caused by various pathological processes involving the chest wall, respiratory muscles, nerves, pleura, and the pulmonary parenchyma and exhibit common pathophysiologic features, including those discussed in the following sections.

Extrapulmonary Restrictive Disorders

Extrapulmonary restrictive disorders don't affect the lungs per se but instead restrict the ability of the lungs to expand normally. Any impairment of lung expansion makes it difficult for the lungs to maintain sufficient air exchange by reducing lung volume and the ability to move air into the lungs. A common physiological adaptation to extrapulmonary restrictive lung disorders is rapid, shallow breathing that over time can lead to atelectasis. Extrapulmonary restrictive disorders include the following:

- Neuromuscular and neurologic disorders
- Muscular muscle disorders (muscular dystrophy, myositis)
- Neural disorders (phrenic nerve paralysis, neuritis)
- Neuromuscular junction disorders (myasthenia gravis, botulism, Eaton-Lambert syndrome)
- Spinal cord disorders such as amyotrophic lateral sclerosis and Guillain-Barré syndrome and those caused by trauma
- Chest wall disorders: kyphoscoliosis, ankylosing spondylitis, thoracoplasty, obesity
- Pleural disorders: fibrosis, effusion

Pulmonary Parenchymal or Interstitial Disorders

This group of disorders is caused by damage followed by inflammation or scarring of the lung parenchyma and connective tissue, resulting in filling of the air spaces with exudate and debris (pneumonitis). There are over 100 different pulmonary parenchymal lung disorders, most of which can be classified according to the cause:

- Inhaled substances: both inorganic (i.e., asbestosis) and organic (hypersensitivity pneumonitis) sources
- Drug induced: antibiotics, antiarrhythmic agents
- Connective tissue disease: lupus, rheumatoid arthritis
- Infection: pneumonia, tuberculosis
- Idiopathic: idiopathic pulmonary fibrosis
- Malignancy

Gas Exchange Abnormalities

In parenchymal lung diseases, alveolar-capillary units are destroyed or replaced by fibrous tissue. In diseases involving the pleura, chest wall, and neuromuscular system, the lung is intrinsically normal but unable to expand normally with respiration. Eventually alveolar units collapse and secondary inflammation and fibrosis develop. The common end result is a loss of alveolar surface area, leading to impaired oxygen diffusion. Diffusion impairment is evidenced by a reduced rate of gas uptake from alveolar air to pulmonary capillary red cells, a decline in arterial oxygen saturation, and a widened alveolar–arterial oxygen tension gradient. Diffusion impairment is commonly measured as lung diffusing capacity for carbon monoxide (DL_{CO}).

Mechanical Ventilatory Dysfunction

Air flow rates are reduced in proportion to the reduction in lung volume. The ratio of forced expiratory volume in 1 s to forced vital capacity (FEV_1/FVC) is normal or elevated. Ventilatory muscle strength, endurance, and mechanical efficiency are reduced especially in neuromuscular and skeletal diseases of the thorax, evidenced from reductions in maximal respiratory muscle strength and ventilatory capacity. Compliance of the lung or thorax is reduced. A more negative airway pressure is required to inflate the stiffer lung with each breath; hence, respiratory muscles must work harder (i.e., work of breathing is elevated). Dead space is increased, so minute ventilation must be higher to maintain a given level of alveolar ventilation, further increasing the work of breathing. A greater fraction of total body metabolic energy must be diverted to respiratory muscles to sustain a given level of ventilation, leaving a smaller fraction available for working limb muscles during exercise. This leads to greater lactic acid production from limb muscles, further stimulating ventilation and increasing work of breathing.

Secondary Hemodynamic and Cardiac Dysfunction

Any pathologic process that obliterates the pulmonary vascular bed increases pulmonary vascular resistance and right ventricular afterload, resulting in a higher pulmonary artery pressure (secondary pulmonary hypertension), right heart strain, and a lower stroke volume during exercise. Because the lungs surround the heart, they form a potential cavity called the cardiac fossa. A stiff lung reduces the compliance of the cardiac fossa and can potentially restrict diastolic ventricular filling, especially during exercise. Cardiovascular deconditioning inevitably develops with progressive pulmonary disease and contributes to disproportional disability out of keeping with the impairment in lung function.

EFFECTS ON THE EXERCISE RESPONSE

Individuals with CRPD experience the following altered exercise responses:

- Reduced exercise tolerance and exertional dyspnea are common manifestations. The typical breathing pattern consists of rapid shallow breaths. Minute ventilation increases mainly via an increased respiratory rate rather than tidal volume.
- DL_{CO} is reduced and alveolar–arterial oxygen tension gradient increased. These abnormalities are more pronounced during exercise and are more sensitive indicators of diffusion impairment than measurements made at rest.
- Normally DL_{CO} increases by 40% to 60% with increasing cardiac output from rest to exercise, primarily as a result of the opening or distension of pulmonary capillaries that increases the surface area for gas exchange. The ability to increase DL_{CO} is essential for maintaining normal arterial oxygen saturation during exercise. Diffuse parenchymal disease such as interstitial pulmonary fibrosis is

characterized by an inability to augment DL_{CO} during exercise, associated with a marked decline in arterial oxygen saturation. In contrast, patients after major lung resection who have normal remaining lung units typically show a small lung volume; however, DL_{CO} increases normally with exercise and arterial oxygen saturation is better maintained.

■ In early extrapulmonary disease, DL_{CO} is typically reduced due to a small alveolar volume (VA), while the ratio of DL_{CO} to VA may be normal. In advanced stages, however, secondary pulmonary fibrosis often develops; then DL_{CO}/VA also becomes impaired. In parenchymal lung disease, DL_{CO}, VA, and DL_{CO}/VA are all reduced. Note that the DL_{CO}/VA ratio does not remain constant at all levels of VA, so the usefulness of the ratio diminishes in individuals with severe lung restriction.

EFFECTS
OF EXERCISE TRAINING

Exercise training can potentially have multiple benefits in restrictive lung disease, including the following:

■ Improved submaximal exercise endurance

■ Improved maximal oxygen uptake, variably, depending on existent fitness level

■ Improved ventilatory endurance, efficiency, and ventilation–perfusion matching

■ Improved cardiovascular conditioning

■ Increased maximal DL_{CO} secondarily if maximal cardiac output increases

■ Improved oxygen extraction, endurance, and efficiency of skeletal muscles

■ Reduced blood flow requirement of respiratory muscles, secondarily increasing blood flow available to working limb muscles

■ Reduced lactic acidosis and minimized stimulation of ventilation during exercise

■ Desensitization to the perception of dyspnea and fear of exertion

Physical training in individuals with CRPD significantly enhances the sense of well being, even if large increases of maximal oxygen uptake do not occur. Training ensures that the subjects are not debilitated more than expected from the pulmonary dysfunction, and that all steps of oxygen transport are matched within the constraints imposed by the primary disorder. Training optimizes the efficiency of oxygen transport—a critical issue, as patients can ill afford any metabolic energy wastage. Careful attention to long-term physical conditioning allows patients to realize the maximum benefit from concurrent specific therapy aimed at correcting the underlying disorder.

MANAGEMENT
AND MEDICATIONS

Restrictive lung disorders are often chronic and progressive; treatment is often empirical. Medical management for the treatment of the underlying physiological disorder includes the following:

■ Corticosteroids: Corticosteroids are prescribed for a wide variety of inflammatory disorders with the intention of reducing inflammation, retarding disease progression, and protecting lung function. Chronic therapy can lead to multiple complications including obesity, skin changes, systemic hypertension, hyperglycemia, loss of bone density leading to pathological fractures, muscle atrophy, gastrointestinal ulcers, immunosuppression, and emotional instability. Steroid-induced respiratory muscle atrophy can aggravate ventilatory insufficiency in severe lung disease.

■ Immunosuppressive agents: These drugs (e.g., azathioprine, cyclophosamide, methotrexate, penicillamine, and chlorambucil) are sometimes used to treat systemic immunological disorders. These agents can depress blood leukocyte count and predispose to opportunistic infections; some can directly cause pulmonary inflammation and fibrosis or aggravate existing fibrosis.

■ Supplemental oxygen is used to correct as necessary.

■ General health maintenance, aimed at optimizing body weight, blood pressure, and nutrition. In obese subjects, weight loss need not be drastic. Even a modest loss of 20 to 30 lb can dramatically relieve shortness of breath as well as improve mobility and the sense of well-being. Exposure to tobacco and environmental irritants should be reduced, and patients should be vaccinated regularly against respiratory pathogens.

RECOMMENDATIONS FOR EXERCISE TESTING

The goals of exercise testing for individuals with CRPD include the following:

- Defining disability due to pulmonary dysfunction
- Detecting coexisting factors that aggravate disability
- Monitoring progression of impairment and response to therapy

Either cycle ergometer or treadmill can be used. Following a resistance-free warm-up period, work rate should be incremented in small steps in accordance with the severity of impairment. Electrocardiogram and transcutaneous oxygen saturation should be monitored. Supplemental oxygen may be needed during testing to maintain the oxyhemoglobin saturation above 90%. Individuals unaccustomed to exercise, particularly on the cycle ergometer, should be coached in the pedaling techniques and allowed several practice runs until they are comfortable with the procedure. Meticulous attention to technical details such as proper seating, mouthpiece fitting, and breathing techniques, as well as verbal reinforcement during testing will greatly reduce subject anxiety and enhance the quality of the measurements (see table 18.1).

Special considerations during exercise testing are as follows:

- Worsening hypoxia may induce angina, dysrhythmias, or both.
- Monitoring of electrocardiogram, blood pressure, and oxygen saturation is essential.
- Spirometry and maximal voluntary ventilation are helpful in defining ventilatory limitations.
- Exercise testing during late morning or early afternoon is preferable.
- Patients should take medications as usual to obtain the best exercise performance.

RECOMMENDATIONS FOR EXERCISE PROGRAMMING

Evaluation and recommendations from the nutrition therapist, physical therapist, and occupational therapist are very helpful for understanding the subject's home environment and occupational and lifestyle constraints before one formulates an individualized exercise program. Simple maneuvers should be implemented first, such as learning efficient breathing techniques and improving ergonomics during daily activities to enhance metabolic energy conservation. Long-term exercise training cannot be sustained unless it is both practical and enjoyable. Maintaining subject motivation for exercise requires creativity and clear communication between the therapist and the subject.

Walking is probably the easiest mode of exercise for most individuals; it requires no special equipment, can be done at a leisurely pace, and is readily integrated into other activities of daily living. Similarly, arm and leg exercises can often be integrated with other sedentary activities such as watching television or reading (see table 18.2).

In sedentary subjects, an initial period of intense training (20-30 min/day, five days a week for six to eight weeks) is helpful in establishing a baseline level of fitness; subsequently, sustained training can be continued three times a week. For subjects with poor exercise endurance, a training session can be divided into several shorter segments with rest periods in between. Regular follow-up assessment of exercise and pulmonary function should provide objective feedback on any improvement or retardation of impairment, which helps to sustain the subject's motivation for continued training.

These are special consideration for exercise programming:

- Ratings of perceived exertion and dyspnea are the preferred methods of monitoring intensity. Patients who are unable to achieve a training heart rate can still show physiological improvement.
- Coexistent coronary artery disease, peripheral artery disease, and musculoskeletal problems (e.g., arthritis, osteoporosis) are common.
- Muscular dysfunction (including respiratory muscles) may be present.
- Clients usually respond to exercise best in mid to late morning.
- Extremes in temperatures and humidity should be avoided.
- Supplemental O_2 flow rate should be adjusted to an oxygen saturation (SaO_2) of >90%.
- Anxiety, depression, and fear are common due to dyspnea and physical disability.

TABLE 18.1

Chronic Restrictive Pulmonary Disease: Exercise Testing

Methods	Measures	Endpoints*	Comments
Aerobic Cycle (preferred) (ramp protocol 10, 15, or 20 W/min; staged protocol 25-50 W/3 min stage) Treadmill (1-2 METs/stage)	■ 12-lead ECG, HR ■ BP ■ RPE, dyspnea scale (0-10) ■ Pulse oximetry/arterial PaO$_2$ ■ Respired gas analysis ■ Blood lactate	■ Serious dysrhythmias ■ >2 mm ST-segment depression or elevation ■ T-wave inversion with significant ST change ■ SBP >250 mmHg or DBP >115 mmHg ■ Maximum ventilations ■ $\dot{V}O_{2peak}$ ■ Lactate or ventilatory threshold	■ Clients with COPD often have coexistent CAD. ■ Breathing pattern analysis may also be helpful.
Endurance 6 min walk	Distance	Note rest stop distance/time, dyspnea index, vitals	Useful for measurement of improvement through conditioning program.
Strength Isokinetic or isotonic	■ Peak torque ■ Maximum number of reps ■ 1RM		
Flexibility Sit and reach	Hip, hamstring, and lower back flexibility		
Neuromuscular Gait analysis Balance	■ Gait speed, distance ■ Berg Balance Scale ■ Ashworth Scale ■ Modified Fatigue Impact Scale		Body mechanics, coordination, and work efficiency are often impaired.
Functional Sit to stand Stair climbing Lifting	Time to 10 reps		

*Measurements of particular significance; do not always indicate test termination.

TABLE 18.2

Chronic Restrictive Pulmonary Disease: Exercise Programming

Modes	Goals	Intensity/Frequency/Duration	Time to goal
Aerobic Large muscle activities (walking, cycling, swimming)	■ Increase $\dot{V}O_{2peak}$ ■ Increase lactate threshold and ventilatory threshold ■ Become less sensitive to dyspnea ■ Develop more efficient breathing patterns ■ Facilitate improvement in ADLs	■ RPE 11-13/20 (comfortable, pace and endurance) ■ Monitor dyspnea ■ 1-2 sessions, 3-5 days/week ■ 20-60 min/session (shorter intermittent exercise sessions may be necessary initially) ■ Emphasize progression of duration more than intensity	2-3 months to ensure completion
Strength ■ Free weights ■ Isokinetic/isotonic machines	■ Increase maximal number of reps ■ Increase isokinetic torque/work ■ Increase lean body mass	■ Low resistance, high reps ■ 2-3 days/week	2-3 months
Flexibility ■ Stretching ■ Tai chi	Increase ROM	1-3 days/week	
Neuromuscular ■ Walking, balance exercises ■ Breathing exercises	■ Improve gait, balance ■ Improve breathing efficiency		

Evidence-Based Guidelines

Ries AL, Bauldoff GS, Carlin BW, et al. Pulmonary rehabilitation: Joint ACCP/AACVPR evidence-based clinical practice guidelines. Chest. 2007;131(5):4S-42S.

Suggested Web Sites

American Association of Cardiovascular and Pulmonary Rehabilitation. www.aacvpr.org/

American Lung Association. www.lungusa.org/

CASE STUDY

Chronic Restrictive Pulmonary Disease

Seven years ago, a 45-year-old African American female complained of episodic fever with sweats, fatigue, and a rash. She was found to have skin nodules and enlarged liver, spleen, and lymph nodes in the chest. Biopsies of these tissues revealed the diagnosis of sarcoidosis, a multisystem granulomatous inflammatory disease. Initially she had no respiratory complaints, but over the years she gradually developed worsening shortness of breath on exertion to the point that she could walk only 0.5 miles (0.8 km) on a flat surface or climb a single flight of stairs without stopping. Her lung volumes and expiratory flow rate (FEV_1) decreased steadily over the years, but diffusing capacity (DL_{CO}) decreased markedly. Although she continued to work full-time as an insurance clerk, she was easily fatigued. She had been treated with oral prednisone continuously since her diagnosis and as a result suffered from the side effects of obesity, hypertension, and hyperglycemia.

S: "I can't get around very well."

O: Vitals

Obese woman at rest, in no acute distress
Multiple flesh-colored skin nodules on face and legs
Bilaterally enlarged parotid glands and cervical lymph nodes
Lung sounds: Clear
Cardiovascular exam normal, no peripheral edema
Enlarged spleen and liver

Labs

Blood counts and electrolytes: Normal
Liver enzymes: Mildly elevated
Angiotensin-converting enzyme and gamma globulins: Grossly elevated
Chest X rays: Reticular interstitial infiltrates in both lungs

Spirometry

FVC: 3.0 L
FEV_1: 3.0 L
DL_{CO}: 12 ml · min^{-1} · mmHg^{-1}

A: 1. Active sarcoidosis involving lung, skin, liver, lymph nodes, and spleen
   2. Progressive deterioration of lung function

P: 1. Start low-dose methotrexate and reduce prednisone.
   2. Conduct exercise tests to measure aerobic capacity, ventilatory response, and arterial O2 saturation.
   3. Initiate a weight loss diet.
   4. Start a regular exercise program.

Exercise Program Goals

1. Aid in weight loss
2. Maintain long-term physical fitness

Mode	Frequency	Duration	Intensity	Progression
Aerobic	5 days/week	20-30 min/session	THR (110 contractions/min) RPE 11/20	Progress as tolerated over 6-8 week program to 13/20 RPE.
Strength (upper and lower extremities)	2 days/week	2 sets of 12 reps	To fatigue	Add resistance until 12 reps achieves fatigue.
Flexibility	3 days/week	Hold 20-60 s/stretch	Below discomfort point	Progress as ROM allows.
Neuromuscular (walk drills, balance drills, breathing exercises)	Daily	5 min	As tolerated	Maintain skill level.
Functional (O.T.)	Daily	Match to ADL tasks as needed	As tolerated	As tolerated.
Warm-up and cool-down	Before and after each session	10 min	RPE <10/20	Maintain.

Asthma

Christopher J. Clark, MD ■ Lorna M. Cochrane, MD

OVERVIEW OF THE PATHOPHYSIOLOGY

Asthma is now a major public health problem in the majority of developed countries worldwide. Asthma is a chronic respiratory disorder, characterized by reversible obstruction to air flow and increased bronchial responsiveness to a variety of stimuli, both allergic and environmental. Essential to the definition of asthma are the following characteristics: recurrent respiratory symptoms, variable air flow obstruction, presence of airway hyperreactivity, and chronic airway inflammation. In 2005, public health surveillance data estimated that 22.2 million Americans had asthma, including 6.5 million children <18 years of age and 15.7 million adults >18 years of age. Of particular concern has been the dramatic rise in asthma prevalence among children, especially those from low-income populations, minorities, and those living in inner cities. From 1980 to 1996, asthma prevalence in U.S. children increased by an average of 4.3% per year. Although the steady rise in the prevalence of childhood asthma has plateaued in recent years, asthma remains one the leading chronic childhood diseases in the United States.

The frequency, severity, length of occurrence, triggers, and symptoms of asthma vary significantly from one individual to another. Asthma can be a chronic respiratory impairment for some; for others, it is marked by symptomatic episodes only when provoked by stimuli such as allergens, stress, or exercise. The most common symptoms associated with an episode of asthma include coughing, chest tightness, shortness of breath (dyspnea), wheezing, and a rapid breathing rate. Although the etiology of asthma is not fully understood yet, both genetics and the environment are primary factors.

EFFECTS ON THE EXERCISE RESPONSE

Although aerobic exercise can by itself trigger an episode of asthma, commonly referred to as exercise-induced asthma (EIA), the majority of the literature suggests that exercise is not only safe and effective for individuals with asthma, but for some, exercise may in fact help control the frequency and severity of asthma attacks. Most studies support the idea that individuals with asthma who participate in an average of 20 to 30 min of aerobic exercise two to three times per week will improve maximal ventilation, oxygen consumption, work capacity, and heart rate. Furthermore, there is little evidence to support the notion that exercise worsens asthma symptoms or that there is any reason for the majority of individuals with asthma to avoid regular physical activity.

EIA is characterized by transient airway obstruction that usually occurs 5 to 15 min following physical exertion. Symptoms consist of wheezing, coughing, shortness of breath, chest discomfort, or a combination of these, lasting up to 30 min following the cessation of exercise. A small percentage of individuals with EIA experience a late reaction (i.e., a further episode of airway obstruction 4-6 h later). The mechanisms of EIA are not completely understood, but are likely related to respiratory heat loss, increased osmolality caused by respiratory water loss, or associated vascular events, all triggered by an increasing minute ventilation during exercise.

Although the prevalence of EIA in the general population is low (3-10%), nearly all individuals with diagnosed asthma will experience EIA at some point. Thus, when one considers exercise for individuals with asthma, it is helpful to group them into one of these categories:

- Exercise-induced asthma without other symptoms
- Mild asthma (ventilatory limitation does not restrain submaximal exercise)
- Moderate-to-severe asthma (ventilatory limitation restrains submaximal exercise)

The amount of physical exertion required to produce asthma symptoms is usually equivalent to a relative work rate of 75% age-predicted maximal heart rate. In individuals with severe asthma, however, very mild exertion can provoke severe air flow obstruction and trigger EIA. Although exercise may provoke an asthma episode, exercise should be incorporated in the treatment and medical management plan for persons with asthma.

When EIA is well controlled, there is no effect on the exercise response. In individuals with asthma who engage in submaximal exercise that is insufficient to induce asthma, the exercise response is essentially unaffected. At higher exercise intensities or with certain modes of exercise that induce an asthmatic response, the exercise response is proportional to the ventilatory limitation imposed by the restriction in air flow. In most cases, the symptoms of breathlessness are sufficient to cause the person to stop exercising. In any event, the induction of an asthma exacerbation signifies a need for more intensive medical management to prevent asthma attacks.

EFFECTS OF EXERCISE TRAINING

When planning an exercise program for individuals with asthma, it is important to know that asthma has intermittent exacerbations and remissions influencing the ability to exercise. The adaptability to training in individuals with asthma is similar to that of a response to a single exercise session. When EIA is well controlled, asthma has no effect on the adaptations to exercise training, and thus it is common to see favorable improvements in fitness when people with asthma adhere to a standard exercise program to improve fitness. When an individual with asthma experiences EIA at submaximal exercise levels, the exercise intensity is usually insufficient to increase fitness but may increase endurance.

Participating in sport can also be safe for individuals with asthma. Mild asthma allows participation in athletic competition even at the highest level, whereas severe asthma can markedly impair physical function. EIA occurs in various types of sports, most often in athletes competing in endurance sports in cold climates and those in sports involving other types of environmental hazards (e.g., swimmers inhale chlorine products in indoor swimming pools), but also among endurance athletes competing in summer sports. The estimated prevalence of EIA in world-class athletes is 2.8% to 14%.

MANAGEMENT AND MEDICATIONS

The use of a short-acting beta$_2$-agonist (e.g., Albuterol) approximately 10 to 15 min before exercise has been shown to reduce the risk of EIA in individuals with asthma. Long-acting beta$_2$-agonists (e.g., salmeterol and formoterol) extend the period of protection, although the length of time the drug remains active after a single dose may decrease. Physicians prescribe salmeterol only if other medications have not controlled a patient's asthma or if the patient's asthma is so severe that two medications are needed for control. Salmeterol should not be the first or the only medication used in a patient's treatment of asthma. A long-acting beta$_2$-agonist might be reserved for individuals who are physically active for more than 30 to 60 min/day and in cases in which objective measures of air flow obstruction demonstrate a late reaction. Effective protection from EIA is also provided by leukotriene receptor antagonists. Although these drugs are slightly less effective than sympathomimetics, leukotriene receptor antagonists have some practical advantages, including an effect lasting over 24 h, single daily-dose administration by mouth, no major adverse effects, and no development of tolerance (decrease in effect with time).

A variety of other agents have variable benefits against EIA. In individuals with asthma at rest who also show manifestations of EIA, prophylactic medication such as inhaled steroids should be used in combination with beta$_2$-agonist. Inhaled steroids reduce susceptibility to EIA when given over one to four weeks. Cromolyn sodium may be effective when given prior to exercise but is largely superseded by the effect of sympathomimetics. The increasing usage of asthma medications by athletes in competitive sport has led to studies of the ergogenic effects of such medications and has resulted in restrictions on their use based on international doping regulations. Both inhaled steroids and beta$_2$-agonist are allowed for use in athletes with "documented" asthma. The International Olympic Committee (IOC) and the committee's national affiliates require methacholine or other challenge testing to confirm the diagnosis of asthma before usage. Systemic sympathomimetics and steroids are not allowed according to IOC policies. Beginning in 1993, only the inhaled beta$_2$-agonist salbutamol and terbutaline were permitted by the IOC. However, subsequent studies demonstrated that additional beta$_2$-agonists (salmeterol, and formoterol) had no effect on performance enhancement and are consequently allowed for use in sport, as are oral leukotriene receptor antagonists. No effect has been found upon performance in cold air conditions in well-trained athletes.

Up to 40% of individuals with asthma experience a refractory period within an hour of a mild asthma attack. Within this refractory period, the resumption of an identical bout of exercise produces an airway response over 50% less than previously observed (i.e., resulting symptoms are either absent or mild). A possible mechanism for this reduction in ensuing symptoms may be due to mediator loss. Therefore mild exercise in the form of a warm-up prior to endurance training may be beneficial in preventing EIA. It should also be noted that any related condition such as sinusitis and nasal polyps should be treated to optimize exercise capability.

RECOMMENDATIONS FOR EXERCISE TESTING

In individuals with well-controlled asthma, standard exercise tests can be used to assess physical fitness and the response to exercise. In persons with asthma that is not diagnosed or not in control, exercise testing can be used to make the diagnosis or assess the quality of control. A common misconception is that EIA is distinct from other forms of asthma. In reality, many asthmatics suffer from EIA when formally given a challenge test. Testing for EIA can be erroneous unless several criteria are fulfilled:

- Intensity (75% predicted maximum heart rate or greater)
- Duration (8 min exercise at that intensity, following a warm-up period)
- Measurement of air flow obstruction 6 to 8 min after cessation of exercise

The delay in measuring air flow allows for the development of an immediate (type I) hypersensitivity response. EIA is defined as

- a fall in FEV_1 of 15% from baseline or
- a fall in peak flow of 20% from baseline.

Some people with asthma experience breathlessness during and after exercise despite medical treatment. These individuals require documentation of pre- to postexercise changes in peak flow, plus a progressive incremental exercise test to determine the specific cause of exercise limitation. However, this type of study is not steady state and thus may not be a substitute for the formal exercise challenge test specifically required to confirm the diagnosis of EIA (see table 19.1).

TABLE 19.1

Asthma: Exercise Testing

Methods	Measures	Endpoints	Comments
Aerobic Cycle Treadmill (constant-load test)	▪ 12-lead ECG, HR ▪ BP ▪ RPE, dyspnea scale (0-10) ▪ Spirometry before and 8 min after exercise	▪ 8 min at ≥75% max HR ▪ Decreased FEV_1 of 15% ▪ Decreased peak flow of 20%	▪ Provide adequate warm-up. ▪ No inhalers or oral bronchodilators.

Methylxanthines, sympathomimetic bronchodilators and loop and thiazide diuretics may improve exercise capacity through bronchodilation, relief of congestive heart failure, and psychotropic effects. However, potential side effects associated with these medications include the following:

- Methylxanthines: May cause tachycardia, cardiac dysrhythmias, and increased dyspnea.

- Sympathomimetic bronchodilators: May cause tachycardia.

- Loop and thiazide diuretics: May cause hypokalemia leading to dysrhythmias and muscle weakness.

Special considerations during exercise testing include the following:

- Running more readily provokes EIA than jogging, which in turn is more asthmogenic than walking.

- Clients have a higher risk for coronary artery disease. Worsening hypoxia during exertion may include angina, dysrhythmias, or both.

- Monitoring of 12-lead electrocardiogram, blood pressure, and oxygen saturation is essential.

- Spirometry, especially maximal voluntary ventilation, is helpful in defining ventilatory limitations.

- Testing in mid to late morning or afternoon is desirable. Chronic asthma patients often have worse symptoms in the early morning.

- Medications should be taken as usual to obtain best exercise performance, especially if test results will be used for exercise prescription purposes.

- Clients may be come more dyspneic when lifting objects. Specific evaluation and training may be necessary.

- Several minutes of warm-up and cool-down may help reduce the likelihood of EIA.

RECOMMENDATIONS FOR EXERCISE PROGRAMMING

An important factor to remember is that individuals with asthma have periods of intermittent exacerbations and remissions influencing their ability to exercise. The exercise professional must identify realistic outcome targets for the exercise program, which may include improvement in one or all of the following (see table 19.2):

- Fitness as judged by usual physiological criteria

- Exercise tolerance (but not necessarily improvement in physiological fitness)

- Musculoskeletal conditioning (i.e., daily kinetic function and activities of daily living)

Improved Fitness

Improving fitness requires participation in a standard aerobic training program, similar to that for sedentary apparently healthy subjects, with intensity, frequency, duration, and longevity prescribed according to American College of Sports Medicine (ACSM) recommendations. In practice, individuals with EIA only, or with mild asthma (American Thoracic Society [ATS]/European Thoracic Society criterion: $FEV_1 = 50\text{-}80\%$ of predicted), can typically participate in such programs. There should be a six-week introductory period during which the client learns to self-monitor exercise intensity.

Another recommendation to help individuals with asthma regulate exercise intensity is to use the Borg CR-10 scale or a visual analog scale to assess the intensity of breathlessness associated with physical activity (the Borg CR-10 scale developed for breathlessness is distinct from that used for perceived exertion and uses a 1 to 10 grading of dyspnea severity; see source in reference section). Familiarization with these self-assessment scales can reduce the fear of difficulty in breathing, especially when combined with optimal premedication and measurement of peak flow. If peak flow measurements indicate that EIA is not fully controlled, changes in medication should be considered before an extensive exercise program is undertaken. The importance of this preparatory process cannot be underestimated.

Improved Exercise Tolerance

Achieving improved exercise tolerance allows for greater flexibility in terms of exercise intensity, and is most appropriate for individuals with moderate to severe asthma. Nevertheless, the objective should be to encourage individuals with asthma to exercise at a work rate that represents a relatively high proportion of their maximal exercise tolerance (e.g., 60% of maximal work rate). Frequency, duration, and length of exercise training program are similar to ACSM recommendations for increased fitness in sedentary healthy persons.

For individuals with some restriction in exercise tolerance caused by ventilatory limitation, use of

TABLE 19.2

Asthma: Exercise Programming*

Modes	Goals	Intensity/Frequency/Duration	Time to goal
Aerobic Large muscle activities (walking, cycling, swimming)	▪ Increase $\dot{V}O_{2peak}$ ▪ Increase lactate threshold and ventilatory threshold ▪ Become less sensitive to dyspnea ▪ Develop more efficient breathing patterns ▪ Facilitate improvement in ADLs	▪ RPE 11-13/20 (comfortable, pace and endurance) ▪ Monitor dyspnea ▪ 1-2 sessions, 3-5 days/week ▪ 30 min/session (shorter intermittent exercise sessions may be necessary initially) ▪ Emphasize progression of duration more than intensity	2-3 months
Strength ▪ Free weights ▪ Isokinetic/isotonic machines	▪ Increase maximal number of reps ▪ Increase isokinetic torque/work ▪ Increase lean body mass	▪ Low resistance, high reps ▪ 2-3 days/week	2-3 months
Flexibility Stretching	Increase ROM	3 sessions/week	Ongoing
Neuromuscular ▪ Walking ▪ Balance exercises ▪ Breathing exercises	▪ Improve gait, balance ▪ Improve breathing efficiency	Daily	

*For individuals with EIA controlled by medications, or those with mild asthma (FEV_1 = 50-80% predicted), use ACSM recommendations for normal sedentary persons. For individuals with moderate asthma (FEV_1 = 30-50% predicted), use this table. For individuals with severe asthma (FEV_1 < 40% predicted), refer to chapter 19 text.

the Borg CR-10 scale for breathlessness allows a comfortable target level of exercise intensity. As a general rule, people with a moderate air flow obstruction (ATS/European Thoracic Society criterion: FEV_1 = 30-50% of predicted) are considered the prime target population for having the option of moving to higher-intensity exercise programs once they achieve tight control of their asthma. Programs should involve aerobic exercise (e.g., brisk walking, jogging, step-ups, rowing) using an intensity determined as "maximal tolerable" for required session duration.

Musculoskeletal Conditioning

The following recommendations are appropriate for musculoskeletal conditioning in individuals with asthma:

- For the most severely asthmatic individuals (ATS criterion: FEV_1 <30% predicted)
- As an introduction to exercise for previously very sedentary individuals
- During recovery from exacerbations that prevent participation in the usual program

Musculoskeletal conditioning can use circuit training exercises for the major limb muscle groups, either unloaded with relatively high-frequency exercises to build endurance and flexibility or loaded to build strength as an addition to endurance training. Both forms of exercise training improve performance in persons with chronic air flow obstruction and provide a range of performance requirements to address the needs of all but the most severe asthmatics.

Special considerations during exercise programming include the following:

- Ratings of perceived exertion and dyspnea are the preferred methods of monitoring intensity. Many patients are unable to achieve a high target heart rate but still show physiological improvement.

- Coronary artery disease, peripheral artery disease, and musculoskeletal problems (e.g., arthritis, osteoporosis) are common in older patients with chronic asthma.

- Muscular myopathy (including respiratory muscles) may be present due to corticosteroids and disuse atrophy.

- Patients usually respond best to exercise in mid to late morning.

- Extremes in temperature and humidity should be avoided.

- Supplemental O_2 flow rate should be adjusted to SaO_2 >90%.

- Anxiety, depression, and fear are common due to dyspnea and physical disability.

- Several minutes of warm-up and cool-down may reduce the likelihood of EIA.

Evidence-Based Guidelines

Joint American College of Chest Physicians/American Association of Cardiovascular and Pulmonary Rehabilitation evidence-based clinical practice guidelines. Chest. 2007;131(5).

Suggested Web Sites

American Lung Association. www.lungusa.org

European Respiratory Society. www.ersnet.org

Global Initiative for Asthma. www.ginasthma.com

National Heart Lung and Blood Institute. www.nhib.nih.gov

CASE STUDY

Asthma

A 22-year-old male city office worker has had a history of asthma since the age of 9 years. His job was sedentary, and he bought a bicycle; he was keen to cycle for leisure and to get to work, but found it difficult to improve his initially modest performance because of breathlessness. He was not clear whether this was due to his asthma or whether he was "quitting when the going got tough" and achieving less than he could if he ignored the breathlessness, considered it a normal response to starting demanding exercise, and kept going.

He was taking a regular steroid inhaler twice daily and had albuterol for episodes of wheezing. He sometimes found this helpful after exercise.

S: "I think my asthma may be limiting my cycling and ability to get fitter."

O: Vitals

Young man at rest, in no respiratory distress
Breath sounds normal, with no rhonchi or wheezes
Chest X ray: Normal lung fields with no evidence of hyper-inflation

Spirometry

FVC, FEV_1, and FEV_1/FVC: Normal
Residual volume: 116% of predicted (mild air trapping, indirect evidence of air flow limitation)
Dl_{CO}: Normal
Diurnal peak flow: <20% variability (night and morning)

Graded Exercise Test

FEV_1 measured after 6-8 min of exercise at ~75% predicted maximum HR

60% decrease in FEV_1 from starting value (98% predicted); repeated on medications (including inhaled albuterol 10 min beforehand)
6% decrease in FEV_1

Maximal Graded Exercise Test

Maximal HR: 184 contractions/min (96% of predicted)
Maximal minute ventilation: 85 L/min (65% of predicted)
$\dot{V}O_{2max}$: 41 ml $\cdot$ kg^{-1} $\cdot$ min^{-1} (57% of predicted)

Dynamic Kinematics

Normal isokinetic quadriceps strength and endurance

A: 1. Severe EIA
2. Moderate aerobic exercise tolerance, capable of improvement
3. Normal quadriceps strength

P: 1. Advise that aerobic activities such as cycling are likely to produce EIA.
2. Take premedication with a sympathomimetic agent such as albuterol at least 10 min prior to exercise.
3. Check peak flow prior to cycling. If symptomatic during cycling, stop and recheck. If peak flow has fallen, repeat sympathomimetic inhalation, and also adjust regular daily medication (by increasing inhaled steroid and/or adding a long-acting sympathomimetic agent or leukotriene antagonist).
4. Continue sporting activities and aspirations.

Exercise Program Goal

Maintain normal ADLs and improve exercise capacity by participation in cycling with self-management plan.

Mode	Frequency	Duration	Intensity	Progression
Aerobic	3-7 days/week	30-45 min/session	RPE 11-14/20	Maintain current level.
Strength	2-3 days/week	1-2 sets of 8-12	To fatigue	Maintain current level.
Flexibility	3-7 days/week	20-60 s/stretch	Maintain stretch below discomfort or pain threshold	Maintain current level.
Warm-up and cool-down	Before and after each session	10-15 min	RPE <10/20	Maintain.

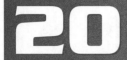

Cystic Fibrosis

Patricia A. Nixon, PhD, FACSM

OVERVIEW OF THE PATHOPHYSIOLOGY

Cystic fibrosis (CF) is the most common inherited life-shortening disease in white populations, occurring in 1 in 3500 live births. The genetic defect causes abnormal epithelial transport of chloride ions, excessive sodium ion resorption, and subsequent extracellular dehydration, resulting in abnormally salty sweat and thick mucus that clogs ducts, tubes, and tubules. The two organs most adversely affected by the mucus blockage are the pancreas and the lungs. In the pancreas, mucus prevents digestive enzymes from reaching the small intestine to digest fats and proteins, leading to malnutrition and poor growth. In the lungs, the thick mucus blocks the airways and leads to infection, inflammation, and eventually fibrosis and an irreversible loss of pulmonary function. The pulmonary involvement accounts for over 90% of the mortality.

EFFECTS ON THE EXERCISE RESPONSE

Many healthier persons with CF have normal aerobic fitness and normal cardiorespiratory responses to a single session of exercise. However, as the disease progresses and pulmonary function deteriorates, exercise tolerance diminishes. During exercise, individuals must use greater minute ventilation to compensate for airway obstruction and increased dead space. Consequently, the ratio of peak minute ventilation to maximal voluntary ventilation ($\dot{V}_E$/MVV) often exceeds the normal range of 60% to 70%, limiting mechanical ventilatory reserve. Most persons with mild to moderate lung disease are able to maintain adequate gas exchange, although those with more severe lung disease may exhibit oxyhemoglobin desaturation and carbon dioxide retention during exercise.

The likelihood that oxyhemoglobin desaturation will fall below 91% during exercise increases in persons with a forced expiratory volume for 1 s (FEV_1) of less than 50% of the predicted value. Peak heart rate may reach age-predicted maximal levels in healthier persons. However, ventilatory factors may prevent the cardiovascular system from being maximally stressed in persons with more severe lung disease, resulting in peak heart rates that are below age-predicted maximal values. In addition, exercise capacity may be limited by peripheral factors associated with deconditioning and malnutrition. In people with very severe lung disease, $\dot{V}_E$/MVV and heart rate (HR) at peak exercise may be well below normal, suggesting that factors such as chest pain, sensations of dyspnea, excessive coughing, or other peripheral factors may limit exercise. During submaximal exercise, oxygen consumption, minute ventilation, and HR may be disproportionately high, possibly as a result of physical deconditioning, airway obstruction, increased dead space, increased work of breathing, hypoxemia, or any combination of these factors.

EFFECTS OF EXERCISE TRAINING

Few randomized controlled trials have examined the effects of exercise intervention in persons with CF. In persons hospitalized for exacerbations of pulmonary infection, short-term aerobic exercise training has been shown to improve FEV$_1$, $\dot{V}O_{2max}$, body mass, fat-free mass, and quality of life. In-hospital strength training has been shown to increase musculoskeletal strength as well as FEV$_1$, body mass, and fat-free mass. Research examining long-term aerobic exercise training suggests that individuals with CF may derive the following benefits:

- Increase in physical work capacity and peak oxygen consumption
- Improvement in cardiopulmonary efficiency for a given submaximal work rate
- Increase in ventilatory muscle endurance
- Enhanced mucus clearance
- Temporary increase or delayed deterioration in some indices of pulmonary function

Higher levels of aerobic fitness have been associated with greater eight-year survival, although it is not known if survival probability can be improved via exercise training. Anaerobic exercise training has also been shown to improve $\dot{V}O_{2max}$, anaerobic performance (mean and peak power), and health-related quality of life.

MANAGEMENT AND MEDICATIONS

Standard treatment for individuals with CF now includes the following:

- Oral pancreatic enzyme supplements to enhance digestion of dietary fats and proteins and improve nutritional status
- Airway clearance techniques to facilitate mucus clearance
- Bronchodilator therapy to open airways
- Antibiotic therapy to fight pulmonary infection
- Yearly influenza vaccine

With a few exceptions, the effects of most of the medications (listed next) on exercise tolerance and responses to exercise have not been studied in persons with CF in a double-blind, randomized controlled trial. Consequently, their potential effects are speculative:

- Pancreatic enzyme supplements may indirectly improve exercise capacity by improving nutrition and growth.
- Inhaled bronchodilator (albuterol, ipratropium) therapy may cause bronchodilation and prevent bronchospasm; may or may not improve exercise tolerance; and may cause tachycardia, cough, and even greater bronchoconstriction.
- Oral bronchodilator (theophylline) therapy may cause tachycardia, ventricular dysrhythmia, and tachypnea.
- Inhaled sodium cromolyn and nedocromil in chronic and acute administration may improve exercise tolerance by diminishing or preventing exercise-induced bronchoconstriction.
- Corticosteroids (oral) used on a long-term basis may improve exercise tolerance by reducing bronchial hyperreactivity and inflammation; but they may retard growth, induce skeletal muscle (including ventilatory muscle) weakness, and myopathy that can reduce exercise capacity and increase blood pressure and blood glucose at rest and during exercise.
- Corticosteroids (inhaled) used on a long-term basis may improve exercise tolerance by reducing bronchial hyperreactivity and inflammation, but may cause effects similar to those of oral corticosteroids if systemically absorbed.
- Mucolytic therapy reduces the viscosity of mucus.
- Recombinant human deoxyribonuclease (DNase) effects on exercise tolerance are not well studied.
- Insulin may improve exercise tolerance in individuals with diabetes.
- Supplemental oxygen improves oxyhemoglobin saturation at rest and during exercise and improves cardiopulmonary efficiency (i.e., lower HR and minute ventilation) during submaximal and maximal exercise, but may not necessarily increase peak oxygen consumption or physical work capacity.

Optimal exercise test results may be obtained if persons undergo testing after airway clearance and bronchodilator therapy. However, some persons with CF have a negative or adverse response to bronchodilator therapy and consequently should not include it as part of their treatment.

RECOMMENDATIONS FOR EXERCISE TESTING

The following are the primary objectives for exercise testing persons with CF:

- To observe cardiorespiratory and metabolic responses to exercise
- To assess physical work capacity and aerobic fitness
- To observe oxyhemoglobin saturation during exercise
- To assess disease severity
- To provide a basis for prescribing exercise within safe limits
- To assess changes in fitness and cardiorespiratory responses to exercise that occur with disease progression or medical intervention (e.g., pharmacologic, exercise, or both)

Physical work capacity and aerobic fitness are ideally evaluated by a progressive maximal exercise test (see table 20.1). Peak HR cannot be estimated from age-predicted equations and therefore must be obtained from a maximal exercise test. Pediatric clients should be tested using a standard pediatric protocol that has established normative data for comparison (e.g., Godfrey protocol). Exercise testing equipment may need to be modified to accommodate children and smaller individuals.

Oxyhemoglobin saturation should be monitored particularly in clients with an FEV_1 less than 50% of the predicted value. If oxyhemoglobin desaturation occurs with the maximal test, a steady-state submaximal test or 6 min walk test should be performed, as it is not uncommon for greater desaturation to occur with sustained submaximal exercise. If the purpose of the exercise test is to provide a basis for prescribing exercise, persons who exhibit oxyhemoglobin desaturation at rest or during exercise should be tested while breathing supplemental oxygen. Termination of the test because of marked oxyhemoglobin desaturation (for instance, <80%) may be overly cautious, since no irreversible or harmful effects of short-term hypoxemia have been

TABLE 20.1

Cystic Fibrosis: Exercise Testing

Methods	Measures	Endpoints	Comments
Aerobic Cycle (preferred) (ramp protocol 10-15 W/min; staged protocol 25 W/3 min stage) Treadmill (1 METs/stage)	■ HR ■ BP ■ Pulse oximetry (SaO_2) ■ Respired gas analysis ■ Spirometry	■ Hypertensive response ■ $\dot{V}O_{2peak}$ ■ $\dot{V}O_{2max}$ ■ $\dot{V}_{Emax}$	SaO_2 <80% may occur
Anaerobic Wingate	■ Peak and mean power output ■ Percent of fatigue	30 s	May reflect nutritional status
Endurance 6 min walk	■ Distance ■ HR, SaO_2	6 min	Most useful in persons with very limited exercise tolerance and in persons who exhibit oxyhemoglobin desaturation with exercise

reported in this population. In severely ill persons for whom a maximal exercise test may be unduly stressful, submaximal steady-state exercise testing or self-paced walk tests (e.g., 6 min) may be useful for examining cardiorespiratory responses and oxyhemoglobin desaturation with exercise, or changes in response to intervention. Exercise may induce excessive coughing in some individuals, causing them to terminate exercise. However, the majority of persons, despite their obstructive lung disease, report leg fatigue as the reason for terminating exercise, particularly on the cycle ergometer.

The following are medications and special precautions to consider during exercise testing:

- Beta agonists have a bronchodilator effect in most persons but may cause tachycardia.
- Inhaled and oral corticosteroids reduce airway inflammation and bronchospasm; oral steroids may cause myopathy, diabetes, and hypertension.
- Cromolyn diminishes or prevents exercise-induced bronchospasm.
- Theophylline has a bronchodilator effect but may cause tachycardia, ventricular ectopy, and tachypnea.
- Ipratropium has a bronchodilatory effect but may cause tachycardia.
- Supplemental oxygen may prevent desaturation, attenuate HR and $\dot{V}_E$, and cause relative hypoventilation.
- Equipment adaptation may be necessary for small persons.
- Supplemental O_2 should be used in persons with hypoxemia if exercise tests are performed for the purpose of exercise programming.
- Premedication with bronchodilator therapy may provide optimal results.

RECOMMENDATIONS FOR EXERCISE PROGRAMMING

The major aims of exercise training are to improve physical functioning and quality of life. Many individuals with CF should be able to engage in continuous aerobic exercise for 20 to 30 min at a moderate intensity (i.e., at 60% to 80% of peak HR). Persons with severe lung disease may need to intersperse rest periods with exercise and may also require supplemental oxygen during training. Training may be better tolerated and optimal benefits gained if training is performed after airway

and bronchodilator therapy (in persons who have a positive response to bronchodilator therapy). Standard exercise equipment may need to be adapted to fit children and smaller individuals. Resistance training should be incorporated to preserve lean body mass. Clients should be encouraged to adopt lifestyle changes that include aerobic activities such as walking, jogging, biking, and swimming (see table 20.2). Exercise intensity may need to be altered during an exacerbation of pulmonary infection, which is commonly experienced by individuals with CF. During such times clients are most likely to attain their target HRs at a less intense workload.

Medications and special precaution to consider during exercise programming include the following:

- Bronchodilator premedication may enhance training effect in persons with a response to bronchodilators.
- Prolonged corticosteroid therapy may cause myopathy, which may not be reversible with exercise training, and may cause elevated blood glucose and blood pressure.
- Supplemental O_2 may enhance the training effect due to increased oxygenation, causing decreased HR.
- SaO_2 should be monitored at the beginning of the program to determine the level of O_2 supplement.
- Severe disease can cause hypertrophic pulmonary osteoarthropathy and bone pain during exercise.
- End-stage lung disease may cause cor pulmonale and severely limit training intensity.

SPECIAL CONSIDERATIONS

Exercise training in a supervised and monitored setting is not necessary for the majority of persons with CF. However, monitoring oxyhemoglobin saturation may be prudent in persons who exhibit hypoxemia in order to determine the desired amount of oxygen supplementation. Some persons with CF may also have asthma- or exercise-induced bronchoconstriction and may require inhaled bronchodilator or cromolyn therapy prior to physical activities that provoke bronchoconstriction. Despite losing excessive salt through sweating, people with CF appear to be able to maintain adequate thermoregulation during shorter periods of exercise in the heat. Longer periods of exercise in the heat may warrant increased fluid and dietary salt intake.

TABLE 20.2

Cystic Fibrosis: Exercise Programming

Modes	Goals	Intensity/Frequency/Duration	Time to goal
Aerobic Large muscle activities (walking, cycling, swimming, jogging)	■ Increase $\dot{V}O_{2peak}$, maximum work rate, and endurance ■ Decrease $\dot{V}_E$, HR, and RPE, and increase SaO_2 at a given work rate ■ Increase respiratory muscle endurance ■ Facilitate mucus clearance	■ 60-85% maximum heart rate (Karvonen) ■ 3-4 days/week; sicker patients may need 2 daily sessions ■ Start at 10 min, build in 1 min increments to 20-30 min ■ Monitor HR, or SaO_2 in hypoxemic persons ■ RPE/dyspnea scales sometimes useful ■ Emphasize duration over intensity	
Strength Large muscle activities	■ Increase strength and endurance ■ Decrease steroid myopathy ■ Decrease air trapping	■ Start with 3 sets of 10 reps, light resistance ■ Optimal programming unknown	
Functional Activity specific	Increase/maintain function and ADLs	Optimal programming not known	

Some persons with more severe lung disease may experience bone or joint pain in the legs, particularly in the knees, which may be attributed to hypertrophic pulmonary osteoarthropathy.

With increasing age, risk of developing impaired glucose tolerance increases, with 6% to 10% of people with CF developing overt diabetes. The risk of diabetes may be exacerbated by oral corticosteroid treatment. Exercise testing and training for these individuals should follow the recommendations outlined in chapter 24.

Finally, some persons with severe or end-stage lung disease may have evidence of cor pulmonale (right ventricular hypertrophy) and even right ventricular failure. For these individuals, submaximal exercise testing may be indicated, and exercise training should be of low intensity and aimed at improving functional capacity with respect to activities of daily living.

Suggested Web Site

Cystic Fibrosis Foundation. www.cff.org

CASE STUDY

Cystic Fibrosis

thin, 22-year-old Caucasian male with CF complained of cessive coughing, shortness of breath, and fatigue when aying basketball with his friends. CF had been suspected at rth, when meconium ileus was detected, and it was subsequently verified by a sweat test. He was pancreatic insufficient d took pancreatic enzyme supplements with meals and acks. He attended the local university full-time and lived the dormitory and had two courses of oral antibiotics for acerbations of pulmonary infections in the past year. He d not been hospitalized since his initial diagnosis as an 'ant. He reported that his cough was sometimes productive, ore so after inhaled hypertonic saline (which he admitted t using routinely due to lack of time). His appetite had t changed, although he thought he might have lost some ight recently.

"I cough and get short of breath and tire more easily hen playing basketball with my friends at school."

Vitals

ight: 5 ft 9 in. (1.75 m)
eight: 140 lb (63.63 kg) (5 lb loss from 3 months ago)
/II: 20.75 kg/m2
R: 90 contractions/min
P: 110/80 mmHg
spiratory rate: 15 breaths/min

Young adult male; coughs infrequently
Pancreatic insufficiency, digital clubbing
Resting oxyhemoglobin saturation: 97% (room air)
FVC: 98% of predicted
FEV_1: 60% of predicted (10% decrease from 3 months ago)
Pseudomonas aeruginosa growth on sputum culture

A: 1. Cystic fibrosis with mild to moderate airway obstruction
   2. Exacerbation of pulmonary infection
   3. Possible exercise-induced bronchoconstriction
   4. Chronic mild undernutrition with recent weight loss

P: 1. Increase airway clearance techniques to TID (three times per day).
   2. Prescribe oral ciprofloxacin 750 mg BID (twice daily) for two weeks.
   3. Prescribe a high-calorie liquid nutrient at snack time BID.
   4. Evaluate exercise tolerance via progressive graded exercise test with spirometry before and after.
   5. Follow up in 3 weeks.
   6. Develop exercise prescription promoting cardio-respiratory endurance.

21

Lung and Heart–Lung Transplantation

David L. Balfe, MD ■ David J. Ross, MD

OVERVIEW OF THE PATHOPHYSIOLOGY

The first human lung transplant operation was performed by James Hardy at the University of Mississippi in 1963. Although the patient survived for only 18 days following the procedure, Dr. Hardy and colleagues confirmed that such a procedure was feasible and that someday such transplantations could help extend the life expectancy and quality of life for end-stage pulmonary patients. The first combined heart–lung transplant operation was performed 18 years later by Stanford University physician Dr. Bruce Reitz. Since 1963, over 8000 lung and heart–lung transplant procedures have been performed, with an average one-year patient survival rate of 75% for both procedures. Following the introduction of the immunosuppressive medication cyclosporine in the early 1980s, lung and heart–lung transplant procedures became clinically successful procedures for numerous end-stage cardiopulmonary diseases. Approximately 900 lung transplant and 40 to 60 heart–lung transplant procedures are performed annually in the United States.

Since May of 2005, the process of allocating donated lungs has been based on the immediacy of need according to a patient's assigned lung allocation score (LAS), which takes into account numerous measures of the patient's health, rather than how long a patient has been on the transplant list. The type of transplant procedure performed is based on several factors, including the native cardiopulmonary disease, recipient age, and scarcity of donor organs. In the United States, approximately 74,000 patients currently await solid organ transplantation, while nearly 4000 specifically require either lung or heart–lung organ donation. Therefore, single lung transplant (SLT) procedures are frequently pursued for older recipients who suffer from the spectrum of diseases associated with interstitial pulmonary fibrosis or emphysema. Conditions associated with significant pulmonary vascular disease (e.g., primary pulmonary hypertension, Eisenmenger's complex, sarcoidosis) are typically treated with either single or bilateral lung transplantation, but generally do not require an en bloc heart–lung transplant except in situations involving complex congenital heart disease. Pulmonary diseases characterized by chronic airway suppuration (e.g.,

Acknowledgment
The editors wish to acknowledge the previous author of this chapter, David J Ross, MD.

cystic fibrosis, bronchiectasis) require bilateral lung transplantation in an effort to lessen the risk of post-transplant infection during immunosuppression. While the number of SLTs performed annually has remained stable, the number of bilateral transplants has consistently increased and as of 2002, surpassed the number of single lung procedures.

The conventional surgical approach to either single or bilateral lung transplantation involves anastomosis of the proximal mainstem bronchus (or bronchi, for bilateral) and pulmonary artery, and the reestablishment of the pulmonary venous effluent by means of anastomosis of a left atrial cuff.

SLT is accomplished via a traditional posterolateral thoracotomy incision, while an extensive transverse bilateral anterior thoracosternotomy (clam shell incision) is utilized for bilateral grafts. Heart—lung transplantation involves the (en bloc) implantation of bilateral lungs and heart via a median sternotomy incision. During these surgical procedures, most centers do not perform revascularization of the bronchial arterial circulation while patients are similarly rendered "extrinsically denervated" from autonomic influences and are devoid of normal pulmonary lymphatic drainage. The physiologic responses observed after transplant may be significantly affected by these fundamental physiologic differences. In addition, the physiologic responses observed posttransplant tend to reflect an admixture of responses determined by the nature of each patient's native lung disease, state of conditioning, and type of transplant procedure (e.g., single or bilateral lung, heart—lung transplant) and not the attributes of the allograft lung. Potential adverse effects of immunosuppressive drugs may affect the physiologic responses to exercise after transplantation as well.

EFFECTS ON THE EXERCISE RESPONSE

Clinical investigations have suggested the following alterations in function that may affect the exercise response observed posttransplantation:

▪ Bronchial hyperresponsiveness to inhaled methacholine, hypertonic saline aerosol, or exercise has been demonstrated in a significant number of lung transplant recipients. Hyperresponsiveness may relate to either extrinsic cholinergic pulmonary denervation or airway inflammation such as that occurring during allograft rejection or infection.

▪ Abnormal mucociliary clearance may relate to a physical impediment imposed by the bronchial

anastomosis. Additionally, studies have suggested bronchial mucosal abnormalities characterized by altered epithelium, decreased ciliary beat frequency, and alteration in mucous rheology.

▪ Cardiac sympathetic denervation after combined heart—lung transplantation, similar to that with isolated orthotopic heart transplantation, can reduce the achieved maximum exercise heart rate, maximum oxygen uptake ($\dot{V}O_{2max}$), maximum oxygen pulse, and lactate threshold. Cardiac reinnervation later occurs in a proportion of such patients and is associated with improved chronotropic and inotropic cardiac responses and enhanced oxygen delivery to exercising skeletal muscles.

▪ Altered pulmonary vascular permeability may occur soon after lung transplantation and relate to "ischemia reperfusion" graft injury or, later in the clinical course, during episodes of rejection and associated perivascular inflammation. Physiologic consequences of an increased pulmonary vascular permeability and interstitial edema may include a decline in spirometric indices, increased wasted ventilation, and increased ventilation—perfusion inequality and gas exchange.

▪ Altered breathing pattern (i.e., disproportionate increase in tidal volume at a reduced respiratory rate), consistent with the absence of vagal-mediated inhibition of inflation (Hering-Breuer reflex), has been detected after combined heart—lung and bilateral lung transplantation. Stable heart—lung recipients with normal graft function, however, manifest an appropriate response of ventilation to exercise or progressive hypercapnia. Furthermore, pulmonary denervation does not impede the normal tachypneic response to either an increased elastic impedance or intrinsic pulmonary restriction. By contrast, the hypercapnic ventilation response may appear blunted relatively soon after lung transplantation when specifically performed for end-stage hypercapnic chronic obstructive pulmonary disease, but subsequently returns toward normal. Further, the detection of inspiratory resistive loads appears normal after combined heart—lung transplantation, despite the absence of pulmonary afferent innervation.

▪ Abnormal pulmonary function tests are frequently observed after both heart—lung and isolated pulmonary transplantation. Heart—lung transplant recipients often have a mild restrictive ventilatory abnormality that may relate to volumetric constraints of the recipient chest cavity and thoracic musculature. The elastic behavior or pressure—volume relationships after uncomplicated lung transplantation appear relatively normal. Values for vital capacity and maximum expiratory flow rates are expectedly less after single (approximately 60% of predicted normal value) versus bilateral or heart–lung transplantation.

EFFECTS OF EXERCISE TRAINING

Despite attainment of higher spirometric values following either single or bilateral lung or combined heart–lung transplantation, cardiopulmonary exercise studies have demonstrated rather ominous results, including the following:

- Values for $\dot{V}O_{2max}$ (approximately 45-55% of predicted) and maximum work rate in these recipients are reduced.

- An abnormally reduced "threshold" for lactate is observed in association with reduction in maximal tolerable exercise capacity, although this cannot be ascribed to factors such as cardiac dysfunction, anemia, or limitations imposed by pulmonary vasculature or lung mechanics.

- Quadriceps muscle biopsies and 31P-magnetic resonance spectroscopy after clinical lung transplantation have suggested a decrease in proportion of type I fibers and reduced skeletal muscle oxidative capacity and reduced intracellular pH. No difference has been detected in the activities of glycolytic enzymes, while transplant recipients demonstrate a higher reliance on glycolytic nonoxidative metabolism. Therefore, alteration in fiber proportion and reduced mitochondrial activity may indeed contribute to the exercise limitation witnessed after lung transplantation.

- Immunosuppressant medications may potentially contribute to an alteration in exercise physiology. Systemic glucocorticoids have well-described adverse effects on peripheral skeletal muscle and are commonly administered to patients suffering from a spectrum of pulmonary diseases prior to transplant, as well as in combination therapies posttransplantation. Glucocorticoids can induce a selective atrophy of type II fibers; however, because these fibers are the major source for lactate production in exercising skeletal muscle, one would not expect corticosteroids to cause inordinate intracellular acidosis. Calcineurin inhibitor-type immunosuppressive medications (e.g., cyclosporine or tacrolimus) have been shown to inhibit skeletal muscle mito-

chondrial respiration in vitro and diminish endurance exercise time in rats. The mechanism involved is not entirely clear but may relate to diminished mitochondrial calcium efflux with subsequent mitochondrial dysfunction. No impact on fiber size has yet been attributed to cyclosporine, although reduction in capillarity of limb musculature may further contribute to the reduction in aerobic capacity.

- The physiologic differences in exercise physiology and aerobic capacity notwithstanding, one preliminary study after lung transplantation has demonstrated significant benefits from formal exercise conditioning. After a six-week program in which training intensity ranged from 30% to 60% of maximum heart rate reserve, improvements were observed in minute ventilation, cardiac reserve, and $\dot{V}O_{2max}$. Congruent with these findings, recent studies of similarly immunosuppressed heart transplant recipients have also highlighted the benefits of structured exercise training. Therefore, to mitigate the potential adverse effects of immunosuppressive medications and the frequent preexistent state of deconditioning, structured exercise rehabilitation programs may offer significant clinical advantages.

MANAGEMENT AND MEDICATIONS

Pulmonary transplantation offers a renewed sense of hope and quality of life for numerous patients with end-stage cardiopulmonary diseases. Nevertheless, the required chronic immunosuppressive medications represent a double-edged sword after transplant. Although decreasing the incidence of acute graft rejection, such medications may heighten the risk of developing opportunistic infection, malignancy, osteoporosis, hypertension, diabetes mellitus, and associated toxicity. The exercise physiologist should be aware of these potential complications and maintain vigilance accordingly. Notable complications for the posttransplant patient may include the following:

- Acute allograft rejection and dysfunction are often heralded by increased subjective sensation of dyspnea, and reduction in spirometric function and pulmonary gas exchange. Expeditious evaluation of the patient for possible trans-bronchoscopic biopsy and therapy is imperative.

- Pneumonia, although often related to typical community-acquired viral or bacterial infections, may be attributed to opportunistic or atypical pathogens caused by chronic immunosuppressive medications. Routine patient vaccinations with polyvalent pneumococcal and annual influenza vaccines are recommended.

- Systemic hypertension is often related to adverse effects of glucocorticoids and calcineurin inhibitor-type medications. Patients often require antihypertensive medications with frequent dosage adjustments. However, significant elevation in blood pressure may indicate a toxic blood level range for either cyclosporine or tacrolimus versus potential worsening renal function related to these medications.

- Osteoporosis, related to both systemic glucocorticoids and calcineurin inhibitor-type immunosuppressants, poses a significant risk for vertebral and hip fracture after transplantation. Newer prophylactic strategies for osteoporosis include calcium supplementation, hormonal replacement therapy, and bisphosphonates, as well as exercise, strength, and balance training.

- Chronic anemia is usually related to suppression of the bone marrow by immunosuppressive medications. However, various viral infections (e.g., Parvovirus B19, herpes virus) may sometimes be responsible. Severe reductions in hemoglobin concentration may affect the patient's maximum exercise tolerance and lactate threshold.

- Bronchiolitis obliterans syndrome (BOS) or chronic graft rejection represents the Achilles heel of lung transplantation and may affect two-thirds of recipients by five years. Progressive small airway fibrosis and obliteration result in an inexorable decay in lung function over time that frequently is refractory to augmented immunosuppressive therapies. Recurrent respiratory tract infections and abnormalities of larger airways (i.e., bronchiectasis) frequently ensue.

- Abnormalities of glucose tolerance and metabolism, related to immunosuppressive medications, may complicate the clinical course of these patients. Excessive weight gain and potential diabetic complications may be favorably affected by regular exercise and nutritional counseling.

- Bronchial anastomosis complications may significantly affect clinical outcomes after lung transplantation. Fortunately, neither dehiscence nor bronchovascular fistula complications are presently common. However, development of bronchial anastomotic stricture or stenosis, usually caused by exuberant scar tissue formation, may impair both spirometric function and the normal "mucociliary escalator." Posttransplant inflammation involving airway cartilage rings may contribute to bronchomalacia, whereupon dynamic airway collapse may limit expiratory flow rates. Potential remedies may include endobronchial laser photoresection of granulation tissue or deployment of a bronchial stent to maintain the bronchial lumen or both. Furthermore, localized infections of the anastomosis (e.g., fungal) may require therapy with systemic or inhaled aerosol antibiotics. Bronchoscopic assessment is generally required to establish a definitive diagnosis and thus direct the appropriate therapies.

RECOMMENDATIONS FOR EXERCISE TESTING

The primary objectives for exercise testing are twofold: (1) to assess the severity of exercise impairment prior to organ transplant or determine progression of disease and urgency for transplantation and (2) to characterize exercise limitations posttransplantation. The assessment of $\dot{V}O_{2max}$ or 6 min walking distance prior to transplantation correlates with the severity of illness for cystic fibrosis, as well as the mortality risk associated with the duration of the waiting period for transplantation. Posttransplant testing may be valuable in determining whether exercise limitation is related to graft dysfunction, occult cardiac disease, peripheral muscle weakness, or a persistent state of deconditioning.

The principal objectives either pre- or posttransplantation for exercise testing are similar (also see table 21.1):

- To assess severity of disease or progression
- To assess maximal physical work capacity and state of aerobic fitness
- To observe cardiorespiratory and metabolic responses to exercise
- To observe oxyhemoglobin saturation during exercise

TABLE 21.1

Lung and Heart–Lung Transplantation: Exercise Testing

Methods	Measures	Endpoints	Comments
Aerobic Cycle (preferred) (ramp protocol 10-15 W/min; staged protocol 25-50 W/3 min stage) Treadmill (1 MET/3 min stage)	▪ 12-lead ECG, HR ▪ BP ▪ RPE, dyspnea scale (0-10) ▪ Pulse oximetry/arterial PaO$_2$ ▪ Respired gas analysis ▪ Blood lactate	▪ Serious dysrhythmias ▪ >2 mm ST-segment depression or elevation ▪ T-wave inversion with significant ST change ▪ SBP >250 mmHg or DBP >115 mmHg ▪ Maximum ventilations ▪ $\dot{V}O_{2peak}$ ▪ Lactate or ventilatory threshold	▪ Atrial dysrhythmias common among early posttransplants ▪ Heart–lung transplant may be associated with cardiac denervation ▪ Lung transplant may be associated with absent Hering-Breuer reflex ▪ Very reduced transitional thresholds for lactate and HCO$_3$
Endurance 6 min walk	Distance	Note rest stop distance/time, dyspnea index, vitals	Useful measure for assessing pretransplant and severity of illness and posttransplant progress
Strength Isokinetic or isotonic	▪ Peak torque ▪ Maximum number of reps ▪ 1RM		Decreased muscle mass/force related to corticosteroids
Flexibility Sit and reach	Hip, hamstring, and lower back flexibility		Postthoractomy pain may restrict flexibility
Neuromuscular Gait analysis Balance	▪ Gait speed, distance ▪ Berg Balance Scale ▪ Ashworth Scale ▪ Modified Fatigue Impact Scale		▪ Tremors and possible myopathy with calcineurin inhibitors ▪ Decreased visual acuity due to cataracts or diabetes
Functional Sit to stand Stair climbing Lifting	Perform tests if clinically indicated		

- To provide a basis for prescribing exercise within safe limits
- To assess changes in fitness and cardiorespiratory responses to exercise that occur with disease progression or medical or surgical interventions

Many of the following medications are used either for immunosuppression or as prophylaxis to prevent potential posttransplant complications:

- Calcineurin-inhibitor immunosuppressive medications (e.g., cyclosporine, tacrolimus), target of rapamycin (TOR) inhibitors (e.g., rapamycin), antimetabolites (e.g., azathioprine, methotrexate, mycophenolate mofetil).
- Loop and thiazide diuretics: May contribute to electrolyte abnormalities and muscle weakness.
- Antihypertensive medications (e.g., beta-blockers, angiotensin-converting enzyme [ACE] inhibitors, calcium channel blockers).
- Antibiotics (e.g., quinolone type [e.g., ciprofloxacin], trimethoprim sulfamethoxazole, antiviral [e.g., ganciclovir sodium, acyclovir]).
- HMG-CoA reductase inhibitor medications (e.g., "statins") for hyperlipidemia posttransplant: May cause muscle pain or severe muscle injury with potential kidney failure.
- Calcineurin inhibitors: May cause tremor, neuropathy or myopathy, electrolyte abnormalities (decreased magnesium and increased potassium), renal tubular metabolic acidosis, or kidney failure.
- TOR inhibitors: May cause bleeding tendency (decreased platelets) and hyperlipidemia.
- Beta-blockers: May reduce heart rate response to exercise.
- Calcium channel blockers: May cause leg swelling or hypotension.
- Quinolone antibiotics: May cause tendinitis and tendon rupture.
- Antiviral medications: May have associated neurotoxicity.
- Many medications may cause anemia or leukopenia. The spectrum of adverse medication effects may influence exercise capacity or muscle function.

RECOMMENDATIONS FOR EXERCISE PROGRAMMING

The principal goals of exercise training, both pre- and posttransplantation, are to improve aerobic fitness and alleviate the sense of dyspnea. Exercise prescriptions should be tailored to the type of native lung disease, level of patient fitness, and posttransplant allograft spirometric function (see table 21.2). Pretransplant patients with pulmonary arterial hypertension, for example, may be predisposed to development of right ventricular ischemia, arterial oxygen desaturation, and syncope during exertion. Exercise of moderate intensity (60-80% of peak heart rate) should be targeted for approximately 20 to 30 min. Resistance training should be encouraged to counteract the effects of steroid treatment both pre- and posttransplantation. Beta-blockers received posttransplant may limit exercise heart rate response; therefore, assessment of perceived exertion may be preferable. Patients should be encouraged to adopt healthy lifestyle modifications that incorporate aerobic activities, balanced diet, and maintenance of appropriate body weight.

Special considerations during exercise programming include the following:

- Ratings of perceived exertion and dyspnea are the preferred methods of monitoring intensity. Many clients are unable to achieve a training heart rate yet demonstrate physiologic improvement.
- Musculoskeletal complaints, postsurgical chest wall pain, and osteoporosis are common posttransplant complications.
- Myopathy involving respiratory and peripheral muscles may be related to calcineurin inhibitors and corticosteroid medications. Severe muscle pain may indicate a serious complication of "statin"-type lipid-lowering medications.
- "Bronchial hyperresponsiveness" posttransplant may contribute to exercise-related bronchospasms and dyspnea.
- Clients usually respond to exercise optimally in mid to late morning, due to adverse effects (e.g., nausea, fatigue) of morning medication schedules.
- Avoid extremes in ambient temperature and humidity, as frequent use of antihypertensive and diuretic medications can increase the

TABLE 21.2

Lung and Heart–Lung Transplantation: Exercise Programming

Modes	Goals	Intensity/Frequency/ Duration	Time to goal
Aerobic Large muscle activities (walking, cycling, swimming)	■ Increase $\dot{V}O_{2peak}$ ■ Increase lactate threshold and ventilatory threshold ■ Become less sensitive to dyspnea ■ Develop more efficient breathing patterns ■ Facilitate improvement in ADLs	■ THR 60-80% of peak HR ■ RPE 11-13/20 (comfortable, pace and endurance) ■ Monitor dyspnea ■ 1-2 sessions/day ■ 3-7 days/week ■ 20-30 min/session (shorter intermittent exercise sessions may be necessary initially) ■ Emphasize progression of duration more than intensity	Variable: 3-12 mo (depending on posttransplant medical/ surgical complication)
Strength Free weights Isokinetic/isotonic machines	■ Increase maximal number of reps ■ Increase isokinetic torque/ work ■ Increase lean body mass	Low resistance, high reps 2-3 days/week	Variable: 3-12 months
Flexibility Stretching Tai chi	Increase ROM	Daily	
Neuromuscular Walking, balance exercises Breathing exercises	■ Improve gait, balance ■ Improve breathing efficiency	Daily	
Functional Activity-specific exercises	■ Restore ADLs ■ Return to work ■ Improve quality of life ■ Restore sexuality	Daily	

incidence of complications under these conditions.

- Supplemental O_2 may be required either early posttransplant or subsequent to graft complications.
- New or worsening SaO_2 responses to exercise may indicate organ rejection or infection and should be communicated to the transplant team.
- Anxiety, depression, and fear are common effects of dyspnea or medications such as corticosteroids.

SPECIAL CONSIDERATIONS

All patients after organ transplantation and certain patients prior to transplant require chronic immunosuppression, which poses an increased risk for serious infection. Isolation of such patients from the general population in rehabilitation programs is generally not warranted, although one should be cognizant of the potential risks for transmission of respiratory pathogens from other clients. Maintaining cleanliness of all exercise equipment and patient avoidance of individuals who are ill during these sessions should be emphasized. Potential for impaired glucose tolerance or systemic hypertension as an adverse effect of immunosuppressive medications should be monitored during exercise and related to the referring physician. Significant deterioration in exercise tolerance or arterial oxygen saturation from prior baseline values may represent a harbinger of allograft rejection, cytomegalovirus, or other posttransplant opportunistic infections. Such data may be of crucial importance to the organ transplant team in determining the need for expeditious clinical evaluation and bronchoscopic lung biopsy. The clinical value of maintaining excellent lines of communication with the transplant team is of paramount importance.

Suggested Web Site

International Society for Heart and Lung Transplantation. www.ishlt.org

---

CASE STUDY

Lung Transplantation

A 45-year-old woman underwent bilateral sequential lung transplantation three years ago for interstitial pulmonary fibrosis complicated by severe secondary pulmonary hypertension with right-sided heart failure. She initially improved quite dramatically with respect to both spirometric lung function and exercise tolerance, and went home (to Kuwait) approximately three months posttransplant on standard triple-drug immunosuppression (i.e., cyclosporine, mycophenolate mofetil, and prednisone). She returned for reevaluation complaining of progressive shortness of breath and recurrent respiratory tract infections with methicillin-resistant Staphylococcus aureus and Pseudomonas aeruginosa. She also complained of severe low back pain after sustaining a "slip and fall" injury.

S: *"I can't breathe again, and my back hurts."*

O: Vitals

Middle-aged woman, on oxygen, breathless and extremely fatigable with minimal exertion
Breath sounds: Bilateral basilar crackles and musical inspiratory and expiratory rhonchi
Thoracolumbar spine: Mildly tender to palpation, with decreased ROM for flexion and extension

Neurologic examination: Normal
Pulse oximetry: 95% arterial oxygen saturation on 3 L/min O2 via nasal prongs
Chest X rays: Bibasilar scarring and probable dilated and thickened larger airways or bronchiectasis
Spirometry: Significant decreases in FVC and FEV_1; severe obstructive ventilatory defect
Spine X rays: Multiple compression fractures of T7, T9, and L1
Spine MRI scan: No evidence of malignancy

A: 1. BOS, or chronic graft rejection
   2. Recurrent respiratory tract infection caused by bronchiectasis and recent exacerbation
   3. Osteoporosis with multiple vertebral compression fractures
   4. Severe exercise intolerance

P: 1. Intravenous antibiotic treatment of current respiratory infection is needed.
   2. Prescribe aerosolized antibiotic prophylaxis for chronic bronchiectasis.
   3. Treat osteoporosis pharmacologically.

(continued)

CASE STUDY Lung Transplantation *(continued)*

4. Additional immunosuppression to prevent further loss of lung function from chronic rejection (e.g., tacrolimus and methotrexate) is necessary.
5. Prescribe outpatient pulmonary rehabilitation after the acute infection is resolved.

Exercise Program Goals

1. Improve functional capacity to increase and maintain ADLs.
2. Alleviate dyspnea; improve strength and balance/coordination.
3. Pulse oximetry during exercise to determine supplemental oxygen requirements.

Mode	Frequency	Duration	Intensity	Progression
Aerobic	3 days/week	20-30 min/session	THR (110 contractions/min) RPE 12/20	Progress as tolerated over 6-week program.
Strength (all major muscle groups)	2 days/week	2 sets of 12 reps	To fatigue	Add resistance until 12 reps achieves fatigue.
Flexibility	Daily	20-60 s/stretch	Below discomfort point	Maintain.
Neuromuscular (walk drills, breathing exercises)	Daily	Individualized as needed	As tolerated	Maintain.
Functional (activity-specific exercises)	Daily	Individualized as needed	As tolerated	Gradual over 3-12 months.
Warm-up and cool-down	Before and after each session	10 min	RPE <10/20	

PART IV

Metabolic Diseases

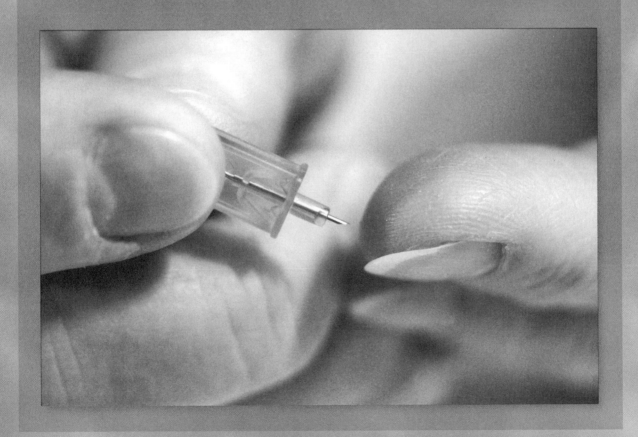

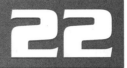

Hyperlipidemia

J. Larry Durstine, PhD, FACSM ■ Geoffrey E. Moore, MD, FACSM
Donna Polk, MD, MPH

OVERVIEW OF THE PATHOPHYSIOLOGY

Lipids are organic macromolecules that include fats, fatty acids, cholesterol, and triglycerides. Lipids play a vital role in the storage of biochemical energy, insulation, structure of cell membranes, and regulation of metabolism. Because lipids are hydrophobic molecules, they must combine with specialized lipid-binding proteins called apolipoproteins to form lipoproteins that are then able move throughout the body. Lipoproteins are spherical, whereas apolipoproteins receive their form by surrounding a lipid core containing triglyceride, phospholipid, and free and esterified cholesterol, which are separated into four different ultracentrifugation gravitational density ranges or classes.

- Chylomicrons are derived from intestinal absorption of exogenous (dietary) triglyceride.
- Very-low-density lipoprotein (VLDL or pre-b-lipoprotein) is synthesized in the liver and is the primary transport mechanism for endogenous triglyceride.
- Low-density lipoprotein (LDL or b-lipoprotein) represents the final stage in the catabolism of VLDL and is the principal carrier of cholesterol. Intermediate-density lipoprotein (IDL) is an intermediate step in the catabolism of VLDL. Other LDL subfractions are lipoprotein(a) (Lp[a]) and small and large LDL particles.
- High-density lipoprotein (HDL or a-lipoprotein) is involved in the reverse transport of cholesterol and is typically studied as two separate subfractions: HDL2 and the denser HDL3.

Triglyceride and cholesterol move between the intestine, liver, and extrahepatic tissue by means of a complex transport system with plasma lipoproteins as the primary transport agent. This system is facilitated by several important enzymes: lipoprotein lipase (LPL), hepatic lipase, lecithin-cholesterol acyltransferase (LCAT), and cholesterol ester transfer protein (CETP). Lipoproteins together with these enzymes interact to create several important metabolic pathways involved in transporting dietary or exogenous fat as well as hepatic or endogenous fat in addition to reverse cholesterol transport. Chylomicrons, VLDL, IDL, and LDL are involved in pathways that move lipids from the intestine or liver to peripheral tissues. High-density lipoprotein, however, is involved in the reverse cholesterol transport (i.e., from the peripheral tissues back to the liver). Various environmental, genetic, and pathologic factors alter these lipoprotein metabolic pathways, influencing blood lipid and lipoprotein concentrations and changing coronary artery disease (CAD) risk. These factors include gender, age, body fat distribution, dietary composition, cigarette smoking, some medications, genetic inheritance, and routine participation in physical activity. When these factors combine to yield elevated blood lipid and lipoprotein concentrations, the condition is referred to as dyslipidemia:

- Hyperlipidemia indicates elevated blood triglyceride and cholesterol.
- Hypertriglyceridemia denotes only elevated triglyceride concentration.
- Exaggerated postprandial lipemia is denoted by prolonged levels of triglycerides in the blood following consumption of dietary fat and failure to return to baseline levels within an 8 to 10 h period.
- Hypercholesterolemia implies only elevated blood cholesterol concentration.
- High LDL-cholesterol (LDL-C) denotes >160 mg/dl LDL-C concentration.
- Low HDL-cholesterol (HDL-C) denotes <40 mg/dl HDL-C concentration
- Hyperlipoproteinemia or dyslipoproteinemia refers to elevated lipoprotein concentrations. Hyperlipoproteinemia is associated with genetic abnormalities or may be secondarily related to an underlying disease such as diabetes mellitus, renal insufficiency, hypothyroidism, biliary obstruction, dysproteinemia, or nephrotic kidney disease.

When one considers CAD and peripheral arterial disease risk, hypertriglyceridemia (elevated VLDL triglyceride), hypercholesterolemia (increased LDL-C), mixed hyperlipidemia (increased LDL-C and VLDL triglyceride), and exaggerated postprandial lipemia must receive appropriate lipid management. The National Cholesterol Education Program Adult Treatment Panel III (NCEP) recommends the following standards for lipid and lipoproteins. The LDL-C goal for all individuals is 100 mg/dl; but in high-risk individuals, an LDL-C of 70 mg/dl is an optional treatment goal.

Triglycerides (mg/dl)

<150 Normal

150-199 Borderline high

200-499 High

≥500 Very high

Total Cholesterol (mg/dl)

<200 Desirable

200-239 Borderline high

≥240 High

LDL-C (mg/dl)

<100 Optimal

100-129 Near or above optimal

130-159 Borderline high

160-189 High

≥190 Very high

HDL-C (mg/dl)

<40 Low for men, (<50 for women)

≥60 High

EFFECTS ON THE EXERCISE RESPONSE

Dyslipidemia alone does not alter the exercise response unless it has contributed to cardiovascular disease and limits the exercise response due to angina or claudication for example. In such cases, attention is given to the exercise response in view of these conditions. Individuals with genetic disorders resulting in excessively elevated cholesterol levels should undergo medical management of the dyslipidemia before they begin an exercise program, and supervised exercise is recommended in these individuals. In addition, prescribed medications for other conditions should be noted before they undergo exercise testing or training.

EFFECTS OF EXERCISE TRAINING

Regular participation in physical activity or exercise results in beneficial changes in persons with normal lipid and lipoprotein concentrations as well as in most persons with dyslipidemia. These changes include the following:

- Lower triglyceride concentrations
- Reduced postprandial lipemia
- Decreased concentrations of small LDL particles
- Increased number of larger-sized LDL particles
- Higher HDL-C concentrations (but not always)
- Increased lipoprotein enzyme activity (LPL, LCAT, and CETP)
- No change in Lp(a)
- Improved glycemic control

These exercise training changes enhance reverse cholesterol transport and are augmented further by a low-fat diet, weight loss, and reduction in adiposity. Thus, exercise training directly (e.g., by increased LPL activity) and indirectly (e.g., by reductions in body weight and body fat) improves blood lipid and lipoprotein profiles. Congenital deficiencies cause abnormal blood lipid and lipoprotein profiles, leading to substantially different responses to physical activity from those seen in healthy individuals. For example, exercise training does not amplify LPL activity in clients with LPL deficiency, nor does HDL-C concentration increase in individuals with low HDL (hypoalphalipoprotein syndrome). The mechanisms responsible for lack of exercise training changes in these conditions are unclear.

MANAGEMENT AND MEDICATIONS

Current treatment guidelines for the management of plasma lipids and lipoproteins are provided by the NCEP. Though dietary modification, weight loss, and exercise are recommended as initial therapy for at least six weeks, pharmacological therapy is the primary modality for reducing lipid and lipoprotein levels and is highly effective and generally well tolerated. In contrast, hygienic therapy (diet, exercise, and weight loss) is limited by patient adherence and effectiveness. Patients can achieve desired lipid levels by hygienic therapy alone; but in clinical practice, this is the exception and not the rule. Nevertheless, because exercise decreases plasma triglycerides while improving glucose intolerance (which contributes to dyslipidemia), daily exercise is recommended for all patients undergoing treatment for lipid disorders. Diet, weight loss, and exercise are considered adjunctive to pharmacological therapy but extremely important for the following reasons.

- Low-calorie diets that cause weight loss decrease total cholesterol and LDL-C and increase HDL-C.

- The effects of low-calorie diets are complex (e.g., low-calorie diets decrease HDL-C in obese women whereas HDL-C is increased in distance runners).

- Very-low-fat and high-carbohydrate diets lower HDL-C and increase triglyceride concentrations (exercise diminishes these diet effects on HDL-C and triglyceride concentrations).

Lipid-lowering medications act by a variety of mechanisms, with rare hemodynamic or electrocardiographic effects. A combinations of lipid-lowering drugs are frequently used and substantially alters dyslipidemia with reductions in cost and side effects. The use of lipid-lowering drug combinations can reduce cost and side effects while also enhances compliance to the medication program. A major risk of combination therapy is muscle damage and toxicity (rhabdomyolysis) with use of fibric acid derivatives in combination with niacin and hepatic hydroxymethylglutaryl coenzyme A (HMG-CoA) reductase inhibitors. Present data suggest that exercise potentates the propensity to develop drug-induced muscle damage.

HMG-CoA reductase inhibitor therapy or statin therapy inhibits the liver enzyme HMG-CoA reductase and is the initial medical therapy for most lipid and lipoprotein disorders. Statins are effective in reducing primary and secondary CAD events in multiple trials and are well tolerated. Six statins are presently available in the United States (atorvastatin, fluvastatin, lovastatin, pravastatin, rosuvastatin, simvastatin). At their maximal doses, statins reduce LDL-C by 20% to 60% and triglycerides by as much as 40% while increasing HDL-C by 6% to 10%. The primary mechanism of action is to reduce liver cholesterol synthesis, which results in a compensatory increase in cellular LDL receptors.

A side effect of statin use is muscle discomfort. Associated with this muscular distress can be elevated blood creatine phosphokinase (CPK). Elevated CPK is also exacerbated by eccentric exercise, making CPK elevations more frequent in cardiac rehabilitation participants who are prescribed statin medications. Though patients rarely experience the breakdown of skeletal muscle tissue referred to as rhabdomyolysis with vigorous exercise, it is important to understand the concomitant role of statins and their potential to exacerbate muscle symptoms in CAD patients participating in exercise programs. Exercise-induced CPK elevations can reach levels as high as 21,000 U/L without significant sequelae. Although no randomized trials have been reported, coenzyme Q-10 (ubiquinone) has been used anecdotally to reduce statin-associated side effects. The incidence of rhabdomyolysis in patients taking statins generally occurs when statins are combined with other medications such as fibric acid derivatives, niacin, cyclosporine, or macrolide antibiotics like erythromycin and azole derivatives. While taking statins, people are cautioned about grapefruit and grapefruit juice consumption as these foods can increase the circulating levels of statins.

Ezetimibe is a cholesterol absorption inhibitor and is also available in combination with the statin drug simvastatin. Ezetimibe acts at the brush border in the intestine to limit absorption of dietary cholesterol and primarily lowers LDL-C. It has little effect on triglycerides or HDL-C.

Bile acid sequestrants are administered as a powdered resin dissolved in liquid or in a synthetic form as tablets. Resins inhibit intestinal bile reabsorption and its transport in the portal circulation to the liver. The loss of bile stimulates the upregulation of hepatic LDL receptor activity, reducing plasma LDL-C levels. These drugs are most effective when given with the fattiest meal because they are most likely to encounter bile in the gut. The major side effects of bile acid sequestrants are constipation, bloating, and flatulence. These medications also interfere with the absorption of fat-soluble vitamins and other medications. The tablet form colesevelam is designed not to interfere with the absorption of other medications and causes fewer gastrointestinal problems.

Fibric acid derivatives are useful in reducing elevated triglyceride levels and raising HDL levels. Gemfibrozil and fenofibrate are currently available in the United States and are well tolerated, with few side effects. Fibric acids may increase LDL-C slightly in patients with hypertriglyceridemia because LPL activity is increased, which facilitates VLDL-to-LDL catabolism. Extreme caution is warranted when fibric acid derivatives are combined, particularly gemfibrozil with statins, because this combination can increase the likelihood of myalgias and rhabdomyolysis. Most physicians should avoid this combination altogether and refer such patients to specialty lipid clinics.

Niacin or nicotinic acid is extremely useful in patients with low HDL-C levels with or without elevated triglycerides. Niacin has multiple potential areas of action, but inhibiting lipolysis is the primary effect. Reduced lipolysis limits plasma free fatty acids and their availability for subsequent synthesis by the liver into triglyceride. Niacin's greatest effects are to increase HDL-C, reduce triglycerides, and reduce LDL-C concentrations. Niacin is the only lipid-lowering agent that has the potential to reduce blood Lp(a) levels.

Because niacin inhibits lipolysis and since lipolysis is greatest during periods of fasting such as overnight, the most important niacin dose is at bedtime. Bedtime dosing helps minimize the discomfort of niacin's side effects such as flushing and itching. Sustained-release formulations of niacin designed solely for nocturnal administration are available and can potentially reduce these side effects. With continued use, the side effects are often minimal. Since flushing is prostaglandin mediated, this effect is also minimized by pretreatment, 30 min prior to niacin intake, with aspirin or other prostaglandin inhibitors. Most patients being treated for lipid disorders are already receiving aspirin. The combination of aspirin and sustained-release niacin is an effective approach to reducing flushing. Other potential side effects of niacin include a reversible hepatitis, activation of gout and peptic ulcers, and glucose intolerance.

All individuals treated with niacin should have liver function tests performed every four months. Hepatitis can occur with both regular-release and sustained-release niacin but is 10 times more frequent with the sustained-release form; therefore nonprescription forms of sustained-release niacin are not recommended. Additionally, "no-flush" niacin is ineffective as a lipid-lowering agent. Patients developing frequent nausea, vomiting, unexpected weight loss, or other potential signs of hepatitis should stop taking niacin and contact their physician.

Combination drug therapy is often utilized. The use of two different drugs is beneficial in that it may allow lower drug doses to reach lipid management goals without the increased risk of toxicity that comes with higher dosage of a single drug. Another benefit is that the two drugs prescribed may affect lipid or lipoprotein levels differently. For example, statins lower LDL-C, but the addition of niacin increases HDL-C.

Stanol esters are food additives approved by the Food and Drug Administration as substitutes for butter and margarine. Stanol esters reduce dietary and biliary cholesterol absorption in a dose-dependent manner. Reduced biliary cholesterol makes these additives effective even among persons on low-cholesterol diets. This plasma cholesterol effect is maximal at three servings daily and is not augmented by additional doses. Stanol esters are stable up to 400° F and are substituted for butter and margarine in cooking.

Several important factors are key in the exercise management of lipids and lipoproteins. One significant element is the total exercise energy expenditure or the weekly exercise volume completed. Training-induced increases in HDL-C and reductions in triglyceride and postprandial lipemia are influenced the most by larger amounts of weekly exercise. Another key issue with respect to training-induced lipid modifications is exercise training status. Exercise-trained individuals must expend greater volumes of energy to cause further lipid and lipoprotein changes. In the future, apolipoprotein E genotyping would be beneficial because some genotypes influence greater exercise lipid and lipoproteins changes than others.

Another medical management issue arises because some of the medications used in treating medical problems also affect plasma lipids and lipoproteins. These include beta antagonists (beta-blockers), thiazide diuretics, oral hypoglycemic agents, insulin, estrogen, and progesterone.

- Beta-blockers may increase triglyceride concentrations and reduce HDL-C concentrations, with the exception of those with intrinsic sympathomimetic activity.
- Thiazide diuretics may increase total plasma cholesterol, VLDL-C, LDL-C, and triglyceride without an effect on HDL-C concentration.
- Oral hypoglycemic agents or insulin therapy may reduce triglyceride and increase HDL-C in people with diabetes. These benefits are secondary to the improvement in blood glucose control.
- Levothyroxine increases hepatic LDL receptor activity and thereby lowers LDL-C in clients who are hypothyroid. This medication may produce elevations of heart rate and blood pressure as well as cardiac dysrhythmias, and can lead to angina in patients with CAD.
- Sex steroids in combination (as in oral contraceptives) tend to increase blood cholesterol depending on the estrogen:progesterone ratio.
- Oral estrogens can raise HDL-C and VLDL triglyceride concentrations especially in postmenopausal women and can reduce Lp(a) levels.
- Progesterone decreases triglyceride as well as HDL-C concentrations.

Few studies have examined the interaction of medications with exercise training. Some results suggest that exercise training may attenuate the increased triglyceride concentration and reduced HDL-C concentrations associated with the use of beta-blockers. Thus, exercise may counteract the adverse effect of some medications.

RECOMMENDATIONS FOR EXERCISE TESTING

When dyslipidemia is considered congenital but the individual does not present with any signs or symptoms of other comorbidities (e.g., CAD or renal insufficiency), exercise testing can follow normal protocols used for populations at risk for CAD. However, if signs or symptoms of comorbidities are present, exercise testing should follow recommendations for the particular disorder in question (see table 22.1). The primary objectives of exercise testing are to

- diagnose CAD,
- determine functional capacity, and
- determine appropriate intensity range for aerobic exercise training.

Medications and special considerations for exercise testing and training include the following:

- HMG-CoA reductase inhibitors and fibric acid used together may cause muscle damage and limit exercise performance.
- Individuals with hyperlipidemia have a high risk of cardiac and arterial insufficiency.
- Xanthomas may cause biomechanical problems.
- High triglyceride or cholesterol may cause intravascular sludging and ischemia.

RECOMMENDATIONS FOR EXERCISE PROGRAMMING

The exercise prescription for dyslipidemia is ancillary to lipid-lowering medications, as well as reduced caloric intake and dietary fat consumption. Present evidence suggests that there may be different energy expenditure thresholds for improved levels of different lipids and lipoproteins. For example, triglyceride concentrations are lower in men with hypertriglyceridemia after two weeks of aerobic exercise (45 min/day) on consecutive days, whereas total plasma cholesterol concentration remains unless body weight is reduced. On the other hand, HDL-C concentrations are frequently increased by exercise regimens requiring 1200 to 1500 kcal of energy expenditure per week (minimal training period of 12 weeks). In any case, inactive persons should expect favorable blood lipid changes within several months (see table 22.2). The primary exercise training goal for beneficial lipids and lipoproteins is to expend calories; thus aerobic exercise is the foundation of the exercise training program. Resistance and flexibility exercise training are adjunct to an aerobic training program designed for the treatment of dyslipidemia primarily because these modes of exercise do not substantially contribute to the overall caloric expenditure. Favorable

TABLE 22.1

Hyperlipidemia: Exercise Testing

Methods	Measures	Endpoints*	Comments
Aerobic Cycle (ramp protocol 17 W/min; staged protocol 25-50 W/3 min stage) Treadmill (1-2 METs/3 min stage)	■ 12-lead ECG, HR ■ BP, rate–pressure product ■ RPE (6-20)	■ $\dot{V}O_{2peak}$/work rate ■ Serious dysrhythmias ■ >2 mm ST-segment depression ■ ST elevation (+1.0 mm) in leads without diagnostic Q-waves ■ Ischemic threshold ■ SBP >250 mmHg or DBP >115 mmHg ■ Hypotensive response ■ Volitional fatigue	
Endurance 6 min walk	Distance	Note time, distance, symptoms at rest	Useful for deconditioned persons

*Measurements of particular significance; do not always indicate test termination.

TABLE 22.2

Hyperlipidemia: Exercise Programming

Modes	Goals	Intensity/Frequency/Duration	Time to goal
Aerobic Large muscle activities	■ Increase work capacity ■ Increase endurance ■ Decrease total cholesterol and triglyceride concentrations ■ Increase daily caloric expenditure ■ Decrease adiposity	■ 40-80% peak work rate ■ 40-80% HRR ■ >5 days/week ■ 20-60 min/session or intermittent sessions (e.g., 2-3 sessions/day of 10-30 min)	■ 4 months (fitness) ■ 9-12 months (lipids)
Strength Free weights Machines	Increase muscle strength and endurance	■ 60-80% of 1RM ■ 2-4 sets of 8-12 reps ■ 2-3 days/week	4-6 months
Flexibility Upper and lower body ROM activities	Decrease risk of injury	■ Static stretches: hold for 10-30 s ■ 2-3 days/week	4-6 months

blood lipid changes are best achieved with exercise that is

- performed at moderate intensities (40-80% of maximal functional capacity);
- performed often (preferably five or more days a week);
- performed once a day, although exercising twice a day may be necessary to increase total energy expenditure and may be useful in persons with time constraints or severe exercise intolerance from chronic disease or morbid obesity; and
- incorporates resistance training as part of the exercise program.

People with dyslipidemia without comorbidities may follow the American College of Sports Medicine's resistance training guidelines for healthy adults.

Medications and special considerations for exercise programming include the following:

- The combined use of HMG-CoA reductase inhibitors and fibric acid—may cause muscle damage and limit exercise performance

- Medication use during exercise training must be taken into consideration (see appendix)
- Obesity—may limit exercise training choices (see chapter 25)

Evidence-Based Guidelines

Executive summary of the third report of the National Cholesterol Education Program (NCEP). Expert Panel on Detection, Evaluation, and Treatment of High Blood Cholesterol in Adults (Adult Treatment Panel III). JAMA. 2001;285(19):2486-2497. [Online]. Available at www.nhlbi.nih.gov/chd.

Fletcher G, Bufalina V, Costa F, et al. Efficacy of drug therapy in the secondary prevention of cardiovascular disease and stroke. Am J Cardiol. 2007;99(6):S1-S35.

Grundy SM, Cleeman JI, Merz CNB, et al. Implications of recent clinical trial for National Cholesterol Education Program Adult Treatment Panel III guidelines. Circulation. 2004;110:227-239.

Suggested Web Sites

Independent Drug Information Service (iDiS). www.rxfacts.org

National Cholesterol Education Program. www.nhlbi.nih.gov/about/ncep/index.htm

---

CASE STUDY

Dyslipoproteinemia

A 51-year-old man with hypertension presented with an acute coronary syndrome. His cardiovascular risk factors were hypertension, tobacco abuse, and sedentary lifestyle. He underwent cardiac catheterization and received a stent in his left anterior descending artery. His ejection fraction was preserved; and he was discharged from the hospital on aspirin, clopidogrel, beta-blocker, and a statin. On presentation to cardiac rehabilitation, he stated that he quit smoking after his hospitalization and began to walk daily. He has been watching his diet and has lost 5 lb (about 2 kg). He appears motivated to do more.

S: "I don't want to have another heart attack."

O: Vitals

Height: 6 ft 1 in. (1.9 m)
Weight: 236 lb (107 kg)
BP: 110/60 mmHg
Heart rate: 72 contractions/min
Well appearing, NAD
Heart and lung exam within normal limits (wnl)

Labs

Total cholesterol: 163 mg/dl
LDL-C: 104 mg/dl
Triglycerides: 148 mg/dl
HDL-C: 29 mg/dl
Glucose: 117 mg/dl
HbA1c: 5.9%
Graded exercise test (Bruce protocol, 6 weeks post event)
Total treadmill time: 6 min 30 s
Rest BP: 120/80 mmHg
Peak BP: 180/76 mmHg
Rest HR: 66 contractions/min
Peak HR: 155 contractions/min
Nonischemic ECG response to exercise

A: 1. Hyperlipidemia with low HDL-C
2. Tobacco abuse
3. Poor exercise tolerance
4. Obesity

(continued)

P: 1. Tobacco cessation
   2. Exercise program
   3. Weight loss

Exercise program goals

1. Consistent exercise
2. Increase exercise duration
3. Goal is 40-60 min of continuous exercise

Follow-Up

The patient attended cardiac rehabilitation and walked on the alternate days. He continued to remain tobacco free. Repeat evaluation 8 weeks later revealed BP 105/65 mmHg, HR 70 contractions/min, and weight 224 lb (about 100 kg). Lipid profile revealed total cholesterol 120 mg/dl, triglycerides 65 mg/dl, LDL-C 68 mg/dl, and HDL-C 39 mg/dl.

The patient remained motivated and continued to increase his exercise duration, and also added resistance training. He was placed on niacin therapy for his low HDL-C. Repeat evaluation 3 months later revealed BP 104/68 mmHg, off all medications, HR 66 contractions/min, and weight 193 lb (88 kg). His repeat lipid profile revealed total cholesterol 124 mg/dl, triglycerides 44 mg/dl, LDL-C 58 mg/dl, HDL-C 57 mg/dl, and fasting glucose 95 mg/dl. He underwent repeat exercise testing and exercised 13:45 min (Bruce protocol). Results of the test were resting HR 54 contractions/min, BP 90/60 mmHg, peak HR 169 contractions/min, and peak BP 140/76 mmHg. He was asymptomatic and had <1 mm upsloping ST-segment changes.

Mode	Frequency	Duration	Intensity	Progression
Aerobic (walking or biking)	4-5 days/week	20 min	THR (60-75% HRR)	Add 5 min of activity every week to 45 min. Increase intensity every 2 weeks to 75%.
Strength (all major muscle groups)	3 days/week		1 set of 10-12 reps	Add weight as needed to maintain comfortable resistance for 10-12 reps.
Flexibility (all major muscle groups)	3 days/week		Maintain each stretch for 15-30 s	
Warm-up and cool-down	Before and after each session	5-10 min	RPE 7-9/20	

End-Stage Metabolic Disease

Chronic Kidney Disease and Liver Failure

Patricia L. Painter, PhD, FACSM ■ Joanne B. Krasnoff, PhD

OVERVIEW OF THE PATHOPHYSIOLOGY

Chronic kidney disease (CKD) refers to the permanent loss of kidney function due to physical injury or disease. The diagnosis of CKD includes the use of pathological abnormalities, markers of damage in the blood, urine tests, or imaging studies. Presence of CKD is clinically confirmed via measurement of the amount of ultrafiltrate formed by plasma flowing through the glomeruli of the kidney, referred to as glomerular filtration rate (GFR). A diagnosis of CKD is made when GFR is <60 ml/min per 1.73 m² for more than three months. An estimated 20 million U.S. adults have CKD, while another 20 million are at increased risk. The loss of kidney function gradually progresses to the point of severe reduction of clearance of necessary waste products from the blood. End-stage renal disease (ESRD) is CKD that has progressed to the point where renal replacement therapy is required. End-stage renal disease results in severe metabolic abnormalities that affect nearly all physiologic systems. Because the kidney, like all vital organs, is essential for life,

ESRD is a life-threatening condition. The following are common consequences of renal failure:

- Metabolic acidosis
- Hypertension
- Left ventricular hypertrophy
- Anemia
- Secondary hyperparathyroidism
- Peripheral neuropathy
- Muscle weakness
- Autonomic dysfunction
- Elevated triglycerides and reduced high-density lipoprotein cholesterol

Over 45% of individuals with ESRD are diabetic and inactive and possess low functional capacities.

End-stage liver disease (ESLD) is characterized by cirrhosis of the liver, which is irreversible, and widespread damage to the hepatocytes. The most common causes of cirrhosis include viral disease (hepatitis), alcoholic liver disease, metabolic diseases, disease of the biliary tract, venous outflow obstruction, toxins, and immunologic disease. Another more recently discovered form of liver disease that leads to ESLD is called nonalcoholic fatty liver disease (NAFLD). This form of liver disease is characterized by a spectrum of liver conditions associated with fat accumulation that ranges from benign, nonprogressive liver fat accumulation (simple steatosis) to severe liver injury in which there is necroinflammation or fibrosis (nonalcoholic steatohepatitis, NASH) or both, cirrhosis, and liver failure. Nonalcoholic steatohepatitis has been associated with the metabolic syndrome (i.e., hepatic manifestation of metabolic syndrome) and disorders with abnormal fat metabolism (i.e., lipodystrophy).

The damaged and permanently destroyed hepatocytes are replaced by fibrous tissue, which leads to fibrosis (scarring). Hepatocytes then regenerate in an abnormal pattern surrounded by fibrous tissue. This abnormal liver structure eventually leads to decreased blood flow to and through the liver. There are many clinical manifestations of cirrhosis, including jaundice, portal hypertension and varices, ascites, hepatic encephalopathy, and ultimately hepatic failure. Individuals with ESLD experience fatigue, muscle wasting, anorexia, and anemia in addition to other symptoms specific to the etiology. Several biochemical markers are monitored, which assess (1) liver function (serum albumin, prothrombin time), (2) excretory function (bilirubin, alkaline phosphatase), and (3) hepatic inflammation (serum aminotransferases: AST, ALT). A liver biopsy is used for determining the etiology of the liver disease, as well as for tracking treatment results and disease progression.

EFFECTS ON
THE EXERCISE RESPONSE

Exercise intolerance is well documented in individuals with CKD who are being treated with dialysis, with average peak oxygen consumption ($\dot{V}O_{2peak}$) of 20 ml · kg^{-1} · min^{-1}. Exercise responses are characterized by a blunted heart rate response and excessive blood pressure increases. The primary reason for termination of exercise is leg fatigue. The limitations to exercise in these individuals could derive from any one of a number of factors, including the following:

■ Reduced peak cardiac output caused by a blunted heart rate response

■ Reduced oxygen-carrying capacity as a result of anemia

■ Subnormal capacity to extract oxygen related to weakness and structural and functional changes in muscle

Individuals with ESLD also have reduced peak oxygen consumption levels, reported to be approximately 55% of age-predicted values. The low $\dot{V}O_{2peak}$ levels in this population may be due to anemia, bed rest or inactivity, protein-caloric undernourishment, metabolic abnormalities related to lipid or carbohydrate metabolism or both, a decrease in muscle mass, and alcoholic myopathy. People with ESLD exhibit a lower maximal heart rate and reduced muscle strength. Electrolyte abnormalities can cause electrocardiographic changes.

EFFECTS
OF EXERCISE TRAINING

Exercise training studies support an effect on persons with ESRD, while few reported studies are available for persons with ESLD.

End-Stage Renal Disease

The level of exercise tolerance that can be achieved by people with ESRD is unclear, and it is probable that some individuals on dialysis will not improve their $\dot{V}O_{2peak}$ levels with training. Thus, the goal of exercise training is to improve or at least maintain exercise capacity. Aerobic exercise training usually improves $\dot{V}O_{2peak}$ by about 20% to 25% as a result of increased oxygen extraction in the muscle versus improvement in stroke volume or cardiac output. Low oxygen delivery to the skeletal muscle is improved by erythropoietin (EPO) therapy that increases hemoglobin as well as $\dot{V}O_{2peak}$ and quality of life. Because $\dot{V}O_{2peak}$ in these individuals correlates with muscle strength more closely than with hemoglobin, it is thought that skeletal muscle dysfunction is a major limiting factor for exercise capacity.

Exercise training improves blood pressure control, lipid profiles, and psychological profiles in some ESRD clients. The peak exercise capacity of many individuals on dialysis is such that the energy requirements of common activities of daily living are significant challenges to them. Thus, increasing exercise capacity is a major objective of exercise therapy for individuals with renal failure. Since limitations may be related to muscle weakness, it is reasonable to try both resistance and aerobic training programs to improve exercise capacity. Exercise counseling for independent home exercise or cycling during dialysis (or both) has been shown to improve physical performance tests (e.g., sit to stand, gait speed) and self-reported physical functioning as measured with the SF-36 questionnaire in patients treated with dialysis.

End-Stage Liver Disease

There is very little exercise training experience in clients with ESLD. One 12-week study (three or four 30 min sessions per week) in persons with chronic hepatitis resulted in a 30% increase in $\dot{V}O_{2peak}$ with no change in liver function tests, indicating no negative training effect on liver function. Improvement in $\dot{V}O_{2peak}$ values has also been demonstrated in individuals with ESLD following liver transplant surgery.

MANAGEMENT AND MEDICATIONS

People with CKD who have reached stage 5 (<15 GFR or on dialysis) require some form of renal replacement therapy for survival. The main form of maintenance therapy is hemodialysis; other treatment options include peritoneal dialysis and renal transplantation. Medical management issues include ensuring adequate dialysis therapy, which is monitored through urea kinetics and other blood testing; adequate blood pressure control, which often requires a variety of antihypertensive agents; control of the anemia using recombinant human EPO; control of secondary hyperparathyroidism through use of phosphate-binding agents; and adequate access for dialysis—that is, either blood access (for hemodialysis via arteriovenous fistula) or peritoneal catheter (for peritoneal dialysis).

End-Stage Renal Disease

Individuals with ESRD may develop any of the following problems:

- Congestive heart failure before the initiation of dialysis (due to fluid overload) or in the case of inadequate dialysis or fluid intake indiscretion
- Accelerated atherosclerosis
- Pericardial effusion resulting from inadequate dialysis and uremia
- Abnormal electrocardiogram caused by electrolyte abnormalities or structural changes
- Dysrhythmias from abnormal electrolytes (rare)

- Cardiomegaly resulting from fluid or pressure overload (or both), coronary artery disease, pericardial disease, uremic toxins, or other conditions
- Renal osteodystrophy resulting from secondary hyperparathyroidism
- Persistent anemia caused by iron deficiency, nonresponse to EPO, or both
- Peritonitis resulting from catheter infection (in clients treated with peritoneal dialysis)

Most people with ESRD are hypertensive and thus are treated with antihypertensive agents. During hemodialysis, a complex interaction of antihypertensive medications and dialysis can lead to either inadequate drug levels or severe hypotension. For this reason, antihypertensive medications are often not taken on dialysis days. Nearly all dialysis clients take recombinant EPO for anemia, although hematocrits are only partially corrected (usually up to 35%). Phosphate binders are prescribed for virtually all dialysis clients to prevent hyperparathyroidism and renal osteodystrophy. Insulin is administered to diabetic clients requiring it, with those on peritoneal dialysis receiving medication in their dialysis fluid. Other medications may be required for coexisting medical concerns.

End-Stage Liver Disease

The management of ESLD focuses on prevention of long-term complications, reduction in mortality, and symptom improvement. Treatment of the underlying liver disease may slow or stop the progression, depending on the etiology. For example, discontinuation of alcohol intake stops the progression of alcoholic cirrhosis. Treatment of metabolic diseases, such as iron overload in hemochromatosis or copper overload in Wilson disease, is also effective in stopping progression. Pharmacological therapy is sometimes effective in chronic viral hepatitis (B, C), autoimmune hepatitis, primary biliary cirrhosis, and sclerosing cholangitis. Complications of cirrhosis are treated using a variety of techniques, including endoscopic sclerotherapy or rubber band ligation for bleeding esophageal varices and low-sodium diet or diuretic therapy for ascites. Coagulation disorders are often responsive to vitamin K. When clients are unresponsive to all treatments and pharmacological therapies, liver transplantation becomes the final treatment option for ESLD. There is no information on how any of these therapies interact with or are affected by exercise training; however, lifestyle modification (i.e., diet and exercise intervention) may prevent the progression of NAFLD (i.e., from simple steatosis to NASH).

RECOMMENDATIONS FOR EXERCISE TESTING

The use of exercise testing for diagnostic purposes is questioned in both these populations since they are limited by muscle fatigue and low functional capacity. Thus, maximal diagnostic exercise testing may not be beneficial for screening before the initiation of an exercise training program; in fact, requiring such testing may present an unnecessary barrier to beginning an exercise program. Since people with ESLD experience continuing and intensive medical care, such testing probably does not provide any additional information. If some evaluation is needed, physical performance testing may be the most appropriate (see table 23.1).

Special considerations during exercise testing include the following:

- Antihypertensive medications should be administered as needed, depending on dialysis schedule and compliance with fluid restrictions.

- Erythropoietin is often used for anemia. Hematocrit should be maintained between 30% and 35%.

- People with ESLD are often on the following medications: interferon, ribavrin (hepatitis antivirals), prednisone, and asathioprine (Imuran) beta-blocker for autoimmune disease; diuretics for edema; Fosamax for low bone mineral density.

TABLE 23.1

ESRD and ESLD: Exercise Testing

Methods	Measures	Endpoints*	Comments
Aerobic Cycle (ramp protocol 17 W/min; staged protocol 25-50 W/3 min stage) Treadmill (1-2 METs/3 min stage)	■ 12-lead ECG, HR ■ BP, rate–pressure product ■ RPE (6-20)	■ $\dot{V}O_{2peak}$/work rate ■ Serious dysrhythmias ■ >2 mm ST-segment depression or elevation ■ Ischemic threshold ■ SBP >250 mmHg or DBP >115 mmHg ■ Hypotensive response ■ Onset of fatigue	Most clients terminate exercise because of skeletal muscle fatigue.
Strength Isokinetic or isotonic	Torque		1RM not recommended.
Flexibility Sit and reach	Distance		Useful in debilitated clients.
Neuromuscular Gait analysis Balance			Indicated for peripheral neuropathy, prosthetic devices, or severe muscle wasting.
Functional Timed sit to stand Gait speed Functional lifting tests	■ 10 reps ■ m/s ■ RPE (6-20)		■ Used for assessment of capacity for ADLs. ■ Useful for ADL assessment.

*Measurements of particular significance; do not always indicate test termination.

- Hemodialysis patients should be tested on a nondialysis day.
- Clients treated with continuous ambulatory peritoneal dialysis should be tested without fluid in the abdomen.
- Do not measure BP in the arm with the arteriovenous fistula (ESRD).
- Spontaneous avulsion fractures are possible in patients with long-standing renal bone disease (usually they have been on dialysis for more than five years).
- 30% of dialysis patients are diabetic (see table on exercise testing in chapter 24).
- Ascites may affect ventilation (ESLD).
- Those who have esophageal or gastric varices should avoid the Valsalva maneuver (ESLD).
- Bleeding and bruising are possible due to coagulation disorders (ESLD).
- Fatigue is a common concern (ESRD and ESLD).

RECOMMENDATIONS FOR EXERCISE PROGRAMMING

There is no guarantee that all individuals on dialysis or those with ESLD will respond to exercise training, including but not limited to increases in $\dot{V}O_{2peak}$ or functional capacity. The optimal program of exercise training has yet to be identified for either of these groups (see table 23.2). Additionally, the interactions between morbidity, the adequacy of dialysis (or treatments for liver disease) and other unknown

TABLE 23.2

ESRD and ESLD: Exercise Programming

Modes	Goals	Intensity/Frequency/ Duration	Time to goal
Aerobic Large muscle activities	▪ Increase aerobic capacity ▪ Increase time to exhaustion ▪ Increase work capacity ▪ Improve BP	▪ 40-80% peak HR or as tolerated ▪ 40-80% $\dot{V}O_{2peak}$ or as tolerated ▪ Monitor RPE ▪ 4-7 days/week ▪ 20-60 min/session or as tolerated	4-6 months
Strength Free weights Weight machines Isokinetic machines	Increase maximal number of reps	▪ Avoid high weights ▪ Concentrate on low-weight/high-rep program	4-6 months
Flexibility Stretching/yoga	▪ Maintain/increase ROM ▪ Improve gait, balance, and coordination		
Functional Activity-specific exercise	▪ Increase ADLs ▪ Increase vocational potential ▪ Increase physical self-confidence		

factors, and the response to exercise training have not been completely defined. The chronic nature of the disease and the multiple medical problems of these individuals often become the focus of the health care professionals who are caring for them. Information about or referral for exercise training in the past has typically not been part of the traditional care routine. Although difficult to integrate an exercise program into an already complex and intensive medical schedule, exercise training does provide the only possible chance to increase or at least maintain functional capacity in persons with these diseases. Increased awareness of the potential exercise benefits for individuals with ESRD or ESLD on the part of the medical community is needed (see table 23.2).

Special considerations during exercise testing include the following:

- Individuals receiving hemodialysis may not tolerate exercise after dialysis treatment.
- Patients treated with continuous ambulatory peritoneal dialysis may be more comfortable exercising without fluid in the abdomen.
- Be aware of the arteriovenous fistula and IV access lines.
- Spontaneous avulsion fractures may occur in patients with long-standing renal bone disease

(usually they have been on dialysis for more than five years).

- 30% of dialysis patients are diabetic (see table on exercise programming in chapter 24).
- Fatigue is a common concern.
- Gradual progression is essential.
- Patients frequently experience medical setbacks; the program may have to be adjusted accordingly.
- Exercise during hemodialysis treatment is recommended and should be encouraged when possible (in conjunction with the dialysis unit staff).

Evidence-Based Guidelines

Ash S, Campbell KL, MacLaughlin H, McCoy E, et al. Evidence based practice guidelines for nutritional management of chronic kidney disease. Nutr Dietetics. 2006;63(S2):S35-S45.

Johnson CA, Levey AS, Coresh J, Levin A, Lau J, Eknoyan G. Clinical practice guidelines for chronic kidney disease in adults: Part I. Definition, disease stages, evaluation, treatment, and risk factors. Am Fam Physician. 2004;70(5):869-876.

Suggested Web Site

American Academy of Family Physicians. www.aafp. org/online/en/home.html

---

CASE STUDY

End-Stage Renal Disease

A 64-year-old African American female with ESRD secondary to hypertension had been treated with hemodialysis for 18 months and referred for exercise training evaluation. She had retired from an office job upon starting dialysis treatments, which were for 3 h three times a week (540 min/week). She tolerated dialysis well and had a synthetic graft in her upper arm as an access for dialysis treatments. The graft had been declotted twice in the past two years and was working well. She had a history of coronary artery disease, which was effectively treated with PTCA three years previously.

On a more recent observation, the client was doing well and was evaluated for a living-related transplant from her daughter. She was not taking part in any regular physical activity and had no exercise history. The daughter was athletic and very interested in getting her mother started on an exercise program.

S: "I have been gradually getting weaker since starting dialysis. My leg muscles are weak and there are times when I am afraid of falling. I have difficulty climbing stairs and tire easily when shopping. I would like to get stronger before my transplant. I have also heard that exercise may help my blood pressure and I would like to take fewer drugs for my blood pressure."

O: Vitals

Height: 4 ft 11 in. (1.5 m)
Weight: 165 lb (75 kg)
BMI: 33.4 kg/m^2
HR: 82 contractions/min
BP: 156/92 mmHg
Elderly, overweight woman, appearing to lack energy
Ambulates slowly, but does not appear short of breath
Medications: EPO, diltiazem, multivitamins, phosphate binders

Labs

Albumin: 3.3 mg/dl
Hematocrit: 32%
Total cholesterol: 148 mg/dl
kT/v (indicator of adequacy of dialysis): 1.6 (average in her
dialysis unit is 1.38)

Graded Exercise Test

6 min walk: 919.5 ft (280 m); 3 rest stops during the test
Sit to stand (10 cycles): 37.58 s (51% age-predicted norm)
Gait speed (20 m): 66.9 cm/s (52.3% of normal for age)

Self-Reported Physical Function (SF-36 Scores)

Physical functioning: 36/100
Physical composite scale: 35.5 (normal: 50.0)

A: 1. ESRD secondary to hypertension, treated with
      hemodialysis
   2. CAD s/p (PTCA 3 years ago)
   3. Exercise intolerance (decreased strength and
      endurance)

4. Hypertension
5. Secondary hyperparathyroidism
6. Renal osteodystrophy

P: 1. Initiate muscular strengthening.
   2. Prescribe a cardiovascular exercise program.

Exercise Program Goals

1. Improved muscular strength, endurance, and
   balance
2. Short-term goals (1 mo):
   • Walk around block at home 3 times con-
     tinuously without stopping
   • Climb 1 flight of stairs without stopping
   • Reevaluate
3. Long-term goals (6 mo):
   • Walk 2 mi (3.2K) continuously
   • Climb 1 flight of stairs 3 times continuously

Mode	Frequency	Duration	Intensity	Progression
Aerobic (walk short distances, bike)	5-7 days/week	As tolerated	As tolerated	Walk 1 block in 1st week; then increase by 1/2 block/week, as tolerated.
Strength (all major muscle groups)	3 days/week	1 set of 10-12 reps	Resistance bands	Increase to 3 sets of 10-12 reps over 4 weeks; increase to stronger color bands as tolerated.
Flexibility (all major muscle groups)	3 days/week	20 s/stretch	Maintain each stretch below discomfort point	
Warm-up and cool-down	Before and after each session	5-10 min	RPE 7-9/20	

24

Diabetes

W. Guyton Hornsby Jr., PhD, CDE, FACSM ■ Ann L. Albright, PhD, RD

OVERVIEW OF THE PATHOPHYSIOLOGY

Diabetes is a chronic metabolic disease characterized by an absolute or relative deficiency of insulin that results in hyperglycemia. The current diagnostic consensus is that anyone with a fasting blood glucose level >125 mg/dl, a random glucose of >200 mg/dl with hyperglycemic symptoms, or a 2 h glucose of >200 mg/dl during an oral glucose tolerance test (OGTT) has diabetes. Blood glucose measurements obtained at initial diagnosis of diabetes reflect a narrow period of metabolic activity, whereas measurement of blood glucose bound to hemoglobin (HbA1c) provides an average blood glucose level over a prolonged period, usually the prior 60 to 90 days. Individuals with diabetes are at risk for developing microvascular complications, including retinopathy and nephropathy; macrovascular disease including heart attack and stroke; and various neuropathies (both autonomic and peripheral). Silent ischemia is common in people with diabetes, particularly if the disease is long-standing (see chapter 6 for management of this problem). Several distinct forms of diabetes are known to exist.

Type 1 Diabetes Mellitus

Individuals with type 1 diabetes have an absolute deficiency of insulin caused by a marked reduction in insulin-secreting beta cells of the pancreas. Con-

sequently, exogenous insulin must be supplied by injection or insulin pump. Individuals with type 1 diabetes are prone to developing ketoacidosis when deficient insulin levels result in hyperglycemia. The cause of type 1 diabetes is thought to involve an autoimmune response affecting the beta cells that ultimately leads to their destruction in genetically susceptible individuals. The factors that trigger the autoimmune response have not been specifically identified but may include viruses or toxins. The precise nature of the genetic influence in the pathogenesis of type 1 diabetes is also unclear, but the histocompatibility (human lymphocyte antigen) types DR3 and DR4 are associated with increased risk for type 1 diabetes. This form of diabetes usually occurs before the age of 30 but can occur at any age. Of the estimated 20.8 million people with diabetes mellitus in the United States, approximately 5% to 10% have type 1 diabetes.

Type 2 Diabetes Mellitus

Individuals with type 2 diabetes are considered to have a relative insulin deficiency, as they can have either elevated, reduced, or normal insulin levels. However, these individuals present with hyperglycemia regardless of their insulin status. Although the pathophysiology of type 2 diabetes remains unclear, possible contributing factors include genetics, the environment, insulin abnormalities, increased glucose production in the liver, increased fat breakdown, and defective hormonal secretions in the intestine. In this form of diabetes, peripheral tissue insulin resistance and defective insulin secretion are common features. With insulin resistance, glucose does not readily enter the insulin-sensitive tissues (primarily muscle and adipose tissue), and blood glucose rises. The increase in blood glucose causes the beta cells of the pancreas to secrete more insulin in an attempt to maintain a normal blood glucose concentration. Unfortunately, this additional endogenous insulin is usually ineffective in lowering blood glucose and may further contribute to insulin resistance. In some people, the beta (β) cells may become exhausted over time and insulin secretion decreases.

The mechanisms underlying insulin resistance remain unclear, although they likely involve defects in the binding of insulin to its receptor and in postreceptor events such as glucose transport. Because the majority of individuals with type 2 diabetes are overweight or obese at onset, obesity is clearly a significant contributor to insulin resistance. Several varieties of abnormalities in insulin secretion have been identified, but virtually all people with type 2 diabetes have lost the first or acute phase of insulin release. Insulin therapy may or may not be required, depending on the degree of functional insulin, or insulin sensitivity or responsiveness (or both), remaining. Individuals with type 2 diabetes do not develop ketoacidosis except under conditions of unusual stress (e.g., trauma). Type 2 diabetes is clearly genetically influenced as well, because it occurs in identical twins with almost total concordance. The onset is insidious, with few or no classic symptoms, and unfortunately many individuals are not diagnosed until organ damage has occurred. Type 2 diabetes affects approximately 90% to 95% of the 20.8 million people with diabetes, yet more than 6.2 million of these cases are undetected. Type 2 diabetes is associated with older age, obesity, physical inactivity, family history of diabetes, history of gestational diabetes, and race or ethnicity. The ethnic groups most commonly affected by type 2 diabetes include African Americans, Hispanic-Latino Americans, American Indians and Alaskan Natives, and some Asian Americans and Native Hawaiians or Other Pacific Islanders. Type 2 diabetes usually occurs after the age of 40, but with the growing rates of obesity and physical inactivity it is developing in young adults and youth.

Gestational Diabetes

Gestational diabetes is defined as glucose intolerance with onset or first recognition during pregnancy. It occurs during pregnancy because of the contra-insulin effects of pregnancy. Gestational diabetes is usually diagnosed by an OGTT performed between 24 and 28 weeks of gestation. Risk factors for the development of gestational diabetes include family history of gestational diabetes, previous delivery of a large-birth-weight baby, and obesity. Approximately 20% to 50% of women who develop gestational diabetes develop type 2 diabetes within 5 to 10 years. Although rates of gestational diabetes have remained relatively stable, the number of women starting their pregnancies with preexisting type 1 or 2 diabetes has more than doubled since 1999, likely due to the rising trend in overweight and obesity.

Other Specific Types of Diabetes

Certain endocrinopathies, genetic syndromes, infections leading to β-cell destruction, reactions to drugs or toxic chemicals, uncommon forms of immune-mediated diabetes, diseases of the exocrine pancreas, and genetic defects in β-cell function and in insulin action can result in rather rare forms of diabetes. Many of these conditions have been identified and are classified as other specific types of diabetes. These types may or may not require insulin treatment, depending on the pathophysiology of the condition and the level of normal insulin secretion and insulin action. These conditions include the following:

- Endocrinopathies such as acromegaly, Cushing's syndrome, glucagonoma, and pheochromocytoma
- Genetic syndromes such as Down syndrome, Klinefelter's syndrome, and Turner's syndrome
- Cell destruction by viruses such as coxsackievirus B, cytomegalovirus, adenovirus, mumps, and congenital rubella
- Reactions to drugs or chemicals such as nicotinic acid, glucocorticoids, thiazides, adrenergic agonists, thyroid hormone, Dilantin, alpha-interferon, and Vacor (rat poison)
- Uncommon forms of immune-mediated diabetes like "stiff man" syndrome and conditions with anti-insulin receptor antibodies
- Diseases of the exocrine pancreas such as pancreatitis, neoplasia, and cystic fibrosis
- Defects in β-cell function such as maturity-onset diabetes of the young (MODY)
- Genetic defects in insulin action such as type A insulin resistance, leprechaunism, and Rabson-Mendenhall syndrome

Impaired Glucose Tolerance and Impaired Fasting Glucose

Impaired glucose tolerance (IGT) and impaired fasting glucose (IFG) are intermediate metabolic conditions between normoglycemia and forthright diabetes. The upper limit of normal fasting glucose has been set at 99 mg/dl, and the value used for the provisional diagnosis of diabetes is any value >125 mg/dl. A confirmed fasting glucose between 100 and 125 mg/dl is recognized as IFG, and a 2 h value on an OGTT falling between 140 and 200 mg/dl may be recognized as IGT. Those with IGT or IFG or both are at an increased risk not only for diabetes but also for cardiovascular disease and for increased mortality from cardiovascular disease.

EFFECTS ON THE EXERCISE RESPONSE

Under normal conditions in individuals without diabetes, a precise coordination of hormonal and metabolic events results in maintenance of glucose homeostasis. Insulin and counterregulatory hormone concentrations in people with diabetes do not respond to exercise in the normal manner, and the balance between peripheral glucose utilization and hepatic glucose production may be disturbed. The effect of diabetes on a single exercise session is dependent on several factors, including the following:

- Use and type of medication to lower blood glucose (insulin or oral hypoglycemic agents)
- Timing of medication administration
- Blood glucose level prior to exercise
- Timing, amount, and type of previous food intake
- Presence and severity of diabetic complications
- Use of other medication secondary to diabetic complications
- Intensity, duration, and type of exercise

EFFECTS OF EXERCISE TRAINING

Exercise is an essential component of diabetes care. An exercise training program has the potential to provide numerous benefits for those with diabetes. These benefits may include the following:

- Possible improvement in blood glucose control. Exercise should be a part of diabetes therapy (in addition to diet and medication) to improve blood glucose control for those with type 2 diabetes. Exercise is not considered a component of treatment or a method for lowering blood glucose in type 1 diabetes Those with type 1 diabetes are encouraged to exercise to gain other benefits such as improving cardiovascular health, but blood glucose must be in reasonable control (<250 mg/dl, no ketones) if the individual is to exercise safely.

- Improved insulin sensitivity, lower medication requirement. Exercise training results in improved insulin sensitivity, and for many with diabetes this translates into a reduction in dose of insulin or oral agents.

- Reduction in body fat. Weight loss increases insulin sensitivity and may allow those with diabetes to reduce the amounts of insulin or oral hypoglycemic agents needed. Exercise coupled with moderate caloric intake is considered the most effective way to lose weight. Exercise is also a critical factor in maintenance of weight loss.

- Cardiovascular benefits. Regular exercise decreases the risk of cardiovascular disease. It is likely that this is true to some extent for persons with diabetes.

- Prevention of type 2 diabetes. Epidemiological studies have indicated that exercise may play a role in preventing type 2 diabetes. Those with IGT, gestational diabetes, or a family history of type 2 diabetes may especially benefit from regular physical activity.

Nearly everyone with diabetes can derive some benefit from an exercise program, although not all benefits will necessarily be realized by each person. Careful monitoring of blood glucose and attention to balancing food intake and medication are necessary in order for the person to participate safely in an exercise program.

MANAGEMENT AND MEDICATIONS

The management of diabetes depends on the form of diabetes, blood glucose goals, and the presence and severity of diabetic complications. One goal of diabetes management is to normalize blood glucose to the extent that it is safe to do so. This regulation of diabetes is accomplished by insulin or oral agents for type 2 diabetes, or both if necessary; by an individual nutrition care plan; and by participation in a habitual exercise program as appropriate.

Insulin therapy for diabetes requires the patient to inject insulin with a syringe one to several times per day or to use an insulin pump. Pumps are small computerized devices that deliver insulin through a catheter inserted beneath the skin. They are set to deliver basal insulin at a slow continuous rate and can deliver larger bolus doses at mealtimes. Because exercise enhances the absorption of exogenous insulin, adjustments in insulin dosage, careful blood glucose monitoring, and attention to diet around the time of exercise are needed to prevent hypoglycemia. Reductions may be needed in both short- or rapid-acting insulin and intermediate- or long-acting insulin. Patients on pump therapy may need to decrease bolus doses by 20% to 50%, and may choose to discontinue basal insulin during exercise and decrease the basal insulin by 25% after exercise. The ability to program changes in basal insulin dosage is a unique advantage of the insulin pump. However, some patients may feel that the use of the pump could limit their ability to perform activities such as contact or water-based sports. During these types of activities the pump must be either removed or worn in a protective casing. Given that pump disconnection ceases all

insulin delivery, patients should go no longer than 1 or 2 h at a time before reconnecting and should also frequently monitor their blood glucose levels. Patients on insulin pumps receive information and educational sessions on their use during exercise. Detailed instructions for the use of an insulin pump are found on the American Diabetes Association Web site.

As the vast majority of morbidity and mortality in diabetes are related to macrovascular disease, medical management must also focus on reducing risk of cardiovascular disease. Medications used in diabetes management not only include glucose-lowering agents but also frequently include aspirin, angiotensin-converting enzyme inhibitors, other antihypertensives, lipid-lowering agents, and pain medications. (See chapter 14 on hypertension and chapter 22 on hyperlipidemia for information on these medications.) Insulin and oral agents are the primary means for proper medical management of diabetes.

- Insulin allows glucose to enter the cells of insulin-sensitive tissue. Several different types of insulin are available pharmaceutically that vary in onset, peak, duration, and source (see table 24.1).

TABLE 24.1

Types of Insulin

Generic name	Trade name	Onset	Peak	Duration
Rapid acting Insulin lispro Insulin aspart Insulin glulisine	Humalog NovoLog Apidra	<15 min	30-90 min	1-3 h
Short acting Regular	Humulin R Novolin R	30-60 min	2-3 h	3-6 h
Intermediate acting NPH Lente	Humulin N Novolin N Humulin L	2-4 h	4-10 h	10-16 h
Long acting Insulin glargine Ultralente	Lantus Humulin U	2-4 h	Does not peak	18-36 h

- Oral and injectable agents for type 2 diabetes are medications that help the pancreas secrete more insulin, alter carbohydrate absorption, reduce liver glycogenolysis, increase insulin sensitivity, or have some combination of these effects (see tables 24.2 and 24.3).

The most significant effect of both insulin and some oral hypoglycemic agents on exercise testing and exercise training is their ability to cause hypoglycemia. Attention to timing of medication, food intake, and blood glucose level before and after exercise is necessary. In addition, blood glucose

TABLE 24.2

Oral Agents Used for Treatment of Type 2 Diabetes

Generic name	Trade name	Concerns with exercise
Biguanides		
Metformin	Glucophage, Glucophage XR	
Metformin (liquid)	Riomet	
Glucosidase inhibitors		
Acarbose	Precose	May produce hypoglycemia with postprandial exercise.
Miglitol	Glyset	
Meglitinides		
Nateglinide	Starlix	May produce hypoglycemia with postprandial exercise.
Repaglinide	Prandin	
Secretagogues		
Acetohexamide	Generic only	Can produce hypoglycemia during or after exercise.
Chlorpromide	Diabinese	
Tolazimide	Tolinase	
Tolbutamide	Orinase	
Glimepride	Amaryl	
Glipizide	Glucotrol, Glucotrol XL	
Glyburide	Diabeta, Glynase, PresTab, Micronase	
Thiazoladinediones		
Pioglitazone	Actos	
Rosiglitazone	Avandia	
Dipeptidyl peptidase-4 inhibitors		
Sitagliptin	Januvia	No hypoglycemia unless given with another drug.
Combinations		
Metformin + glyburide	Glucovance	See concerns for individual drugs.
Metformin + rosiglitazone	Avandamet	
Metformin + glipizide	Metaglip	
Sitagliptin + metformin	Janumet	

TABLE 24.3

Other Injectable Medications Used in Treatment of Diabetes

Generic name	Trade name	Comments and concerns with exercise
Exanitide*	Byetta	Exanitide is used in treatment of type 2 diabetes and is found to increase postprandial insulin response, delay gastric emptying, suppress glucagon secretion, and reduce appetite.
Pramlintide*	Symlin	Pramlintide is a synthetic hormone similar to human amylin. It may be used in combination with insulin therapy for treatment of either type 1 or type 2 diabetes. Pramlintide works by suppressing glucagon secretion and delaying gastric emptying.

*Both exanitide and pramlintide are used to reduce postprandial increases in blood glucose and may assist with weight loss. The timing of exanitide and pramlintide injections can be an important consideration in exercise therapy, as they may reduce absorption of oral medications such as antihypertensives. They may also interfere with absorption of dietary carbohydrate when one is attempting to treat hypoglycemia.

should be checked periodically during exercise of long durations (i.e., >60 min).

RECOMMENDATIONS FOR EXERCISE TESTING

Recommendations for exercise testing depend on age, duration of diabetes, and presence of diabetic complications (see table 24.4). Exercise testing using protocols for populations at risk for coronary artery disease (CAD) is recommended in individuals who

- have type 1 diabetes and are over the age of 30,
- have had type 1 diabetes longer than 15 years,
- have type 2 diabetes and are over age 35,
- have either type 1 or type 2 diabetes and one or more of the other CAD risk factors,
- have suspected or known CAD, or
- have any microvascular or neurological diabetic complications.

Impaired chronotropic response during exercise testing (achievement of <80% heart rate reserve) in individuals with diabetes is associated with an increased risk of all-cause mortality, myocardial infarction, and coronary revascularization procedures.

TABLE 24.4

Diabetes: Exercise Testing

Methods*	Measures	Endpoints**	Comments***
Aerobic Cycle (ramp protocol 17 W/min; staged protocol 25-50 W/3 min stage) Treadmill (1-2 METs/stage)	■ 12-lead ECG, HR	■ Serious dysrhythmias ■ >2 mm ST-segment depression or elevation ■ Ischemic threshold ■ Significant T-wave change	High risk for CAD
	■ BP	■ SBP >250 mmHg or DBP >115 mmHg	
	■ RPE (6-20)	■ Onset of peripheral pain	

*Methods of exercise testing are conservative because of the high risk of underlying cardiovascular disease and other chronic complications. More aggressive methods may be indicated for athletes or active patients without complications.

**Measurements of particular significance; do not always indicate test termination.

***Exercise testing is contraindicated if blood glucose is <70 mg/dl.

People with diabetes who do not meet any of these criteria may be tested with use of protocols for the general healthy population. The primary objectives of exercise testing in those with diabetes are to

- identify the presence and extent of CAD, and

- determine appropriate intensity range for aerobic exercise training.

RECOMMENDATIONS FOR EXERCISE PROGRAMMING

The exercise prescription for people with diabetes must be individualized according to medication schedule, presence and severity of diabetic complications, and goals and expected benefits of the exercise program. Physical activity for those without significant complications or limitations should include appropriate endurance and resistance exercise for developing and maintaining cardiorespiratory fitness, body composition, and muscular strength and endurance (see table 24.5). Food intake with exercise must be considered for anyone on a hypoglycemic medication. In general, 1 h of exercise requires an additional 15 g of carbohydrate either before or after exercise. People should consume an additional 15 to 30 g of carbohydrate every hour when performing vigorous or long-duration (>60 min) exercise. Exercise is contraindicated under the following circumstances:

- Active retinal hemorrhage is present or the person has received recent therapy for retinopathy (e.g., laser treatment).

- Illness or infection is present.

- Blood glucose is above 250 mg/dl and ketones are present (blood glucose should be lowered before initiation of exercise).

- Blood glucose is less than 70 mg/dl—because the risk of hypoglycemia is great (if pre- or

TABLE 24.5

Diabetes: Exercise Programming

Modes	Goals	Intensity/Frequency/Duration	Time to goal
Aerobic Large muscle activities	▪ Increase aerobic capacity ▪ Increase time to exhaustion ▪ Increase work capacity ▪ Improve BP response to exercise ▪ Reduce cardiovascular risk factors	▪ 50-80% peak HR* ▪ 50-80% $\dot{V}O_{2peak}$* ▪ Monitor RPE** ▪ 4-7 sessions/week ▪ 20-60 min/session	4-6 months
Strength Free weights Weight machines Elastic tubing or bands	▪ Increase maximal number of reps ▪ Improve performance for patients interested in competition	▪ Low resistance, high repetitions for most clients ▪ High resistance OK for patients with well-controlled diabetes	4-6 months
Anaerobic High-intensity intervals	Only for athletes in good diabetic control	Same as for nondiabetic athletes	

Modes	Goals	Intensity/Frequency/ Duration	Time to goal
Flexibility Stretching/yoga	■ Maintain/increase ROM ■ Improve gait	Limited data available; 2-3 sessions/week may suffice	4-6 months
Neuromuscular Yoga	■ Improve balance ■ Improve coordination		
Functional Activity-specific exercise	■ Increase ADLs ■ Increase vocational potential ■ Increase physical self-confidence	Individualized to each client	

*Lower-intensity activity may be advisable if complications are present or if diabetes is of long duration. The majority of persons with type 2 diabetes will benefit from low- to moderate-intensity physical activity of 40-70% $\dot{V}O_{2max}$.

**RPE is especially useful in persons whose HR has been altered by autonomic neuropathy or medications.

postexercise blood glucose is less than 100 mg/dl, carbohydrate should be eaten and blood glucose allowed to increase before initiation of exercise).

Exercise precautions include the following:

■ During exercise, a source of carbohydrate (that does not also contain fat) should be readily available

■ Consuming adequate fluids before, during, and after exercise

■ Practicing good foot care by wearing proper shoes and cotton socks, and inspecting feet after exercise

■ Carrying medical identification

Evidence-Based Guidelines

American Diabetes Association. Clinical practice recommendations 2008. Diabetes Care. 2008;31:suppl 1.

American Diabetes Association. Evidence-based nutrition principles and recommendations for the treatment and prevention of diabetes and related complications. Diabetes Care. 2002;25:202-212.

Suggested Web Sites

American Diabetes Association. www.diabetes.org/home.jsp

National Diabetes Information Clearinghouse (NDIC). http://diabetes.niddk.nih.gov/

CASE STUDY

Diabetes Mellitus

A 47-year-old woman with hypertension, hyperlipidemia, obesity, and type 2 diabetes presented for weight loss and improvement in glycemic control. She had undergone a cardiac catheterization, which showed diffuse diabetic coronary artery disease, especially at the left anterior descending with a proximal 70% stenosis at the first diagonal, 80% ostial stenosis, and a 90% mid left anterior descending coronary stenosis. Subsequently she had undergone a percutaneous transluminal coronary angioplasty with stent placements at the proximal, mid, and distal left anterior descending coronary artery. She denied chest pain, shortness of breath, or nausea. Her past medical history was pertinent for bilateral fourth finger Dupuytren's contracture and adhesive capsulitis of the right shoulder.

S: "I'm here because they tell me I need to exercise."

O: Vitals

Height: 5 ft 5 in. (1.65 m)
Weight: 231 lb (105 kg)
BMI: 38.57 kg/m^2
HR: 66 contractions/min
BP: 130/76 mmHg
Obese female in no acute distress
Nodularity overlying fourth flexor tendon sheaths of both hands
Decreased active and passive ROM in all fields in right shoulder
Medications: Insulin glargine, insulin lispro, metformin, valsartan and hydrochlorothiazide, metoprolol, amlo-dipine, nitroglycerin, acetylsalicylic acid, clopidogrel bisulfate, ezetimibe, gemfibrozil, sertraline, gabapentin

Labs

Fasting glucose: 199 mg/dl
A1c: 10.2% (normal range: 3.8-6.3%)
Triglycerides: 222 mg/dl
Total cholesterol: 170 mg/dl
HDL: 41 mg/dl
LDL: 99 mg/dl

Graded Exercise Test (Modified Balke Protocol)

Peak $\dot{V}O_{2peak}$: 14.7 · kg^{-1} · min^{-1}
Peak RPE: 18/20
Peak HR: 122 contractions/min
Peak BP: 204/74 mmHg
ECG: Sinus rhythm at rest and throughout exercise and recovery
No dysrhythmias and no report of chest discomfort

Body Composition

Fat: 46.2% (BodPod)

A: 1. Type 2 diabetes mellitus
2. CAD
3. Obesity
4. Dupuytren's contracture
5. Decreased ROM of the right shoulder

P: 1. Initiate comprehensive exercise and lifestyle modification.

Mode	Frequency	Duration	Intensity	Progression
Aerobic (recumbent bike, elliptical walker, rower)	3 sessions/week	10 min/apparatus	RPE 11-13/20 HR 94-105 contractions/min	Add 1 min/week up to 15 min/apparatus.
Strength (all major muscle groups)	3 sessions/week	2-3 sets of 10-15 reps	~40-50% 1RM	Increase to 18-20 reps, then to ~50-60% 1RM.
Flexibility (all major muscle groups)	Daily	Hold each stretch for 6-10 s	Maintain stretch below discomfort point	Increase to 20 s as tolerated. Add rotator cuff stretch.
Neuromuscular				
Functional				
Warm-up and cool-down	Before and after each session	5-10 min	Below talk test level RPE 7-9/20	

2. Prescribe a comprehensive diabetes program including diabetes management and cardiovascular risk reduction.
3. Refer for individualized medical nutrition therapy.

Exercise Program Goals

1. Increase aerobic capacity
2. Increase strength
3. Increase ROM, especially in right shoulder
4. Reduce body weight by at least 7%
5. Educate client on glucose management during exercise

Follow-Up

- Conduct blood glucose tests before and after exercise.
- Beware of hypoglycemia during and after exercise.
- Practice proper foot care and teach inspection of feet.

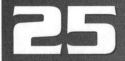

Obesity

Janet P. Wallace, PhD, FACSM ■ Shahla Ray, PhD

OVERVIEW OF THE PATHOPHYSIOLOGY

Obesity is defined as an excessive accumulation of body fat and is associated with numerous comorbidities, many of which are life threatening. Prevalence estimates of the number of obese children and adults vary depending on variations in obesity classification systems and ethnic origins within population samples, as well as other factors. In 2006, population-based estimates revealed that 33.3% of U.S. adult men and 35.3% of women aged 20 years and older were obese (body mass index [BMI] >30 kg/m^2); this included notably higher rates of obesity in Hispanic and non-Hispanic black women in particular. A BMI level above the 95th percentile for age and sex, or exceeding 30, whichever is smaller, is the standard by which obesity is classified in children and adolescents. In 2006, population-based estimates indicated that 11.3% of U.S. children and adolescents had a BMI at or above the 97th percentile for age and sex while 16.3% were at or above the 95th percentile. Despite the unfortunate trend of more than two decades of steadily increasing rates of obesity, it appeared that since the end of 2006, obesity rates for U.S. children and adults have stabilized, at least for the time being.

Obesity is a complex multifaceted disease involving, among other factors, hypothalamic, endocrine, and genetic disorders; the environment; and behavior. A common misconception is that the primary cause of obesity is overeating. In fact, most evidence suggests that energy imbalance resulting from the consumption of excess total calories (especially a diet high in fat and refined sugar), or from a sedentary lifestyle, or from a combination of the two is the primary cause of obesity in the United States. In the United States, as well as many other industrialized countries, the rapid appearance of obesity has been largely fueled by the exploitation of accessible, abundant, and inexpensive energy-dense foods and the substantial reduction in average daily energy expenditure required for survival. Further complicating the matter is the evolutionary adaptation theory. According to this theory, even though our bodies have evolved over millions of years, we have inherited the genetic makeup of our nomadic hunter-gatherer forefathers, who expended large amounts of energy to survive in periods of feast and famine without becoming overweight or obese.

The human body has difficulty adapting to chronic periods of energy imbalance, as indicated by the altered physiological responses associated with obesity, including the following:

- Increased fasting insulin
- Increased insulin response to glucose
- Decreased insulin sensitivity
- Decreased growth hormone
- Decreased growth hormone response to insulin stimulation
- Increased adrenocortical hormones
- Increased cholesterol synthesis and excretion
- Decreased hormone-sensitive lipase

Altered insulin function may be a primary mechanism in the etiology and maintenance of obesity.

The primary difference between the identification, definition, and classification of obesity and of overweight is the assessment of body fat. In addition to the percentage of body fat, factors to consider in determining the degree to which obesity impairs health are the location of fat deposits and other comorbidities. Ideally, obesity should be classified based on body composition assessment, although this rarely occurs, especially in large population samples. Since the National Institutes of Health recommended using BMI to define and classify obesity in 1988, BMI has become the accepted international standard for classifying obesity and overweight for large population-based studies. Although BMI is a crude measurement that doesn't quantify body composition, from a public health standpoint it correlates fairly well with the subcutaneous body fat in the majority of individuals and is easy and very convenient to obtain. Obesity has been defined with the use of many systems, most commonly height/weight tables, BMI, and body fat percentage. More recently, in addition to calculation of BMI, body fat distribution has been estimated using waist circumference (WC).

Current population-based BMI and WC classification levels are shown in tables 25.1 and 25.2.

The body fat percentages in table 25.3 for men and women 18 years and older can additionally be used to identify obesity and stratify obesity-related health risks.

Obesity can also be classified based on phenotype, fat cell morphology, and overall health status, although these methods constitute more theoretical versus practical applications:

Phenotype

Type I: Excess body mass or percentage fat

Type II: Excess subcutaneous truncal-abdominal fat (android)

Type III: Excess abdominal visceral fat

Type IV: Excess gluteal-femoral fat (gynoid)

Cell Morphology

Hyperplastic obesity

Hypertrophic obesity

Health Status

Mild obesity

Morbid obesity

Obesity increases the overall risk and severity of numerous diseases. The distribution of body fat may contribute more to disease than total body fat alone. Upper body fat distribution (android obesity)

TABLE 25.1

Classification of Disease Risk Based on Body Mass Index (BMI) and Waist Circumference

	BMI (kg · m²)	Disease risk[†] relative to normal weight and waist circumference	
		Men, ≤102 cm Women, ≤88 cm	Men, >102 cm Women, >88 cm
Underweight	<18.5	—	—
Normal	18.5-24.9	—	—
Overweight	25.0-29.9	Increased	High
Obesity, class			
I	30.0-34.9	High	Very high
II	35.0-39.9	Very high	Very high
III	≥40	Extremely high	Extremely high

[†]Disease risk for type 2 diabetes, hypertension, and cardiovascular disease. Dashes (—) indicate that no additional risk at these levels of BMI was assigned. Increased waist circumference can also be a marker for increased risk even in persons of normal weight.

Reprinted from Expert Panel, 1998 "Executive summary of the clinical guidelines on the identification, evaluation, and treatment of overweight and obesity in adults," *Archives of Internal Medicine* 158: 1855–1867.

TABLE 25.2

Criteria for Waist Circumference in Adults

Risk category	Waist circumference in centimeters (inches)	
	Females	Males
Very low	<70 cm (<28.5 in)	<80 cm (31.5 in)
Low	70-89 (28.5-35.0)	80-99 (31.5-39.0)
High	90-109 (35.5-43.0)	100-120 (39.5-47.0)
Very high	>110 (>43.5)	>120 (47.0)

Adapted, by permission, from G.A. Bray, 2004, "Don't throw the baby out with the bath water," *American Journal of Clinical Nutrition* 70(3): 347-349.

TABLE 25.3

Classification of Disease Risk Based on Body Fat Percentages

	Men	Women
Minimal fat	5%	8%
Below average	5-15%	14-23%
Above average	16-25%	24-32%
At risk	>25%	>32%

is strongly correlated with increased risk of coronary artery disease (CAD), hypertension, hyperlipidemia, and diabetes, as well as hormone and menstrual dysfunction. Truncal adipocytes are unique in that they are metabolically more active and secrete proteins called adipocytokines that control various metabolic functions. The higher metabolic activity of these adipocytes is associated with insulin resistance, hypertension via increased sodium retention, sympathetic nervous system activation, increased intracellular calcium, and hypertrophy of smooth muscle vessels. Abdominal adipocytes are also associated with increased very-low-density lipoprotein, triglyceride, and adipose lipoprotein lipase activity. Thus it is clear that excess fat accumulation in specific body areas likely contributes more to increased disease risk than the classification of obesity alone. Another body fat distribution assessment technique, waist-to-hip ratio, also correlates with disease risk prediction, especially CAD risk, although risk varies with age and sex. The recommended technique for assessing waist-to-hip ratio is to measure the minimal waist (at or above the umbilicus) and divide by the circumference of the hips at the widest gluteus level. Standards for the waist-to-hip ratio are as follows:

- Lower body fat distribution for men: <0.776
- Lower body fat distribution for women: <0.776
- Upper body fat distribution for men: >0.913
- Upper body fat distribution for women: >0.861

EFFECTS ON THE EXERCISE RESPONSE

Besides the overall low functional status of this population, one of the most discernible effects of obesity on the exercise response involves the ways in which obesity adds stress to the joints, affects movement, affects gait, increases foot pressure, decreases strength, and subsequently increases the risk of osteoarthritis. Apart from the biomechanical effects, other common comorbidities of obesity, including diabetes, hypertension, CAD, and sleep apnea, increase the overall risk of exercise and can affect the exercise response. Social and behavioral factors associated with obesity, such as past experiences with and current fears of exercise should also be considered. Prior to any formal exercise, including exercise testing, a comprehensive health history and, if possible, a medical history should be obtained from all obese clients.

EFFECTS OF EXERCISE TRAINING

Exercise training, alone or in combination with caloric restriction, is an effective intervention for reducing body weight and favorably altering body composition, especially in mildly to moderately obese individuals. In morbidly obese individuals, however, exercise and caloric restriction as a primary intervention is typically ineffective, although it later becomes important in weight maintenance. The benefits of regular physical activity and exercise in the treatment of obesity are numerous; these include preservation of lean body mass despite caloric restriction, improved insulin sensitivity, favorable changes in metabolic rate and lipid profiles, reduced blood pressure, improved mood, possible effects on satiety, and overall reduction in comorbidity risk.

Physical activity also promotes loss of regional fat, especially abdominal fat deposits. A number of research studies have confirmed that exercise alone or in combination with caloric restriction is more effective in reducing abdominal fat cell size than diet alone. Thus the most efficient means of reducing abdominal fat is through exercise. Physical activity may be one of the most important factors in the maintenance of weight loss because of the resultant increase in energy expenditure or because thispositive behavior change indirectly influences caloric intake.

Research has clearly shown that energy expenditure following exercise remains elevated above pre-exercise levels, the degree of elevation depending primarily on the type and intensity of exercise and to a lesser extent the duration. The elevated energy expenditure following exercise can have a significant impact, in some cases, on the total number of calories expended (beyond those expended during exercise). Although highly trained endurance athletes can exhibit higher overall resting metabolic rates (RMR), there is little evidence that the type and intensity of exercise performed by untrained obese individuals produce any significant lasting increases in RMR. Metabolic rate, including the caloric cost of physical activity, does not appear to decline with weight reduction. In the starvation state, however, the maintenance of metabolic rate through exercise may not always counteract the reduction mediated by food restriction.

Exercise training also has profound effects on glucose metabolism, in both moderately and morbidly obese persons. These include

- decreased fasting glucose,
- decreased fasting insulin,
- increased glucose tolerance, and
- decreased insulin resistance.

These changes can occur with and without changes in body weight or body fat, with the most dramatic changes occurring in those who have exhibited the greatest reduction in visceral fat.

MANAGEMENT AND MEDICATIONS

Reduction of fat weight with the preservation of lean body weight is the primary objective of obesity management. Those who are most likely to be successful in weight loss include people who

- are slightly or moderately obese,
- have upper body fat distribution,
- have no history of weight cycling,
- have a sincere desire to lose weight, and
- became overweight as an adult.

The most common and widely accepted intervention for the treatment of obesity is behavioral change focused on dietary and activity habits toward weight reduction; more invasive interventions may be more appropriate in morbid or extreme obesity (BMI >40).

Pharmacology

The most common Food and Drug Administration (FDA)-approved drugs for the treatment of obesity are based on reducing fat absorption, suppressing appetite, and stimulating the central nervous system. These drugs are shown in table 25.4.

Bariatric Surgery

The FDA has approved two invasive methods for treating obesity that are based on reducing the size of the stomach and lowering the absorption of nutrients in the intestine. Individuals with a BMI of >40, or between 35 and 40 with comorbidities such as diabetes mellitus and hypertension, are eligible for bariatric surgery. The surgical treatment of obesity has been shown to address most of the obesity-related comorbidities and reduce excess body weight by an average of 50% to 60%. Laparoscopic

TABLE 25.4

Common FDA-Approved Medications for the Treatment of Obesity

Drug	Mechanism of action	Exercise-related precautions
Adipex-P (phentermine)[1]	Appetite suppressant	Increase in blood pressure
Meridia (sibutramine hydrochloride)[1]	Appetite suppressant	Increase in blood pressure
Dexedrine (dextroamphetamine saccharate)[1]	Central nervous system stimulant	Possible cardiovascular risks
Alli (orlistat)[2] Xenical (orlistat)[1]	Reduction in fat absorption via inhibition of pancreatic lipase activity in intestine	–

[1]Prescription; [2]over the counter.

gastric banding (Lap-Band) is a minimally invasive surgery that involves the placement of an adjustable silicone band around the top portion of the stomach, creating a small gastric pouch that reduces the capacity of the stomach and produces a feeling of fullness shortly after eating. The Lap-Band has numerous benefits, including less surgical trauma and pain, faster recovery rate, and rare operative mortality. The Roux-en-Y gastric bypass (RYGBP) is a more invasive surgical procedure that reduces the capacity of the stomach. A small pouch is created at the top of the stomach that is then connected directly to the middle portion of the small intestine, bypassing the rest of the stomach and the upper portion of the small intestine. The RYGBP procedure has a higher mortality and complication risk than gastric banding because the surgery is more invasive.

RECOMMENDATIONS FOR EXERCISE TESTING

Standardized exercise protocols may be appropriate for people who are obese once they have been cleared for testing; however, low-level protocols are recommended because of the low functional capacity of most individuals in this group. The exercise testing protocol should also take into consideration any comorbidities, orthopedic limitations, and current medications. Arm or leg ergometry may be more appropriate for some patients, depending on orthopedic limitations and weight limits of treadmills. Test sensitivity for CAD may be low in this population due to associated comorbidities, orthopedic limitations, current medications and poor motivation.

Exercise testing may not always be necessary for obese adults who want to start an exercise program. In many cases, the initial exercise intensity is far below the point at which cardiac risk is a concern during exercise. Nevertheless, exercise testing plays an important role in the optimal management of exercise treatment for individuals who are obese. The primary objective of exercise testing for this group is ultimately to develop a safe and effective exercise prescription. Disease diagnosis is a secondary, yet essential, objective as well. Determining physical work capacity is important for selecting the intensity of exercise for obese individuals; one can make this determination in a number of ways, including exercise testing using the 12 min walk or treadmill or cycle ergometer testing, for example (see table 25.5).

Important considerations regarding obese individuals during exercise testing include the following:

- An increased risk of orthopedic injury
- An increased risk of cardiovascular disease
- An increased risk of heat intolerance

RECOMMENDATIONS FOR EXERCISE PROGRAMMING

The exercise prescription for obese individuals must optimize energy expenditure yet minimize potential for injury. Exercise should also be enjoyable and practical and should fit into the person's lifestyle. One should consider the energy expenditure of the actual exercise, as well as that of the recovery period, in determining the total energy expenditure for a single exercise session. In some cases, two or more short sessions a day is more tolerable and can result in the same or even higher total energy expenditure than one longer session of the same intensity. The use of two or more shorter sessions has been recommended because the elevated energy expenditure of recovery may be sustained for a longer period of time than after a single session. However, a single longer exercise session may have an advantage for substrate utilization and for ease of incorporation

TABLE 25.5

Obesity: Exercise Testing

Methods	Measures	Endpoints*	Comments
Aerobic			
Cycle (ramp protocol 17 W/ min; staged protocol 25-50 W/3 min stage) Treadmill (1-2 METs/3 min stage)	■ 12-lead ECG, HR	■ Serious dysrhythmias ■ >2 mm ST-segment depression or elevation ■ Ischemic threshold ■ T-wave inversion with significant ST change ■ SBP >250 mmHg or DBP >115 mmHg	■ Clients are at higher than normal risk for ■ CAD/hypertension. ■ Increased risk of orthopedic injury. ■ Increased risk of cardiovascular disease. ■ Increased risk of heat intolerance.
	■ BP, rate–pressure product		
	■ RPE (6-20) ■ METs		
Flexibility			
Goniometry			Used to determine joints that need stretching.
Neuromuscular			
Gait analysis Balance			

*Measurements of particular significance; do not always indicate test termination.

into some people's lifestyles. More recently the accumulation of physical activity during the day has been promoted; this may distribute the caloric energy expenditure throughout the day in the absence of formal exercise sessions.

The focus of substrate utilization in weight reduction may not be that important compared to the total calories expended. The American College of Sports Medicine recommends accumulating 200 to 300 min/week or >2000 kcal/week of physical activity for weight loss and weight maintenance. Progression to the longer duration and total calories should be gradual. Because the initial exercise intensity and duration levels are low for people who are obese, the exercise recommendations are fairly general (see table 25.6):

- Mode: Non-weight-bearing exercise; walking; increase in activities of daily living; resistance training
- Frequency: Daily or at least five sessions per week
- Duration: 200 to 300 min/week (i.e., 30-60 min/day)
- Intensity: 40% to 60% of peak oxygen consumption ($\dot{V}O_{2peak}$); exercise intensities of 60%

to 75% of $\dot{V}O_{2peak}$ can be prescribed providing the risk of injury is minimal
- Accumulating >2000 kcal/week

Exercise programs that include high-resistance activities (i.e., free weights, resistance machines) can lead to preferential retention of lean body weight. However, aerobic activity has more potential to decrease fat weight than does resistance training because it can be sustained for a longer time, allowing expenditure of more energy.

SPECIAL CONSIDERATIONS

Exercise is not as effective if the obese individual is not motivated or ready to make the necessary changes. Motivational strategies are often required to help clients move into readiness for change. These strategies can include

- goal setting and
- decision or balance sheets.

Injury prevention is another important consideration in exercise for obese individuals. In fact, physical injury may be one of the primary reasons for discontinuation of exercise. Excess body weight

TABLE 25.6

Obesity: Exercise Programming

Modes	Goals	Intensity/Frequency/Duration	Time to goal
Aerobic Large muscle activities (walking, rowing, cycling, water aerobics)	■ Reduce weight ■ Increase functional performance ■ Reduce risk of CAD	■ 40-60% $\dot{V}O_{2peak}$ (up to 75% if low risk) ■ Monitor RPE and HR ■ 5 or more days/week ■ 30-60 min/session (or 2 sessions/day of 20-30 min) ■ Emphasize duration rather than intensity	■ 9-12 months ■ Increase duration over intensity
Flexibility Stretching	Increase ROM	Daily or at least 5 sessions/week	
Functional Activity-specific exercise	■ Increase ease of performing ADLs ■ Increase vocational potential ■ Increase physical self-confidence		

may exacerbate existing joint conditions. Another concern is thermoregulation. The following considerations and guidelines are relevant for exercise programming in obese populations:

- Prevention of overuse injury
- Injury history
- Adequate flexibility, warm-up, and cool-down sessions
- Gradual progression of intensity and duration
- Use of low-impact or non-weight-bearing exercises
- Thermoregulation
- Neutral temperature and humidity
- Times of day (e.g., should be cool)
- Adequate hydration
- Clothing (e.g., should be loose fitting)

Other considerations may depend on diseases that coexist with obesity.

Evidence-Based Guidelines

National Institutes of Health. The practical guide: Identification, evaluation, and treatment of overweight and obesity in adults. 2000. Available at www.nhlbi.nih.gov/guidelines/obesity/.

National Institutes of Health (NIH) and National Heart, Lung, and Blood Institute (NHLBI). Clinical guidelines on the identification, evaluation, and treatment of overweight and obesity in adults: Evidence report. Bethesda, MD: NIH NHLBI; 1998. [Online]. Available at www.nhlbi.nih.gov.

Orzano AJ, Scott AG. Diagnosis and treatment of obesity in adults: An applied evidence-based review. J Am Board Fam Med. 2004;17:359-369.

Suggested Web Site

National Heart, Lung, and Blood Institute. www.nhlbi.nih.gov

CASE STUDY

Obesity

A 33-year-old woman had entered a medical fitness facility 10 years earlier wanting to lose weight, feel better, improve her health, and have more energy. She had been overweight for 12 years and wanted to lose 100 lb (45 kg) as a long-term goal. Her attitude was optimistic. She went through periods of weight cycling in the program. Her beginning weight was 350 lb (159 kg). Over six months of exercise and nutritionally balanced caloric restriction, she lost 8 lb (3.6 kg). Within nine months she had lost an additional 4 lb (1.8 kg). At the one-year mark she had gained back to 350 lb. She continued to cycle between 337 and 370 lb (153 and 168 kg) for the next 10 years. During this time, her adherence to exercise and diet was not remarkable. Finally, her health and inability to lose weight made her a candidate for the Roux-en-Y gastric bypass surgery.

S: "I've just had bariatric surgery and now need exercise supervision.

O: Vitals

Past history: Hypertension (onset at 34 years), worsening PAT, and hospitalization for sinus node surgery three months ago.

Family history: Heart disease and diabetes; mother died at age 40 years from heart disease and father had heart disease and diabetes at age 40.

Social history: Her usual day is moderately stressful as a university administrator.

Medications: Norvasc 5 mg daily, but not adhering

24-hour diet recall and 2-day diet diary: Vegetarian

Total caloric intake: 1690 kcal/day

Protein intake: 52 g/day (12% of total calories)

Carbohydrate intake: 329 g (76% of total calories)

Fat intake: 24 g (12% of total calories)

Vitamin and mineral intake: 40-435% of dietary goals

Variable	Presurgery	Postsurgery
Height	5 ft 4 in.	–
Weight (pounds)	370.7	290.8
BMI (kg/m^2)	61.8	49.3
Percent body fat (%)	45.8	–
Waist circumference (in.)	54.25	48.3
Waist:hip ratio	0.80	0.81
Total cholesterol (mg/dl)	163	174
HDL -cholesterol (mg/dl)	45	48
Triglycerides (mg/dl)	208	110
Glucose (mg/dl)	139	125
Blood pressure (mmHg)	148/98	132/86
Resting heart rate (contractions/min)	78	74
Vital capacity (L)	4.08	–
FEV$_1$ (% of VC)	77%	–
Physical work capacity (ml · min^{-1} · kg^{-1})	$\dot{V}O_{2max}$ = 18.82	3/4 mile in 12 min
Maximal heart rate (contractions/min)	170	–
Exercise ECG	Supraventricular beats in recovery	–

(continued)

Psychometric Evaluations

Internal locus of control
Self-efficacy good for walking 1 mi (1.6K)

Diet Readiness Assessment

May be close to being ready to begin a program but should think about ways to boost preparedness before she begins.

Some or most of her eating may be in response to thinking about food or exposing herself to temptations to eat.

Does not seem to let unplanned eating disrupt her program.

Binge eating is not a problem.

Sometimes eats in response to emotional highs and lows.

A: 1. Morbid obesity with good eating and physical activity habits

2. Recent surgery for weight loss; progressing well
3. Low aerobic capacity
4. Possible PAT arrhythmia during and following exercise

P: 1. Prescribe a diet program for weight loss.
2. Institute an exercise program to increase caloric expenditure.
3. Identify multiple psychological support systems.

Exercise Program Goals

1. Increase physical activity without injury to maintain weight loss
2. Precautions for malnutrition and dehydration from surgery
3. Weekly support sessions; monthly meetings with dietitian and/or support group

Mode	Frequency	Duration	Intensity	Progression
Aerobic (stationary cycling, water aerobics)	At least 5 sessions/week	To start: 15-20 min session	Talk test limit (must be able to carry on a conversation)	Increase as tolerated to 30-40 min/session. Gradually increase ADLs to 30 min/day. Possibly consider 2 sessions/day.

Frailty

Constance Mols Bayles, PhD, FACSM ■ Selena Chan, BS
Joseph Robare, MS, RD, LDN

OVERVIEW
OF THE PATHOPHYSIOLOGY

Physical decline associated with aging can be attributed to a number of complex interactions, including normal aging and disease. Frail health can be found across the entire age spectrum; but elderly adults, typically those older than 65 years of age, have a greater risk of becoming frail. Although frailty is a common term, especially in the field of geriatrics, there is no consensus on its definition. One of the accepted standards for the diagnosis of frailty is based on the presence of muscle weakness, low physical activity, slow walking speeds, physical exhaustion, and unintentional weight loss. According to a more holistic definition of frailty, this syndrome involves an increased vulnerability to stressors that results from decreased physiological reserves and multisystem dysregulation, as well as limited capacity to maintain homeostasis and to respond to internal and external stresses. Frailty in older adults usually manifests itself as a disability associated with other chronic diseases or geriatric syndromes. Compared to nonfrail older adults, frail older adults are more dependent, display a slower recovery from illnesses, undergo more falls and injuries, have more acute illnesses, and are more often institutionalized or hospitalized. All these factors can result in increased mortality. With an estimated 20% to 30% of the population over 75 years of age affected by frailty, and the 85+-year age group growing rapidly, frailty is a significant

current public health concern that will most likely attract greater attention in the future.

Many older adults who are considered frail tend to be vulnerable to the most serious health conditions and disabilities, or are functionally impaired, or both. Functional impairment for the elderly means a restriction in activities of daily living or a lack of ability to perform them. Elderly individuals are often confronted with disease that results in disuse of the affected body parts and may accelerate the development of frailty, such as sarcopenia, osteopenia, balance disorders, and nutritional problems. The body is in a constant state of change throughout life, with changes occurring in the cardiovascular, respiratory, nervous, musculoskeletal, renal, and metabolic systems as part of the normal aging process (table 26.1). Sarcopenia, or age-related loss of skeletal muscle mass, is especially associated with increasing physiological and functional vulnerability related to frailty. Along with normal aging, the presence of multiple chronic medical conditions, specifically inflammatory and neuroendocrine diseases, also contributes to increased functional decline (table 26.2).

EFFECTS ON
THE EXERCISE RESPONSE

Persons who are elderly and frail are faced with a variety of medical conditions that can place them at risk for a medical emergency during exercise testing.

TABLE 26.1

Physiological Changes Associated With Aging

System	Function	Change
Cardiovascular	Resting HR	No change
	Maximal HR	Decrease
	Resting cardiac output	Decrease
	Maximal cardiac output	Decrease
	Resting SV	Decrease
	Maximal SV	Decrease
	Resting BP	Increase
	Exercise BP	Increase
	$\dot{V}O_{2peak}$	Decrease
Respiratory	Residual volume	Increase
	Vital capacity	Decrease
	Total lung capacity	No change
	Respiratory frequency	Increase
Nervous	Reaction time	Decrease
	Nerve conduction time	Increase
	Sensory deficits	Increase
Musculoskeletal	Muscular strength	Decrease
	Muscle mass	Decrease
	Flexibility	Decrease
	Balance	Decrease
	Bone density	Decrease
Renal	Kidney function	Decrease
	Acid–base control	Decrease
	Glucose tolerance	Decrease
	Drug clearance	Decrease
	Cellular water	Decrease
Metabolic	Basal metabolic rate	Decrease
	Lean body mass	Decrease
	Body fat	Increase

As a result, the following should be considered with respect to exercise testing in persons who are frail:

- Preliminary tests such as Independent Activities of Daily Living (IADL), Activities of Daily Living (ADL), Mini Mental State, the Geriatric Depression Scale, and the Nutritional Risk Index may be helpful to review before exercise testing.

- Medical history, including any comorbidities, as well as present medications should be reviewed before the person undergoes testing.

- Exercise tests should be individualized, starting at low work rates, and in many cases should incorporate longer warm-up periods. Various modes of testing should be considered to meet the needs of the client.

- Older frail persons usually take a longer time than others to reach steady state during exercise. Testing should focus on longer work stages with increases in grade rather than speed.

- Caution is warranted regarding the length of exercise stages. One should ensure that stages are short because older frail individuals

TABLE 26.2

Common Medical Disorders That Contribute to Frailty in Elderly Individuals*

System	Medical Disorder
Cardiovascular	Hypertension, hypotension, coronary artery disease, valvular heart disease, heart failure, dysrhythmias, peripheral arterial disease
Pulmonary	Asthma, chronic pulmonary disease, pneumonia
Musculoskeletal	Arthritis, degenerative disc disease, polymyalgia rheumatica, osteoporosis, degenerative joint disease
Metabolic/endocrine	Diabetes, hypercholesterolemia
Gastrointestinal	Dental disorder, malnutrition, incontinence, diarrhea
Genitourinary	Urinary tract infection, cancer
Hematologic/immunologic	Anemia, leukemia, cancer
Neurological	Dementia, Alzheimer's disease, cerebrovascular disease, Parkinson's disease
Eye and ear	Cataracts, glaucoma, hearing disorders
Psychiatric	Anxiety disorders, hypochondria, depression, alcoholism

*May be taking one or more of the following medications (see appendix for effects): diuretics, antihypertensives, antianginal agents, antiarrhythmic agents, psychotropic medications, insulin, anticoagulants.

fatigue more quickly than others, and this could serve as negative reinforcement. If the test is needed for diagnostic purposes, however, a more aggressive protocol may be used.

- Older frail individuals are susceptible to dehydration and insulin insensitivity, and care should be taken to identify physiological features associated with these conditions.

EFFECTS OF EXERCISE TRAINING

Physical activity appears to be of critical importance for delaying the metabolic and inflammatory disorders associated with aging, such as sarcopenia and osteoarthritis. In older populations, physical activity improves muscle strength, endurance, and maximal aerobic power. Flexibility, balance, motor control, and coordination are also improved, resulting in decreased risk of falling while enhancing mobility. Exercise has also been shown to prevent or delay cognitive impairment while increasing socialization and self-esteem. These benefits improve functional limitations and have important implications for maintaining or promoting independence in daily living activities.

MANAGEMENT AND MEDICATIONS

The frail elderly usually take more medications than any other segment of the population. In fact, increased risk for developing comorbid diseases and the complexity of medication regimens invite less predictable responses to medications. Additionally, since renal excretion of chemicals is reduced in the elderly, drugs remain in the body for longer periods of time. This increases the importance of recognizing conditions such as polypharmacy, self-medication, and therapeutic compliance. It is estimated that two-thirds of the older adult population use over-the-counter dietary supplements. Exercise professionals working with this group must be able to identify individuals who do not follow medication instructions. Before developing an exercise program for an elderly person, review the client's medications, since all medications can have side effects (table 26.3). Specifically, psychotropic medications are associated with increased risk for falls, while medications with anticholinergic properties may affect visual and cognitive functions.

TABLE 26.3

Common Side Effects* of Medications in Frail Elderly Individuals

Side effect	Medications
Dizziness	Sedatives, hypnotics, anticonvulsants, tricyclic antidepressants, antipsychotics
Confusion, depression, or both	Sedatives, hypnotics, anticonvulsants, antipsychotics, antidepressants, diuretics, antihypertensives
Fatigue and weakness	Beta-blockers, diuretics, tricyclic antidepressants, antipsychotics, barbiturates, benzodiazepines, antihistamines, antihypertensives
Postural hypotension	Tricyclic antidepressants, antipsychotics, antihypertensives, diuretics, nitrates, narcotic analgesics, vasodilators, levodopa
Involuntary muscle movements	Antipsychotics, levodopa, tricyclic antidepressants, adrenergics
Urinary incontinence	Benzodiazepines, barbiturates, phenothiazines, chlorpromazines, anticholinergics, diuretics
Increases in heart rate	Antiglaucoma agents/miotics, bronchodilators/antiasthmatic agents

*Recognizing medication side effects is important before development of an exercise program.

RECOMMENDATIONS FOR EXERCISE TESTING

Cardiorespiratory, strength, neuromuscular, flexibility, and functional performance tests enable the exercise professional to assess current functional levels of clients and develope an appropriate exercise program. Frail individuals with a history of cardiac problems or those who exhibit coronary artery disease risk factors should be assessed by graded exercise testing. The use of various testing modalities, including treadmill and cycle tests, depends upon the client's medical status. A simple 6 or 12 min test or a 20 ft (6.1 m) walk test, or a 400 m test, is recommended for clients who are free from any coronary heart disease and who have physician clearance (see table 26.4). Heart rate, blood pressure, ratings of perceived exertion, and distance walked should be monitored and recorded to ensure a proper exercise prescription and to decrease complications.

Maintaining or improving muscle strength may improve functional ability in persons who are elderly. A handheld dynamometer is often used to assess muscle strength because it is easy to use and is a reliable means of obtaining an objective measurement of strength. Baseline measures of strength enable the exercise professional to chart and assess progress and provide feedback to clients as they progress in an exercise program. Neuromuscular and functional performance tests are also important for evaluating progress in these frail individuals before developing an exercise program. Information obtained from gait, balance, and coordination tests enables the exercise professional to plan appropriate intervention programs, to target those individuals who are at risk for falling, and to assess needs for assistive devices. Flexibility training may increase joint flexibility and mobility. The goniometer is an important tool for measuring flexibility, and information gained from such tests can be employed as feedback that individuals may use to track improvements.

Medications and special considerations for exercise testing and training people who are frail include the following:

- Monitor balance difficulties (to prevent falls)
- Fractures caused by osteoporosis may be present
- Assess for cardiovascular and cerebrovascular diseases
- Low tolerance for hot and cold environments may be exhibited
  - Reduced effectiveness of sweating
  - Increased susceptibility to heat cramps, exhaustion, stroke, and dehydration
- Note prescribed medication schedule
- Be aware of possible cognitive deficits
- Adaptation of the test if client is using an assistive device

TABLE 26.4

Frailty: Exercise Testing

Methods	Measures	Endpoints*	Comments
Aerobic			
Cycle (ramp protocol 17 W/min; staged protocol 25-50 W/3 min stage) Treadmill (low-level protocol such as Naughton, Balke, Ware)	■ $\dot{V}O_{2peak}$ ■ 12-lead ECG, HR	■ Serious dysrhythmias ■ >2 mm ST-segment depression or elevation ■ Ischemic threshold ■ T-wave inversion with significant ST change	■ $\dot{V}O_{2peak}$, METs, and RPE are often best for exercise prescription because of possible cardiovascular dysautonomia.
	■ BP, rate–pressure product ■ RPE (6-20) ■ METs	■ SBP >250 mmHg or DBP >115 mmHg	■ Attenuated BP response may occur.
Endurance			
6 or 12 min walk	■ Distance ■ Speed	■ Volitional fatigue ■ Unsteadiness	6 or 12 min walk is good for measuring progress in exercise programs.
Strength			
Handheld dynamometer	3RM		■ Used to determine intensity of strength training and progress in strength training programs. ■ Sometimes contraindicated in people with osteoporosis.
Flexibility			
Sit and reach Goniometer	■ ROM ■ Distance		
Neuromuscular			
20 ft (6.1 m) walk Chair stand One-legged stance 8-step tandem gait 360° turn	Time and distance	■ Volitional fatigue ■ Unsteadiness	Walk tests are good for measuring gait and balance disorders.

*Measurements of particular significance; do not always indicate test termination.

RECOMMENDATIONS FOR EXERCISE PROGRAMMING

The exercise prescription for elderly frail individuals should reflect medical and social needs. Past exercise experience and goal setting are major contributors to program success. In many instances, the choice of activity for elderly individuals is very important, especially when they have lost the freedom to make choices on their own. Compliance to exercise programming is enhanced when the exercise professional and the client work together. If tailored appropriately to be pleasurable, specific, realistic, and safe, some degree of physical activity is always better than a sedentary lifestyle. Lastly, it is important to stress that advanced age is not a barrier to exercise; instead, the health care practitioner may focus on individualized therapeutic effects of physical activity.

Care must be taken when prescribing the mode of exercise for persons who are elderly. The primary goal for this population is to increase functional capacity and independence. A multidimensional approach for improved health is important. Specifically, physical activity can be integrated into daily routines in short bouts, multiple times a day, and be just as effective as one single continuous bout of exercise. Medical history and past exercise experience are important indicators of the type of exercise to be recommended to a client. Finally, monitoring changes in health status and subsequently reevaluating the exercise program are important to keep the activity plan both effective and safe.

Although walking is the easiest and least expensive form of exercise, this activity may not be best for everyone (see table 26.5). Cycling, swimming, and chair activities are most appropriate for people with degenerative joint disease, gait abnormalities,

TABLE 26.5

Frailty: Exercise Programming

Modes	Goals	Intensity/Frequency/Duration	Time to goal
Aerobic Large muscle activities (walking, cycling, rowing, swimming; chair exercise may be indicated for some clients)	Increase functional capacity and independence	■ Monitor RPE (intensity should not be the main focus) ■ 3-5 days/week ■ 5-60 min/session	
Strength Low-level, progressive resistance exercise (free weights, weight machines, isokinetic machines) Ball machines	■ Increase overall muscular strength ■ Decrease risk of falling ■ Increase hand strength	■ Start program without weight; add weight slowly ■ 3 days/week ■ Approximately 20 min/session	
Flexibility Stretching/yoga			
Neuromuscular One-foot stand Stair climbing Practice falling techniques Balloon activity Tandem gait Chair stand exercise	■ Increase neuromuscular coordination, gait, balance, flexibility, and lower body strength ■ Prevent falls ■ Increase hand–eye coordination and reaction time		

hip replacements, and knee replacements. Low-level strength training programs in the frail elderly can incorporate ankle and wrist weights as an essential component. Strengthening exercises for the lower extremities are especially important for fall prevention. Flexibility, eye–hand coordination, reflex training, balance, and fall prevention activities such as tai chi are also important.

Special considerations for exercise programming include the following:

- Target heart rate should not be the main focus.
- Avoid ballistic exercises.
- Avoid neck circumduction.
- Avoid isometric and static resistance exercises (see table 26.4).

Evidence-Based Guidelines

Moreland J, Richardson J, Chan DH, et al. Evidence-based guidelines for the secondary prevention of falls in older adults. Gerontology. 2003;49(2):93-116.

Suggested Web Sites

Center for Healthy Aging. www.healthyagingprograms.org

Center for Healthy Aging University of Pittsburg Prevention Center. www.healthyaging.pitt.edu

Centers for Disease Control and Prevention. www.cdc.gov/index.htm

Centers for Disease Control and Prevention. www.cdc.gov/prc/research-projects/core-projects/promoting-health-preventing-disease-pittsburgh-older-adults.htm

National Institutes of Health Senior Health. http://nihseniorhealth.gov/exercise/benefitsofexercise/01.html

---

CASE STUDY

Frailty

A Caucasian widowed 84-year-old female volunteered to participate in a Center for Healthy Aging research project focusing on the "10 Keys to Healthy Aging" (see www.cdc.gov/prc/research-projects/core-projects/promoting-health-preventing-disease-pittsburgh-older-adults.htm). She lived alone in an underserved community, attended a teacher's college, worked as a teacher, and is currently retired. She recently lost her husband but tried to keep busy with her best friend, who lived next door. Her past medical history included left breast cancer (partial mastectomy) and diabetes. She maintained a youthful appearance but on arrival to the clinic complained of headaches and dizziness. She also noted that she frequently became tired upon exertion and that it was difficult for her to regulate her diet. She was not a smoker and denied any alcohol use. She had never participated in any formal exercise program and was interested in learning about the "10 Keys to Healthy Aging."

S: *"I need help because I would like to have more energy, and I am frequently tired and dizzy. I am interested in beginning a regular exercise program and learning more about what foods are best for me to eat. I have been a little lonely since my husband died and would like to socialize with people my own age."*

O: Vitals

Height: 64.5 in. (1.64 m)
Weight: 120 lb (54.5 kg)
BMI: 20.3 kg/m²
Resting BP: 158/72 mmHg
Nonsmoker

Labs

LDL-cholesterol: 174 mg/dl
Fasting blood glucose: 88 mg/dl
Exercise testing: Muscle weakness, able to sit to stand for 5 min
Physical activity: not physically active (i.e., 0 hours/wk)
Center for Epidemiologic Studies Depression Scale (CES-D) (<16): 15

Medications

Synthroid, 125 mg, QD (once per day)
Glucophage, 500 mg, BID (two times daily)
Actos, 30 mg, QD
Lipitor, 20 mg, QD
Fosamax, 70 mg, QD
Baby aspirin, 81 mg, QD

A: 1. Blood sugar out of control for many years
2. Hypertension was diagnosed at baseline
3. Exercise intolerance caused by deconditioning

P: 1. Begin supervised walking and weight training program.
2. Begin nutritional counseling with diabetes education.
3. Learn the 10 Keys to Healthy Aging and set goals for the next year based on the 10 Keys™.
4. Reevaluate 10 Keys™ at 12 and 24 months.

(continued)

Mode	Frequency	Duration	Intensity	Progression
Aerobic	5-6 days/week	As tolerated to start	As tolerated	Increase over 1 month to 40 min/session.
Strength (all major muscle groups)	3 days/week	1 set of 10 reps	Resistance bands	Achieve 1 set of 10 reps for all muscle groups.
Flexibility (all major muscle groups)	3 days/week	20-60 s/stretch	Maintain stretch below discomfort point	
Warm-up and cool-down	Before and after each session	10-15 min		

Exercise Program Goals

1. Work with participant's physician to balance diabetic medications, exercise regimen, and eating plan
2. Focus on compliance to an exercise and nutrition intervention
3. Reevaluate 10 Keys™ goals short-term (every month) and long-term (12 and 24 months)

Follow-Up

Participant was randomized to the Lifestyle Plus intervention group, which included an exercise program intervention of walking and weightlifting, nutritional counseling, and an educational program to learn about the 10 Keys to Healthy Aging. Adherence to intervention programming proved to be a challenge. The 400 m walk, performed at baseline and at years 1 and 2, showed a maintenance of gait speed with an average of 1.16 m/s. Increases in physical activity did occur throughout the time period with coaching but did not meet goal requirements of 2.5 h/week. Balance decreased throughout the two years, but chair strength remained the same. Her Nutritional Risk Index, Independent Activities of Daily Living, and Activities of Daily Living were slightly below standards at baseline but improved through time. The participant's cognitive status remained high throughout the two-year period (3 MSE = mean score of 95, total 100 points). The Center for Epidemiological Studies Depression Scale (CESD) scores showed borderline depression and remained the same from baseline through year 2 (CESD mean score = 14). With reference to her baseline vitals, the participant improved her systolic and diastolic blood pressure in the two-year period (from 158/72 to 138/56 mmHg) and decreased low-density lipoprotein cholesterol level (from 174 to 92 mg/dl). Despite notifying her doctor, blood glucose levels continued to fluctuate throughout the two years. However, the participant admitted that she did not monitor blood glucose levels. It was felt that she was possibly not following her medication regimen and eating plan. At year 1, dizziness and fatigue tended to subside. It was recommended that this participant continue a structured and monitored exercise and nutrition intervention to maintain and improve her 10 Keys Healthy Aging goals.

PART V

Immunological and Hematological Disorders

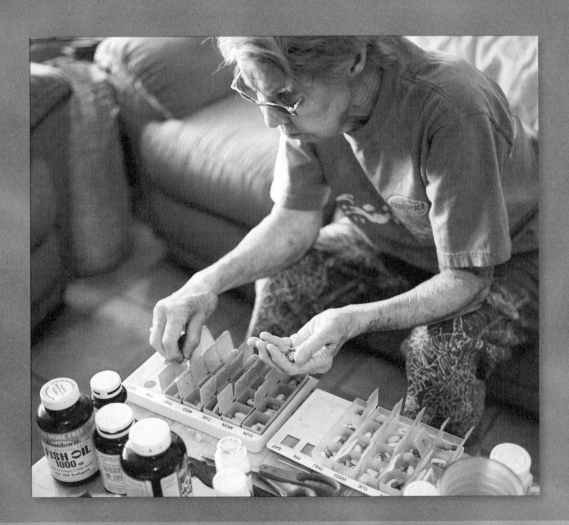

Cancer

Anna L. Schwartz, PhD, ARNP, FAAN

OVERVIEW OF THE PATHOPHYSIOLOGY

Cancer is a term used to describe hundreds of diseases that share the common feature of uncontrolled, abnormal growth and proliferation of cells, which in some cases can spread to distant anatomical sites (metastasis). The initial symptoms of cancer can be localized, as in the cough of the person with lung cancer, or systemic, as in the drenching night sweats of Hodgkin's lymphoma. Following treatment, the symptoms of cancer can result from the progression of the illness or from the side effects of the treatment itself. Treatment options for cancer include surgery, radiation, chemotherapy, and immunotherapy, either singly or in combination, and can be designed to achieve a cure or to control the disease and relieve symptoms. Cancer is considered cured when a remission is thought to be permanent, but many cancers are considered cured if the patient does not have a recurrence within five years after treatment. Recurrence of cancer occurs when one or more cancer cells survive following treatment and subsequently proliferate over time.

Virtually all individuals with cancer can benefit from rehabilitation and exercise. The goals of exercise therapy vary depending on whether an individual is receiving initial treatment for a new diagnosis, is in remission, or is receiving treatment for a recurrence. Moreover, the response to exercise and adaptability to training are influenced by whether the individual has local or metastatic disease and by the side effects of the particular form of treatment. The specific roles and applications of exercise programming for individuals with cancer are complex and require a thorough understanding of the person's past and current medical history, treatments, medications, signs and symptoms, and functional capacity as well as consideration of comorbidities. Exercise management for persons with cancer requires extensive individualization by the exercise professional. The key to recovery for people with cancer is to have hope. Perhaps there is no greater example of hope for cancer survivors than Lance Armstrong's five victories in the Tour de France, which proved that it is indeed possible to have advanced cancer, undergo extensive treatment, and go on to achieve extraordinary levels of human performance. While most individuals with cancer will not exhibit the athletic prowess of Lance Armstrong, they will achieve a variety of health benefits from formal exercise programming and by adopting an active and fit way of living.

EFFECTS ON THE EXERCISE RESPONSE

Individuals with cancer, as well as cancer survivors, often have disease- or treatment-specific physical limitations that pose challenges to exercise. Tumors can involve any part of the body, and their effect on the exercise response is directly related to the tissues affected. Pain is common when a tumor involves the musculoskeletal system; shortness of breath is common with lung involvement; neural deficits and seizures are common when the central nervous system and brain are involved; and anemia is common when bone marrow is affected. Easy fatigability is common during treatment, in the recovery following treatment, and in advanced cancer. The specific effects of cancer on the exercise response are determined by the tissue(s) affected and by the extent of involvement. The result is often exercise intolerance, but the limiting factors can be varied.

The side effects of anticancer therapy also affect the exercise response. Some side effects may occur early during treatment and then resolve once treatment ends, whereas other side effects may occur late during the treatment period and may persist for some time thereafter or may be permanent (see table 27.1). Amputations result in permanent disability; radiation and chemotherapy can cause permanent scar formation in joints and lung and heart tissues; and drug-induced cardiomyopathies and anemia can cause a permanent limitation in cardiovascular function.

EFFECTS OF EXERCISE TRAINING

Exercise training is safe and beneficial for cancer patients when the exercise is individualized to suit the characteristics of the person. For those undergoing therapy for cancer, exercise training should have the objectives of maintaining strength, endurance, and level of function. For cancer survivors who have completed treatment, exercise training should have the objective of returning them to their former level of physical and psychological function. Studies have shown that regular, moderate-intensity aerobic exercise during cancer therapy results in reduced levels of fatigue, greater body satisfaction, maintenance of body weight, improved mood, less side effect severity, improved aerobic capacity, and a higher quality of life.

Aerobic and resistance exercise programs have the potential to improve balance and bone remodeling and to reduce muscle weakness and the muscle-wasting effects of glucocorticoids that are often part

TABLE 27.1

Acute and Chronic Treatment Effects

Treatment	Acute effects	Chronic effects
Surgery	Pain Lymphedema Fatigue Limited ROM	Pain Loss of flexibility Nerve damage
Radiation	Pain Fatigue Skin irritation Pulmonary inflammation	Scar tissue buildup at radiation site, including cardiac and lung scarring Loss of flexibility Fractures
Chemotherapy	Fatigue Nausea Anemia Nerve damage Muscle pain Weight gain Neuropathy	Cardiomyopathy Lung scarring Nerve damage Fatigue Bone loss Leukemia Neuropathy
Immunotherapy	Weight gain or loss Fatigue Flu-like symptoms Nerve damage Skin changes	Nerve damage Myopathy

of the treatment regimen. Significant improvements in aerobic capacity, as measured by a 12 min walk, have been observed in clients who participated in an aerobic exercise programs, both home based and supervised. In contrast, people who followed the motto of "get more rest" showed declines of as much as 25% in aerobic capacity during treatment. Individuals undergoing intensive cancer therapy benefit from low- to moderate-intensity aerobic and resistance exercise. Despite the significant fatigue that cancer patients experience, exercise reduces fatigue and improves aerobic capacity, mood, and quality of life.

The effects of exercise in individuals with cancer have been studied in patients receiving many different forms of therapy for different cancers. Results of exercise studies during and following cancer treatment have shown improvements in

- shoulder range of motion,
- flexibility,
- muscle strength,
- balance,
- treatment-related side effects (e.g., nausea, pain, fatigue),
- aerobic capacity,
- weight control,
- body image,
- sense of control,
- depression and mood, and
- quality of life.

The effects of exercise on children receiving cancer treatment have not been extensively studied. However, survivors of childhood leukemia have been observed to have mild, persistent cardiovascular compromise as a result of therapy. This does not usually impair function during exercise of moderate intensity but may hinder elite-level athletic performance. Nonetheless, aerobic capacity and submaximal performance of both children and adults should significantly improve after a scientifically sound, step-by-step exercise training program. A concern with adult cancer survivors is that they often have comorbid conditions such as coronary artery disease, hypertension, diabetes, or hyperlipidemia. Some cancer treatments also increase risks for cardiovascular disease and death from myocardial infarction. These comorbid conditions may actually influence exercise prescription and management more than the history of cancer does.

MANAGEMENT AND MEDICATIONS

Cancer treatment usually includes some combination of surgery, radiation therapy, chemotherapy, and immunotherapy. While many treatments have become more targeted to the type of tumor, most continue to cause significant side effects.

Surgery can cause many side effects that clients need to learn to accommodate to within their exercise routine. In the acute stage, pain and loss of flexibility may be the primary side effects. Adequate pain control is critical for the client to be able to begin a basic flexibility and exercise program. Light exercise helps to hasten recovery. Long-term side effects of surgery can be related to pain from amputation and from motor and sensory nerve damage. Exercise programs may need to be adjusted for these physical changes and the client educated in how to move and maximize his or her abilities.

Radiation is given in multiple doses, usually over several weeks. The effects of radiation therapy are cumulative over time. Fatigue gradually increases during the course of radiation therapy. Skin changes such as radiation dermatitis usually become evident toward the middle or end of treatment. These side effects are generally mild to moderate and manageable with clinical intervention. Radiation dermatitis can be irritated with perspiration, and the area may need to be covered with gauze or a bandage to keep it dry. More serious side effects are uncommonly seen; these can include loss of flexibility in irradiated joints and cardiac or lung scarring, or both.

Chemotherapy and immunotherapy are generally given in combinations of drugs that have different mechanisms of action and side effect profiles. The severity of side effects depends on the dose of drug, the pharmacological profile, and to some extent the individual characteristics of the person. Most chemotherapy and immunotherapy drugs cause anemia, fatigue, and nausea, and many cause myopathies and neuropathies (e.g., vincristine, paclitaxel, docetaxel). Some medications have dose-limiting toxicities (i.e., doxorubicin, bleomycin) that limit the amount of drug that can be given to prevent cardiomyopathy and pulmonary fibrosis. Corticosteroids are commonly given with chemotherapy to reduce some of the side effects or reduce tumor volume. Glucocorticoids (decadron, prednisone) contribute to muscle weakness, wasting, and changes in body composition that undoubtedly also influence balance and gait.

The exercise prescription needs to take into account where an individual is in his or her treatment cycle, how well the side effects are being managed, and any physical changes that may put the person at risk during exercise. If chemotherapy is causing neuropathy, balance safety issues need to be considered. Individuals on treatment are often limited by muscle weakness and pain from the tumor, the surgery, or the therapy itself. People are often in a debilitated state, and their ability to walk or perform other functional tests may be limited by the disease or treatment and may necessitate alternative modes of testing and training. Exercise prescription should include slow progression, flexibility surrounding medical management, and adaptability to changes in the client's health status.

RECOMMENDATIONS FOR EXERCISE TESTING

Exercise testing is appropriate for cancer survivors during and following treatment. Individuals actively receiving treatment are generally capable of completing exercise testing and then of following an exercise prescription calibrated to functional capacity and individual limitations that may be disease or treatment related. For clients who have completed therapy, regular exercise is important to maintain or improve function and prevent the development of diseases associated with inactivity (e.g., cardiovascular disease, overweight, diabetes).

Formal exercise testing should be individualized to the client with attention to the type and stage of cancer, type of treatment, and physical limitations (see "Management and Medications"). For example, persons actively receiving treatment who are anemic have reduced aerobic performance because of reduced oxygen-carrying capacity. Exercise testing is useful to quantitatively monitor progress during training and rehabilitation in order to help both the exercise specialist and the survivor track and see progress.

Depending on the functional capacity of a client, exercise testing can usually be performed using standard protocols. Persons who are receiving treatment or who have recently completed treatment may be extremely deconditioned or may have experienced significant changes in body weight (either increases or decreases), and may require low-level exercise protocols. Submaximal and subjective symptom-limited treadmill tests are well tolerated, even by debilitated clients, and provide information on aerobic capacity. Use of 12-lead electrocardiography may be indicated in some patients whose clinical profile places them at increased risk of obstructive coronary artery disease (see table 27.2).

Special considerations for exercise testing include the following:

- Obtain basic history of diagnosis and treatment.
- Assess for adverse acute, chronic, and late effects of cancer treatment.
- Evaluate other comorbidities that may influence ability and safety to exercise.
- Consider how cancer and its treatments may affect balance, agility, speed, flexibility, endurance, and strength and select, modify, and interpret fitness tests accordingly.
- Determine if medical clearance is required prior to exercise testing.
- Consider relative and absolute contraindications to exercise testing.

RECOMMENDATIONS FOR EXERCISE PROGRAMMING

Recommendations for exercise programming are dependent on whether the individual is actively receiving cancer treatment, is a survivor cured or in remission, or is being treated for recurrent or metastatic disease (see table 27.3). For people receiving treatment or with recurrent, localized disease, the goal is to preserve and possibly even improve function. For survivors, the goal is to return to a healthy, active lifestyle and make exercise an integral part of everyday life. For those with recurrent or metastatic disease, the goals need to be tailored to the person's current level of function. In the setting of metastatic cancer, the goal may be to maintain mobility and independence in the home. Many persons have disease- or treatment-specific limitations to exercise that necessitate accommodating the mode of exercise to the client's limitation (e.g., needs of amputees, requirement for portable oxygen).

The optimal frequency, duration, and time course of adaptation to aerobic and resistance exercise training in cancer patients are not known. There appears to be a dose–response relationship of exercise to fatigue, with less fatigue experienced in persons who exercise for durations of more than 10 min and in clients who exercise at least every other day. More study of the dose-response of exercise in cancer survivors is needed to further determine important prescribing guidelines. Longitudinal exercise stud-

TABLE 27.2

Cancer: Exercise Testing

Methods	Measures	Endpoints*	Comments
Aerobic Cycle (ramp protocol 17 W/min; staged protocol 25-50 W/3 min stage) Treadmill (1-2 METs/3 min stage)	■ 12-lead ECG, HR	■ $\dot{V}O_{2peak}$/work rate ■ Serious dysrhythmias ■ >2 mm ST-segment depression or elevation ■ Ischemic threshold ■ T-wave inversion with significant ST change	
	■ BP, rate–pressure product ■ RPE (6-20)	■ SBP >250 mmHg or DBP >115 mmHg ■ Exaggerated or hypotensive response	
Endurance 6 to 12 min walk	Distance	Volitional fatigue	
Strength Isokinetic or isotonic	■ 1RM ■ 3RM	Volitional fatigue	
Flexibility Goniometry Sit and reach		■ Angle of flexion/extension ■ Distance	
Functional ADLs Sit to stand Stair climbing			Use to determine level of assistance needed.
Neuromuscular Gait analysis Balance	Gait and balance measures as appropriate for client		Use to determine level of assistance needed.

*Measurements of particular significance; do not always indicate test termination.

ies of women with breast cancer, survivors receiving peripheral stem cell transplant, and survivors with malignant melanoma and colon cancer all demonstrate that persons adapt to exercise, become more physically fit, and experience less mood disturbance and an improved quality of life.

The side effects of anticancer treatment can be acute or delayed in onset. Therefore, distinct issues must be addressed in exercise programming for persons who are actively receiving treatment versus survivors. During radiation therapy, for example, a client may experience radiation dermatitis, a reddening of the skin that is painful and often limits motion. Radiation therapy can also cause an acute inflammatory response in lung tissue that can impair oxygen transfer. The effects of radiation can

TABLE 27.3

Cancer: Exercise Programming

Modes	Goals	Intensity/Frequency/Duration	Time to goal
Aerobic Large muscle activities (walking, rowing, cycling, water aerobics)	■ Improve/maintain work capacity ■ Control body weight ■ Improve mood ■ Reduce fatigue ■ Improve quality of life	■ Symptom limited; moderate intensity (40-60% VO$_2$R or HRR) ■ 3-5 days/week ■ 20-60 min/session	
Strength Free weights Weight machines Isokinetic machines Resistance bands Circuit training	■ Maintain or improve strength in arms, legs, and trunk ■ Increase maximal voluntary contraction, peak torque, and power	■ Symptom-limited intensity ■ 40-60% of 1RM ■ 2-3 days/week for 20-30 min ■ 1-3 sets of 3-5 reps, building to 8-15 reps ■ Add RPE 11-13/20	
Flexibility Stretching	■ Increase/maintain ROM ■ Decrease stiffness from disuse	■ 20-30 s/stretch ■ 2-4 reps/stretch ■ 5-7 days/week	
Functional ADLs Gait and balance exercise	■ Maintain as much independence as possible ■ Return to work ■ Improve gait ■ Improve balance	Daily	

also have a delayed onset, occurring months to years after therapy. For example, radiation can cause lung scarring many months after therapy (which also impairs lung function). In addition, chemotherapy and immunotherapy have acute and long-term side effects that one needs to consider when planning exercise prescriptions. Virtually all anticancer drugs cause fatigue and declines in blood cell counts. Exercise prescriptions should take into account where a client is in treatment and accommodate for periods of increased fatigue and for cycles of treatment. Since most people are treated with combinations of surgery, radiation, chemotherapy, and immunotherapy, the exercise specialist is likely to encounter a combination of treatment-related problems.

When survivors are actively receiving treatment, it is important to assess their general health status. Persons with uncontrolled vomiting, pain, or diarrhea should postpone the exercise session. Individuals with neutropenic fever should postpone the exercise session until the source of infection is determined and appropriate therapy has been started. Exercise prescription for clients with thrombocytopenia (platelet count <50,000/mm^3) must consider the risk of bleeding (see chapter 33), and appropriate steps should be taken to prevent falls and increases in blood and intracranial pressure. Exercise should probably be limited to low-intensity walking, stationary cycling, and flexibility exercises. Although no studies have examined the effects of exercise in cancer survivors with clinically manifested coronary artery disease, logic would suggest that these persons may have to lower their exercise intensity to accommodate a lower oxygen-carrying capacity during periods of anemia (e.g., when hemoglobin levels reach 10 g/dl). Exercise programs may need to be adjusted for changes in the individual's condition and treatment plan.

The following are special considerations for exercise programming:

- Assess client's current medical condition, functional ability, and general health before each exercise session.
- Consider relative and absolute contra-indications to exercise.
- Develop an exercise program to accommodate to changes from cancer and its treatment that may alter balance, agility, speed, flexibility, endurance, and strength.
- Know where a client is in the treatment schedule and adapt the exercise program to the person's ability at each session.
- Recognize when to refer clients back to their physician for evaluation of new or worsening symptoms.
- Know cancer-specific emergencies (e.g., sudden loss of limb function, fever in immune-incompetent patients, superior vena cava syndrome, spinal cord compression) and plan for handling an emergency situation.
- Assess risks for adverse late effects of treatment that could increase risks associated with exercise (e.g., heart failure).
- Adjust program for the presence of a central line (e.g., a peripherally inserted central catheter [PICC] or port).
- Modify exercise program based on current medical condition if the client is actively receiving treatment or has completed treatment.

Evidence-Based Guidelines

Humpel N, Iverson DC. Review and critique of the quality of exercise recommendations for cancer patients and survivors. Supp Care Cancer. 2005;13(7):493-502.

Kamidono S, Ohshima S, Hirao Y, et al. Evidence-based clinical practice guidelines for prostate cancer (summary—JUA 2006 edition). Int J Urol. 2006;15:1-18.

Mock V. Evidence-based treatment for cancer-related fatigue. JNCI Monographs. 2004;32:112-118.

Suggested Web Sites

Breast Cancer Watch. http://breastcancer.evidence-watch.com

National Cancer Institute. www.cancer.gov

CASE STUDY

Cancer

A 57-year-old male with stage III colon cancer received surgical adjuvant chemotherapy with leucovorin, fluorouracil, and oxaliplatin (FOLFOX). He was an executive in a large company and continued to work during treatment. Patient complained of feeling tired, weak, and having worsening numbness in his feet and fingers, and had a poor appetite. During the chemotherapy weeks, his fatigue was worse. On treatment weeks, he was well enough to work 3 to 4 h in the morning but quit early because of mild nausea, diarrhea, and fatigue of 7/10 (0 = no fatigue; 10 = extreme fatigue). He reported that even on nontreatment weeks he noticed that he got tired quickly with simple activities such as house cleaning and daily chores. He had recently become so tired and weak that he was unable to do much after work and relied on his family to prepare meals and do basic things around the house, like his laundry. He wanted to get strong enough to resume playing golf, which he said was key to networking and working with his colleagues and made him happy. He requested guidance in setting up an exercise program but was too busy to attend regular supervised sessions.

S: "I feel OK, but too weak and tired to do the things I'd like to do, like play golf."

O: Vitals

HR: 78 contractions/min
BP: 128/70 mmHg
Weight: 199.0 lb (90.45 kg)
Lungs clear, heart regular rate and rhythm
Moderate peripheral neuropathy feet and hands
Pale
No lymphedema
Fatigue: 7/10 on a 0 = no fatigue to 10 = worst imaginable fatigue scale

(continued)

Labs

Hemoglobin: 11.2 g/dl
White blood cells: 5000/mcl
Absolute neutrophil count (ANC): 1000/mm^3
Platelets: 200,000/mm^3
CEA: 21 ng/ml

Exercise Testing

12 min walk: 1215 ft (370.3 m)
Peak HR: 154 contractions/min
Peak BP: 175/88 mmHg
Peak RPE: 19
No complaints of chest pain, light-headedness, pain, or other discomfort
Overhead press 1RM: 23 kg
Leg press 1RM: 52 kg

A: 1. Stage III colon cancer postsurgical resection; receiving FOLFOX chemotherapy for 2 more cycles. Labs within safe range for exercise.
   2. Deconditioning with easy fatigability. Moderate exercise intolerance (low endurance and weakness).

P: Prescribe an aerobic exercise program 3-4 days per week and resistance exercises 2 days a week. Both aerobic and resistance programs will progress slowly with short- and long-term goals. Neuropathy in feet will necessitate special precautions related to risk of falls and potential instability on feet.

Exercise Program Goals

1. Short-term (1 mo): Increase endurance to be able to walk 20 min (1.6 km); increase muscle strength to be able to complete 3 sets of 12 repetitions at 50% of 1RM
2. Long-term (6-mo): Regain functional capacity and muscle strength to resume playing a full game of golf

Follow-Up

After six weeks patient reported lower levels of fatigue, 5 on a 0 to 10 scale. His weakness is improving and he is now able to walk over 1.6 km with resting in less than 20 min. Patient is exercising at least four days/week (one day supervised and three days on his own). At the 12-week follow-up, both his aerobic capacity and strength had improved, and he reported that he is starting to play a few holes of golf but still gets tired. He reports feeling inspired by the gains that he's seen in his fitness in the past few weeks and is focused on his goal to be able to play a full game of golf.

Mode	Frequency	Duration	Intensity	Progression
Aerobic	3-4 days/week	15-30 min	RPE 11-13/20 (avoid exhaustion)	Gradually increase to 30-45 over 8 weeks.
Strength (all major muscle groups)	3 days/week	1 set of 10-12 reps	To fatigue, but avoid exhaustion	Increase as tolerated.
Flexibility (all major muscle groups)	3 days/week	20-30 s/stretch	Maintain stretch below discomfort point	
Warm-up and cool-down	Before and after each session	10-15 min	RPE 11-12/20	

28

Acquired Immune Deficiency Syndrome (AIDS)

Gregory A. Hand, PhD, FACSM ■ G. William Lyerly, MS
Wesley D. Dudgeon, PhD

OVERVIEW OF THE PATHOPHYSIOLOGY

Acquired immune deficiency syndrome or acquired immunodeficiency syndrome (AIDS) is a group of symptoms and infections caused by the human immunodeficiency virus (HIV). The first definition of AIDS appeared in the September 24, 1982 issue of *Morbidity and Mortality Weekly Report*, published by the Centers for Disease Control (CDC). Since 1982, the definition of AIDS has evolved as scientists and public health experts understand more about the etiology and epidemiology of AIDS. The most current and widely accepted definition of AIDS is the CDC AIDS case definition, which states that an individual has AIDS if he or she is infected with HIV and

- presents with a CD4+ T-cell count below 200 cells/µl (or a CD4+ T-cell percentage of total lymphocytes of less than 14%) or

- presents with one of 25 different AIDS-defining illnesses.

The CDC's AIDS case definition is used to monitor trends in the number and distribution of AIDS cases in the United States and severe morbidity due to infection with HIV.

Twenty-five years after the first cases of AIDS were reported in the United States, prevalence rates worldwide continue to increase, especially in African countries. By the end of 2007, an estimated 40 million people were living with HIV/AIDS worldwide. In less developed countries the AIDS epidemic has resulted in a drop in life expectancies from 60 years to only about 40 years. In developed countries with access to antiretroviral therapy, including highly active antiretroviral therapy (HAART), the time of progression from HIV infection to AIDS diagnosis has increased by three years, and life expectancy of those with AIDS has increased by 15 years. Antiretroviral therapy has transformed HIV infection from an acute disease

Acknowledgment
The editors wish to acknowledge the previous authors of this chapter, Arlette C. Perry, PhD, FACSM; Arthur LaPerriere, PhD, FACSM; and Nancy Klimas, MD.

to a chronic condition. Unfortunately, though, even with aggressive medical therapy such as HAART, further HIV-related side effects continue to occur despite an increase in life expectancy. Conditions such as atherosclerosis, heart disease, and diabetes are occurring in HIV-infected persons 20 to 30 years prior to their usual onset with aging in the non-infected population.

Human immunodeficiency virus infection weakens and reduces the function of the immune system. The body's nonspecific defense mechanism, secondary to structural barriers such as skin and tissue acidity, includes immune system functions such as inflammation and cells that attack and destroy infectious agents. The cells that make up the nonspecific immune system, such as macrophages, neutrophils, and natural killer cells, are activated when cell surface receptors encounter and recognize a foreign microbe. The nonspecific immune response is relatively short-lived, as the response dissipates when the infective agent is eliminated. The specific, or adaptive, immune system is the most complex component of immune function. A unique aspect is that immune function is activated by antigen-specific mechanisms that provide long-term immunological "memory" of the foreign antigen. The adaptive immune system is dependent on the function of small lymphocytes; the most common of these are T-lymphocytes and B-lymphocytes (T-cells and B-cells, respectively). T-cells are associated with cell-mediated immunity that enlists immune cells to physically attack and destroy infected cells, while B-cells neutralize microbes through production of antibodies that coat the foreign body. Most pertinent to HIV infection, the CD4+ T-cell (identified by the CD4 coreceptor on the T-cell surface) releases cytokines and growth factors; these generate antigen-specific cellular responses that destroy infected cells. These cells are critical in regulating the specific immune response to infection and are a primary target of HIV virus. The most common immunological abnormalities observed in HIV infections occur in cell-mediated immunity: (1) a marked decrease in total T-cells; (2) a marked decrease in the number of regulatory CD4+ T-cells and reduced response to infectious agents, which is strongly associated with risk of progression to AIDS and death; (3) a normal or slight increase in the CD8+ T-cells (those cells that destroy virally infected cells and cancer cells); and (4) a decrease in natural killer cell activity.

The progression from initial HIV infection to AIDS moves through delineated stages, the boundaries of which have been distorted to some degree by HAART therapy. These progressive stages include:

1. Seroconversion. Immediately postinfection; a large production of HIV virus with initial immune response; often manifests as flu-like symptoms.

2. Asymptomatic (World Health Organization [WHO] Stage 1). Can last for many years; significant HIV activity in the lymph nodes and glands.

3. Symptomatic (WHO Stage 2). Characterized by multisymptom disease; emergence of opportunistic infections and cancers.

4. AIDS (WHO Stage 3). Severe weight loss and muscle atrophy; recurring or continuous infection of multiple organ systems, especially the respiratory, digestive, and nervous systems, as well as the skin.

Adding to the difficulty of managing the health of HIV-infected individuals in this new era is the prevalence of medication-related physical and psychological side effects. The most common drug-related physical side effects involve the gastrointestinal tract. These include abdominal cramps, nausea, vomiting, and diarrhea. Neurological complications are also frequent side effects of anti-HIV medications, the most common being peripheral neuropathy. Other conditions such as lethargy, malaise, fatigue, anemia, mitochondrial toxicity, and myopathies are all common complaints of those taking various anti-HIV drugs. A metabolic complication that has arisen with HAART is lipodystrophy, which is a redistribution of fat stores from the arms, legs, and face to the abdomen and lower cervical region. This condition, which encompasses fat wasting (lipoatrophy) and fat accumulation (lipohypertrophy), is also characterized by dyslipidemia. All of these symptoms can lead to an extremely sedentary lifestyle that often exacerbates the viral and medication-related symptomatology.

EFFECTS ON THE EXERCISE RESPONSE

The response to graded exercise testing in both trained and untrained HIV-infected individuals is typically an abbreviated test resulting from poor functional aerobic capacities. The tests are usually voluntarily terminated due to fatigue or exhaustion. It is unknown currently if the typical HIV-associated changes are due to the infection or associated disease symptoms. The following list illustrates potential HIV-associated changes from age-adjusted norms for a graded exercise stress test.

Asymptomatic

- Normal graded exercise test with physiological parameters within normal limits
- Potentially reduced exercise capacity related to sedentary lifestyle

Symptomatic

- Significantly reduced time on treadmill or bike, peak oxygen consumption ($\dot{V}O_{2peak}$), and ventilatory threshold
- Increased heart rate at absolute submaximal work rate

AIDS

- Dramatically reduced time on treadmill or bike and peak oxygen consumption ($\dot{V}O_{2peak}$)
- Possible failure to reach ventilatory threshold
- Potential abnormal neuroendocrine responses at moderate- and high-intensity test stages

EFFECTS OF EXERCISE TRAINING

Evidence suggests that exercise is safe for individuals with HIV and AIDS who are medically stable. Aerobic exercise at low to moderate intensities does not increase the prevalence of additional infections, does not increase viral load, and does not decrease CD4+ T-cell count; in fact, it increases CD4+ T-cell count. Additionally, adverse side effects to relatively high-intensity exercise interventions have not been reported. Several studies have indicated exercise-enhanced immune function, particularly in asymptomatic participants; however, these activity-related changes to immunity are controversial and contradicted by other research. In any case, one should consider immunosuppression associated with overtraining when prescribing physical activity for the HIV-infected individual.

As with other clinical populations, aerobic and resistance exercise are beneficial for HIV-infected individuals. Almost without exception, studies involving the effects of aerobic exercise training in HIV-infected individuals demonstrate enhanced functional capacity, cardiovascular and muscular endurance, and general well-being. Although there is less evidence to support strength training in HIV-infected individuals, those studies that have been published have demonstrated that progressive resistance exercise programs increase lean tissue mass and improve strength in HIV-infected individuals both with and without muscle wasting.

MANAGEMENT AND MEDICATIONS

Currently, 29 drugs are approved by the Food and Drug Administration for treatment of HIV infection. These drugs are categorized by mode of function, as follows:

- Nucleoside reverse transcriptase inhibitors (NRTIs) and non-nucleoside reverse transcriptase inhibitors (non-NRTIs) that work at different stages of the retroviral replication process to inhibit the conversion of HIV RNA to DNA
- Protease inhibitors (PIs) that stop the processing of HIV genetic material within the infected cell
- Fusion inhibitors (FIs) that inhibit HIV virus from attaching to targeted cells, thus inhibiting initial infection
- Integrase inhibitors that prevent HIV from integrating its genetic material into the infected cell's DNA

Typical treatment regimens include drugs from three or more of these categories. Due to the number of drugs, in addition to medications for the treatment of specific opportunistic infections and HIV symptoms, there are significant issues with side effects and drug interactions. One must consider and monitor these adverse conditions, which are constantly changing, when prescribing an exercise regimen. Many of them, including hyperglycemia, diabetes, hyperlipidemia, and lipodystrophy, are responsive to exercise training. As with other clinical populations, it is recommended that exercise prescription be used in conjunction with nutritional interventions. A number of generally accepted nutritional strategies are accepted for HIV infection and its comorbidities. While exercise and diet have been shown to be beneficial for many of the conditions associated with HIV infection and drug side effects, it should be noted that there is virtually no information on the interaction of medications with exercise training.

RECOMMENDATIONS FOR EXERCISE TESTING

Regardless of disease status, it is important to assess the individual's current level of fitness prior to developing an exercise prescription. While it is understood that a majority of HIV+ individuals have lower functional capacities than others, the majority of standard physical fitness tests are applicable to the HIV+ population. The process of exercise testing HIV+ individuals, therefore, does not differ greatly from that for testing apparently healthy populations; this includes a strict adherence to blood-borne pathogen protections (see table 28.1).

Cardiorespiratory Fitness Testing

A wide array of tests are available to assess cardiovascular fitness in HIV+ individuals; the majority either predict or directly measure peak or maximal $\dot{V}O_2$. Given the common finding of lower than normal peak $\dot{V}O_2$ in this population, the recommendation is to choose a test that is lower in intensity and is submaximal. For example, since people with HIV+ have been shown to have very low $\dot{V}O_{2max}$ values, the modified Bruce protocol may be more appropriate than the standard Bruce protocol for this population. A submaximal cycle ergometry test such as the YMCA protocol would also be appropriate. Field tests for assessing cardiovascular fitness, such as the Rockport walk test or the Cooper 1.5-mile walk/run, from which $\dot{V}O_{2max}$ is predicted, are also applicable to this population.

Muscular Fitness Testing

Assessing muscular strength, endurance, and flexibility in HIV+ individuals should not differ significantly from testing apparently healthy individuals. Because this population is generally untrained and likely unfamiliar with resistance training, using a

TABLE 28.1

AIDS: Exercise Testing

Methods	Measures	Endpoints*	Comments
Aerobic			
Cycle (ramp protocol 17 W/min; staged protocol 25-50 W/3 min stage) Treadmill (1-2 METs/stage)	■ 12-lead ECG, HR, rate–pressure product ■ BP ■ RPE (6-20)	■ Serious dysrhythmias ■ >2 mm ST-segment depression or elevation ■ T-wave inversion with significant ST change ■ SBP >250 mmHg or DBP >115 mmHg	■ Increased prevalence of cardiovascular impairments requires monitoring of ECG and BP. ■ Exercise technician should pay strict attention to blood-borne pathogen protection and universal precautions.
Strength			
Isotonic	3-, 6-, or 10RM		May be necessary to test muscular strength on multiple occasions given the general deconditioning and inexperience of this population.

*Measurements of particular significance; do not always indicate test termination.

3-repetition maximum (RM), 6RM, or 10RM protocol may be more appropriate than 1RM for assessing muscular strength. Muscular strength testing on multiple occasions may be necessary given the general deconditioning and inexperience of this population. The tests commonly used to assess muscular strength closely match the tests used to assess muscular endurance.

RECOMMENDATIONS FOR EXERCISE PROGRAMMING

Regardless of stage of disease progression, all HIV-infected individuals should obtain medical clearance before participating in an exercise program. They should be evaluated for standard physical function, including functional aerobic capacity, muscular strength, body composition, and flexibility. Neuromuscular function should also be assessed, as peripheral neuropathy is a common symptom of HIV infection and can dictate appropriate modes of training. The following are principles for prescribing exercise programs to HIV-infected individuals (see table 28.2).

▪ Though the initial recommendations are for lower levels of exercise in HIV+ individuals than those presented by the American College of Sports Medicine (ACSM), the ultimate goal is to eventually meet the ACSM recommendations for aerobic and resistance exercise. However, because many of the medications prescribed to people with HIV+ have side effects, the final goals of exercise may need to be modified or adjusted.

▪ Aerobic exercise programs for this population should begin at lower volumes, and progression may occur at slower rates than in uninfected, apparently healthy populations.

▪ The design of a resistance exercise program, in addition to taking into account disease and medication limitations, should also adhere to the ACSM

TABLE 28.2

AIDS: Exercise Programming

Modes	Goals	Intensity/Frequency/Duration	Progression
Aerobic Cycling Walking/jogging Swimming Rowing	Increase/maintain cardiovascular function	▪ 40-60% $\dot{V}O_2R$ or HRR ▪ 3-4 days/week ▪ 30-60 min/session	▪ Increasing frequency, duration, intensity. ▪ Severe HIV/AIDS and presence of comorbidities may require restriction on intensity range.
Strength Free weights Isotonic machines		▪ 2-3 days/week ▪ 2 sets of 8-10 reps ▪ 10-12 separate exercises targeting major muscle groups ▪ ~60% 1RM	▪ Frequency and reps remain constant, increasing resistance based on the 2+2 method. ▪ Severe HIV/AIDS and presence of comorbidities may require restriction on intensity range.
Flexibility Stretching	Increase/maintain ROM	▪ Perform after each session ▪ Hold 15-30 s, stretch to point of tightness, avoid discomfort	ROM will increase over time.

guidelines for exercise testing and prescription. The contraindications for participation in resistance exercise are the same as those for aerobic exercise. Participants are recommended to choose a form of resistance training that is comfortable and provides pain-free range of motion with appropriate progression.

SPECIAL CONSIDERATIONS

Continually monitoring the general health of the HIV-infected exercise participant is critical. This is especially true for the novice participant. Those who are untrained are at increased risk for opportunistic infections generally, and especially so if they are training at a level that is too high for their fitness status. The exercise provider should emphasize the importance of reporting increased feelings of tiredness or exhaustion, changes in lower gastrointestinal function (especially diarrhea), shortness of breath, or a sense of increased effort in performing everyday activities. Staff members must have training in universal precautions and must follow universal precaution practices.

Evidence-Based Guidelines

Centers for Disease Control. Updated compendium of evidence-based interventions for HIV/AIDS. www.cdc.gov/hiv/topics/research/prs/evidence-based-interventions.htm.

Hammer SM, Saag MS, Schechter M, et al. Treatment for adult HIV infection: 2006 recommendations of the International AIDS Society–USA panel. JAMA. 2006;296(7):827-843.

Lyles CM, Kay LS, Crepaz N, et al. Best-evidence interventions: Findings from a systematic review of HIV behavioral interventions for US populations at high risk, 2000–2004. Am J Public Health. 2007;97(1):133-143.

Touger-Decker VR, Matheson P, Perlman A, et al. Professional practices of registered dietitians regarding complementary and alternative medicine use for individuals with HIV/AIDS. J Am Diet Assoc. 2004;104(S2):22 Abstract.

Suggested Web Site

Centers for Disease Control. www.cdc.gov/hiv/

CASE STUDY

Human Immunodeficiency Virus

A 37-year-old man, infected with HIV for five years and symptomatic, recently began a highly active antiretroviral therapy (HAART) regimen of dapsome, Truvada, and Kaletra. He had a CD4 count of 300 cells/mm³, which was slowly dropping, and he suffered from osteoporosis. Before starting HAART he experienced frequent diarrhea and muscle weakness, but was recently feeling less gastrointestinal distress and put on weight in his abdomen, neck, and chest. He had become more sedentary because it was "hard to do the things I used to do." He stated that he was "tired more often" and was "having trouble keeping up with my friends like I used to."

S: "I would like to get in better shape, feel more energetic about doing daily activities, and feel like my old self."

O: Vitals

Height: 5 ft 10 in. (1.78 m)
Weight: 170 lb (77.27 kg)
BMI: 24.38 kg/m²
HR: 72 contractions/min
BP: 138/90 mmHg
Central adiposity; waist circumference 34.1 in. (76.45 cm)

Medications: Dapsome, Truvada, Kaletra, Toprol XL, and Lipitor

Labs

CD4 count: 300 cells/mm³
Viral load: 5500 RNA copies/ml
Hemoglobin: 14.4 g/dl
Hematocrit: 41%
Fasting glucose: 96 mg/dl
Total cholesterol: 290 mg/dl
Triglyceride: 180 mg/dl

Graded exercise test (modified Bruce protocol)

Peak work rate: 2.5 mph at 12% grade
Total treadmill time: 6.5 min
Test termination from volitional exhaustion
Peak RPE: 18 out of 20
Peak HR: 183 contractions/min
Peak BP: 190/95 mmHg
$\dot{V}O_{2peak}$: 15.84 ml · kg^{-1} · min^{-1}
ECG: Sinus rhythm at rest and throughout exercise and recovery
No dysrhythmias observed or reported

No report of chest discomfort
Body composition: 22.7% fat (DEXA)
Bone density: 1.27 g/cm^2

A: 1. Deconditioned; fatigues easily
   2. Hyperlipidemic
   3. Hypertensive

P: 1. Begin a combined moderate-intensity aerobic and resistance training regimen in an attempt to increase functional aerobic capacity and muscular strength while also increasing lean body mass and reducing body fat.
   2. After 6-8 weeks, monitor performance and body composition outcomes, assess subjective progress, and update the regimen as needed.

Exercise Program Goals

1. Short-term goals (1-2 mo):
   • Attend majority (~90%) of exercise sessions
   • Walk/jog for 30 min at a moderate intensity without terminating exercise due to fatigue
   • Increase muscular strength on all exercises
   • Increase lean tissue mass
   • Decrease fat mass, specifically central obesity
2. Long-term goals (6 mo):
   • Walk/jog for 60 min at a moderate intensity without terminating exercise due to fatigue
   • Increase muscular strength
   • Increase lean tissue mass
   • Decrease fat mass, specifically central obesity
   • Improve subjective QOL

Mode	Frequency	Duration	Intensity	Progression
Aerobic (walking, jogging)	3-4 days/week	10 min to start, increasing to 30 min	40% $\dot{V}O_2R$ or HRR, increasing to 60% $\dot{V}O_2R$ or HRR	Add 5 min every 1-2 weeks. Increase intensity after 2 months.
Strength (all major muscle groups)	3 days/week		2 sets of 8-10 reps at 60% 1RM	
Flexibility (all major muscle groups)	After each session		Hold 15-30 s, stretch to point of tightness, avoid discomfort	
Warm-up and cool-down	Before and after each session	5-10 min	RPE 6-8/20	

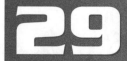

Abdominal Organ Transplant (Kidney, Liver, Pancreas)

Patricia L. Painter, PhD, FACSM ■ Joanne B. Krasnoff, PhD

OVERVIEW OF THE PATHOPHYSIOLOGY

The most common organ transplants performed in the United States are kidney, liver, heart, and pancreas. Abdominal organ transplant surgery is performed on individuals with end-stage liver or kidney failure, whereas pancreas transplant is performed on individuals with type 1 diabetes (usually simultaneously with kidney transplant). End-stage diseases severe enough to require a transplant are due to a variety of causes.

Liver Transplant

Individuals in need of a liver transplant have no other therapies for survival, which is why the liver is one of the most commonly transplanted major organs, second only to the kidney. Cirrhosis is the most common cause of liver failure resulting in the need for a liver transplant. Although there are many causes, in the United States cirrhosis is almost always the result of either chronic alcoholism or hepatitis C. Cirrhosis is a chronic, potentially life-threatening liver disease characterized by the development of fibrous scar tissue leading to progressive loss of liver function over time. The one- and five-year survival

rates for liver transplantation in the United States are 85% and 75%, respectively. Despite the potential risks and complications of liver transplant surgery, including organ rejection and the surgery itself, the majority of transplant patients return to a normal lifestyle and activity within three months following the transplant.

Kidney Transplant

The most common causes of kidney failure in adults are the result of complications associated with diabetes and hypertension. Other less common causes of kidney disease or failure include systemic lupus erythematosus, polycystic kidney disease, and glomerulonephritis. Unlike people with liver failure, those with end-stage renal disease are typically treated with dialysis until a transplant can be performed. The waiting times for transplant vary from months to several years and are increasing because of a shortage of organs available from cadaveric sources. (Living donors are possible for those in need of a kidney and in some centers for those needing a liver transplant.) Severe deconditioning can occur during the waiting period for transplant. The one- and five-year survival rates for kidney transplantation in the United States are 90% and 85%, respectively.

Pancreas Transplant

A pancreas transplant is an option for individuals who have advanced type 1 diabetes with end-stage renal disease. The majority of pancreas transplantations (>90%) are simultaneous pancreas–kidney transplants because a pancreas transplanted along with a kidney is less likely to fail than a pancreas transplanted alone. The one-year survival rate following pancreas transplantation is >90%. After a successful pancreas transplant, the majority of patients no longer require insulin injections and blood glucose monitoring.

Following successful transplantation, most concerns relate to side effects or complications of immunosuppression medications. Except in the case of primary nonfunctioning or rejection of a transplanted organ, a patient's clinical status following transplant surgery is primarily related to the side effects of medications and infection. Other side effects include hypertension, hyperlipidemia, corticosteroid-induced diabetes, muscle weakness, and reduced bone mineral density. Many people experience significant and often excessive weight gain following transplant surgery that is frequently attributed to increased appetite related to corticosteroid use. However, accumulating evidence suggests that weight gain may be more strongly related to lifestyle factors, specifically increased caloric intake with minimal physical activity, and not necessarily to increased appetite induced by the medication. Following transplant surgery, most individuals experience increased feelings of well-being and have few, if any, dietary restrictions.

Persons presenting for abdominal organ transplant are typically deconditioned due to the progression of their disease and lack of pretransplant rehabilitation opportunities or counseling, which results in significant physical inactivity. Following transplantation, lifestyle issues are rarely addressed as part of the post–abdominal transplant medical therapy despite a high prevalence of cardiovascular risk factors and incidence of cardiovascular complications in the long-term posttransplant course.

EFFECTS ON THE EXERCISE RESPONSE

Peak oxygen consumption ($\dot{V}O_{2peak}$) in kidney transplant recipients averages 26 to 30 ml · kg^{-1} · min^{-1} and is close to normal sedentary values. Liver transplant recipients have improved $\dot{V}O_{2peak}$ compared to pretransplant values, but remain 10% to 20% lower in this regard than age-matched controls. Pancreas–kidney transplant recipients are reported to have $\dot{V}O_{2peak}$ values similar to those of nondiabetic kidney transplant recipients. With the exception of diabetic kidney transplant recipients, transplant recipients who participate in regular physical activity have higher exercise capacity than those who remain sedentary. Transplant recipients often exhibit exaggerated blood pressure responses to a single session of exercise. Generally, heart rate responses to exercise are normal except in diabetic kidney-only transplant recipients, who exhibit a blunted heart rate response to exercise. After liver transplant, 6 min walk distances and measures of muscle strength increase but remain low compared to age-expected values. $\dot{V}O_{2peak}$ and self-reported physical functioning improve posttransplant and are significantly higher in recipients who are physically active compared to those who remain sedentary.

EFFECTS OF EXERCISE TRAINING

Organ transplant recipients are able to achieve normal or above-normal levels of exercise capacity with training. Participants in competitive events at the U.S. and International Transplant Games show impressive performances in a variety of athletic events. The number of exercise training studies involving various transplant populations is limited, however. Two exercise training studies involving kidney transplant recipients indicated significant improvements in exercise capacity (by 25% to 28%). In addition, improved blood pressure control, indications of bone remodeling, and increased muscle strength have been reported. Although muscle weakness may continue to persist, specific resistance training programs increase muscle strength and reduce the fat-to-muscle ratio, presumably counteracting the muscle-wasting effects of glucocorticoid therapy.

MANAGEMENT AND MEDICATIONS

Following organ transplant surgery, virtually all individuals are treated with immunosuppression therapy to prevent rejection. The medications currently used include glucocorticoids (prednisone), cyclosporine, tacrolimus, mycophenolate mofetil, and sirolimus. Although new immunosuppressive medications are continually being developed that are more specific to the rejection response, transplant recipients are always at risk for organ rejection. In addition to the medications, many individuals are on prophylactic therapy to reduce infections, antihypertensive therapy, and lipid-lowering medications (see chapters 14 and 22). Liver transplant recipients with recurrent hepatitis C may be treated with antiviral therapies such as interferon or ribavirin, which often result in excessive fatigue. Interferon has also been associated with ST-segment depression and cardiac dysfunction.

RECOMMENDATIONS FOR EXERCISE TESTING

Standard exercise testing protocols are acceptable for transplant recipients. Low-level exercise testing protocols are indicated early posttransplant. The high prevalence of cardiac risk factors and high incidence of cardiovascular disease posttransplantation indicate that a 12-lead electrocardiogram (ECG) should be used during exercise testing (see table 29.1). Because skeletal muscle weakness is prevalent and may result in submaximal performances, exercise tests may be of limited diagnostic use. Performance-based testing such as the 6 min walk may be appropriate early posttransplant but later may not accurately reflect exercise capacity or changes with training. A shuttle walk, which is a progressive exercise test, may be more useful over time after transplant surgery.

Important medications and special considerations during exercise testing include the following:

- Prednisone may cause muscle weakness and wasting, as well as some joint discomfort, and is associated with excessive weight gain and truncal obesity.

- In rare incidences, immunosupressants (e.g., cyclosporine, azathioprine, FK506): can cause drug-induced myopathies.

- For antihypertensive agents, see chapter 14 and appendix.

- For lipid-lowering agents, see chapter 22 and appendix.

- Clients typically present in a deconditioned state.

- Most clients are limited by muscle weakness.

- Be aware of steroid-induced diabetes that occurs after transplant (~30% of cases).

RECOMMENDATIONS FOR EXERCISE PROGRAMMING

Exercise training should begin soon after transplant, and transplant recipients should be encouraged to incorporate physical activity and healthy lifestyle activities into their "new life" routines. After transplant, many recipients present in a significantly deconditioned state and may need strength training prior to participating in aerobic activities (see table 29.2). Once aerobic activities are tolerated, gradual progression should be implemented. Joint discomfort may be experienced by those on high doses of prednisone and during the "taper" phase of the immunosuppressive management. Non-weight-bearing activities may be best tolerated by some, while many recipients are able to progress to jogging and other sporting activities without difficulty.

Some low-level activities are recommended during rejection episodes to maintain a pattern of activity and counteract muscle-wasting effects of the prednisone doses. Prednisone affects muscle metabolism, so a longer period is necessary for strength gain; strength training programs may have to incorporate a slower rate of progression to allow for this longer adaptation time. Liver transplant recipients may experience delayed wound healing and back pain and are at risk for incisional hernias. Liver transplant recipients being treated for recurrent hepatitis C may also experience extreme fatigue. Motivation and adherence to exercise programs remain the major challenges following transplantation.

The following are special considerations for exercise programming:

- Most persons present in a deconditioned state and are limited by muscle weakness.

- Progression with resistance training may need to be slower because of prednisone-induced muscle wasting.

- Exercise intensity should be reduced to mild levels during rejection episodes.

- Vigorous training for competition is possible for those with a good baseline of regular activity.

- Steroid-induced diabetes occurs in about 30% of patients.

- Low-impact activities may be most appropriate for persons on high doses of prednisone or those with joint disease.

- Caloric reduction must be a part of the weight management strategy.

- Motivation and adherence are major challenges.

TABLE 29.1

Abdominal Organ Transplant: Exercise Testing

Methods	Measures	Endpoints*	Comments
Aerobic			
Cycle (ramp protocol 5-20 W/ min; staged protocol 15-25 W/3 min stage) Treadmill (0.5-2 METs/stage)	■ 12-lead ECG, HR, rate–pressure product ■ BP ■ RPE (6-20) ■ METs	■ Serious dysrhythmias ■ >2 mm ST-segment depression or elevation ■ T-wave inversion with significant ST change ■ SBP >250 mmHg or DBP >115 mmHg ■ Leg fatigue	■ Submaximal fitness testing may be appropriate for most clients because cardiac status is, in most cases, known prior to acceptance for transplant. ■ Leg fatigue is typically the reason for test termination. ■ Some immunosupression medications may cause hypertensive responses. ■ Interferon has been associated with ST-segment depression and cardiac dysfunction.
Endurance			
6 min walk	Distance	Note time and distance at rest stops	Mainly useful early after transplant.
Strength			
Isokinetic or isotonic	■ Maximal number of reps ■ Isokinetic work/peak ■ Torque at fast speeds	Maximum ROM	Be aware of prior long-standing bone disease in kidney transplant recipients and other persons who have been on long-term glucocorticoid therapy; 1RM test may not be appropriate.
Flexibility			
Sit and reach Other ROM tests (e.g., Thomas, Active knee extension test)			Pretransplant inactivity may predispose to decreased ROM.

*Measurements of particular significance; do not always indicate test termination.

Evidence-Based Guidelines

Carithers RL. AASLD practice guidelines—liver transplantation. Liver Transpl. 2000;6(1):122-135.

Demartines N, Schiesser M, Clavien P-A. An evidence-based analysis of simultaneous pancreas-kidney and pancreas transplantation alone. Am J Transpl. 2005;5:2688–2697.

Suggested Web Sites

American Diabetes Association. www.diabetes.org

American Liver Foundation. www.liverfoundation.org

National Kidney Foundation. www.kidney.org

TABLE 29.2

Abdominal Organ Transplant: Exercise

Modes	Goals	Intensity/Frequency/Duration	Time to goal
Aerobic Large muscle activities	• Increase aerobic capacity • Increase time to exhaustion • Increase work capacity • Improve BP • Assist with weight management • Reduce risk of cardiovascular disease	• 50-90% peak HR • 50-85% $\dot{V}O_{2peak}$ • 4-6 days/week • 20-60 min/session • Monitor RPE	3-6 months
Strength Free weights Isokinetic machines	• Increase maximal number of reps • Reverse steroid-induced muscle wasting and weakness • Maintain bone mineral density	• 1 set of 8-15 reps • 2-3 days/week • Monitor RPE • Avoid Valsava	4-6 months
Anaerobic Interval training	Improve performance for those interested in competition		
Flexibility Stretching Yoga	Maintain/increase ROM	• 20-30 s/stretch • 2-3 days/week	
Functional Activity-specific exercise	• Increase ADLs • Recreation/fun		

CASE STUDY

Organ Transplantation

A 52-year-old Caucasian man with ulcerative colitis had been sedentary for two months after an orthotopic liver transplantation for sclerosing cholangitis. He also had a history of diabetes mellitus. His convalescence was complicated by hepatic artery thrombosis that necessitated a retransplant six days after the first transplant, as well as by polymicrobial sepsis/intra-abdominal abscess three weeks after the second transplant. After that, he was generally well but had a low energy level and muscle weakness, slept quite a bit at home, and had "enormous" cravings for sweets. He had a 16-year-old son and a 19-year-old daughter, so he was anxious to get back to work as a financial planner.

S:*"I am turning into fat. I am afraid of falling down the stairs as my balance is not great and my legs are weak. I purchased a commode for the downstairs bathroom because getting on and off the toilet was too much work for my little legs."*

O: Vitals

Height: 5 ft 10 in. (1.78 m)
Weight: 140.6 lb (63.8 kg)
BMI: 20.12 kg/m^2
HR: 92 contractions/min
BP: 106/62 mmHg
Tired appearance (bags under eyes), cachectic
Gait slow and unstable
Notably short of breath after walking 500 ft (152.4 m) down the hallway for examination
Medications: Prograf, CellCept, prednisone, acyclovir, Prilosec, dapsone, NPH insulin

Labs

Hemoglobin: 10.2 g/dl
Hematocrit: 30.0%
Fasting glucose: 125 mg/dl
Total cholesterol: 181 mg/dl
HDL: 29 mg/dl
LDL: 92 mg/dl
Triglycerides: 302 mg/dl

Graded exercise test (ramp protocol)

Peak work rate: 3.0 mph at 10% grade
Test termination from leg fatigue
Peak HR: 149 contractions/min
Peak BP: 166/70 mmHg
Peak RPE: 19/20
$\dot{V}O_{2max}$: 21.3 ml · kg^{-1} · min^{-1}
Peak respiratory exchange ratio: 1.15

ECG: Sinus rhythm at rest and throughout exercise and recovery, no ST changes or dysrhythmias
No symptoms of cardiac ischemia
Bone densitometry: 1.109 g/cm^2 with a T-score of −2.7 (> −2.5 is indicative of osteoporosis)
Body composition:
Fat: 19.3% (skinfolds)
DEXA: 20.1% fat

Muscle strength

Isokinetic knee extension: 20 reps at 180°/s
Peak torque/body weight: 41% (normal: 58-75%)

A: 1. Deconditioning with muscle atrophy, weakness, and fatigue
2. Status: post liver transplantation (sclerosing cholangitis)
3. Multiple concomitant diseases:
   - Ulcerative colitis
   - Diabetes mellitus
   - Osteoporosis

P: 1. Complete a comprehensive rehabilitation program, including muscle strength and cardiovascular exercise.
2. Prescribe nutrition counseling for diabetes/cardiovascular risk.

Exercise program goals

1. Short-term goals (1 mo):
   - Be able to walk 4 laps (1 mi [1.6K]) around the track in 20 min
   - Climb 1 flight of stairs 3 consecutive times
   - Discontinue use of the commode
   - Improve glucose regulation
2. Long-term goals (6 mo):
   - Return to work part-time
   - Be able to walk 3 mi (4.8K)
   - Improve glucose regulation

Special Precautions

- Carry/wear medical alert with transplant, diabetes, and medication information.
- With incisional hernia, avoid Valsalva maneuver.
- Check blood sugars before and after exercise.
- Inject insulin into nonworking muscles.
- Carry glucose tablets.
- Keep well hydrated and avoid exercise in hot environments.

(continued)

CASE STUDY Organ Transplantation *(continued)*

Mode	Frequency	Duration	Intensity	Progression
Aerobic	4-5 days/week	20 min/session	THR (98-112 contractions/min 65-75% $\dot{V}O_{2peak}$) RPE 13-15/20	Add 5 min/week to a target of 45 min. Increase intensity every 2 weeks to a THR 75-85% of maximum.
Strength (all major muscle groups)	3 days/week	1 set of 10-12 reps	<12RM	Add weight as needed to maintain comfortable resistance for 10-12 reps.
Flexibility (anterior chest, hip flexors, plantarflexors)	3 days/week	20 s/stretch	Maintain each stretch below discomfort threshold	
Warm-up and cool-down	Before and after each session	5-10 min	RPE 7-9/20	

Chronic Fatigue Syndrome

Stephen P. Bailey, PhD, PT, FACSM

OVERVIEW OF THE PATHOPHYSIOLOGY

Chronic fatigue syndrome (CFS), also known as chronic fatigue and immune dysfunction syndrome (CFIDS), is a puzzling and complex idiopathic condition defined only by its symptoms because of the absence of any known confirming diagnostic criteria. Chronic fatigue syndrome is characterized by persistent debilitating fatigue, not relieved by rest and not accounted for by any specifically identified medical or psychiatric condition. Although the etiology and pathophysiology of CFS remain unknown, possible causes include viral infection, immunologic dysfunction, abnormal hypothalamic-pituitary-adrenal (HPA) axis activity, neurally mediated hypotension, nutritional deficiency, and profound psychological stress. Chronic fatigue syndrome likely represents a common endpoint of disease resulting from multiple precipitating causes.

In addition to fatigue, symptoms of CFS may include frequent sore throats, painful lymph nodes, headache, difficulty with concentration and memory, and a low-grade fever. Chronic fatigue syndrome and fibromyalgia have similar symptomatic characteristics; however, individuals with fibromyalgia also experience diffuse nonarticular soft tissue pain. Chronic fatigue syndrome has been thought to disproportionately afflict well-educated Caucasian women, but recent evidence suggests that CFS affects all racial and ethnic groups and both sexes. Current estimates are that approximately half a million people in the United States have a CFS-like condition.

In 1988 the Centers for Disease Control (CDC) published a set of criteria for defining cases of CFS. The case definition of CFS was revised in 1993 and again in 2003 in an effort to address some ambiguities in the previous version. As currently defined, CFS is considered a subset of chronic fatigue (unexplained fatigue of six months duration or more). In turn, chronic fatigue is considered a subset of prolonged fatigue (fatigue lasting one month or more). Cases of unexplained chronic fatigue can be defined as CFS if they meet both of the following criteria (taken from CDC Web site):

- Clinically evaluated, unexplained persistent or relapsing chronic fatigue of new or definite onset (i.e., not lifelong) that is not the result of ongoing exertion, not substantially alleviated by rest, and results in substantial reduction in previous levels of occupational, educational, social, or personal activities

- The concurrent occurrence of four or more of the following symptoms*:
  - Substantial impairment in short-term memory or concentration
  - Sore throat
  - Tender lymph nodes
  - Muscle pain
  - Multijoint pain without swelling or redness
  - Headaches of a new type, pattern, or severity
  - Sleep that is not refreshing
  - Postexertional malaise lasting more than 24 h

To confirm a diagnosis of CFS, all other conditions that may precipitate similar symptoms must be excluded. Conditions that often exclude a CFS diagnosis include hypothyroidism, sleep apnea, hepatitis B or C, major depressive disorder with psychotic or melancholic features (including bipolar affective disorder, schizophrenia, delusional disorders, dementia, anorexia nervosa, and bulimia nervosa), alcohol or other substance abuse within two years of the onset of chronic fatigue, and severe obesity.

Because the diagnosis of CFS is based solely on symptomatology and exclusion of other conditions, there are no recommended specific laboratory tests. Laboratory tests should be directed toward confirming or excluding other possible conditions. Recently it has been suggested that CFS can be more empirically identified and monitored with the use of three questionnaires: SF-36, the Multidimensional Fatigue Inventory (MFI), and the CDC Symptom Inventory.

EFFECTS ON THE EXERCISE RESPONSE

Exercise testing is not a routine action when one is establishing a diagnosis of CFS because there are no unique diagnostic findings. Individuals with CFS are found on average to have mild reductions in both peak oxygen consumption ($\dot{V}O_{2peak}$) and ventilatory threshold compared to normal subjects, but findings in individual clients vary considerably. It is presently not known whether the reduction in exercise capacity commonly seen in this population is attributable in part to CFS itself or to the deconditioning that accompanies a reduction in activity level. Although there are occasional reports to the contrary, the consensus of findings from studies of individuals with CFS is that cardiac, pulmonary, muscular, metabolic, immune, and endocrine responses to acute exercise are similar to those seen in normal individuals with profound deconditioning. The symptom of fatigue is therefore viewed as "central" (neurological) in nature. While exercise testing does not establish a CFS diagnosis, it may be requested as part of a client's evaluation for excluding other conditions, such as cardiovascular diseases. Exercise testing may also be used for designing an individualized exercise program for clients who have a diagnosis of CFS.

EFFECTS OF EXERCISE TRAINING

A common complaint among individuals with CFS is that their fatigue and other symptoms are noticeably worse in the days following any amount of physical exertion. The basis for this phenomenon is currently not well understood. Attempts at exercise conditioning may be frustrated by this circumstance, and a successful exercise prescription needs to respect this observation. Despite the initial aggravation of symptoms caused by exercise, some overall improvement in symptoms has been reported for clients with CFS. Similarly, individuals with CFS who are educated on the benefits and are encouraged to participate in regular physical activity at home tend to show significant improvement in functional capacity and quality of life. In most cases, the physiological and functional changes seen in individuals with CFS following exercise training are relatively modest, while improvements in perceived outcomes (e.g., quality of life) can be dramatic.

MANAGEMENT AND MEDICATIONS

Because the etiology and pathophysiology of CFS remain unknown, treatment is directed at reduction of symptoms rather than reversal of the underlying condition. Medications and other interventions therefore vary according to which symptoms are

---

*These symptoms must have persisted or recurred during six or more consecutive months of illness and must have predated the fatigue.

predominant, and may also vary with the experience and judgments of the primary physician. Medications commonly used to treat individuals with CFS include analgesic, antidepressant, gastrointestinal, immunosuppressive, and endocrine agents; sleep aids; stimulants; and muscle relaxant agents. Individuals with CFS often do not tolerate standard doses of many medications; as a consequence it is advisable to begin at lesser than usual dosages and then gradually increase the dosage to the therapeutic range. People with CFS often seek relief of their symptoms through remedies that are available outside of the traditional medical model, such as dietary manipulation, vitamin and mineral supplementation, herbal preparations, massage therapy, and aroma therapy.

RECOMMENDATIONS FOR EXERCISE TESTING

Incremental exercise testing with monitoring of standard cardiovascular and ventilatory responses (electrocardiogram, blood pressure, heart rate, respiratory gas exchange, and ventilation) may be indicated as a screening test for individuals whose diagnosis is not yet established. If a myopathic disease is suspected as an alternative diagnosis, appropriate screening for metabolic intermediates in blood or muscle samples might also be incorporated into the study. Individuals with long-standing symptoms are very likely to have had a low level of exercise activity and have undergone significant deconditioning. Work rate increments used in testing will therefore usually be low relative to the levels that would be predicted for age, size, and gender. For example, protocols initiated at work rates below 2 METs (metabolic equivalents) and increasing 0.5 to 1 MET per stage have been effective (see table 30.1).

Important considerations during exercise testing include the following:

▪ Clients with CFS often seek remedies for symptom relief that are available outside of the traditional medical model.
▪ Testing should be scheduled for a day when the client does not have other activities scheduled.

RECOMMENDATIONS FOR EXERCISE PROGRAMMING

Little is known about the clinical effect of exercise training in this population. Thus, general recommendations regarding exercise programming for individuals with CFS are difficult to make (see table 30.2). Reports of clinical improvement resulting from exercise conditioning could reflect a systematic bias, in that clients who do not tolerate exercise may be underrepresented in such studies and therefore not be fully reflected in the outcome measurements. To date, however, there does not appear to be any

TABLE 30.1

Chronic Fatigue Syndrome: Exercise Testing

Methods	Measures	Endpoints*	Comments
Aerobic Cycle (ramp protocol 1-20 W/min; staged protocol 25-50 W/3 min stage) Treadmill (1-2 METs/3 min stage)	▪ 12-lead ECG	▪ Serious dysrhythmias ▪ >2 mm ST-segment depression or elevation ▪ Ischemic threshold ▪ T-wave inversion with significant ST change	▪ Maximal aerobic power test may be indicated for exclusion of other diagnoses. ▪ Respired gas analysis may be useful.
	▪ BP	▪ SBP >250 mmHg or DBP >115 mmHg	
	▪ RPE (6-20) ▪ METs ▪ Other measures as clinically indicated		

*Measurements of particular significance; do not always indicate test termination.

TABLE 30.2

Chronic Fatigue Syndrome: Exercise Programming

Modes	Goals	Intensity/Frequency/Duration	Time to goal
Aerobic Large muscle activities	▪ Prevent deconditioning ▪ Maintain functional work capacity	▪ RPE 9-12/20 ▪ Intensity not main focus ▪ 3-5 days/week ▪ 1-2 sessions/day ▪ 5 min/session, progressing to 60 min sessions as tolerated	~3 months
Strength	▪ Maintain strength ▪ Avoid muscle soreness		
Flexibility	Maintain ROM		
Functional Activity-specific exercises	Increase ease of performing ADLs		

evidence of adverse outcomes from prospectively studied exercise trials in clients with CFS.

For those who wish to undertake an exercise program, the following general guidelines offer a conservative approach to exercise programming that takes into account some of the unique difficulties characteristic of this population:

- The goal of exercise programming in this condition should be, first and foremost, to prevent further deconditioning that could compound the disability of chronic fatigue. Individuals and trainers alike should resist the temptation to adopt a traditional method of training aimed at optimization of aerobic capacity and should focus instead on modest goals of preventing progressive deconditioning.

- Individuals should be warned that they might feel increased fatigue in the first few weeks of an exercise program.

- Exercise should generally be initiated at very low levels, based on the client's current activity tolerance.

- Aerobic exercise should utilize a familiar activity, such as walking, that can be started at a low level.

- Flexibility exercises may be prescribed to preserve normal range of motion.

- Strength training should focus on preservation of levels of strength commensurate with daily living activities and should attempt to avoid activities and intensities that induce delayed-onset muscle soreness (DOMS).

- The progression of exercise activity should focus primarily on increasing the duration of moderate-intensity activities in preference to increasing exercise intensity. Identification of the appropriate magnitude of progression from one exercise session to the next is the most challenging aspect of exercise programming for individuals with CFS. They should be "coached" to not overexert themselves on days when they are feeling well and to reduce their exercise intensity when their symptoms are increased.

SPECIAL CONSIDERATIONS

Several psychological considerations are relevant to exercise in individuals with CFS:

- Chronic fatigue syndrome is often accompanied by depression, although it is now clear that depression itself does not precipitate the disease process.

- Because misunderstanding abounds concerning CFS, some clients may express frustration and disillusionment with both lay and medical communities, which may have been less than sympathetic to their problems.

- A supportive and understanding environment is important in evaluation and counseling of clients with CFS.

- Clients who have CFS cope with their symptoms in part by planning their activities so as to "budget" their energy. Providing advance information about what they can anticipate when referred for exercise testing or training will help them to do so.

Evidence-Based Guidelines

Evidence based guideline for the management of CFS/ME (chronic fatigue syndrome/myalgic encephalopathy) in children and young people. Royal College of Paediatrics and Child Health. 2004. Available from www.rcpch.ac.uk/Research/CE/Guidelines/appraisals-details.

Whiting P, Bagnall AM, Sowden AJ, et al. Interventions for the treatment and management of chronic fatigue syndrome: A systematic review. JAMA. 2001;286:1360-1368.

Working Group of the Royal Australasian College of Physicians. Chronic fatigue syndrome. Clinical practice guidelines—2002. Med J Aust. 2002 May 6;176 suppl:S23-56.

Suggested Web Sites

Centers for Disease Control: Chronic fatigue syndrome. www.cdc.gov/cfs

CFIDS Association of America. www.cfids.org

IACFS/ME International Association for CFs/ME. www.iacfsme.org/

CASE STUDY

Chronic Fatigue Syndrome

A 28-year-old Caucasian woman was referred to an exercise specialist by a psychiatrist because she had become deconditioned secondary to CFS. She stated that her fatigue started dramatically 14 months ago after she was involved in an auto accident. She reported that she did not experience panic attacks and had no history of substance abuse. She lived with her husband in a two-story house, but she left the house only occasionally (approximately two times a week) due to profound fatigue and a fear of not being able to return. She believed that starting an exercise program would help her "get her life back," but when she attempted to exercise on her own she typically experienced more profound fatigue for several days after a single exercise session. Prior to her accident she worked as an intensive care nurse.

S: "I just feel out of it all the time. I used to be very active, now I can't do anything. I try to get outside and work in the garden, but I work for 10 to 15 minutes and then I have to stop and rest for an hour. I seem to end up sitting in front of the television or computer and not really thinking about anything."

O: Vitals

Height: 5 ft 3 in. (1.60 m)
Weight: 148 lb (67.3 kg)
BMI: 26.3 kg/m²
HR: 82 contractions/min
BP: 102/52 mmHg
Caucasian female with normal muscle tone and bulk
Physical exam: Unremarkable
Psychiatric exam: Difficulty concentration on immediate question
Labs (all routine blood tests): Within normal limits
Medications: Prozac, Advil, Ritalin-SR, Cortef

Graded Exercise Test (Low Level; 6 min 15 s on Treadmill)

Peak work rate: 2.5 mph @ 1% grade
Peak HR: 114 contractions/min
Peak BP: 128/58 mmHg
$\dot{V}O_{2peak}$: 21 ml^{-1} · kg · min^{-1}
RPE: 19/20

(continued)

Flexibility: Normal
Declined to perform other tests because of fatigue

A: 1. CFS
   2. Aerobic exercise intolerance

P: 1. Continue psychiatric treatment, including trial of Florinef.
   2. Prescribe an exercise program.

Exercise Program Goals

1. Walk on a treadmill at 3 mph at 1% grade for 20 continuous minutes

2. Do upper extremity strengthening exercises (3 sets of 10 reps):
   - Shoulder flexion, protraction, retraction, and abduction
   - Elbow flexion and extension
   - Latissimus pulldown
3. Do a home exercise program twice/wk.

Follow-Up

The client never met any of these goals. She frequently canceled appointments and discontinued participation after only three sessions.

Mode	Frequency	Duration	Intensity	Progression
Aerobic	2-3 days/week	Two 5 min sessions with 5-10 min recovery between	2-2.5 mph, 0% grade	Increase until 20 min continuous at 4 weeks.
Strength (focus on antigravity and postural/ trunk muscles)	2-3 days/week	1 set of 10 reps	Green Theraband	Advance to 3 sets of 10 reps in 4 weeks.
Flexibility	2-3 days/week	20-60 s/stretch		
Neuromuscular				
Functional				
Warm-up and cool-down	Before and after each session			

Fibromyalgia

Kathy Lemley, PT, MS ■ Barbara B. Meyer, PhD

OVERVIEW OF THE PATHOPHYSIOLOGY

Fibromyalgia (FM) or fibromyalgia syndrome (FMS) is a chronic disorder characterized by widespread musculoskeletal pain in addition to a variety other multisystemic symptoms. An estimated 5 to 10 million people in the United States are diagnosed with FM, making it the third most prevalent rheumatologic disorder in the country. Although the disease affects both men and women, 80% of those afflicted are women between 20 and 55 years of age. Fibromyalgia is a complex multidimensional condition characterized by the presence of chronic diffuse pain and tenderness at specific anatomic locations referred to as "tender points." Additional symptoms include sleep disturbance, chronic fatigue, morning stiffness, paresthesia in the extremities, altered perception of physical exertion, depression, and anxiety. The primary FM symptoms precipitate secondary symptoms of the disease, including impaired functional ability, poor physical fitness, social isolation, low self-esteem, and poor quality of life. The etiology of FM remains elusive, though theories on the causal mechanisms include muscle abnormalities (e.g., muscle microtrauma, local muscular ischemia), neuroendocrine and autonomic system regulation disorders (e.g., stage IV sleep disturbance, hypothalamic-pituitary-adrenal [HPA] axis disturbance, diminished local muscular glucose metabolism), central augmentation of pain processing (serotonin metabolism abnormality, decreased activity of the descending antinociceptive pathways), and genetic predisposition. Another theory relates to the origin of onset versus the cause of FM in suggesting that certain events, such as physical or emotional trauma or disturbance in brain chemistry or sleep patterns, could trigger the onset of FM by activating some unknown physiological abnormality already present in individuals who develop FM.

EFFECTS ON THE EXERCISE RESPONSE

The symptoms associated with FM directly and indirectly affect the acute response to exercise. Pain associated with basic activities of daily living, general fatigue, and altered perception of exertion contribute to the fact that individuals with FM are largely sedentary and deconditioned. Reports of morning stiffness, exaggerated delayed-onset muscle soreness (DOMS) response with poor recovery from exercise, and difficulty with use of the arms in elevated positions may limit the timing of exercise as well as the type of activities that individuals with FM should attempt. Specifically, eccentric muscle contractions, sustained overhead activities, and vigorous or high-impact activities are poorly tolerated.

EFFECTS OF EXERCISE TRAINING

Exercise training has been shown to be both safe and effective in producing the same general benefits for individuals with FM as it does for apparently healthy individuals (i.e., improved cardiorespiratory function, reduced coronary artery disease risk factors, decreased cardiovascular mortality and morbidity, and improved psychosocial function). The majority of subjects participating in studies on exercise and FM who achieved some health-related benefits typically engaged in aerobic exercises for at least 20 min a day, two days a week, and performed strength training two or three times a week utilizing 8 to 12 repetitions per exercise for an average of 12 weeks. Less clear, however, is the exact dose of exercise required to improve specific FM symptoms. The main goal of exercise training in this population is not to enhance cardiopulmonary fitness but rather to restore and maintain functional ability. Specific benefits to individuals with FM as reported in published training studies include the following:

- Reduced number of tender points and decreased pain at tender points (reduced myalgic score)
- Decreased general pain
- Improved sleep and less fatigue
- Fewer feelings of helplessness and hopelessness
- More frequent and meaningful social interactions
- Lessened impact of the disease on daily activities

Because individuals with FM tend to be physically inactive and fearful of the pain associated with exertion, they may be unwilling or unable to participate at the same level as healthy individuals. Thus they may need to begin at lower levels of intensity, duration, and frequency and proceed in a more gradual fashion than typically prescribed.

MANAGEMENT AND MEDICATIONS

The American College of Rheumatology (ACR) has established specific criteria that are used by physicians to make a definitive diagnosis of FM (see ACR criteria for classification of FM in this section). As with the majority of chronic health conditions, medical personnel should guide management of the disease, and clients themselves should assume responsibility for symptom management. Evidence exists to support a variety of treatment options for FM, including pharmacological intervention (e.g., medications for pain, sleeplessness, depression, anxiety). In contrast to opioid therapy, which has poor clinical efficacy, positive results with serotonin-norepinephrine reuptake inhibitors (SNRIs) and the antiepileptic drug pregabalin have been shown in the literature. Other treatment options include exercise programs, client education programs, cognitive behavioral therapy, hypnosis, and acupuncture. There has been little control or standardization to date in the empirical study of FM treatment; however, multidisciplinary approaches that include some form of exercise (e.g., exercise combined with medication, cognitive behavioral therapy combined with physical activity) may be better than any single approach. Additionally, all approaches appear to have the greatest efficacy when medical management is optimal.

The following criteria were developed by the ACR for classification of FM.

Widespread pain for at least three months, defined as the presence of all of the following:

- Pain on the right and left sides of the body
- Pain above and below the waist (including shoulder and buttock pain)
- Pain in the axial skeleton (cervical, thoracic, or lumbar spine or anterior chest)
- Pain on palpation with a force of 4 kg (approximately 9 lb) in the following 11 sites (nine bilateral sites):

Occiput at the insertions of one or more of the following muscles:
- Trapezius
- Sternocleidomastoid
- Splenius capitis
- Semispinalis capitis

Low cervical (at the anterior aspect of the interspaces between the transverse processes of C5-C7):
- Trapezius (at the midpoint of the upper border)
- Supraspinatus (above the scapular spine near the medial border)
- Second rib (just lateral to the second costochondral junctions)

- Lateral epicondyle (2 cm distal to the lateral epicondyle)
- Gluteal (at the upper outer quadrant of the buttocks, at the anterior edge of the gluteus maximus muscle)
- Greater trochanter (posterior to the trochanteric prominence)
- Knee (at the medial fat pad proximal to the joint line)

From Wolfe F., Smythe HA, Yunus MB et al. The American College of Rheumatology 1990 criteria for the classification of fibromyalgia. *Arthritis Rheumatology.* 1990;33:160-72.

RECOMMENDATIONS FOR EXERCISE TESTING

Individuals with FM tend to be sedentary and deconditioned, with poor ability to sustain exercise for extended periods. Therefore, tests of muscular endurance (e.g., 6 min walk test; see table 31.1) may be useful for developing an exercise prescription. Aerobic exercise testing is usually symptom limited rather than metabolically limited in the FM population, and thus people with FM tend to reach peak rather than maximal aerobic effort. Symptom

TABLE 31.1

Fibromyalgia: Exercise Testing

Methods	Measures	Endpoints*	Comments
Aerobic			
Cycle (ramp protocol 1-20 W/min; staged protocol 25-50 W/3 min stage) Treadmill (0.5-1.0 METs/3 min stage)	■ 12-lead ECG, HR	■ Serious dysrhythmias ■ >2 mm ST-segment depression or elevation ■ Ischemic threshold ■ T-wave inversion with significant ST change	■ Gluteal trigger points may limit usefulness of cycling.
	■ BP	■ SBP >250 mmHg or DBP >115 mmHg	
	■ RPE (6-20) ■ METs ■ Time to exhaustion		■ RPE may be inaccurate.
Strength			
Handgrip	■ MVC	■ 3 attempts	May reflect functional strength.
Isotonic	■ 1RM	■ MVC with full ROM	
Endurance			
6 and 12 min walk	Distance	Total distance/stops	May be more useful than aerobic tests.
Flexibility			
Sit and reach Goniometry		Full flexion and extension	Identify specific joints for stretching exercise.
Functional			
Lifting-specific activities			Useful for program to maintain ADLs.

*Measurements of particular significance; do not always indicate test termination.

limitations and low intrinsic motivation tend to favor submaximal testing, including graded exercise protocols with smaller increments (i.e., Naughton, Balke-Ware) or ramp protocols. Walking or cycle tests are also recommended, although individuals with gluteal tender points may find it difficult to tolerate cycling on a standard ergometer. A recumbent cycle ergometer should be considered in these cases. Exercise testing should take place on a day when no other activities are scheduled to minimize its impact on later function, since the client is likely to be worn out by the testing.

Flexibility programs have been shown to result in short-term improvements in FM symptoms. Simple flexibility testing can identify specific areas that would benefit from routine stretching. Strength training has consistently been shown to lead to improvement in strength in the FM population comparable to that of healthy sedentary individuals. A grip strength test and 1-repetition maximum tests may give some indication of functional strength as well as identify starting weights for a strengthening program.

During exercise testing, several medications and factors should be considered:

- The majority of commonly used agents are unlikely to alter test results. These include the following (clients with multiple physical symptoms may take many medications):
  - Analgesics
  - Antidepressants (Tricyclic antidepressants [TCAs], Selective serotonin reuptake inhibitors [SSRIs], Serotonin and norepinephrin reuptake inhibitors [SNRIs])
  - Anxiolytics or benzodiazepines
  - Antiepileptics (pregabalin)
- Subjects may be extremely deconditioned.
- Perception of increased exertion may alter rating of perceived exertion.
- Avoidance of early morning testing will help prevent morning stiffness.
- It is best to test on a day when other activities are not scheduled.
- Postexertional muscle pain may be severe 24 to 48 h after testing.

RECOMMENDATIONS FOR EXERCISE PROGRAMMING

Methodological inconsistencies and high attrition rates among participants in published studies on exercise and FM make it difficult to provide defini-

tive recommendations for exercise programming in this population. However, it appears that exercise programming for individuals with FM should primarily consist of low- to moderate-intensity aerobic activities (see table 31.2). Muscular endurance or aerobic exercise testing should be conducted prior to exercise prescription so that individual programs, which may facilitate adherence, can be developed. Programs should consist of non- or low-impact activities that minimize eccentric contraction. Because the small muscles of the shoulder do not tolerate sustained overhead activities, exercise programs involving the lower body (e.g., water exercise, walking, cycling) are recommended. Warm water aquatic exercise programs longer than 12 weeks have demonstrated consistent improvement in physical function similar to that for land-based exercise and may have greater benefits on mood than land-based programs. Activities such as tai chi and yoga have also been shown to be beneficial and should be considered in the design of exercise programs for individuals with FM. While stretching may minimize muscle microtrauma and improve tolerance of aerobic exercise, few if any long-term benefits have been reported from participation in flexibility programs alone. Likewise, strength training activities alone have not been found to consistently improve pain and impact of FM; nevertheless, due to the general deconditioned state of individuals with FM, strength training should be considered as part of the overall exercise program to improve fitness. Since people with this disease have a poor tolerance for eccentric movements, exercises should be designed to minimize the eccentric component.

The optimal dose of aerobic exercise is currently unknown; however, psychophysiological responses to activity indicate the need to begin slowly and increase work rate gradually. Researchers and clinicians alike suggest that despite requests to exercise three times a week, people with FM prefer or self-select exercise twice a week. Thus it may be worthwhile to try to gradually increase duration of exercise from the typical 20 to 30 min per session to 30 to 40 min.

Empirical and anecdotal evidence suggest poor adherence rates among individuals with FM. Thus, it is advisable to conduct exercise sessions under supervised conditions or in a group setting. People with this disease should be encouraged to combine exercise with other symptom management techniques such as medication, support groups, and client education programs. Cognitive behavioral therapy with an emphasis on increasing self-efficacy may be especially helpful, as self-efficacy has been found to be the most powerful construct in predict-

TABLE 31.2

Fibromyalgia: Exercise Programming

Modes	Goals	Intensity/Frequency/Duration	Time to goal
Aerobic Large muscle activities (walking, cycling, aquatics)	■ Restore/maintain functional ability* ■ Decrease pain ■ Decrease anxiety/depression ■ Increase $\dot{V}O_{2max}$ ■ Decrease CAD risk ■ Go faster/longer ■ Increase time to exhaustion	■ 50-75% HRR ■ 20-40 min ■ 2-3 days/week ■ Monitor pace and HR ■ Favor duration over intensity	Progress very gradually.
Strength Handgrip Isotonic	Maintain or improve muscle strength	■ 1 set of 8-12 reps ■ Begin 40% of 1RM ■ Progress to 60-70% of 1RM ■ Pause between reps ■ Minimize eccentric phase	Progress very gradually.
Flexibility Sit and reach Goniometry	■ Increase ROM (especially in shoulders, hips, knees, and ankles) ■ Decrease risk of injury	As tolerated	Maintain.
Functional Lifting-specific activities Individualized activities (O.T.)	■ Increase ADLs ■ Restore work potential ■ Improve quality of life	■ As tolerated ■ Minimize eccentric contractions	

*Other major goals not ascribed to specific exercises include the following:

Reduce the number of tender points/myalgic score

Reduce general pain

Improve sleep

Improve psychological well-being

Avoid exhaustion (i.e., budget activities/exercise)

ing exercise initiation and maintenance in the FM population.

Important medications and special considerations for exercise programming include the following:

■ Most commonly used agents should be unlikely to alter test results (see section on exercise testing).

■ Gluteal trigger points may limit the usefulness of cycling with a standard cycle.

■ Morning exercise should be avoided because of morning stiffness.

■ Supervision or group exercise may increase adherence.

■ Clients may experience an increase in symptoms.

- Sustained overhead activities should be avoided.
- Eccentric movements should be minimized.

SPECIAL CONSIDERATIONS

Often characterized as a "difficult" or "needy" population, individuals with FM may require more time and attention than the generally healthy population with respect to obtaining good adherence to a program. Clients with FM are usually hesitant to exercise or to increase the intensity of activity when they do exercise. Avoiding or limiting early morning exercise, eccentric movements, and repetitive overhead activities may help to minimize attrition. Offering choices about the mode and timing of exercise, offering simple methods of assessing progress such as the use of a pedometer, and yielding to weather-related complaints may help to maximize participation in and adherence to the exercise program. Because symptoms may worsen initially, it is important for participants to budget exercise in conjunction with other activities and obligations. Concomitantly, the importance of self-efficacy to exercise adoption and adherence reinforces the need to begin with exercise activities that are easily mastered and to progress slowly toward those of greater intensity or frequency. A supportive and understanding environment will also foster adherence to programs of exercise and ultimately the utilization of a comprehensive treatment program.

Evidence-Based Guidelines

Carville SF, Arendt-Nielsen S, Bliddal H, et al. EULAR evidence based recommendations for the management of fibromyalgia syndrome. Ann Rheum Dis. 2008;67:536-541.

Wood PB. Symptoms, diagnosis, and treatment of fibromyalgia. Virtual Mentor. 2008;10(1):35-40.

Suggested Web Sites

American College of Rheumatology. www.rheumatology.org

Centers for Disease Control and Prevention. www.cdc.gov/arthritis/arthritis/fibromyalgia.htm

Mayo Clinic. www.mayoclinic.com/health/fibromyalgia/DS00079

National Fibromyalgia Association. www.fmaware.org

CASE STUDY

Fibromyalgia

A 44-year-old woman complained of a two-year history of pain, including aches and pains in the neck, upper and lower back, arms, and legs. Her pain was usually worse later in the day. She awakened unrefreshed and occasionally experienced morning stiffness. She also had carpal tunnel syndrome in her right hand, which was on her dominant side.

S: "I don't sleep well. I wake still feeling tired and I ache all over."

O: Vitals

Height: 5 ft 2 in. (1.6 m)
Weight: 131 lb (59.4 kg)
BMI: 23.2 kg/m²
HR: 82 contractions/min
BP: 128/84 mmHg
Middle-aged woman; no notable joint inflammation/activity
Tender point assessment: Positive in 12 of 18 sites
Graded exercise test (modified Balke protocol): Completed 4 stages (12 min), terminated from fatigue
ECG: No abnormalities
Peak exercise capacity: 5.4 METs
Peak HR: 130 contractions/min (74% of age predicted); normal pressor response
Medications: Paxil daily, trazodone as needed

Questionnaires

Fibromyalgia impact questionnaire (FIQ): Score of 47.86/100 Beck Depression Inventory (BDI): 13/63 (mild depression) State Anxiety Inventory (SAI): 51 (score range 20-80)

A: 1. Fibromyalgia with nonarticular pain
   2. Low aerobic capacity and deconditioning (decreased tolerance for ADLs resulting from pain and fatigue)

P: 1. Start a walking program.
   2. Prescribe stretching exercises as warm-up and cool-down activities.

Exercise program goals

1. Decrease myalgic pain
2. Improve ability to perform ADLs
3. Improve physical fitness

Follow-Up

At week 12, the client's tender points had decreased to 6 out of 18, and she completed 5 stages of a modified Balke protocol. Heart rate at stage IV decreased to 110 contractions/min. Her BDI had increased to 18. FIQ and SAI scores, however, improved (FIQ = 40.95; SAI = 39). Beginning at approximately 16 weeks, her logs revealed a reduction in compliance with the exercise program due to family-related issues. After 24 weeks, she had increased to 8 out of 18 tender points, and her questionnaire scores showed a general regression (FIQ = 50.72; BDI = 15; SAI = 66). She was able to complete 4 stages of the modified Balke protocol prior to fatigue with a peak heart rate of 125 contractions per minute.

Mode	Frequency	Duration	Intensity	Progression
Aerobic	2-3 days/week*	12 min/session	Start at 25% of HRR	Slowly progress to 30-40 min. Increase intensity 5%/week to 50-75% of HRR.
Strength	2 days/week	1 set, 8 reps	40% 1RM	Progress to 12 reps. Slowly progress to 60-70% 1RM.
Flexibility (all major muscle groups)	2-3 days/week			
Warm-up and cool-down	Before and after each session	See flexibility suggestions in table 31.2		

*May self-select 2 days/week (all modes included).

32

Anemia

Kirsten L. Johansen, MD

OVERVIEW OF THE PATHOPHYSIOLOGY

Anemia is one of the most common blood disorders in the United States, affecting an estimated 3.5 million Americans from all age, racial, and ethnic groups. Anemia is defined as the condition in which the number of red blood cells per cubic millimeter, the amount of hemoglobin in 100 ml of blood, and/or the volume of packed red blood cells per 100 ml of blood is less than normal, thereby reducing the oxygen-carrying capacity of the blood. Although both men and women can develop anemia, women of childbearing age are more at risk for anemia than men. Other populations at risk for anemia include adults with other medical conditions and infants <2 years of age. Major risk factors for anemia include the following:

- Poor or inadequate diets low in iron, vitamins, and minerals.
- Blood loss from surgery or injury.
- An intestinal disorder that affects the absorption of nutrients in the small intestine, such as Crohn's disease or celiac disease. Surgical removal of or surgery to the parts of the small intestine where nutrients are absorbed can lead to nutrient deficiencies and anemia.
- Pregnancy. Pregnant women are at an increased risk of iron deficiency anemia because their iron stores have to serve their own increased blood volume and also serve as a source of hemoglobin for the growing fetus.

- Chronic or serious illnesses such as kidney disease, cancer, diabetes, rheumatoid arthritis, HIV/AIDS, inflammatory bowel disease (including Crohn's disease), liver disease, and thyroid disease.
- Being female. In general, women are at greater risk of iron deficiency anemia than men because they lose blood (and therefore iron) each month during menstruation.
- Chronic infections.
- Family history of inherited anemia, such as sickle cell anemia or thalassemia.

A defect in any one or more of the key components in red blood cell metabolism can result in anemia. The following are specific mechanisms of anemia and their causes:

- Reduced red blood cell production
- Reduced serum ferritin levels
- Marrow damage by drugs or tumor infiltration
- Failure of erythropoietin response to anemia (inflammatory disorders, renal failure)
- Abnormal red blood cell precursor maturation
- Iron, B12, or folate deficiency
- Thalassemia
- Drug toxicity (e.g., chemotherapeutic agents)
- Increased red blood cell destruction or loss

- Hemolysis (autoimmune defects, hemoglobinopathies such as sickle cell disease)
- Blood loss (e.g., menstruation, gastrointestinal bleeding, or other source)

The signs and symptoms of anemia depend on how fast it develops, its severity, the age of the individual, and the presence of underlying medical conditions such as atherosclerosis. The primary symptoms of anemia are easy fatigability, shortness of breath with exercise, and decreased work capacity. Anemia can also be associated with worsening of angina (chest discomfort), claudication (leg pain with exercise), or heart failure in clients with these conditions. Symptoms are related primarily to the low oxygen-carrying capacity of anemic blood, but severe iron deficiency may also reduce the activity of iron-containing muscle enzymes and impair the intrinsic ability of skeletal muscle. In the setting of rapid blood loss, symptoms may be more severe because low blood volume further reduces tissue oxygen delivery.

A common question among sport coaches is whether or not to take preparticipation measures and screen their athletes for anemia. Screening for anemia among male athletes is of no value, as the incidence of false positives is high due to the low hemoglobin levels frequently observed in this population. Hemoglobin levels are commonly low because aerobic exercise expands baseline plasma volume (a marker for physical fitness), which dilutes hemoglobin concentration.

Screening for anemia in female athletes, however, is warranted. Anemia is common among female athletes (approximately 10% of young women have iron deficiency anemia) because dietary iron often fails to meet physiologic needs. Athletes with the highest risk include those with heavy menses who avoid eating red meat. Anemia testing in females is justifiable, as the financial burden for detecting anemia is low, the remedy is simple, and the benefits for the athlete with respect to overall health and sport performance are extensive.

EFFECTS ON THE EXERCISE RESPONSE

At rest, the anemic individual may feel few side effects as the cardiovascular system compensates for low oxygen- and carbon dioxide-carrying capacity by increasing cardiac output and breathing rate. In addition, there is often a rightward shift of the oxyhemoglobin dissociation curve (Bohr effect) to facilitate a higher percentage of oxygen extraction by the tissues. During submaximal exercise, cardiac output and muscle blood flow increase at a faster rate in anemic individuals and remain higher for the duration of the exercise. Thus, oxygen delivery to exercising muscle is preserved at near-normal levels under submaximal exercise conditions. However, during peak exercise, the low hemoglobin levels associated with anemia cannot be compensated for by cardiac output, muscle blood flow, or oxygen extraction; consequently energy production and performance are limited.

Individuals with sickle cell anemia and thalassemia are severely limited by their low hemoglobin, but it is reported that they can exercise to exhaustion without precipitating any complications (such as sickle pain crisis). On the other hand, persons with sickle cell trait (heterogeneous hemoglobin S) are not limited because their hemoglobin levels are normal. In fact, the percentage of African American professional athletes with sickle cell trait is about the same as in the general population. However, this does not mean that sickle cell trait is benign, as there have been numerous sudden deaths in young men with sickle cell trait. These incidents seem to have occurred after sudden increases in activity; a rapid increase in altitude; or prolonged, very-high-intensity exercise. Dehydration may also have played a part in these tragic deaths.

EFFECTS OF EXERCISE TRAINING

While persons with chronic anemia will always have their peak aerobic performance limited by the anemia, data gathered from animals suggest that aerobic exercise training in anemic individuals can improve exercise endurance to levels superior to those of nonanemic sedentary persons. Moreover, submaximal performance, which is largely a parameter of skeletal muscle function, can be markedly improved by endurance training. Women who are iron deficient but not yet anemic can also experience reduced endurance capacity, but this is easily corrected with iron supplementation.

MANAGEMENT AND MEDICATIONS

When treatment results in complete correction of anemia, exercise capacity usually returns to normal. Restoration of normal hemoglobin levels is often possible for anemia related to a deficiency state or to blood loss, but is not always possible or even desirable for clients with other conditions such as thalassemia, sickle cell disease, renal failure, or bone marrow abnormalities. In fact, because of recent studies showing a higher risk of heart problems or death in patients with cancer who are treated with erythropoietin-stimulating agents (ESAs) and a similarly increased risk in patients with chronic kidney disease treated more aggressively with these agents, the Food and Drug Administration recently issued an alert and health advisory about the use of ESAs in the treatment of anemia. Physicians are now advised to adjust the ESA dose to maintain the lowest hemoglobin level needed to avoid the need for blood transfusions and to monitor patients' hemoglobin levels to ensure that they do not exceed 12 g/dl. Thus, individuals with these conditions may have chronic anemia and reduced exercise capacity despite appropriate treatment. In addition, exercise limitations may persist even after normalization of hematocrit in persons with conditions that are associated with other exercise limitations, such as chronic renal failure.

Exercise capacity improves with erythropoietin treatment in clients with renal failure, but not as much as would be expected based on observed increases in hematocrit, and normal exercise capacity is not achieved. This has led investigators to conclude that renal failure causes muscle abnor-malities that also limit exercise capacity. Similarly, clients with underlying heart failure, lung disease, or other conditions may have exercise limitations not related to anemia. However, since anemia can exacerbate the exercise intolerance associated with all of these conditions, treatment is usually associated with improvement.

RECOMMENDATIONS FOR EXERCISE TESTING

The exaggerated heart rate response to exercise and limited peak performance in individuals with anemia suggest that aerobic exercise tests will be likely to end sooner than predicted by age and gender. Thus, one should consider choosing a low-level exercise protocol. Submaximal endurance testing may also be helpful in monitoring the response to training or to treatment for anemia (see table 32.1).

RECOMMENDATIONS FOR EXERCISE PROGRAMMING

The main goal of exercise in this population is to improve endurance. Any form of large muscle exercise is acceptable (see table 32.2), although intensity should be moderate. The optimal frequency

TABLE 32.1

Anemia: Exercise Testing

Methods	Measures	Endpoints	Comments
Endurance 6 min walk	Distance covered	Note time and distance at rest stops	Useful throughout exercise training program

TABLE 32.2

Anemia: Exercise Programming

Modes	Goals	Intensity/Frequency/Duration	Time to goal
Aerobic Large muscle activities	Increase $\dot{V}O_{2max}$, $\dot{V}O_{2peak}$, work rate, and endurance	■ 40-70% peak HR ■ RPE 11-14/20 ■ 3-7 days/week ■ 30-60 min/session ■ Emphasize duration over intensity	4-6 months

and duration of training sessions are not known. Adaptability is not known, but the time course of improvement in performance is presumably normal after anemia is corrected.

The following are special considerations in the exercise testing and training of persons with specific medical conditions:

- Sickle cell anemia or trait: High-intensity exercise and dehydration may increase the risk of sickle cell crisis. Therefore, moderate exercise and liberal fluid intake are especially recommended for these individuals.

- Known or suspected coronary artery disease or peripheral vascular disease: Vigorous exercise, especially in combination with anemia, may cause angina (chest discomfort) or may unmask claudication. For this reason, exercise testing and training should be carefully monitored until the cause of anemia has been identified and treated or until tolerance of the exercise program has been established.

- Peripheral vascular disease: Vigorous exercise may elicit or unmask claudication.

CASE STUDY

Anemia

53-year-old woman complained of reduced exercise toler-nce over several months. She was training for a marathon nd noted she had gone from a 9.5 to 10 min/mile pace to a 1.5 to 12 min/mile pace, and her heart rate during running d increased from the 140s to the 150 to 160 range despite e slower pace. Because it was more difficult to exercise, she duced the frequency from five to six sessions per week to ree to four sessions. She had not experienced menopause d was having extremely heavy menstrual flow. Iron supple-ents had been poorly tolerated, and laboratory testing did t indicate imminent menopause.

"It's become very hard to exercise."

Vitals

R: 60 contractions/min
P: 110/60 mmHg
b: Hemoglobin 8.8 g/dl
ndometrial biopsy normal

A: 1. Chronic anemia secondary to menorrhagia

P: 1. Continue to encourage iron intake in diet and in supplemental form.
2. Monitor hormones for evidence of impending menopause; consider hysterectomy.
3. Continue training at lower intensity while reducing distance as little as possible.

Exercise Program Goal

Continue to train for marathon distances

Follow-Up

The client struggled unsuccessfully to increase iron stores and hemoglobin for two years in the setting of ongoing heavy menstrual blood loss. At that point, she underwent hysterectomy. Since that time, hemoglobin has risen into the normal range, and her exercise tolerance has returned to baseline. She continues to train for and to run marathons at age 59.

33

Bleeding and Clotting Disorders

Geoffrey E. Moore, MD, FACSM ■ Michael Lockard, MA

OVERVIEW OF THE PATHOPHYSIOLOGY

Physical activity causes trauma to the circulatory system, and thus bleeding and clotting are normal consequences of exercise. The blood hemostatic system serves to counteract this trauma, minimizing blood loss and maintaining normal blood flow. Hemostasis involves a complex balance of platelet aggregation, coagulation, and clot dissolution (fibrinolysis). These three processes involve many proteins and enzymes, continually working to maintain the integrity of the vascular system. In addition, the inflammatory response is an essential component of the initiation and resolution of hemostasis.

When a vessel is torn or cut, the open ends spasm, reducing blood flow and allowing blood platelets to aggregate at the site of injury. This aggregate of platelets forms a plug in the damaged area of the vessel. Simultaneously, pro-inflammatory substances released from the damaged tissue initiate a series of reactions known as the extrinsic pathway of the coagulation cascade. The coagulation cascade consists of proteolytic enzymes called coagulation factors that are suspended in blood. Upon damage to the vessel, these activated factors precipitate to form a web-like tangle of a protein called fibrin. The combination of platelet aggregation and the acti-

vated coagulation cascade produces a durable clot at the site of injury. As injured tissue heals, the fibrin in the clot is gradually disintegrated by the enzyme plasmin in the process known as fibrinolysis.

Diseases of hemostasis present clinically either as inadequate clotting (hemorrhage) or as excessive clotting (thrombosis). Abnormalities occur in each of the three phases: platelet plug formation, fibrin formation and development of a clot, and fibrinolysis and resolution of the clot.

Abnormalities of Platelet Function

Platelet disorders can produce inappropriate bleeding or inappropriate clotting. The most common platelet bleeding disorder is thrombocytopenia, which is an insufficient number of platelets. The hemorrhages of thrombocytopenia, called petechiae, are pinpoint-sized red spots in the skin that are too small to feel. Petechiae resemble a rash, but are in fact small pools of blood that have leaked out of broken capillaries. Normally, platelet counts range from 120,000 to 600,000/mm^3. It is commonly advised that exercise be avoided if the platelet count is less than 50,000/mm^3.

The most common disorder associated with activated platelet aggregation is probably atherosclerosis. Platelet aggregation disorders alone rarely cause a clinically meaningful obstruction of blood flow.

Abnormalities of the Coagulation Cascade

Coagulation disorders generally cause excess bleeding. Bleeding disorders from factor deficiencies can be congenital or acquired. The most common congenital bleeding disorders are factor VIII deficiency (classic hemophilia), factor IX deficiency (Christmas disease), and von Willebrand disease. Acquired factor deficiencies can also be caused by autoimmune illnesses and some cancers such as lymphoma. Also, many people have medically induced factor deficiencies from taking anticoagulant drugs such as warfarin. The purpose of medical anticoagulation is to prevent blood clots in persons who are at high risk for forming them. Fortunately, medical anticoagulation very rarely causes spontaneous bleeding, although there is increased risk of bleeding after an injury.

Abnormalities of Anticoagulation and Fibrinolysis

Although coagulation disorders generally cause excessive bleeding, some disorders in the coagulation cascade involve anticoagulation factors designed to keep coagulation in check. Such disorders cause excessive clotting because coagulation is insufficiently countered by anticoagulant activity. Common congenital deficiencies of the anticoagulant system include deficiency of protein S or protein C. Again, autoimmune illnesses can cause acquired forms of thrombotic disorders.

Likewise, abnormalities in fibrinolysis may result in inadequate dissolution of a fibrin clot, causing excessive clotting. Common abnormalities include deficiency in tissue plasminogen activator (tPA) and overexpression of plasminogen activator inhibitor (PAI-1).

In sum, the general clinical manifestations of bleeding disorders include the following:

- Thrombocytopenia: petechial bleeding
- Hemophilia: hemarthrosis (i.e., bleeding into joints or into muscle); retroperitoneal bleeding
- von Willebrand disease: prolonged bleeding after minor trauma; gastrointestinal bleeding; heavy menses
- Medical anticoagulation: easy bruising ability; gastrointestinal bleeding

General clinical manifestations of clotting disorders include the following:

- Thrombocytosis: deep venous thrombosis (DVT)
- Anticoagulant deficiencies: arterial occlusion and tissue infarction; DVT

EFFECTS ON THE EXERCISE RESPONSE

Disorders of bleeding and clotting have little effect on the exercise response, but exercise markedly alters function of the thrombotic and fibrinolytic pathways. Moreover, the preponderance of evidence suggests that exercise has dose-dependent effects on platelet aggregation, thrombosis, and fibrinolysis. Therefore, it is less important to know how these disorders affect the exercise response than to know how exercise can trigger bleeding or clotting in persons with these disorders.

Exercise causes a complex mechanical and biochemical stimulation of platelet aggregation and fibrin formation that promotes the formation of a thrombus. Sympathetic stimulation (i.e., release of epinephrine) activates platelet aggregation and binding of fibrinogen receptors on platelets. In addition, shear stress from increased blood flow stimulates both the endothelium-dependent and platelet-dependent activation of the coagulation cascade. The interaction of the platelet plug with the coagulation cascade potentiates the binding of platelet glycoprotein (GP) IIb/IIIa receptors to fibrinogen and increased P-selectin activity. Platelet glycoprotein IIb/IIIa activity is dependent on its binding with von Willebrand factor.

Exercise also causes a transient increase in fibrinolysis, as reflected by an increase in fibrinolytic enzymes and serum fibrin degradation products. The risk of a clinically meaningful bleed or clot is therefore determined by a change in the balance of thrombogenesis and fibrinolysis. If thrombogenesis is insufficient to match the vascular trauma of exercise, the risk of a bleed increases. In contrast, if exercise causes excessive thrombogenesis, the risk of an arterial or venous clot increases. Likewise, an insufficient increase in fibrinolysis would increase the risk of a clot. Despite recent advances in our knowledge of the exercise effects on various aspects of coagulation and fibrinolysis, there are not sufficient data to allow full characterization of the balance of these systems during exercise. Table 33.1 summarizes the expert opinion regarding these independent effects.

After exercise, thrombotic pathway activity remains increased long after the fibrinolytic activity

TABLE 33.1

Exercise Effects on Various Aspects of Coagulation and Fibronolysis

Exercise intensity	Platelet aggregation	Coagulation	Fibrinolysis
Light (<60% HR$_{max}$)	No effect	No effect	Increased
Moderate (60-80% HR$_{max}$)	Decreased	No effect	Increased
Hard (>80% HR$_{max}$)	Increased	Increased	Much increased

has returned to baseline. Interestingly, the incidence of myocardial infarction is increased in the hours shortly after physical activity, and myocardial infarction has been anecdotally reported in a patient with an activated protein C (APC) deficiency. Many experts believe that exercise-induced increases in thrombogenesis can cause myocardial infarctions.

The major risks for exercise in persons with low platelet counts or coagulation factor deficiencies are bleeding from trauma or from high blood pressure associated with exercise. Unfortunately, the quality of data to guide the exercise specialist in recommending exercise in persons with thrombocytopenia is mixed. Exercise specialists must use their best judgment and are advised to err on the conservative side. Taking evidence from sedentary persons as a guide, bleeding from a low platelet count is rarely a problem in sedentary persons unless the count is well below 100,000/mm^3. Occasionally, intracranial (inside the skull) bleeds occur spontaneously when the platelet count is markedly low (<20,000/mm^3). There are no controlled studies on exercise in clients with low platelets; but a conservative approach is recommended and vigorous exercise is probably contraindicated when platelet counts are below 50,000/mm^3. In persons with platelet counts between 20,000 and 50,000/mm^3, exercise should probably be limited to use of elastic bands, stationary cycles, range of motion exercises, and ambulation.

A few circumstances deserve special mention. First, since lifting heavy weights dramatically increases blood and intracranial pressures, the risk of an intracranial bleed probably outweighs the benefits in persons with platelets between 50,000 and 100,000/mm^3. Second, in persons with hemophilia or von Willebrand disease, the mode of testing should minimize joint trauma and weight bearing. Additional limitations may be imposed by preexisting joint contractures from prior bleeds. Of course, these contractures may be good targets for flexibility testing and stretching exercises.

In addition to the effect of exercise on hemostasis, it is important to be familiar with the consequences of hemorrhages and thrombosis, as well as the effects of these complications on the exercise response.

The most common bleeding disorder is classic hemophilia, and about 20% persons with hemophilia have experienced exercise-related intra-articular bleeds. The most commonly affected joints are the knees and hips. In addition, it is common for persons with hemophilia to have intramuscular bleeds, typically in the back and lower extremity. Both intra-articular and intramuscular bleeds cause contractures that lead to loss of range of motion, balance, and proprioception skills.

In another common circumstance, a person has suffered a DVT and subsequently resumes physical activity. Typically, DVT alters venous return in the affected limb, and the muscles distal to the DVT have altered venous drainage. This increases venous pressure, reduces muscle pump effects, causes extravasation of fluid (edema), and is commonly painful or uncomfortable. This discomfort is frequently sufficient to limit exercise tolerance, as the client stops exercising due to pain.

EFFECTS OF EXERCISE TRAINING

The effects of exercise training on the blood hemostasis system are complex and not well understood. Regular exercise is protective against myocardial infarction and sudden cardiac death during physical activity, but this information does not imply that clotting is the precise mechanism guarding against an MI and sudden death during exercise.. Exercise training studies examining the balance of thrombosis and fibrinolysis have not provided consistent results, in part because different responses in various populations make it a little unclear how exercise training affects blood hemostasis. Markers of hemostasis appear to correlate with several risk factors for heart disease that are known to be altered with exercise training. As mentioned earlier, inflammation is an important aspect of atherosclerosis; and recent data suggest that C-reactive protein (a marker of inflammation) is increased in coronary artery disease. Exercise training often reduces blood pressure and may reduce C-reactive protein, so the compound effects of exercise training on all the factors that influence hemostasis are extremely complex. The effects of exercise training on the thrombotic and fibrinolytic cascades in persons with disorders of these cascades have not been well researched.

Persons with hemophilia benefit from regular exercise but consequently are at some risk of bleeding into joints and developing joint contractures. Neither aerobic nor strength training alters the underlying disorder of hemophilia, but non-weight-bearing aerobic exercise, as well as strength and flexibility training, can be of immense functional and psychological benefit.

A number of case reports exist regarding DVT in athletes. Deep venous thromboses are potentially life threatening because of their potential to break loose and create a pulmonary embolus. For this reason, continued training is contraindicated in an athlete who has developed a DVT. The duration of convalescence prior to resumption of sporting activities has not been objectively studied, but most sources advise an extended layoff of six months or more, until the thrombus has clearly resolved on vascular imaging studies.

MANAGEMENT AND MEDICATIONS

The management of bleeding disorders is determined by whether the problem predisposes to bleeding or to clotting and also by the cause of the disease. Anticoagulants are used much more commonly than natural and recombinant biologic factors because these latter medications are expensive. We will consider in turn persons with platelet disorders, those with coagulation factor disorders, and finally those with prosthetic heart valves.

In persons with low platelets caused by an overly rapid destruction of platelets (most often by the immune system), the goal of treatment is to decrease the rate of platelet destruction with immunosuppressive medicines, such as prednisone, and sometimes through splenectomy. Platelet transfusion works only for a very short while and is therefore limited to hospitalized persons. In persons with high platelets resulting from overproduction of platelets, the treatment is to decrease the rate of platelet formation, usually through chemotherapy.

In persons with coagulation factor deficiencies, a variety of medicines can be used to raise factor concentrations. Purified factor transfusions are available for some factor deficiencies. Mild von Willebrand disease can be treated to increase the level of von Willebrand factor. Unfortunately, as with platelet disorders, treatment for coagulation factor deficiencies is temporary. Nonetheless, regular home infusions of factor VIII, up to three times a week, are now commonly used in young persons with hemophilia to prevent hemarthroses and intramuscular bleeds. This approach is expensive but has proven to be less expensive than not replacing factor VIII.

Persons at risk for inappropriate clot formation because of mechanical heart valves, dilated hearts, or DVT require some form of anticoagulation. These inappropriate clots are highly dangerous because they can either grow in place and block blood flow or break off and lodge downstream in blood vessels critical to vital organs such as the brain or lungs. For this reason, such individuals are given anticoagulants, usually either warfarin or heparin derivatives. It is worth noting that these medications are commonly called "blood thinners," though they do not alter the viscosity of blood.

Aspirin is commonly used for prophylaxis against stroke and myocardial infarction. The antiplatelet effects of aspirin at rest are, however, acutely overwhelmed by the pro-thrombotic effects of exercise. The longer-term interaction of aspirin and exercise, including postexercise recovery, is not known.

Some have recommended the use of medications in athletes who have had a clotting disorder, such as DVT caused by protein C or protein S deficiencies or both. Persons with such deficiencies who are genetically heterozygous are usually not detected unless a thorough family history is known or until they present with a clot. Since such cases seem to be relatively rare, even though these deficiencies are common in the general population, prophylaxis with anticoagulants has not been recommended. Treatment for an acute case of DVT and prophylaxis against future episodes are commonly recommended for individuals who have had a clot. Persons with homozygous factor deficiencies should be treated with the appropriate factor replacement or anticoagulant (e.g., warfarin or heparin).

RECOMMENDATIONS FOR EXERCISE TESTING

When exercise testing a person with bleeding or clotting disorders, adhere to the following recommendations (also see table 33.2):

- Persons with hemophilia have historically been advised to avoid weight-bearing exercise; recently many sports physicians have been recommending all kinds of exercise except contact sports, coupled with factor VIII replacement prophylaxis. It is worth noting that these recommendations are based on case report experience, not randomized trials.

- Range of motion testing will help in managing flexibility exercises for persons with hemophilia.

- Strength training has been piloted in young persons with hemophilia and may be beneficial. No large-scale randomized strength training studies have been published; most rehabilitation experts support emphasis on core stability training.

- No high-resistance strength testing should be performed by persons with low platelet counts (risks intracranial bleed).

- Presence of an acute DVT is a contraindication to exercise; pilot walking training studies have been initiated within four weeks of diagnosis, but larger-scale randomized trials have not been completed.

RECOMMENDATIONS FOR EXERCISE PROGRAMMING

The goal of exercise training is to improve endurance, strength, and flexibility. Swimming or stationary cycling has historically been recommended for persons with hemophilia, but more and more sports physicians have been recommending all kinds of activity except for high-contact sports. Outdoor cycling is a non-weight-bearing activity in relation to joints but risks trauma, though data have shown that up to 55% of Germans with hemophilia commute by bicycle. About one in five German youths with hemophilia reports a history of hemarthrosis, even with factor VIII therapy. Flexibility exercises may help restore joint mobility and proprioception in persons with hemophilia who are affected with contractures. The optimal frequency and duration of training are not known, but most investigators have used common strength training paradigms (e.g., 30 min, three times a week, 8-15 repetitions maximum,

TABLE 33.2

Bleeding and Clotting Disorders: Exercise Testing

Methods	Measures	Endpoints	Comments
Strength Free weights Weight machines Elastic bands			Avoid high resistance in persons with platelets <50,000/mm^3 and bleeding disorders.
Flexibility Goniometry		Asymmetrical or limited ROM	Clients with hemophilia or von Willebrand disease may have decreased ROM, atrophy of shoulders, elbows, wrists, hips, knees, and ankles secondary to old hemarthroses.
Functional Gait analysis		Assess effect of hemarthrosis or surgery on walking ability	

emphasis on core strength and lower extremities). Adaptability is not known but is presumably normal (see table 33.3).

Exercise training should be curtailed in individuals who have had a recent DVT. The necessary duration of exercise restriction has not been thoroughly studied. Historically, resumption of training has been advised sometime after three to nine months of treatment, with optional follow-up vascular studies to demonstrate resolution of the thrombus. Recent studies have challenged that notion and suggest that the resumption of light walking as early as four weeks after diagnosis is beneficial. Theoretical rationale for early return to walking includes the notion that increased flow may help with recanalization or growth of collateral vessels (or both) and thus reduce muscular edema and symptoms in the long term. Larger studies continue to examine this theory, and until these studies are complete the exercise therapist is advised to proceed with caution in order to avoid embolic complications.

SPECIAL CONSIDERATIONS

Special considerations that should be taken into account in work with patients who have bleeding or clotting disorders (or both) include the following:

- Aspirin and other nonsteroidal anti-inflammatory drugs (e.g., ibuprofen) render platelets partially inactive, and their use is dangerous in individuals who have concomitant bleeding or platelet disorders.
- Persons who have any bleeding disorder or who are receiving medical anticoagulation are advised to avoid circumstances in which collisions are possible, for example contact sports (e.g., football, hockey, basketball).
- Persons with low platelet counts are advised to avoid high-resistance strength training.
- Low-resistance strength training and low-intensity endurance exercise are probably quite safe in the vast majority of persons with platelet, coagulation, or fibrinolysis disorders.
- Persons with hemophilia A are advised to use factor VIII therapy as part of their exercise program.
- Nonsteroidal anti-inflammatory drugs should not be used either as analgesics or as thrombosis prophylaxis.

TABLE 33.3

Bleeding and Clotting Disorders: Exercise Programming

Modes	Goals	Intensity/Frequency/Duration	Time to goal
Aerobic Program should follow ACSM guidelines for normal sedentary persons			
Strength Circuit training	Reverse secondary atrophy	■ Mix of high reps/low resistance and low reps/high resistance ■ Program should follow ACSM guidelines for normal sedentary persons	4-6 months
Flexibility Stretching	Normalize ROM in hemarthritic joints		

CASE STUDY

Deep Venous Thrombosis

A 20-year-old female track athlete presented to the emergency department after five to six days of swelling and tightness in the left thigh and calf. She had a history of a synovial sarcoma in the left hip 3 1/2 years prior to admission, which was surgically excised and treated with six months of radiation therapy. A CT scan three weeks prior to admission showed no recurrence of cancer. She did not use tobacco or oral contraceptives and did not recall a recent injury. She denied family history of bleeding or clotting disorders. Venous ultrasound revealed a DVT extending from the iliac vein to the popliteal vein.

S: "My leg is swollen."

O: Vitals

HR: 53 contractions/min
BP: 110/62 mmHg
Temp: 99.1° F (37.3° C)
Left leg/thigh: Warm, red
2+ nonpitting edema
Good posterior tibial pulses
Neurological: Intact in both lower extremities
Doppler ultrasound: DVT from iliac to popliteal vein in left leg

    A: 1. DVT in a track athlete
       2. History of synovial sarcoma with surgical excision, lymph node dissection, radiation therapy

P: 1. Lovenox and Coumadin
    2. Lovenox
    3. No running or other forms of heavy exertion.
    4. Advise on the bleeding risks of Coumadin therapy.

Follow-Up

Six days later, she had improved symptoms and no bleedin[g]. Coagulation studies were followed weekly to biweekly. Repe[at] Doppler ultrasound revealed that the DVT had resolved. T[he] plan:

1. Continue Coumadin.
2. Monitor coagulation status (via INR).
3. Evaluate for etiology of DVT prior to resuming sports. Consider the following:
   - Vascular injury secondary to treatment for cancer, factor V Lyden, protein C, protein [S], lupus, anticoagulant, etc.
   - After diagnosis and stable prophylaxis for recurrent DVT, gradually resume activity over next 6 months, progressing from nor[mal] weight-bearing activities (e.g., cycling, po[ol] exercise) to slow jogging.

PART VI

Orthopedic Diseases and Disabilities

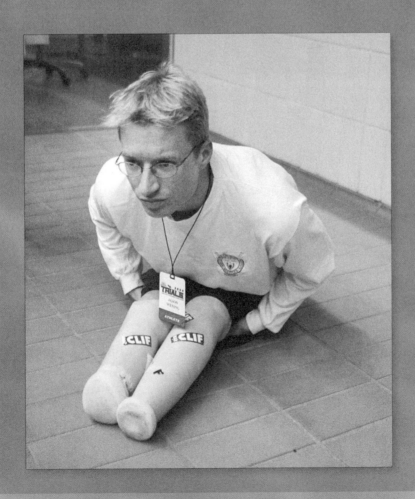

Arthritis

Marian A. Minor, PhD, PT ■ Donald R. Kay, MD

OVERVIEW OF THE PATHOPHYSIOLOGY

Arthritis is a chronic and often debilitating disease caused by inflammation of one or more joints, resulting in pain, swelling, stiffness, and limited movement. An estimated 46 million U.S. adults currently have at least one of the more than 100 different forms of arthritis (see table 34.1 for the most common rheumatologic diseases), including the two most common: osteoarthritis arthritis (OA) and rheumatoid arthritis (RA). Individuals with arthritis tend to be physically inactive and deconditioned, which tends to accelerate the progression of their disease and increase their risk for associated comorbidities. Arthritis is now the leading cause of disability in individuals older than 55 years; but depending on the duration and severity of an individual's disease, disability may develop at a much earlier age. To date, there is no known cure for arthritis, but tremendous advances have been made in treatment and control that include evidence-based guidelines for disease management and recommendations for exercise.

Osteoarthritis, which is also known as degenerative joint disease (DJD), is the oldest and most prevalent form of arthritis, affecting an estimated 27 million Americans. Osteoarthritis results from the deterioration or loss of cartilage in synovial joints, particularly in weight-bearing joints, followed by formation of bone spurs and subchondral cysts. Osteoarthritis is further characterized by its etiology; primary OA is associated with the normal wear and tear of aging whereas secondary OA is associated with injury, heredity, obesity, or other cause. Age is the strongest predictor of OA, in addition to obesity, injury, and heredity. Besides being the leading cause of disability in adults, OA accounts for 25% of visits to primary care physicians and half of all nonsteroidal anti-inflammatory drug prescriptions. Early diagnosis of OA improves treatment options and prognosis. In addition to taking prescribed medications for relieving symptoms, individuals with OA are encouraged to make lifestyle changes, manage stress and depression, avoid joint damage, and balance rest and activity to help control symptoms and improve prognosis.

Rheumatoid arthritis is a chronic and debilitating disease characterized by inflammation and swelling of the synovial membrane; the formation of pannus tissue within the joint; and the eventual deterioration of bone and cartilage, which causes swelling, pain, deformity, and loss of movement within the joint. Although the etiology of RA is not completely understood, RA is associated with higher than normal levels of the antibody rheumatoid factor (RF) and as such is referred to as an autoimmune disease. There is no cure for RA, but the disease can be well controlled for most individuals with the right combination of medications, exercise, joint protection techniques, and other self-management techniques.

TABLE 34.1

Most Common Rheumatologic Diseases With Joint Involvement

Diagnosis	Disease type	Commonly affected joints	Features related to exercise
Osteoarthritis	Local degeneration	Hands, spine, hips, knees	Joint pain, stiffness Osteophytes Cartilage degeneration
Rheumatoid arthritis	Inflammatory, systemic	Wrists, hands, knees, feet, cervical spine	Morning stiffness lasting >30 min Acute and chronic inflammation Chronic pain and loss of joint integrity
Ankylosing spondylitis Lupus Psoriatic arthritis	Inflammatory, systemic	Hands, knees, elbows, feet, spine	Arthralgia Fatigue
Gout Pseudogout	Crystal deposition	Great toe, ankles, knees, wrists	Acute joint inflammation Pain Tophi

EFFECTS ON THE EXERCISE RESPONSE

Inflammatory rheumatic diseases can affect cardiac and pulmonary function, as well as causing widespread vasculitis, which must be considered before individuals with systemic rheumatic disease are allowed to exercise. Vigorous exercise is contraindicated in the presence of acute joint inflammation (red, hot, swollen, painful) or uncontrolled systemic disease. However, the more common presentation of an individual with inflammatory rheumatic disease is subacute or chronic joint symptoms combined with possible sequelae of previous systemic inflammation. In the absence of acute flare-ups in people with systemic forms of arthritis (e.g., rheumatoid, lupus), the degenerative and inflammatory joint diseases have similar effects on exercise, whether musculoskeletal, biomechanical, or cardiovascular. There are few differences among the various systemic forms of arthritis in terms of effects on the response to moderate exercise. In persons having an acute flare-up of systemic illness, the exercise response can be quite blunted.

- Individuals with joint involvement tend to be less active and less fit than their unaffected peers.
- Resting energy expenditure may be elevated in people with systemic inflammatory disease, even when the disease clinically appears inactive or under control.
- Pain, stiffness, biomechanical inefficiency, and gait abnormalities can increase the metabolic cost of physical activity by as much as 50%.
- Joint range of motion may be restricted by stiffness, swelling, pain, bony changes, fibrosis, and ankylosis.
- Inability to perform rapid, repetitive movements may affect exercise performance in terms of walking speed and cycle revolutions per minute.
- Site and severity of joint involvement determine exercise mode for aerobic and strength tests.
- Deconditioned and poorly supported joints are at high risk for injury from high-intensity exercise or poorly controlled movement.

EFFECTS OF EXERCISE TRAINING

Individuals with either inflammatory or degenerative joint disease are able to participate in regular, moderate exercise to improve cardiovascular status, neuromuscular fitness, flexibility, and general health status. Improved aerobic capacity, endurance, strength, and flexibility are associated with improved function, decreased joint swelling and pain, increased social and physical activity in daily life, and reduced depression and anxiety. Disease-specific patterns of joint involvement should be considered during exercise prescription, monitoring, and follow-up assessments.

The most immediate benefit of conditioning exercise in this population may be to diminish effects of inactivity. Loss of flexibility, muscle atrophy, weakness, osteoporosis, elevated pain threshold, depression, and fatigue, which are problems common to both inflammatory and degenerative conditions, respond favorably to a low to moderate, gradually progressed exercise program. Improved pain and function are found consistently in well-controlled clinical trials. The potential for conditioning exercise to have a therapeutic effect on the disease process itself has yet to be determined.

MANAGEMENT AND MEDICATIONS

Joint protection, exercise, and education for self-management are essential components of comprehensive management. The goals are to decrease impairment, maintain or restore function, protect joint structures from further damage, and maintain healthful levels of physical activity. Ideally, care is coordinated in a multidisciplinary setting that offers preventive and rehabilitative care as well as medical management. To meet individual needs in an integrated program, the exercise component should incorporate joint protection and therapeutic exercise as needed. Health, safety, and successful exercise experiences for persons with joint disease can best be achieved by ongoing consultation with health care providers experienced in rheumatologic care and rehabilitation.

The major therapeutic goal in treatment of inflammatory rheumatologic disease is to control the destructive inflammatory process. Medications prescribed to achieve this goal range from aspirin and other nonsteroidal anti-inflammatory drugs (NSAIDs) to disease-modifying drugs (DMARDs) and biologic response modifiers (BRMs), which are designed to target specific immune processes believed to cause inflammation and tissue damage. Oral corticosteroids may be used when other drugs do not control inflammation. Combination therapy with two or more slower-acting DMARDs is commonly used to provide maximum inflammation and disease suppression. Drug therapy is usually continued indefinitely except when all signs of disease activity or progression disappear. In OA, NSAIDs or acetaminophen is prescribed to manage

symptoms of pain and stiffness. Local joint injections may be effective in both inflammatory and noninflammatory diseases to alleviate inflammation or provide pain relief within specific joints or at other specific sites. Intra-articular corticosteroid injections should be given no more often than every four to six months, because frequent injections can cause tissue destruction. The need to restrict activity following an injection is debated; however, vigorous weight-bearing activities are probably best avoided for at least one week.

Common Medications

Analgesics—acetaminophen

Nonsteroidal anti-inflammatory drugs, including these:

- Salicylates (both acetylated, such as aspirin, and nonacetylated)
- Traditional NSAIDs (e.g., ibuprofen, ketoprofen, and naproxen)
- COX-2 inhibitors

Corticosteroids (e.g., methylprednisolone and prednisone)

Disease-modifying antirheumatic drugs (DMARDs), including the following:

- Azathioprine
- Cyclosporine
- Hydroxychloroquine
- Gold sodium thiomalate
- Leflunomide
- Methotrexate
- Sulfasalazine

Biologic response modifiers, including the following:

- Tumor necrosis factor (TNF) blockers (etanercept [Enbrel], infliximab [Remicade], adalimumab [Humira])
- Anakinra (Kineret) (interleukin-1 inhibitor)
- Abatacept (Orencia) (T-cell costimulation modulator)
- Rituximab (Rituxan) (targets B-cells)

RECOMMENDATIONS FOR EXERCISE TESTING

In spite of the challenges presented by joint pain and dysfunction in arthritis, exercise testing is safe and should be performed when indicated. Submaximal and subjective symptom-limited treadmill tests requiring less than 3 mph (4.8 km/h) walking speed and common cycle ergometer protocols are well tolerated in this population. Early-onset muscle fatigue may reduce the prognostic value regarding cardiopulmonary disease; thus if someone is suspected of having coronary artery disease, other diagnostic tests are recommended. Standardized tests of functional muscle strength and endurance are most commonly used to establish a baseline for exercise prescription, including 1-repetition maximum tests if performed correctly. Range of motion measurements (goniometry) are useful for persons who have limited flexibility and need stretching programs. Gait analysis may be necessary for those who have severe disease, altered biomechanics, and a need for orthoses (see table 34.2).

Special considerations for exercise testing include the following:

- Pain or swelling may reduce performance.
- Vigorous, highly repetitive exercise should not be performed with unstable joints.
- Some arthritides involve cardiopulmonary systems, which may decrease performance.
- Spinal involvement may cause radiculopathy.
- Morning exercise should be avoided in clients with RA because of morning stiffness.

- Variable-speed protocols should be available. Cycle ergometers should have loose-fitting toe straps to accommodate genu valgum.

RECOMMENDATIONS FOR EXERCISE PROGRAMMING

The major impact of joint disease on exercise programming is the need for joint protection. Thus, the following recommendations apply:

- Select low-impact activities and functional exercises for strengthening when possible.
- Stair climbing, contact sports, and activities requiring prolonged one-legged stance or rapid stop-and-go actions should be avoided in individuals with symptomatic hip or knee involvement.
- Muscles should be conditioned before exercise intensity is increased.

TABLE 34.2

Complications in Exercise Programming

Osteoarthritis

Spinal stenosis	▪ Localized and radiating back pain; spinal cord compression; neurologic deficits; claudication-like symptoms; worsening with spinal extension and weight bearing
Spondolysis	▪ Localized and radiating back pain

Rheumatoid

Cervical spine subluxation	▪ Cervical instability; spinal cord compression; neurologic deficits (numbness, tingling weakness)
Foot disease	▪ Metatarsalgia; subluxation of metatarsal heads; midfoot pain/instability; calcaneal valgus; overpronation on weight bearing; gait deviation
Wrist/hand disease	▪ Joint pain/instability; loss of grip strength (Avoid power grip, ulnar deviation, joint stress at wrist.)

Systemic lupus erythematosus

Necrosis of femoral head	Hip pain (also associated with long-term corticosteroid use)

Ankylosing and psoriatic spondylitis

Enthesopathy	Acute and chronic plantar fasciitis; Achilles tendinitis, costochondritis

- Include flexibility and joint range of motion as key exercise components.
- Overstretching and hypermobility should be avoided.
- If pain or swelling appears or persists, reduce load on joint (reduce exercise duration or intensity; exercise in a pool, or cycle or row).
- Shoes and insoles should be selected for maximum shock attenuation during weight-bearing activities; and if hip or knee pain occurs with weight bearing activities, evaluate for rigid or semirigid arch supports for mechanical support or joint unloading.

Exercise programs should also be designed with an individualized progression of intensity and duration (see table 34.3):

- Use low intensity and duration during initial phase of programming.
- If necessary, exercise dose should be accumulated during several sessions throughout the day.
- Recommend alternate exercise modes and interval or cross-training methods to allow for changes in disease status.
- Set time goals, rather than distance goals, to encourage self-management to pace activity.
- Choose an appropriate exercise or fitness goal, and recommend that the person not exceed intensity, duration, and frequency guidelines for training.

Encourage exercise as a component of a fitness routine that is part of self-management:

- Stretching and warm-up should be performed daily, even on days when the disease flares and vigorous activity is undesirable.
- Use aerobic activities that incorporate alternative forms of exercise (weight bearing, partial

TABLE 34.3

Arthritis: Exercise Testing

Methods	Measures	Endpoints	Comments
Strength Repetition maximum (1, 8 or 12) Isometric knee extension Standardized functional measures	▪ Timed chair rise ▪ Timed up and go		
Endurance 6 min walk Aerobic capacity test	▪ HR ▪ RPE (6-20)		
Flexibility Goniometry	▪ Functional range of motion ▪ Assess symmetry		Helpful in preventing contractures and injury
Functional Balance Gait	▪ Berg Balance Test ▪ Short Physical Performance Battery ▪ Observe for symmetry; speed		

weight bearing, and nonweight bearing) to allow for migrating joint symptoms and changes in disease activity.

- Recommend that individuals learn a strengthening routine.
- Avoid activities that cause increased joint pain.
- Some postexercise soft tissue discomfort may be expected.

See table 34.4 for complications related to exercise programming for people with various forms of arthritis.

Evidence-Based Guidelines

American College of Rheumatology Subcommittee on Rheumatoid Arthritis Guidelines. Guidelines for the management of rheumatoid arthritis—2002 update. Arth Rheum. 2002;46(2):328-346.

Ottawa panel evidence-based clinical practice guidelines for therapeutic exercises and manual therapy in the management of osteoarthritis. Phys Ther. 2005;85(9):907-971.

Zhang W, Moskowitz RW, Nuki G, et al. OARSI recommendations for the management of hip and knee osteoarthritis, part II: OARSI evidence-based, expert consensus guidelines Osteoarth Cartil. 2008;16:137e162.

Suggested Web Sites

American College of Rheumatology. www.rheumatology.org

Arthritis Foundation. www.arthritis.org

Osteoarthritis Research Society International. www.oarsi.org

TABLE 34.4

Arthritis: Exercise Programming

Modes	Goals	Intensity/Frequency/ Duration	Time to goal
Aerobic Large muscle activities (walking, cycling, rowing, swimming, water aerobics, dance)	Increase $\dot{V}O_{2max}$, peak work, work rate, and endurance	■ 60-80% peak HR or 40-60% $\dot{V}O_{2max}$ ■ RPE 11-16/20 ■ 3-5 days/week ■ 5-10 min/session building to 30 min/session ■ Emphasize progression of duration over intensity	3-6 months
Strength Circuit training Free weights Weight machines Elastic bands Isometric exercises	■ Increase 1-, 8-, or 12 Repetition maximum ■ Increase repetitions and resistance ■ Increase peak torque, or power	■ 1 or more sets of 2-3 reps initially, building to 10 reps ■ 2-3 days/week training	3-6 months
Flexibility Stretching	■ Increase/maintain pain-free range of motion ■ Decrease stiffness	Before aerobic or strength activities	
Functional Addresses functional needs; simulates daily activity	■ Improve balance ■ Improve ADLs ■ Improve gait		

CASE STUDY

Arthritis

A 65-year-old woman was referred to a community-based cardiac rehabilitation program as follow-up to a recent cardiovascular workup ordered by her primary care physician. Although she was asymptomatic at the time, she was obese and had high blood pressure and elevated blood glucose. She was sedentary and ascribed her inability to exercise to her knee OA, which had been diagnosed about eight years earlier following an X ray that had been done after she had fallen on a hiking trip. Before the diagnosis she had walked regularly, played tennis, and gone backpacking with her family. Following the injury and diagnosis she had limited physical activity in order to avoid pain and in the belief that rest would protect her knees from further damage. Over the past several years she noticed increased knee stiffness in the morning and after prolonged periods of sitting. Pain had increased from mild discomfort after strenuous activity to moderate to severe pain with stair climbing, squatting, and arising from a chair. She knew she needed to exercise for health benefits, but wondered how she could do anything beneficial with such weak and painful knees.

S: "I am frustrated that I am so heavy and out of shape and now I'm worried about heart disease. I've just gone downhill these past few years. My knees are terrible and I hurt all over when I try to do any exercise at all."

O: Vitals

Height: 5 ft 3 in. (1.6 m)
Weight: 170 lb (77.3 kg)
BMI: 30.2 kg/m^2
HR: 80 contractions/min BP: 160/90 mmHg
Tender knees, bilaterally, with notable crepitus
Decreased range of motion bilateral: knee flexion, hip extension and internal rotation, ankle dorsiflexion
Strength deficits bilateral: knee flexion and extension, hip abduction, ankle dorsiflexion

X rays: Some narrowing of the medial joint space bilaterally; no osteophytes or bony deformities observed

Graded exercise test: $\dot{V}O_{2peak}$: 24.3 ml · kg^{-1} · min^{-1}

Sit-to-stand test: 31.3 s (age predicted: 15.9 s)
Sit and reach: 20.8 in. (52.8 cm) (normal for age)

A: 1. Painful knees limit physical activity (pain and fear avoidance behavior)
2. Low cardiovascular fitness
3. Lower extremity weakness and limited range of motion
4. Significant postexercise discomfort (joint and muscle)
5. Obese

P: 1. Pain self-management with the following:
- Heat/cold/topical agents
- Acetaminophen (OTC)
- Joint protection techniques (athletic shoes, shock-absorbing insoles)
- Limit standing or sitting with knees flexed (≤1 h)
- Pain evaluation (0-10 visual analog scale)
2. Improve lower extremity neuromuscular fitness and flexibility.
3. Prescribe an aerobic exercise program.
4. Provide nutritional counseling for weight loss.

Exercise Program Goals

1. Decrease knee pain
2. Improve neuromuscular fitness
3. Increase cardiovascular fitness
4. Teach self-management skills for self-directed exercise

Mode	Frequency	Duration	Intensity	Progression
Aerobic Walking on level; cycling, no resistance; water aerobics	3-4 days/week	■ Three 10-min sessions if needed for pain ■ Initial exercise- specific warm-up	Low to moderate	■ 30 min continuous, ■ 4-5 days/week as tolerated; low to moderate intensity as tolerated.
Neuromuscular Isometric quad exercise (flexion and extension); leg press; wall squats; step-ups	2 days/week	■ 3-5 exercises, ■ 5-10 reps as tolerated	8-12 reps max, to moderate fatigue	Increase speed and/ or resistance after 4-6 weeks; increase number of reps as tolerated.
Flexibility	Daily; use as warm-up and cool-down	Hip, knee, and ankle range of motion exercise for 5-10 min	Static, to point of tension (not pain); hold 10-30 s	Greater motion and flexibility will increase pain-free range of movement.

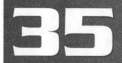

Lower Back Pain Syndrome

Maureen J. Simmonds, PhD, PT, MCSP ■ Tamar Derghazarian, PT

OVERVIEW OF THE PATHOPHYSIOLOGY

Lower back pain (LBP) is one of the most widely experienced health-related problems in the world. The lifetime prevalence of LBP is between 58% and 70% of the population in industrial countries, and the yearly prevalence rate is between 15% and 37%. Low back pain is defined as pain and discomfort, localized below the costal margin and above the inferior gluteal folds, with or without leg pain. Nonspecific low back pain, the most common form, is defined as low back pain not attributed to recognizable, known specific pathology (e.g., infection, tumor, osteoporosis, ankylosing spondylitis, fracture, inflammatory process, radicular syndrome, or cauda equina syndrome). Lower back pain may occur suddenly and be unclear in onset, and may result from major trauma or multiple episodes of microtrauma. It is characterized by variability in terms of its impact and recurrent episodes. Pain may stem from a variety of spinal structures, including muscle, joint, or disc (or more than one of these) and may have inflammatory, nociceptive, and neuropathic components. The consensus belief regarding the chronic neuropathophysiological state is that chronic pain is the pathology rather than the symptom. Regardless of whether pain is the primary pathology or the symptom of acute injury, the consequences of pain are important for the individual and society. The consequences of pain include the problem of recur-

rence, including severity and disability, loss of work, increased use of health care services, and reduced health-related quality of life.

The importance of low back pain in health care is widely recognized, and concerns have been raised about evidence of significant variation in the care provided for this condition, inappropriate and excessive use of diagnostic techniques and therapeutic interventions, and huge costs regarding its management. Evidence-based guidelines for LBP consistently suggest that individuals with LBP should be reassured and educated about pain and activity; they should also be given explicit information and advice that not only is it safe to remain active and to continue working with appropriate temporary modifications but that doing so improves long-term outcomes.

EFFECTS ON THE EXERCISE RESPONSE

In and of itself, LBP does not have an effect on the exercise response. However, exercise positions involving standing or sitting may exacerbate pain and prevent individuals from reaching their best effort or may contribute to a variation in effort. Therefore, people with LBP should be allowed to practice a variety of exercise modalities using different positions while noting any limiting factors. Limiting factors may be physical (e.g., pain or fatigue), psychological (e.g., fear of reinjury), or sociological (concern about who is watching them during exercise).

EFFECTS OF EXERCISE TRAINING

Individual beliefs about LBP will influence the approach to exercise. Some people will consider LBP minor or inconvenient, ignore it, and go about performing their usual exercise regimen. Others will stop their daily activities immediately and seek professional advice. If pain is aggravated by certain exercise activities, some persons with LBP may avoid these specific activities or may even avoid those activities that they anticipate will cause pain. Therefore, the ability to exercise may be greatly compromised by the degree to which people respond to LBP based on their beliefs.

Most episodes of LBP require no specific treatment and, if necessary and at most, minor modification of heavy physical activities for a couple of days. For significant acute LBP (less than three months in duration), in which pain and injury are somewhat related, it is reasonable to modify activity temporarily, potentially treat the pain with analgesics or a physical modality such as ice, and be guided by pain intensity and duration as normal exercise is resumed (after one or two days). However, the period of inactivity should be limited by time, not pain. An early return to normal exercise activities should be encouraged. Any advice to rest must be accompanied by advice about the exact time for exercise resumption.

For chronic or recurrent LBP (more than three months in duration), pain frequently persists but is not indicative of ongoing tissue injury and therefore cannot be used as a guide to adjust exercise management. Indeed, as noted earlier, in some cases pain is the pathology rather than the symptom. This does not imply that practitioners should focus on pain and pain behavior, but rather that they should address misconceptions or inappropriate fears about exercise or activity as a cause of further pain and reinjury. It is appropriate to motivate and guide the individual to resume activity. For chronic nonspecific LBP, exercise and activity are strongly recommended.

MANAGEMENT AND MEDICATIONS

Nonsteroidal anti-inflammatory medications (NSAIDs; e.g., aspirin, ibuprofen, indomethacin, nabumetone) or nonnarcotic analgesics (acetaminophen, tramadol), and sometimes both, are commonly used by individuals with LBP. These medications should have no effect on the individual's exercise capacity. Muscle relaxants and antidepressants are sometimes used and may cause drowsiness. Opiates and oral steroids are occasionally used for short-term management (one to three weeks) of acute back pain. Such short-term use of oral steroids should have no adverse effect on exercise capacity.

RECOMMENDATIONS FOR EXERCISE TESTING

Individuals with LBP should be able to perform all exercise tests (i.e., aerobic, anaerobic, endurance, strength, flexibility, coordination, and functional) recommended by the American College of Sports Medicine (ACSM), although some tests may not be necessary. Individuals with LBP may be limited in exercise test performance by an actual or anticipated increase in pain. Therefore, allowing practice time on different test modalities in order to select the best modality is essential, and one should identify the limiting factor (i.e., pain or fatigue) so that the data can be interpreted accurately. Symptom-limited maximal exercise tests using a treadmill, upper extremity ergometer, or bicycle ergometer can be used, although results may differ. The preferred modality for assessing aerobic fitness levels in patients with chronic LBP is the treadmill. Treadmill testing yields the highest peak oxygen consumption compared with other tests and comes closest to measuring maximal oxygen consumption (see table 35.1).

RECOMMENDATIONS FOR EXERCISE PROGRAMMING

Little is known about the level of aerobic fitness in patients with chronic LBP, although many rehabilitation programs emphasize aerobic exercise as an important part of their therapy. Other rehabilitation programs focus on muscle strength, muscle coordination, or flexibility, especially of core trunk muscles, or some combination of these, as key components of rehabilitation. A number of studies and systematic reviews have shown that exercise is significantly more effective than rest for LBP. There is also strong evidence that no one specific exercise regimen is superior. Exercise guidelines for individuals with LBP are therefore similar to the guidelines established by ACSM for apparently healthy populations, with appropriate adjustments.

The goals for exercise programming in individuals with LBP are to improve health and well-being,

TABLE 35.1

Lower Back Pain Syndrome: Exercise Testing

Methods	Measures	Endpoints	Comments
Aerobic Maximal and submaximal testing unnecessary			Testing may be warranted if risk factors/symptoms of CAD are present.
Strength Isometric trunk testing			Measure isometric strength in multiple positions to find true peak torque.
Flexibility Straight leg stretch Inclinometry	Angle to elicit pain or radiating symptoms		

increase exercise tolerance, and prevent debilitation caused by inactivity. Exercise modalities that minimize stress to the lower back should be started during the first two weeks of acute LBP. During the acute stage of severe LBP only, exercises for hip and back muscles could be delayed for at least two weeks and the intensity should be low, with gradual increases in intensity and duration (see table 35.2). For those with chronic LBP, exercise intensity and

duration should also be graded, gradual in progression, and time rather than pain contingent. This is particularly important in individuals who are debilitated or fearful of reinjury. Finally, given that adherence to any exercise or activity regimen is essential if benefits are to accrue, and given that no one exercise regimen is superior, it is essential that exercise or activity prescriptions consider client preference.

TABLE 35.2

Lower Back Pain Syndrome: Exercise Programming

Modes	Goals	Intensity/Frequency/Duration	Time to goal
Strength Resistance: abdominal strengthening Back extensions	■ Increase abdominal strength ■ Increase lumbar extensor strength	■ Under age 50: 10-15 reps/day ■ Over age 50: 8-12 reps/day ≥2 days/week	2-4 weeks
Flexibility Any standard flexibility exercise that does not increase LBP	Increase trunk and hip flexor and extensor ROM	2 min/muscle group; hold position for 3 reps, 10 s/stretch	
Functional 5 min walk 1 min chair sit to stand	Increase/maintain ADLs	■ Brisk walk, 3-5 days/week ■ Chair sit and stand, 2-3 days/week	2-4 weeks

Evidence-Based Guidelines

Airaksinen O, Brox JI, et al. European guidelines for the management of chronic nonspecific low back pain. Eur Spine J. 2006;15 suppl 2:S192-300.

Chou R, Qaseem A, Snow V, et al. Diagnosis and treatment of low back pain: A joint clinical practice guideline from the American College of Physicians and the American Pain Society. Ann Int Med. 2007;147(7):478-491.

Suggested Web Sites

American Academy of Spine Physicians. www.spine-physicians.org

American Association of Neurological Surgeons. www.aans.org

Congress of Neurological Surgeons. www.neurosurgeon.org

North American Spine Society. www.spine.org

CASE STUDY

Lower Back Pain

A 32-year-old male presented with a two-year history of frequent episodic LBP. The onset of the recent symptoms occurred two weeks prior to examination. Over the two years, he saw several different health care providers (family physician, orthopedic surgeon, physical therapist, chiropractor, and massage therapist). He was treated with home exercise, passive stretching, supervised exercise, manipulations, medications (NSAIDs and muscle relaxants), and pool therapy. None of these treatments provided more than temporary symptomatic relief. X rays, magnetic resonance imaging (MRI), and CT scans all yielded negative findings.

S: *"I have pain in my left leg, and I'm numb below the knee."*

O: Vitals

Adult male, in no acute distress

Spine: Normal lordosis, low lumbar tenderness, pain with percussion

Neurological: Reflexes normal, motor strength normal

Straight leg raise (SLR): Limited on the symptomatic side by back pain

Back flexion: Caused symptoms to move further down his leg

Back extension: Relieved the leg symptoms

Gait: Antalgic (i.e., decreased time of weight bearing on left leg)

Heel and toe walking: Done with some difficulty

Inclinometer: Greatly decreased lumbar inclination angle

Isokinetic lumbar spine function:

Strength: 100 foot-pounds (ft-lb) (13.83 kg-m) (65% of predicted)

ROM: 39° (normal: 72°)

A: 1. Low back pain
   2. Osteoarthritis of the lumbar spine

P: 1. Prescribe a strengthening/retraining program.
   2. Instruct on postural training exercises.
   3. Learn self-management.

Exercise Program Goals

1. Reduced pain
2. Increased strength and flexibility
3. Improved posture/gait
4. Ability to self-manage future episodes

Follow-Up

Following eight weeks of rehabilitation, the client's symptoms were completely abolished. His lumbar strength had increased to 211 ft-lb (29.18 kg-m) with a ROM of 7°. He also became well educated in self-treatment during flare-ups of LBP.

Mode	Frequency	Duration	Intensity	Progression
Aerobic				
Strength (multifidi, erector spinae, latissimus dorsi, rhomboids)	Daily	1-2 sets of 10-20 reps	Antigravity	Increase to 2 sets of 10-20 reps, as tolerated
Flexibility	Daily			Incorporated into strength and postural exercises
Neuromuscular	Daily	1-2 sets of 10-20 reps		
Warm-up and cool-down				

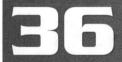

Osteoporosis

Susan S. Smith, PT, PhD, CCD ■ Che-Hsiang Elizabeth Wang, PT, MS
Susan A. Bloomfield, PhD, FACSM

OVERVIEW OF THE PATHOPHYSIOLOGY

Bone-forming cells decline in activity after the age of 35 years; therefore, all humans incur a small loss of bone mass every year. This phenomenon has been observed in multiple races, geographical locations, and historical periods. Dietary habits and physical activity patterns over the life span may alter the timing or rate of bone loss, but nearly all elderly men and women in industrialized countries have some degree of low bone mass, or osteopenia. Low bone mass is of concern because bone strength and resistance to fracture, key functional attributes of bone, are determined in large part by bone mass. Once low bone mass becomes severe enough to result in fractures from minimal trauma, such as a fall from standing height, it is clinically defined as osteoporosis. Bone status for most individuals over the age of 60 years is somewhere on the continuum from benign, age-related low bone mass to bone loss severe enough to make fracture imminent.

Osteoporosis is a condition in which the bones become weak and can break from a minor fall or, in serious cases, from a simple action such as a sneeze. The National Institutes of Health (NIH) Consensus Development Panel on Osteoporosis defines osteoporosis as "a skeletal disorder characterized by compromised bone strength predisposing to an increased risk of fracture. Bone strength reflects the integration of main features: bone density and bone quality." The standards of the World Health Organization (WHO) for diagnosing low bone mass and osteoporosis are based on bone mineral density (BMD) levels at the hip and spine as measured by central dual-energy X-ray absorptiometry (DXA). The WHO standards are widely adopted to establish the diagnosis, assist in determining fracture risk, and help the individual and the health care provider decide whether treatment is warranted. Osteopenia is defined as BMD between 1.0 and 2.5 standard deviations below that of a "young normal" adult value (T-score = –1.0 and –2.5 SD). Osteoporosis is defined as BMD 2.5 standard deviations below the "young normal" adult value (T-score at or below –2.5 SD).

An estimated 34 million Americans have low bone mass, and 10 million more have osteoporosis. Women over the age of 50 have a 50% likelihood of having an osteoporotic fracture in their lifetime, whereas men of equivalent age have a 25% likelihood. Women tend to begin losing bone earlier in life and may experience a three- to five-year acceleration of bone loss after menopause because the effects of estrogen withdrawal are temporarily superimposed on age-related loss. Women can lose up to 20% of their bone mass in the five to seven years after menopause. This fact, in addition to a lower peak bone mass in young adulthood, largely explains the greater incidence of osteoporotic fractures in women as compared to men.

Primary osteoporosis can occur in both genders at all ages but often follows menopause in women aged 50 to 75 years. Estrogen deficiency at menopause results in altered bone resorption and bone formation such that the rate of bone resorption exceeds the rate of bone formation. Primary osteoporosis occurs later in life in men, typically aged 70 years and older. Secondary osteoporosis can result from various medications (e.g., chronic glucocorticoid therapy), certain diseases (e.g., cystic fibrosis, organ transplant), or other conditions (e.g., athletic amenorrhea [female athletic triad]).

The most commonly cited risk factors for osteoporosis include heredity, estrogen deficiency, and exogenous factors affecting bone metabolism. The loss of lean body mass over several decades of chronic physical inactivity may be a strong contributor to the development of osteoporosis. Individuals with low muscle mass and strength are more likely than others to have lower bone mass. A detailed list of risk factors for osteoporosis includes the following:

- Gender (females have a higher incidence)
- Older age
- Certain races and ethnicities: Caucasian, Asian, Hispanic/Latino (although African Americans are also at risk)
- Family history of osteoporosis or fractures
- Low body mass index (BMI), thinness, low body weight for height (in general, individuals that weigh less than 127 lb [58 kg] are at an increased risk)
- Low estrogen levels in women (risk factor includes menopausal women)
- History of fractures
- Amenorrhea (missed periods)
- Low sex hormones, including low testosterone and estrogen in men
- Inadequate physical activity and immobilization
- Smoking
- Alcohol consumption (three or more drinks per day)
- Low dietary calcium intake
- Vitamin D insufficiency
- Excessive intake of protein, sodium, caffeine, and vitamin A
- Certain medications causing bone loss (e.g., glucocorticoids, anticonvulsants, antacids containing aluminum, depo-medroxyprogesterone)
- Certain diseases and conditions (e.g., anorexia, bulimia, asthma, cystic fibrosis, celiac disease, rheumatoid arthritis)
- Loss of height (may suggest spinal fracture)

Fractures resulting from osteoporosis are most likely at the hip, spine, and wrist, but any bone can be affected. In 2005, the cost associated with osteoporosis-related fractures was estimated at $19 billion; and by 2025, the costs are expected to rise to approximately $25.3 billion. Compression or wedge fractures of the vertebrae are common in older individuals with osteoporosis. Several may accumulate without obvious symptoms before they are detected, often as a chance finding with a chest radiograph performed for other purposes. A significant functional limitation imposed by multiple vertebral fractures is the severe increased thoracic kyphosis that can result. In extreme cases, this spinal deformity can impede normal ventilatory function by altering respiratory muscle function and decreasing vital capacity. Kyphosis can produce a shift in the center of gravity as well, increasing the risk of falls. Evidence also suggests that depression, reduced quality of life, and increased mortality are associated with an osteoporosis-related severe kyphotic deformity. About one-third of individuals with vertebral fractures experience significant back pain in the acute phase of recovery. Weakness of the back extensor muscles may be associated with this kyphotic deformity.

The most serious and potentially life-threatening osteoporosis-related fractures are those of the hip and femoral neck. Approximately 24% of individuals with hip fractures over the age of 50 will die within the first year after the fracture, while others may lose functional ambulatory ability and require nursing home care. Six months after a hip fracture, only 15% of individuals will be able to walk unaided. An average American woman's risk of hip fracture is equivalent to her combined risk of developing breast, uterine, and ovarian cancer.

Although risk factors for falls are numerous, the WHO absolute fracture risk assessment algorithm for predicting the probability of a major osteoporotic fracture narrows to the following risk factors:

- Current age
- Gender
- Personal history of a fragility (low trauma) fracture

- Femoral neck BMD
- Low BMI (kg/m²)
- Use of oral glucocorticoid therapy
- Secondary osteoporosis (e.g., rheumatoid arthritis)
- Parental history of hip fracture
- Current smoking
- Alcohol intake of three or more drinks per day

This fracture prediction model was calibrated to U.S. population parameters. The WHO Fracture Risk Assessment Tool (FRAXTM), available online, can be used to determine the 10-year probability of a major osteoporotic fracture (hip, cervical spine, forearm, or proximal humerus) using the BMD T-score at the femoral neck, age, and the number of clinical risk factors (CRFs) from the preceding list. In addition, in the absence of DXA-determined BMD results, the 10-year risk can be estimated using BMI, age, and the number of CRFs. Identifying and reducing the modifiable risks factors and other risk factors for falls (e.g., checking and correcting vision and hearing, evaluating neurological problems and medications that may affect balance, and modifying the environment to improve safety) may be indicated. Wearing hip protectors is advised for those individuals who are at especially high risk.

EFFECTS ON
THE EXERCISE RESPONSE

The primary consideration relative to people with osteoporosis is the degree of orthopedic limitation imposed by bony fractures, if they have occurred, or by coexisting conditions such as osteoarthritis. Some individuals have limited locomotor abilities after a hip fracture, which directly affects the ability to perform exercise testing. The primary clinical goals include appropriate physical therapy to maximize balance, muscle strength, and mobility and to prevent further falls. Physician-approved exercise testing can be performed as usual for individuals with diagnosed vertebral fractures unless severe kyphosis is present. For those whose only complication is low bone mass, standardized exercise testing with precautions to minimize the risk of falls during the test is appropriate. Fear of falling often leads to reduced physical activity in the elderly, which exacerbates their risk of developing coronary artery disease (CAD). Therefore, electrocardiographic monitoring for ischemic responses to exercise is always advised.

EFFECTS
OF EXERCISE TRAINING

Because people with osteoporosis are more likely to be deconditioned than average, a low-intensity exercise training program is recommended initially. In addition, orthopedic limitations may slow progress or mandate the use of additional supports during walking. There is no evidence in the literature to support the claim that osteoporosis, in and of itself, should alter the usual cardiovascular and skeletal muscle responses and adaptations with chronic exercise training. One exception that could be a limiting factor during exercise training is the mechanical limitations imposed on respiratory muscle function in individuals with severe thoracic kyphosis. Regular aerobic, weight-bearing, and resistance exercise training has been shown to have a positive effect on the BMD of the spine in postmenopausal women. Walking is also effective for hip BMD. Therefore, long-term commitment to these forms of exercises is essential for people with low bone mass and osteoporosis.

There is no support for the concept that exercise training can provide an effective alternative to medication and dietary supplements in preventing bone loss in the early menopausal years. Nonetheless, evidence does suggest that regular exercise training can significantly slow the age-related decline in bone mass and thereby delay the time point at which low bone mass progresses to clinically significant osteoporosis. However, increasing BMD, and therefore bone strength, is only part of the equation in reducing fragility fractures. What exercise training provides that dietary supplements or medications cannot, are improvements in muscle strength, mobility, and balance—all of which have been shown to improve quality of life and to minimize the risk of falling, thereby reducing the risk of fractures.

MANAGEMENT
AND MEDICATIONS

Although there is no cure for low bone mass and osteoporosis, successful management is possible. The National Osteoporosis Foundation suggests the following five steps that together optimize bone health and help prevent osteoporosis:

1. Obtaining the recommended, age-related amounts of calcium and vitamin D per day
2. Engaging in regular weight-bearing and muscle strengthening exercise training
3. Avoiding tobacco use and excessive alcohol intake
4. Becoming educated about bone health
5. Having a bone density examination and taking medication when recommended

Once osteoporosis has been diagnosed, with confirmation of low BMD or fractures incurred with little or no trauma, the primary form of treatment is the use of medications to slow bone resorption or to increase bone formation. Should significant spinal deformities develop, bracing of the torso may be recommended to prevent worsening of the deformity, along with appropriate physical therapy to symptomatically treat back pain and to improve trunk muscle strength. In addition, hip, knee extensor, and ankle muscle strength may be low, along with poor static and dynamic standing balance, requiring focused exercise or physical therapy regimens.

Medications are used for prevention, treatment, or both. Some of these medications have side effects such as gastrointestinal irritation. According to the National Osteoporosis Foundation, common medications prescribed to individuals with osteoporosis include the following:

Antiresorptive Medications: Bisphosphonates

Bisphosphonates include alendronate and alendronate plus vitamin D3 (brand names Fosamax and Fosamax plus D). Alendronate is Food and Drug Administration (FDA) approved for the prevention and treatment of osteoporosis in postmenopausal women and for the treatment of osteoporosis in men. Alendronate is also approved for the treatment of glucocorticoid-induced osteoporosis in men and women. Risedronate (brand name Actonel) is also approved by the FDA for the prevention and treatment of postmenopausal osteoporosis and treatment of osteoporosis in men. Ibandronate (brand name Boniva) is approved for the prevention and treatment of osteoporosis in postmenopausal women. Ibandronate can be taken in a once-a-month dose. Zoledronic acid (brand name Reclast) is approved for treatment of osteoporosis in postmenopausal women.

Other Antiresorptive Medications

Selective estrogen receptor modulators (SERMs) or estrogen agonists/antagonists are other antiresorptive medications. Raloxifene (brand name Evista) is approved by the FDA for the prevention and treatment of osteoporosis in postmenopausal women. Raloxifene is advertised as having few to none of the undesirable side effects of hormone replacement therapy (e.g., there is no increased risk of uterine cancer). Calcitonin (brand names Fortical and Miacalcin) is FDA approved for the treatment of osteoporosis in women who are at least five years past menopause, and may have an analgesic effect in relieving pain associated with bone fractures. Calcitonin must be administered via subcutaneous injection or as a nasal spray. Hormone replacement therapy was formerly the most commonly prescribed medical regimen for bone loss in postmenopausal women. Estrogen (multiple brand names available) therapy (ET) and estrogen with progesterone hormone therapy (HT) are approved for the prevention of osteoporosis in postmenopausal women. However, according to the FDA, postmenopausal women should consider other medications before taking ET or HT to prevent osteoporosis because of risks associated with these forms of therapy.

Bone Forming (Anabolic) Medications

Teriparatide (brand name Forteo) is a form of parathyroid hormone approved for a limited time only for the treatment of postmenopausal women and in men with very low BMD who are at a high risk for fracture.

RECOMMENDATIONS FOR EXERCISE TESTING

The exercise testing protocols typically used with older individuals at risk for CAD are appropriate for individuals with diagnosed osteoporosis. In the presence of comorbidities (e.g., osteoarthritis with joint pain), testing must be modified to accommodate these additional limitations. For those with severe kyphosis, treadmill exercise is likely to be unsafe if forward vision is limited or if the neck is affected. In addition, a significant shift in the center of gravity may occur that could affect balance. Stationary bicycle ergometry, provided that it results in no compression of the anterior aspect of the spine, is a safer alternative to treadmill testing.

Supplementary testing in addition to standardized graded exercise testing could be extremely beneficial for this population (see table 36.1). Assessment of muscle strength to identify particularly weak muscle groups (especially trunk and lower extremity musculature) would also assist in exercise prescription. Neuromuscular function, such as balance, should be assessed by standardized tests like the Berg Balance Scale or timed single-leg stance test or both. Functional tests such as functional reach , timed up and go , and 3 s chair stand test are appropriate to evaluate function as well as

TABLE 36.1

Osteoporosis: Exercise Testing

Methods	Measures	Endpoints*	Comments
Aerobic			
Cycle (ramp protocol 5-20 W/min; staged protocol 25-50 W/3 min stage) Treadmill (1-2 METs/stage)	▪ 12-lead ECG, HR	▪ Serious dysrhythmias ▪ >2 mm ST-segment depression or elevation ▪ Moderate to severe angina ▪ T-wave inversion with significant ST change	▪ Most clients will be at a high risk for CAD.
	▪ BP	▪ SBP >250 mmHg or DBP >100 mmHg ▪ Failure of SBP to rise with increases in exercise intensity	▪ Helpful to check for hyper- or hypotensive response.
	▪ RPE (6-20)	▪ Volitional fatigue	▪ Useful for clients who have difficulty with HR measurements.
	▪ METs		▪ Helpful in determining exercise intensity.
Strength			
Weight machines Free weights	1- to 10RM	▪ Pain ▪ Fatigue	▪ Helpful in determining resistance training intensity. ▪ Decline in muscle strength common in persons with declining bone mass and osteoporosis.
Handheld dynamometer			▪ Consider using a "make test" versus a "break test" with a handheld dynamometer with persons with low bone mass and osteoporosis.**
Neuromuscular			
Gait analysis Balance	▪ Observation or instrumentation ▪ Time ▪ Force plate ▪ Balance scales (e.g., Berg)	▪ Pain ▪ Fatigue	▪ Especially useful for symptomatic clients and those at risk for falls.

Methods	Measures	Endpoints*	Comments
Functional			
6 min walk	■ Distance	■ Pain	
Tandem gait speed	■ Speed	■ Fatigue	
Step test	■ Count		
Timed chair sit to stand test	■ Try without use of arms		■ Sit-to-stand test provides easy practical evaluation of lower extremity strength. If arms are required for standing, this indicates weak hip/knee extensors and increased fall risk.
ADL/functional performance tests			
Posture	■ Flexicurve to determine the index of kyphosis (IK)		■ Useful for documenting kyphotic curve.
Quality of life scales			■ Useful in goal setting.

*Measurements of particular significance; do not always indicate test termination.

**In break tests, the examiner pushes against the client's limb until the client's maximal muscular effort is overcome and the joint being tested gives way. In make tests, the examiner holds a dynamometer stationary while the subject exerts a maximal force against it.

fall risk. The 30 s chair stand test, in particular, is a quick and simple test to reliably identify weakness of lower extremities and fall risk. Fewer than eight chair-stands in 30 s indicates an elevated risk of falls. A thorough quantitative and qualitative assessment of kinematic parameters of gait biomechanics may also be appropriate in some cases. In addition, the index of kyphosis (IK) can be determined using a flexicurve; the ability to perform activities of daily living (ADLs) can be determined using various tests or simulations; and quality of life using condition-specific measures should be determined to assist in goal setting and tracking progress.

RECOMMENDATIONS FOR EXERCISE PROGRAMMING

Currently, no definitive exercise training studies exist; however, current knowledge indicates that one should emphasize a well-balanced exercise training program focusing on both aerobic and strength activities for individuals with low bone mass and osteoporosis. In those with osteoporosis, the individual's physician, ideally in consultation with a physical therapist experienced with the limitations of persons with osteoporosis, should make the initial decision regarding the safety of a proposed exercise training program. There is little information in the literature regarding the safety of

various forms of exercise training for individuals with osteoporosis except for the recommendation that they should avoid exercises involving trunk flexion.

Evidence suggests that appropriate exercises and activities, specific to the individual, are required to assist in maintaining and preventing bone loss. In general, aerobic weight-bearing activity (four sessions a week) and resistance training (two or three sessions a week) are recommended, with the more vigorous, impact-oriented activities reserved for those not yet classified as severely osteoporotic. Specific exercises focusing on improving balance and modification of ADLs can also be helpful in individual cases. Improving muscle strength helps to conserve bone mass and improve dynamic balance. Best results are obtained when exercisers can progress to using relatively high intensities (>75% of 10-repetition maximum) and fewer repetitions. Adaptations in bone are site specific; therefore, any program should include exercise for upper and lower body and trunk muscles, particularly the extensors. Floor calisthenics and some lifting activities need to be modified to avoid forward flexion and twisting of the spine, especially in combination with stooping. Regular performance of flexion exercises such as crunches and sit-ups increases the risk of causing vertebral fractures in people with established osteoporosis. If an individual presents with multiple vertebral fractures, severe low bone mass, or back pain, participation in weight-bearing exercise training should be limited; and shifting to swimming, walking in the water, water aerobic programs, or chair exercises should be considered. Although these non-weight-bearing activities are not as optimal in affecting bone as strength training and weight-bearing activities, these programs are likely to improve muscle strength and balance and contribute to a lowered risk of CAD. See table 36.2 for more information.

SPECIAL CONSIDERATIONS

Individuals with osteoporosis have a heightened degree of fear and anxiety about falling. Careful attention must be made to ensure that the exercise environment is free of hazards such as loose floor tiles or mats and exercise equipment strewn over the floor. Wall railings in exercise areas would be helpful for exercises performed during standing, and side rails are helpful on treadmills. Close

TABLE 36.2

Osteoporosis: Exercise Programming

Modes	Goals	Intensity/Frequency/ Duration	Time to goal
Aerobic Large muscle activities (depending on BMD and client factors: walking, cycling, elliptical, swimming, water walking, running, sports)	■ Improve/maintain work capacity ■ Maintain bone mass	■ 40-70% peak HR, METs ■ 3-5 days/week ■ 30-60 min/session	■ 2-6 months ■ 9-24 months to see effect on BMD
Strength Dumbbells Weight machines Cuff weights Floor calisthenics Vibration machines	■ Improve strength of trunk, upper and lower extremities; emphasis on hip musculature (especially hip extensors), knee extensors, back extensors, lower abdominal muscles, and ankle dorsiflexors ■ Improve posture; emphasis on postural muscle strength ■ Maintain bone mass ■ Decrease fall risk	■ 75% of 1RM, 8-12 reps ■ 2 sets of 8-10 reps ■ 2-3 days/week for 20-40 min	≥6 months to reach maximum
Flexibility Stretching Chair exercises	Increase/maintain ROM, especially hip, knee, and pectoral muscles	5-7 days/week with prolonged holding (30 s as tolerated)	
Functional Activity-specific exercises Brisk walking Chair sit to stand Balancing exercises	■ Increase/maintain ADLs ■ Improve balance ■ Decrease fall risk	■ 3-5 days/week ■ 2-3 days/week	2-6 weeks

monitoring by staff, particularly when balance training is used (e.g., heel-to-toe walks, balancing on a single foot), should help prevent unintended injuries during exercise sessions. As low bone mass and osteoporosis are long-term chronic conditions, an ongoing, regular home or gym program should be encouraged, with periodic follow-up to correct exercise performance, vary the program, progress the intensity, and enhance compliance.

Evidence-Based Guidelines

Boonen S, Body J, Boutsen Y, et al. Evidence-based guidelines for the treatment of postmenopausal osteoporosis: A consensus document of the Belgian Bone Club. Osteoporos Int. 2005;16(3):239-254.

Brown JP, Josse RG, Scientific Advisory Council of the Osteoporosis Society of Canada. 2002 clinical practice guidelines for the diagnosis and management of osteoporosis in Canada. CMAJ. 2002 Nov 12;167(10 suppl):S1-34.

North American Menopause Society. Management of postmenopausal osteoporosis: Position statement of the North American Menopause Society. Menopause. 2002 Mar-Apr;9(2):84-101.

Suggested Web Sites

International Osteoporosis Foundation. www.iofbone-health.org

International Society for Clinical Densitometry. www.iscd.org

National Osteoporosis Foundation. www.nof.org

CASE STUDY

Osteoporosis

The client was an 83-year-old woman, a retired teacher with a history of back, hip, leg, and bilateral foot pain and numbness that had increased over the preceding three years. She also had a history of frequent falling. Pain was rated 6/10 and was aggravated with standing and walking; with rest the pain eased, but she experienced more stiffness. She lived alone in a three-story house. She walked with a single-point cane. She was unable to drive but performed most ADLs independently and volunteered weekly at the local arboretum. She was unable to lie prone or supine without two pillows. The client reported the following fracture history: right elbow (1952), right heel (1976); right hip with open reduction and internal fixation (1983). She had been diagnosed with osteoporosis, with DXA −3.1 SD below the young adult T-score. Concomitant medical problems included osteoarthritis in multiple joints (responsible for the pain), mixed urinary incontinence, carpal tunnel syndrome, difficulty sleeping, hypertension, and history of cervical cancer with hysterectomy.

S: Client complained of pain, loss of mobility, generalized weakness, falling, and difficulty with walking and ADLs. She reported fear of loss of independence. Her goals were to relieve pain; improve activity level, strength, balance, posture, and bone health; and continue living independently in her own home.

O: Vitals

Resting HR: 62 contractions/min
Sitting BP: 130/70 mmHg
Inspiratory force: 16.7 cm H_2O
Posture (Observation): Thoracolumbar scoliosis, increased thoracic kyphosis; forward head; rounded shoulders

Anthropometrics

Height: 5 ft 2 in. (157.5 cm)
Arm span: 5 ft 7 in. (171.2 cm)
Arm span − height: 5 in. (12.7 cm)
Weight: 144 lb (65.4 kg)
BMI: 26.2 kg/m²
Index of kyphosis (IK): 20.5
Dominance: Right

A: Problems:
1. Back/right hip/bilateral foot pain
2. Increased kyphotic posture
3. Decreased stability/balance
4. Decreased leg and trunk strength
5. Decreased flexibility
6. Difficulty with ADLs
7. Low bone mineral density
8. General deconditioning
9. Falling

Potential factors limiting progress

1. Pain, especially with walking
2. Compliance
3. Concomitant medical problems
4. Stamina

Goals (expected 1-year outcomes with estimated 60% compliance with follow-up at 3 and then 6-month intervals)

1. Reduce pain to 3/10
2. Decrease IK
3. Stability of 5 s in single-leg stance (eyes open)

(continued)

Muscle Performance and Strength (Dynamometers)			
	Left	Right	Units
Trunk extensors		38.5	N-m
Hip flexors	16.6	8.1	
Hip extensors	13.8	8.9	
Hip abductors	14.3	5.4	
Hip adductors	26.9	14.8	
Hip internal rotators	17.7	10.2	
Hip external rotators	4.7	2.3	
Knee extensors	35.6	29.4	
Knee flexors	23.0	16.6	
Ankle dorsiflexors	2.0	1.6	
Ankle plantarflexors	2	1	reps
Handgrip		21	kg
Flexibility/Muscle length			
Hip flexors	−10 to neutral	−13 to neutral	degrees
Rectus femoris	89/120	91/120	
Hamstrings	30/80	35/80	
Gastrocnemius	5/20	0/20	
Pectoralis minor shortness	0.5	0.4	cm
Range of motion (goniometer)			
Shoulder flexion	134/180	119/180	degrees
Hip flexion			
Balance			
Single-leg stance (eyes open)	Unable	Unable	s
Berg Balance Scale		29 (med. risk)	Score
Function			
Chair stand test		0/9-14	Number of stands
Functional reach (standing)		18 (7.1 in.)	cm
Fitness			
Timed 10 m walk test		15.4 (with cane)	s
Quality of life			
Fear of falling		21/48	Score
Self-reported health status		Good	
Qualeffo-41		46.5/100	Transformed score
SF-36		47	Total score

4. Trunk & leg strength to 60% age-norm referenced data
5. Flexibility to 60% normative values
6. Continued independent management of personal ADLs

7. Loss of bone mineral density <1%
8. 10 m walk test (with cane) 12 s
9. No report of falls

P: One educational session followed by training in a home-based program at facility 1 day/wk for 8 wk with home exercise performed 2 days/wk. Exercise plan:

Follow-Up

At 3 mo (10th visit): With moderate to good compliance, client reported increased mobility, continuing volunteer work, ability to lie supine with 1 pillow, no falls, and ability to progress all exercises. She reported hip/back pain as 3-4/10. Recheck in 3 mo, remeasure, and continue to upgrade the program.

Mode/Activity	Frequency	Initial duration	Initial intensity	Progression
Aerobic Stationary bicycling Walking (weather permitting (monitor HR/RPE)	• 2 days/week • 1 day/week	20 min	Self-selected	• 2 days/week, 30 min • 2 days/week, 30 min
Strength Sitting hip flexion Side-lying hip abductors with hip and knee flexion Bridging Standing partial wall squats Standing hip extensions Standing hip abductions Toe raise Heel raise Abdominal draw-in Back lateral Bent-over row Upright row Standing biceps curl Triceps kick-back Sitting back extension	2 days/week	25 min	• 0 lb, 10 reps • 0 lb, 10 reps • 10 reps • 15 reps • 0 lb, 10 reps • 0 lb, 10 reps • 0 lb, 5 reps • 0 lb, 5 reps • 10 reps, 10 s holds • 1 lb, 10 reps • 2 lb, 10 reps • 2 lb, 10 reps • 2 lb, 10 reps • 1 lb, 10 reps • 15 reps	• 2 days/week, 40 min; increase to 2 sets • Elastic band resistance • 15 reps, 2 sets
Flexibility Hip extensors (supine) Hip flexors (prone lying) Hamstrings (supine) Heel cords (standing)	2 days/week	5 min (total)	2 reps, 15 s holds	• 2 days/week, 1 rep, 30 s holds • Prone lying 1 min, 2 days/week
Balance Static stork standing Sitting reaching	2 days/week	• 10 s • 10 s	• 5 reps/leg • 5 reps	• Goal: 1 rep, 3 s • Goal: increase reach distance
Functional Chair stand from elevated chair (3 pillows)	Daily		5 reps	
Warm-up and cool-down Sitting reverse arm circles	2 days/week	15 s	10 reps	• Standing reverse arm circles • 20 reps, 15 s

37

Lower Limb Amputation

Kenneth H. Pitetti, PhD, FACSM ■ Mark H. Pedrotty, PhD

OVERVIEW OF THE PATHOPHYSIOLOGY

Amputation is the removal of a body extremity through trauma or surgery. Surgical amputations are typically performed due to disease that affects a specific limb. Within the United States, an estimated 1.9 million individuals are living with an amputation. Each year approximately 135,000 amputations are performed in the United States; of those, the majority are lower limb amputations due to complications of the vascular system as a result of diabetes, peripheral vascular disease, or atherosclerosis. Amputation trends in the United States show that amputations due to vascular disease-related complications are on the rise. Loss of a limb results in a permanent disability that can have a profound effect on an individual's self-image, relationships, employment, self-care, mobility, and capacity to exercise. Following a lower limb amputation, people are encouraged to participate in rehabilitation and develop the skills necessary to engage in normal daily activities including regular physical activity. Advances in prosthetic technology, disease management, and rehabilitation strategies have enhanced long-term outcomes for individuals with lower limb amputations.

The main causes of lower limb (LL) amputation are as follows:

- Vascular and circulatory diseases caused by either type 2 diabetes or peripheral vascular disease, 82%

- Trauma (e.g., traumatic amputation; massively crushed limbs; massive fractures causing ischemia and irreparable vasculature; thermal, chemical, and electrical burns; and frostbite), 22%

- Curative treatment of tumors (e.g., a malignant osteogenic sarcoma that has not yet metastasized), 4%

- Congenital deformities (i.e., a prosthetic limb replaces the amputated deformed limb to allow for improved ambulation), 4%

The majority of individuals requiring LL amputation are over the age of 55, and their amputations are primarily the result of neuropathies and peripheral vascular disease secondary to either type 2 diabetes or atherosclerosis; these persons are classified as vascular amputees. Individuals with LL amputation from trauma, tumors, or congenital deformities are usually less than 50 years of age (e.g., children, adolescents, and young adults), and are classified as nonvascular amputees.

Determining the specific classification for an LL amputee is important because the purpose of exercise differs between these classifications. The main purpose of exercise management for vascular amputees is to preclude or abate the pathogenesis of diabetes, atherosclerosis, or both. On the other hand, exercise management for nonvascular LL amputees is similar to that for nondisabled persons. That is, exercise management focuses on risk reduction for developing secondary disabilities such as cardiovascular disease, diabetes, high blood pressure, and obesity. In fact, LL amputees have a higher risk for developing secondary cardiovascular-related disabilities than nondisabled individuals because of the LL amputee's predisposition toward living a sedentary lifestyle.

There are several classifications of LL amputees:

- Symes (amputation of the forefoot or midfoot, usually leaving the heel bones intact and therefore allowing full weight bearing onto the heel of the foot)
- Transtibial (below-knee amputation)
- Transfemoral (above-knee amputation)
- Hip disarticulation (removal of the leg at the femoral hip joint)
- Unilateral amputation (involvement of only one leg, as in amputation of one leg below the knee or above the knee)
- Bilateral amputation (involvement of both legs, as in amputation of one leg below the knee and the other above the knee)

EFFECTS ON THE EXERCISE RESPONSE

The appropriate exercise modality for nonvascular unilateral amputation above or below the knee, unilateral hip disarticulation, bilateral amputation below the knee, or bilateral amputation above and below the knee (one leg amputated above the knee, the other below the knee) should incorporate a sufficient amount of muscle mass (e.g., for aerobic and anaerobic testing) to elicit exercise responses similar to those of nondisabled individuals. However, for bilateral above-knee amputation or bilateral hip disarticulation, individual responses will be limited by the muscle mass and work capacity of the upper body musculature (i.e., arms, shoulders, chest, and trunk), similar to the situation in persons with paraplegia lesions below the L1 vertebra. The same precepts hold true for vascular amputees but are further complicated by medications and the extent of the primary disease (e.g., type 2 diabetes).

EFFECTS ON EXERCISE TRAINING

The effect of exercise training is dependent on the modality used and amount of musculature involved for LL amputees. For instance, a unilateral below-knee, above-knee, or hip disarticulation amputee will involve enough muscle mass exercising on a sitting arm-leg ergometer (e.g., Schwinn Air-Dyne) to see an improvement in cardiovascular fitness similar in magnitude to that of a nondisabled person on the same modality. However, a bilateral above-knee amputee, limited to modalities such as arm ergometry or swimming that incorporate a smaller muscle mass, will elicit cardiovascular improvements but of a smaller magnitude than obtained by the unilateral amputee exercising on an arm-leg ergometer.

In addition, the modalities of walking or jogging are not viable or feasible long-term exercise regimens for many LL amputees for the following reasons:

- Energy expenditure (i.e., physical effort) of walking is higher for LL amputees compared to nondisabled individuals and is directly related to the level of amputation (i.e., energy cost for a unilateral above-knee amputee is greater than for a unilateral below-knee amputee).
- The potential painful consequences of skin breakdowns or infections can further exacerbate a disability, acutely limiting all exercise, recreational activities, work-related activities, or activities of daily living.
- Any additional trauma and painful consequences to the amputated limb(s) as well as a noninvolved limb (e.g., overuse injuries) will impair the ability to walk or jog.

The combination of additional energy expenditure, the painful consequences of skin breakdown or infections, and the high risk of overuse injuries precludes walking or jogging as a physical activity pattern that can be maintained or easily integrated into the daily activities of most LL amputees.

MANAGEMENT AND MEDICATIONS

A large majority of LL amputations are the direct result of peripheral arterial disease and diabetes (see chapters 15 and 24), which require specific medications. The types of medications specific to these conditions and their exercise effects are covered in the respective chapters.

Most amputees experience the so-called phantom pain phenomenon (i.e., pain that seems to come from the amputated body part). Phantom pain can range from mild to severe. When it is severe, relief is often obtained from drugs that are also given to counteract epilepsy or depression and are thought to have little or no exercise effect. Some amputees find that their phantom pain is eased by a combination of antidepressants and narcotics (e.g., methadone). Antidepressants can cause drowsiness. Amputees using narcotics for their phantom pain should consult their physician before continuing an exercise program.

RECOMMENDATIONS FOR EXERCISE TESTING

In aerobic and anaerobic exercise testing, unilateral above- or below-knee amputees, bilateral below-knee amputees, and bilateral amputees having one below-knee and one above-knee amputation should use an arm-leg ergometer such as the Schwinn Air-Dyne or SciFit Pro II Power Trainer. Lower limb amputees who are unable to involve their lower extremities when using an arm-leg ergometer (e.g., bilateral above-knee amputees) should be tested with either an arm crank ergometer (e.g., Monark Rehab Trainer model 881), Cybex upper body ergometer, or the arm mechanism of an arm-leg ergometer.

For safety purposes, weight machines rather than free weights should be used in testing for muscle strength and endurance. Trunk (e.g., sit-ups, back extension) and upper body strength (e.g., sitting military press, bench press, biceps curl) tests can be performed using the same protocols as for nondisabled individuals. Lower body strength and endurance testing should use both the noninvolved limb (if the amputation is unilateral) and the muscles of the amputated leg. For instance, an above-knee amputee may not be able to perform knee extension and flexion with the amputated limb but could perform hip extension and flexion. Appraising flexibility, especially of the joints of the lower extremities (e.g., hip, knee) of both involved and noninvolved legs, is also recommended (see table 37.1).

The most important functional evaluation for LL amputees is walking capacity (i.e., time to walk a given distance) because research has established that exercise programs improve the walking efficiency of LL amputees. The distance of the walk test will depend on the level of amputation and the physical condition of the individual. For instance, a physically fit unilateral above- or below-knee amputee should be tested in distances of 500 to 600 yd (457.2 to 548.6 m), whereas distances of 100 to

TABLE 37.1

Lower Limb Amputation: Exercise Testing

Methods	Measures	Endpoints*	Comments
Aerobic Submaximal Maximal (for athletes)	▪ HR ▪ BP ▪ Work rate ▪ RPE (6-20)	▪ RPE 16/20 ▪ Volitional exhaustion (athletes)	Use measure to prescribe exercise intensity.
Strength Weight machines	1RM		Use 1RM to prescribe exercise intensity (e.g., 60% 1RM).
Flexibility Goniometry	Abduction, adduction, flexion, extension of available ankle, knee, hip joints		Over time, loss of flexibility suggests reassessing stretching program.
Functional 100 to 600 yd (91.4 to 548.6 m) walk	▪ Time (s) ▪ Number of steps		Walk at a "comfortable" walking speed; should not be a race.

*Measurements of particular significance; do not always indicate test termination.

200 yd (91.4 to 182.9 m) would be appropriate for deconditioned unilateral and bilateral amputees or amputees with a hip disarticulation. Walking tests should be performed on gymnasium floors, indoor tracks, tennis courts, or any smooth, level surface.

RECOMMENDATIONS FOR EXERCISE PROGRAMMING

In general, individuals with a LL amputation can follow the same exercise guidelines (i.e., frequency, intensity, and duration) as the apparently healthy population. For aerobic exercise, LL amputees should use a mode that (1) incorporates enough muscle mass to produce improvements in cardiovascular fitness and (2) will not cause overuse injuries, skin breakdowns, and joint pain or inflammation in the nonamputated or amputated limbs. Based on the level of amputation, the following modalities are recommended (see table 37.2):

- Sitting arm-leg ergometer (e.g., Schwinn Air-Dyne), arm ergometer, swimming, and rowing ergometer for all amputees
- Cycle ergometer, reclined or sitting, for all except bilateral below-knee amputees (who may not utilize sufficient muscle mass with this mode) and bilateral above-knee amputees (who will most likely be unable to use the bike)
- Standing arm-leg ergometer (e.g., Reebok Body Trec) for unilateral below-knee amputees, although unilateral above-knee and bilateral below-knee amputees may be capable of using this apparatus

Strength and stretching regimens, as well as exercise progression (i.e., frequency, duration, and intensity), would follow the same guidelines as for nondisabled individuals or individuals with only type 2 diabetes or cardiovascular disease.

TABLE 37.2

Lower Limb Amputation: Exercise Programming

Modes	Goals	Intensity/Frequency/Duration	Time to goal
Aerobic Ergometers: ■ Sitting arm-leg ■ Arm ■ Rowing ■ Cycle ■ Standing arm or leg ■ Swimming	■ Increase cardiovascular fitness and endurance of uninvolved and involved limbs ■ Increase efficiency of ADLs and ambulation	■ 40-80% $\dot{V}O_2R$ or HRR ■ RPE 11-16/20 ■ 4-7 days/week ■ 30-60 min/session	■ Duration should be 10-20 min initially, with a goal of 30-60 min.
Strength Weight machines	■ Increase strength of trunk, hip, and involved and uninvolved leg ■ Increase efficiency of ADLs and ambulation	■ 1-2 sets at 60-80% 1RM or a weight that allows for 8 reps ■ 2-3 days/week ■ Perform ≥5 separate exercises/session	■ Initial weight used until 12 reps can be performed, then increase weight 5-10 lb (2.3-4.5 kg) and return to 8 reps. ■ Do not lift 2 days in a row. ■ 2 upper body, 1 trunk, and 2 lower body exercises/session.
Flexibility Stretching (target trunk, hip, and available lower limb joints)	Maintain ROM		

Evidence-Based Guidelines

Broomhead P, Dawes D, Hale C, Lambert A, Quinlivan D, Shepherd R. Evidence based clinical guidelines for the physiotherapy management of adults with lower limb prostheses. British Association of Chartered Physiotherapists in Amputation Rehabilitation. 2003 (cited 2008 June 18). Available from www.csp.org.uk.

Burgess EM, Rappoport A. Physical fitness: A guide for individuals with lower limb loss. Darby, PA: DIANE; 1993. p. 245.

Vestering MM, Schoppen T, Dekker R, Wempe J, Geertzen JH. Development of an exercise testing protocol for patients with a lower limb amputation: Results of a pilot study. Int J Rehabil Res. 2005;28(3):237-244.

van Velzen JM. Physical capacity and walking ability after lower limb amputation: A systematic review. Clin Rehabil. 2006;20(11):999-1016.

Suggested Web Site

National Center on Physical Activity and Disability. www.ncpad.org

CASE STUDY

Lower Extremity Amputation

A 14-year-old female had her left leg amputated (Symes amputation) because of a congenital deformity (5-in. [12.7-cm] discrepancy between her lower left and right leg) at the age of 4. She also had congenital short femurs, hip dysplasia, and proximal femur focus deficiency and had undergone an osteotomy of the right hip at age 8. She was referred for a multidisciplinary weight loss program involving diet, exercise, and psychiatric evaluation and counseling. She expressed a desire to lose weight and to be involved in an activity program that would help her ambulate on her prosthetic leg (she was restricted to a wheelchair). She also wanted to discuss the circumstances and her feelings about her amputation. Her parents agreed to participate.

S: "I wish I could get around like everyone else."

O: Vitals

Height: 5 ft 1 in. (1.55 m)
Weight: 235 lb (106.6 kg)
BMI: 44.4 kg/m^2
Morbidly obese young woman, flat affect, in wheelchair
Left leg amputation below the knee
Psychological evaluation: Axis I (major depression)
Poor ambulation; hip on the involved side unable to support weight for more than a few steps

A: 1. Left leg amputation below the knee
   2. Major depression
   3. Morbid obesity

P: 1. Orthopedic evaluation (prosthetic/surgical modification) is necessary.
   2. Medically manage weight loss and depression.
   3. Individual psychotherapy (cognitive behavioral therapy/increase self-esteem) is needed.
   4. Group counseling on the family culture that produced her situation would be helpful.
   5. Prescribe a weight loss diet (1500 kcal/day).
   6. Formulate an exercise program.

Exercise Program Goals

1. Ambulation without crutches
2. 25 lb (11 kg) weight loss
3. Improved ADLs

Follow-Up

By 6 months, the client had lost 17.5 lb (7.9 kg). Psychotherapy was slowly progressing with her many issues. She was ready to focus medically on lifestyle changes specific to exercise and diet. She had begun ambulating at school without crutches, using the crutches only as a backup for muscle and stump fatigue. She participating in an adapted physical education program focused on improving walking capacity.

Mode	Frequency	Duration	Intensity	Progression
Aerobic (arm ergometer)	3 days/week	10-20 min	RPE 12/20	Increase as tolerated to 30-60 min/session.
Strength (upper and lower body)	3 days/week	1 set of 8-12 reps	Versus gravity	Increase to 2 sets. Full recovery between sets.
Flexibility (upper and lower body)	3 days/week	20-60 s/stretch	Maintain stretch below discomfort point	
Warm-up and cool-down	Before and after each session	5 min	As tolerated/low	

PART VII

Neuromuscular Disorders

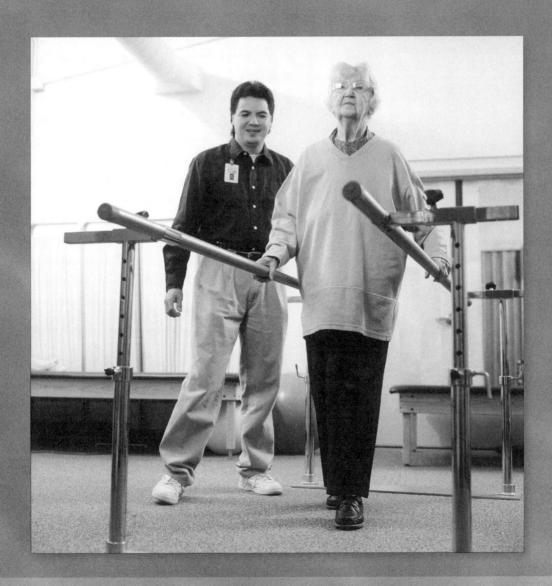

Stroke and Brain Injury

Karen Palmer-McLean, PhD, PT ■ Kimberly B. Harbst, PhD, PT

OVERVIEW OF THE PATHOPHYSIOLOGY

A stroke occurs when blood flow to a region of the brain is obstructed, resulting in a rapid loss of brain function lasting for 24 h or more or until death. The majority of strokes (87%) are ischemic, resulting from a thrombosis or embolism; 10% are hemorrhagic, caused by rupture of a vessel in the brain and consequent leaking of blood into brain tissue or cerebrospinal fluid. Stroke is the third leading cause of death in America and the number-one cause of adult disability. During an ischemic stroke, a phenomenon called the ischemic cascade occurs as diminished blood flow to the brain initiates a series of events that can result in additional, delayed damage to brain cells. The more immediately medical intervention is received following the first warning signs of stroke, the better are the chances that the process can be halted and the risk for irreversible complications reduced. Stroke is often referred to as a cerebrovascular accident (CVA) or brain attack; however, the preferred term is stroke, because the event may not necessarily be cerebrovascular or accidental.

Approximately 780,000 Americans, the majority of them over the age of 60, suffer a new or recurrent stroke each year. Males are 1.25 to 1.5 times more likely to have a stroke than females until the age of 74, when the incidence rate equalizes. Modifiable risk factors for stroke include hypertension (the most important risk factor for stroke), hyperlipidemia, cigarette smoking (increases risk twofold), diabetes mellitus, cardiac or arterial disease, atrial fibrillation, metabolic syndrome, poor diet, physical inactivity, and alcoholism. In addition, one of the strongest predictors of a stroke is transient ischemic attacks (TIAs). Transient ischemic attacks, often called "mini-strokes," produce stroke-like symptoms but cause no lasting damage. An individual who has had one or more TIAs is nearly 10 times more likely to have a stroke than someone of equivalent age and sex who hasn't ever had one. Approximately 23% of stroke victims have a previous stroke history. The 30-day survival rate is 88% for ischemic and 62% for hemorrhagic strokes. Approximately 25% of stroke victims die as a result of the event itself or its complications, and roughly 50% will have moderate to severe health impairments and long-term disabilities. Only 26% of stroke victims recover most or all of their prestroke health and function.

The lack of blood flow to the brain during a stroke causes both primary neuronal cell death and secondary impairments. The resulting neurological impairment depends on the size and the location of the lesion, as well as the speed with which the lesion occurs. Collateral blood flow formation occurs with slowly forming lesions, and less impairment occurs as a result. After a stroke, individuals may experience the following problems:

- Paralysis or problems controlling movement (motor control): Paralysis is one of the most common disabilities resulting from a stroke. The paralysis is usually on the side of the body opposite the side of the brain damaged by the stroke and may affect the face, an arm, a leg, or the entire side of the body.

Damage to a lower part of the brain, the cerebellum, can affect the body's ability to coordinate movement, a disability called ataxia, leading to problems with body posture, walking, and balance.

▪ Sensory disturbances including those involving pain: Stroke survivors may lose the ability to feel touch, pain, temperature, or position.

▪ Problems using or understanding language (aphasia): At least one-fourth of all stroke survivors experience language impairments, involving the ability to speak, write, and understand spoken and written language.

▪ Problems with thinking and memory: Stroke survivors may have dramatically shortened attention spans or may experience deficits in short-term memory.

▪ Emotional disturbances: Many stroke survivors experience fear, anxiety, frustration, anger, sadness, and a sense of grief for their physical and mental losses.

Acquired traumatic brain injury (TBI) results from a blow or jolt to the head, from a penetrating head injury, or from being violently shaken. Traumatic brain injury causes permanent damage to the brain, resulting in total or partial functional disability or psychosocial impairment, or both. After a TBI, impairments in one or more of the following are common: cognition; language; memory; attention; reasoning; abstract thinking; judgment; problem solving; sensory, perceptual, and motor abilities; psychosocial behavior; physical functions; information processing; and speech. Approximately 1.4 million new cases of TBI occur each year in the United States; 50,000 of these people die and 85,000 have long-term disability. The typical ages of onset for a TBI are between 0 and 4 years, between 15 and 19 years, and then later in life (75 years plus). Falls and motor-vehicle-related accidents are the most common causes of TBI.

When an individual sustains a blow to the head, primary damage occurs directly beneath (coup) and opposite (countercoup) the site of impact. Rapid acceleration and deceleration of the gelatinous brain within the hard skull results in neural tissue laceration by sharp, irregular bony structures or dural edges, as well as stretching and breaking of axons within the myelin sheath (diffuse axonal injury). Additional secondary damage accompanies both TBI and stroke and can result in more extensive permanent brain damage. Secondary neurological damage occurs when edema compresses the uninvolved surrounding tissue (i.e., the tissue that was not affected by direct trauma), resulting in the disruption of metabolic processes due to a reduction in oxygenated blood supply to the compressed tissue.

Damage from TBI is typically more diffuse, with more generalized impairments, than from stroke. After moderate TBI, physical disabilities affecting movement and control of all four extremities, neck, and trunk are prominent. Upper motor neuron damage may result in spasticity, clonus, and atypical involuntary posturing. The brainstem and cranial nerves may be involved, affecting vital functions. The cerebellum may be affected, resulting in imbalance, incoordination, and difficulty controlling the extent and timing of movements. Finally, primary factors limiting a person's independence even after mild brain injury include behavioral and cognitive disturbances such as agitation, confusion, impulsiveness, inattention, disturbed memory, apathy, poor judgment, and learning deficits.

EFFECTS ON THE EXERCISE RESPONSE

Overall functional capacity is typically low in individuals who have recently sustained a TBI or stroke. Following a stroke, submaximal oxygen uptake is increased and peak oxygen uptake is decreased. $\dot{V}O_{2peak}$ is approximately half that of age-matched healthy counterparts, resulting in lower maximal workloads. Following TBI, aerobic capacities are typically 67% to 74% below predicted levels based on height and age. The impaired cardiac response and exercise performance in this population may in part be due to the lack of motor function following trauma to the brain. Only 20% to 34% of individuals with stroke are able to achieve 85% of age-predicted maximal heart rate. Because of associated physical impairments, people with TBI have much higher submaximal heart rates during cycle ergometry than age-matched controls. Even with minimal to no physical deficits, response to exercise is significantly less efficient after TBI as indicated by submaximal $\dot{V}_E/\dot{V}O_2$, oxygen pulse, maximal heart rate, $\dot{V}O_2$, and $\dot{V}_E$.

The functional implications for stroke or TBI survivors are that they tend to breathe harder with exertion, fatigue approximately 2.5 times more rapidly, and are less efficient in mobility skills and activities of daily living. Thus, they are more likely to adopt a sedentary lifestyle with increased risk of negative secondary conditions. Fatigue and lack of endurance may have significant functional consequences, including potential of decreased job productivity and employability.

EFFECTS OF EXERCISE TRAINING

Recurrent stroke and coronary artery disease (CAD) are leading causes of death following stroke; however, recent studies have confirmed that exercise alone can reduce mortality by 20% or more. After stroke, leg cycling exercise has resulted in 60% greater $\dot{V}O_{2peak}$, and treadmill training has improved peak oxygen consumption, workload response, blood pressure, resting heart rate, and cholesterol levels. Exercise after a stroke is also associated with increased walking speed, decreased ambulation assistance, and improved functional mobility.

Specific exercise programs may have limited benefits. For example, aerobic training improves fitness and gait without improving activities of daily living. The American Heart Association (AHA) recommends stretching, flexibility, balance, and coordination exercises two or three times per week. Muscle weakness frequently results from stroke, so the AHA recommends strength training with light resistance two or three days per week. Strengthening after a stroke is associated with improved activities of daily living and increased walking speed and distance. Care should be taken to avoid overtraining, as overtraining has been identified as a potential detriment in at least one study involving gait and strength training in stroke survivors.

Although most individuals with TBI are young, their physical capacities and endurance may be severely limited by multisystem trauma. Exercise can significantly improve $\dot{V}O_{2peak}$, endurance, and muscle strength in individuals with TBI, resulting in greater independence, more efficient locomotion, and greater employability. In addition, post-TBI individuals who exercise are typically less depressed and report fewer cognitive symptoms.

MANAGEMENT AND MEDICATIONS

Medical treatment for stroke survivors includes the following:

- Short-term use of anticoagulants and long-term use of platelet-inhibiting agents, such as heparin, Coumadin, and aspirin
- Vasodilators, such as hydralazine, clonidine, or Isordil, if vasospasm of the cerebral arteries is suspected
- Antihypertensive medications after hemorrhagic stroke requiring strict control of blood pressure, including angiotensin-converting enzyme inhibitors (ACE inhibitors), beta-blockers, calcium channel blockers, diuretics, and sympathetic nerve inhibitors

Some people with a brain injury may require more intensive postacute medical management. Seizures and spasticity may necessitate long-term anticonvulsant and antispasmodic medications. Cognitive slowing may be a side effect of these drugs. Seizure medications may be withdrawn after one or more seizure-free years. The following are medications that may be used for prevention of seizures:

- Phenobarbital
- Clonazepam
- Gabapentin
- Carbamazepine

In addition, some individuals may receive medical therapy for the treatment of depression or anxiety after TBI, which can cause dizziness, hypotension, and altered arousal states. Drugs used for depression or anxiety include the following:

- Venlafaxine
- Amitriptyline
- Desipramine
- Nortriptyline
- Fluoxetine
- Sertraline
- Lorazepam
- Diazepam
- Alprazolam

Hypertonia is a condition marked by an abnormal increase in muscle tension and a reduced ability of a muscle to stretch. Hypertonia may significantly impair movement in individuals who have experienced either a stroke or TBI. Oral medications (e.g., baclofen, diazepam, tizanidine) may reduce hypertonia but may be intolerable due to diminished arousal and cognitive slowing. Alternatives to oral medications include intrathecal baclofen pumps and injections that block local motor activation. The following are medications that are typically used to address hypertonia or other movement-related issues after TBI:

- Dantrolene
- Diazepam
- Baclofen

Finally, some drugs may be used to combat cognitive deficits in people with TBI or stroke, such as the following:

- Tacrine
- Sinemet
- Aricept
- Ritalin
- Dexedrine
- Cylert

The use of some medications may affect acute physiologic response during graded exercise tests:

- Vasodilators may increase the cool-down period required after exercise to prevent postexercise hypotension.
- Medications that limit cardiac output by reducing heart rate may cause lower peak heart rates.
- Diuretics reduce fluid volume and may alter electrolyte balance, causing dysrhythmias.

RECOMMENDATIONS FOR EXERCISE TESTING

Because many stroke survivors either currently have, or are at risk for, cardiovascular disease, their exercise tests should be supervised by a physician and monitored with a 12-lead electrocardiogram (ECG). Endpoints for exercise testing in this population are the same as with high-risk individuals and those with known or suspected CAD (see *ACSM's Guidelines for Exercise Testing and Prescription, 8th edition*). Exercise testing in individuals with neurologic deficits can be more challenging than in able-bodied persons. For this reason, instructions on how to perform specific tests must include extra emphasis prior to conducting an exercise test on an individual with a neurological deficit (see table 38.1). The mode of exercise testing depends on the severity of physical impairments.

Leg Cycle Ergometry

A standard leg cycle ergometer can be used if sitting balance on the cycle can be safely maintained. A ramp protocol can be used with workload increases of 5 to 10 W/min or 20 W/stage. Semirecumbent cycle ergometry can be used if imbalance is a problem, with modified $\dot{V}O_{2max}$ guidelines to reflect decreased work produced on recumbent equipment. Test protocols should be individualized based on strength. A pedaling rate of 50 rpm and a starting power output of 20 W with 20 W stage increments are suggested guidelines.

Treadmill

Treadmill testing using a Balke protocol may be appropriate in individuals with minimal motor impairment, good standing balance, and independent unassisted ambulation. Treadmills should have a "zero start" feature to avoid abrupt speed changes that could cause a fall. Individuals with weakness, loss of movement, or balance deficits may be unsafe on a treadmill. Treadmill testing could still be conducted with use of a harness system to prevent a fall or to support some body weight. Treadmill speed may need to be decreased to accommodate the slower preferred speed in this population. Energy expenditure at a specific work rate can be expected to be 55% to 64% greater than in someone who has not had a stroke. Exercise protocols with a very gradual increase in exercise intensity, such as the Naughton-Balke or modified Balke, should be used with increases of 0.5 to 2 METs/3 min stage.

Combined Arm and Leg Ergometry

If affected extremity spasticity or muscle weakness interferes with pedaling during leg cycle testing, and use of only the unaffected leg results in inability to achieve a work rate that can stress the heart, a combination arm-leg ergometer (Schwinn Air-Dyne or PowerTrainer) is useful. Subjects can use only the unaffected extremities or can assist with the affected extremities if spasticity and weakness do not interfere. An intermittent protocol is suggested to avoid upper extremity muscle fatigue.

Steppers

Mechanical steppers or stair climbers are another option for exercise testing and training. A suggested protocol begins at 25 steps per minute with incremental increases of 7 steps per minute. Assistance may be required for appropriate foot placement. Another mode combining arm and leg exercise is the seated stepper (NuStep) with reciprocating arm levers. Some models include a seat with back support and optional seat belt for additional trunk stability. Some seats swivel and have flip-up armrests facilitating transfer onto the device. In contrast to the pronated forearm position for most other ergometers, these devices employ a grip midway between pronation and supination. This neutral position is easier for clients with limited range of motion and encourages a more upright trunk posi-

TABLE 38.1

Stroke and Brain Injury: Exercise Testing

Methods	Measures	Endpoints*	Comments
Aerobic Cycle ergometer (5-10 W/min using ramp protocol) Treadmill (0.5-2 METs/stage) Combination arm-leg ergometer Seated stepper Arm ergometer	▪ 12-lead ECG, HR ▪ BP, rate–pressure product ▪ RPE ▪ $\dot{V}O_{2peak}$	▪ Serious dysrhythmias ▪ >2 mm ST-segment depression or elevation ▪ Ischemic threshold ▪ SBP >250 mmHg or DBP >115 mmHg ▪ Volitional fatigue	▪ CAD is a major risk factor for CVA. ▪ Hypertension is a major risk factor for CVA. ▪ Useful in prescribing exercise intensity. ▪ Necessary only if conducting research.
Endurance 6 or 12 min walk Leg cycle ergometer (or combination arm-leg ergometer)	▪ Distance walked ▪ Time of exercise at 60% peak power	Note, time, distance, symptoms at rest stops	Use with ambulatory clients (with/without assistive devices).
Strength Manual muscle test with/without handheld dynamometer Computerized dynamometer (e.g., isotonic, isokinetic, isometric)	▪ Force generated on dynamometer ▪ Peak torque normalized to body weight ▪ Total work normalized to body weight	▪ Pounds, kilograms, number of repetitions ▪ Max torque	Valid only if client can isolate movement.
Flexibility Handheld goniometer	▪ ROM in shoulder, elbow, wrist, knee, ankle, and other joints of affected limbs ▪ Distance reached	▪ Degrees of full flexion/extension ▪ Total arc	
Neuromuscular Gait analysis Berg Balance Functional reach Tinetti (performance-oriented mobility assessment)	▪ Gait speed ▪ Symmetry of movement		Useful in assessing safety and efficiency of movement.
Functional Duke mobility Functional Independence Measure (FIM) Individualized criterion-referenced tests			Useful in overall progress of ADLs.

*Measurements of particular significance; do not always indicate test termination.

tion. Finally, instead of the traditional bike pedal, the foot plate supports the entire sole with raised lateral and posterior borders and optional foot straps to maintain foot placement.

Exercise Equipment Modifications

Exercise devices may be adapted to accommodate a client's motor impairments. An extended backrest can be added to upright ergometers to accommodate balance impairments. Seat belts and chest straps can add trunk stability. A strap, mitt, or ACE wrap may be used to secure the affected hand or foot to the handgrip or pedal of any ergometer. Many products are commercially available to customize exercise devices to clients' unique needs. Clients should be closely supervised if a strap is used to secure an extremity on a handle or pedal because the individual will be unable to stop a fall by extending the arm or leg. Finally, a step stool may be required in order to get on and off a cycle ergometer. The client should step up onto the stool with the unaffected leg and step down with the affected leg.

Muscle Strength Tests

Muscle strength can be measured using computerized dynamometers (e.g., Cybex, Biodex). A handheld dynamometer can also be used to measure the amount of resistance applied as the individual maintains the testing position. Reliability of strength measures may be affected by inability to isolate joint motions.

Flexibility Tests

Flexibility is a particularly important component of fitness that should be tested in both the post-CVA and post-TBI populations. As noted earlier, 80% of stroke patients are in their 60s, 70s, and 80s, a time when arthritic complaints are much more common. Following TBI, an individual is likely to demonstrate limited joint range of motion caused by the multiple joint traumas that may have accompanied the TBI, reduced mobility during the acute phase of recovery, and have an increased risk of heterotopic ossification. Brain injury that results in muscle weakness or hypertonia also has the potential to limit joint range. Joint range of motion can be measured with a handheld goniometer.

Endurance Tests

Endurance can be estimated using a 6 or 12 min walk.

Neuromuscular Tests

Neuromuscular testing can involve gait analysis, Berg Balance Scale, functional reach, Tinetti Assessment Tool, and the NIH Stroke Survivor Scale.

The following are special considerations for exercise testing:

- A large percentage of clients who have had a CVA are on hypertension and cardiovascular medication (see appendix).
- Seizure-prone clients may be on anticonvulsant medication.
- Clients with hypertonia may use medications to reduce muscle tone.
- Arthritis is common in clients with CVA.
- Reduced motor control of a limb may necessitate using only the uninvolved limb in arm, leg, or arm-leg bicycle ergometry.
- An exercise device may need to be modified (e.g., using hand mitts on arm ergometer, adding toe clips to bicycle ergometer).
- Clients who have had a CVA are also at risk for CAD, so close monitoring of ECG is essential.
- Sensation may be impaired, so careful observation is necessary to prevent injury.
- Clients who have had a CVA may also have peripheral arterial disease, which may impair their ability to ambulate or cycle.

RECOMMENDATIONS FOR EXERCISE PROGRAMMING

The AHA recommends endurance training programs for individuals with brain lesions, citing documented physiological, psychological, and functional benefits. Although both populations tend to be deconditioned, some of the exercise considerations following stroke and TBI differ. The majority of recent stroke survivors are elderly and also have comorbidities, such as osteoarthritis and additional cardiovascular disease, that may limit function more than their stroke. Experts suggest a three-tier exercise training approach months to years after the initial insult. Immediately following a stroke, the goal of exercise is to return to function (see table 38.2). The goal of the second phase is to decrease the risk of additional strokes and cardiovascular disease by influencing glucose regulation, decreasing weight and blood pressure, and managing blood lipid levels. The third-phase goal is to improve aerobic

TABLE 38.2

Stroke and Brain Injury: Exercise Programming

Modes	Goals	Intensity/Frequency/ Duration	Time to goal
Aerobic Upper and lower body ergometer Cycle ergometer Treadmill Arm ergometer Seated stepper	▪ Increase independence of ADLs ▪ Increase walking speed ▪ Decrease risk of cardiovascular disease	▪ 40-70% $\dot{V}O_{2peak}$* ▪ 3-5 days/week ▪ 20-60 min/session (or multiple 10 min sessions)	2-4 months
Strength Isometric exercise Weight machine Free weights	Increase independence of ADLs	▪ 3 sets of 8-12 reps ▪ 1-2 sets ▪ 2 days/week	2-4 months
Flexibility Stretching	Increase ROM of involved extremities Prevent contractures	2 days/week (before or after aerobic or strength activities)	2-4 months
Neuromuscular Coordination and balance activities	Improve levels of safety during ADLs	2 days/week (consider performing on same day as strength activities)	2-4 months

*$\dot{V}O_{2max}$ is undefined in stroke, brain injury, and many other neurological pathologies.

fitness and decrease stroke risk by exercising 20 to 60 min, three to seven days a week. The time can be divided into 10 min intervals.

Aerobic Training

An aerobic conditioning program can alter several of the risk factors associated with the incidence of stroke by reducing blood pressure, enhancing glucose regulation, improving blood lipid profile, and reducing body fat. Training mode depends on the individual's ability, but the various modes described for exercise testing could also be employed for exercise training. In addition, if safety can be assured given the client's cognition and judgment, endurance exercise can take place in a regular or rehabilitation or conditioning pool. Buoyancy assists limb movement and gait, which may be difficult on land. For individuals with cardiovascular disease, care should be taken to monitor pulse, blood pressure,

and subjective reports as hemodynamic responses change with an increased depth of immersion. In general, cardiac performance can actually improve as both stroke volume and cardiac output increase while heart rate decreases or remains constant with immersion. However, difficulties can arise in individuals with breathing problems because increases in external pressure resist inspiration, as well as in those with disorders of left ventricular function due to increased left ventricular filling pressure. In addition, sustained immersion can lead to alterations of hormone levels and diuresis.

Suggested frequency is three to five days a week. Exercise intensity and duration depend on the subject's initial fitness level. In highly deconditioned individuals, exercise intensities may need to start at an equivalent of 40% to 50% $\dot{V}O_{2peak}$. Intermittent training may be needed initially until the client can perform rhythmical exercise for 12 min continuously. The goal should be at least 20 min of aerobic activity per day. As tolerance increases, the duration should be gradually increased until the individual can complete an exercise session equivalent to a caloric expenditure of 300 kcal. Cardiovascular status may be monitored using pretest, working, and 1 min recovery heart rates in conjunction with ratings of perceived exertion.

Strength Training

Resistance training for TBI and stroke survivors has been shown to be both safe and effective. Resistance exercises should be used three times per week to address any muscle weakness identified during the fitness assessment. Individuals with neurological impairments may have difficulty with preparatory postural adjustments and recruiting strength quickly enough to combat the loss of balance. Thus, some of the positions typically used for weight training may need to be modified. For example, upper extremity strengthening exercises typically performed with dumbbell weights in stance may be safer with the client seated, supported by a stable object, or on a machine that supports the weights. Each repetition should be performed slowly without any breath holding.

Flexibility Training

Various methods can be used daily to improve joint, muscle, and soft tissue flexibility following stroke or TBI. Regardless of the method, prolonged stretch or positioning without rapid changes of muscle length is crucial. Ballistic motions increase the risk of tissue damage. Muscle contraction followed by relaxation can be used if the client can comprehend and follow the directions. Prolonged passive stretch can be achieved with nighttime bracing or splinting.

Exercise Environment

One should consider behavioral factors (e.g., impulsivity, a tendency to display outward aggression, lack of judgment, misunderstanding of directions) following TBI when selecting the most appropriate environment for exercise. A client who lacks judgment may need close supervision, while someone who displays outward aggression may not succeed in group settings. A client who is easily agitated or frustrated or highly distractible might be scheduled to exercise at a quieter time or in a less distracting area. The client who lacks initiative might be more successful in a group setting.

General Exercise Considerations

Depression and apathy are common following a stroke or TBI and might interfere with long-term adherence to an exercise program. After TBI, cognitive deficits such as memory loss and slowed processing, as well as behavioral sequelae including impulsivity, agitation, and lability, may interfere with the ability to follow directions in testing and training. Frontal lobe involvement can result in lack of initiative, apathy, frustration, disinhibition, and impaired higher cognitive functions. Temporal lobe lesions may inhibit new learning, impair memory, and result in aggressive outbursts. Involvement of cortical association areas may cause problems for people to screen out irrelevant environmental input and focus on important cues. Receptive aphasia, mental confusion, or apraxia (or some combination of these) may interfere with the ability to understand and follow directions during exercise testing or training sessions. These deficits may be addressed by cognitive retraining, behavioral management, and medication. Close supervision, alternative methods of communication, and modification of the environment to allow exercise in a quieter time and space may be necessary for clients after TBI.

In individuals with TBI or stroke, weakness, inflexibility, and imbalance can hinder exercise and functional mobility. Orthopedic injuries and immobilization can significantly limit flexibility. Hypertonia and clonus can influence functional range of motion, affecting balance and limb positioning. Seizures are more common following TBI and pose safety concerns during exercise If the impairment cannot be eliminated, exercise position or equipment must be modified. Weakness, inflexibility, or impaired sensation may preclude independent ambulation or exercise in standing. Harness-assisted body weight support allows upright exercise despite weakness, imbalance, and diminished flexibility. Inadequate family or social and societal support can limit participation in a routine exercise program. Examples include lack of accessible transportation, poor financial support, and inaccessibility of the exercise facility.

Evidence-Based Guidelines

The evidence-based review of moderate to severe acquired brain injury (ABIEBR). [Online]. 2007 Nov 22 (cited 2008 Mar 27). Available from www.abiebr.com.

Roth EJ, Shephard T, Gordon NF, Gulanick M, Costa F, Fletcher G, Franklin BA. Physical activity and exercise recommendations for stroke survivors: An American

Heart Association scientific statement from the Council on Clinical Cardiology, Subcommittee on Exercise, Cardiac Rehabilitation, and Prevention; the Council on Cardiovascular Nursing; the Council on Nutrition, Physical Activity, and Metabolism; and the Stroke Council. Circulation. 2004;109:2031-2041. [Online]. 2008 Jan 16 (cited 2008 Mar 27). Available from http://circ.ahajournals.org/cgi/reprint/109/16/2031.

Teasell R, Foley N, Salter K, Bhogal S, Jutai J, Speechley M. Evidence-based review of stroke rehabilitation. 10th ed. [Online]. 2007 (cited 2008 Mar 27). Available from www.ebrsr.com.

Suggested Web Sites

American Heart Association. www.americanheart.org

National Stroke Association. www.stroke.org

CASE STUDY

Traumatic Brain Injury

A 15-year-old high school student sustained a severe TBI in an accident two years earlier while in-line skating. He was hit by a motor vehicle that was traveling at 45 mph (72 km/h), and was thrown 30 ft (9 m). He sustained a left frontal intracerebral contusion and had massive intracranial edema; increased intracranial pressure; and right acetabular, proximal tibial-fibular, and pelvic ramus fractures. He initially had a 4 on the Glasgow Coma Scale; he was unconscious for two weeks and at a significantly decreased state of consciousness for six weeks, during which time a decompressive craniotomy was performed. He was hospitalized for acute and rehabilitative care for five months. Blood pressure was initially elevated for a period of four months after injury, and heterotopic ossification developed outside the right knee joint at approximately three months. Surgical hip flexor, hamstring, and Achilles tendon lengthenings were performed at approximately one year postinjury. His family sought organized exercise opportunities as well as home programming at 15 months postinjury to enable him to return to recreational activities and improve fitness and endurance. He returned to his sophomore year of high school six months after his injury.

S: "I want to walk normally again and skate."

O: Vitals

Young male high school student

Medications: Baclofen; weaned over the first six months of exercise

Graded exercise test: Unable to complete secondary to extreme fatigue

No ECG abnormalities

Peak HR with exertion: 135 contractions/min

Peak BP with exertion: 160/82 mmHg

Strength: Left upper and lower extremities 5/5 strength throughout available range of motion; right upper and lower extremities 3+ to 4-/5 strength indicating ability to move limb fully against gravity with mild resistance

Flexibility

Hip extension: Right 5°; left 0°

Hamstring length with hip at 90°: Left -30°; right -10

Ankle dorsiflexion: Right 10°; left 5°

Shoulder elevation: Right 155°; left 180°

Intention tremor and ataxia present in the left upper extremity. Tremor increases in intensity with stress or fatigue and disturbs standing balance.

Neuromuscular

Gait: Walks using right ankle-foot orthosis (AFO) and single-tipped cane held in right hand due to left upper extremity tremor; loses balance and cannot regain without moderate external support when changing direction or when encountering other people in a hallway. His strategy is to abruptly stop walking and wait for others to pass.

Gait speed: 0.2 m/s

Single-limb stance: Right leg 3 s; left leg <1 s

Requires close supervision to contact guard assistance ascending and descending stairs using a cane and one handrail for support. Unsafe to climb stairs at school or in other crowded stairways.

Major limitations

Unable to walk without physical assistance secondary to imbalance

Unable to walk for functional distances at functional rates of speed

Unable to walk over uneven surfaces without losing balance; requires contact guard assistance to safely step over 4 in. (10 cm) obstacles

Requires assistance, assistive devices, and controlled environments to ascend/descend stairs independently

Cannot step over an obstacle in walking path

Cannot come to an abrupt stop without stumbling or grabbing

(continued)

CASE STUDY Traumatic Brain Injury *(continued)*

Cannot turn while walking without staggering or falling

A:
1. Low aerobic capacity due to TBI and resultant immobilization and inactivity leading to easy fatigue; multiple complaints of fatigue after school day and after exercise
2. Weakness in bilateral extremities with ataxia in right arm and leg that worsens with fatigue
3. Poor balance resulting in close supervision to assist with balance or falls—worsens with stress and fatigue especially when others are observing
4. Decreased left ROM on left
5. Slow gait speed precludes functional ambulation; requires use of a cane and/or handheld assistance for 75 ft (23 m), or without the cane with close supervision and occasional assistance for 30 ft (9 m)
6. Dependent for most ADLs or modified to perform in sitting position
7. Impulsive with impaired inhibition

P:
1. Exercise to increase strength, endurance, balance, and gait speed.
2. Adapt devices to facilitate exercise/independent function.

Exercise Program Goals

1. Improve balance to allow safe transitions between postures and independent gait
2. Increase speed, endurance, and safety of gait
3. Be able to climb and descend stairs independently

Exercise Program

For aerobic training, stationary cycling and upper extremity ergometer work were introduced. The client initially required assistance in securing his foot to the stationary cycle and contact guard assistance to maintain balance on the bicycle.

He had two sessions per week of aquatic exercise in a SwimEx pool with variable resistance. Initially, this required the assistance of two people and progressed to independence with exercises at a resistance level of 4. He performed lower extremity exercises, resisted swimming, and resisted walking in this setting. Weights were added as tolerated to the client's legs and increased to 5 lb (2 kg). Resistance bands were also used to resist lower extremity motion when weights were not strapped to the client's legs.

Two sessions per week of land exercise included work on upper and lower extremity strengthening with weight machines and free weights. Modifications had to be made for differing strength, range of motion, and balance between

Mode	Frequency	Duration	Intensity	Progression
Aerobic Recumbent stepper (NuStep), walking on indoor track lightly touching rail	3-5 days/week	7-10 min	• THR (60-75% HR_{max}) • RPE 11-13/20	• Increase to 30 min at 65-80% HR_{max}. • RPE 12-14/20. • Increase walking speed/distance.
Strength (focus on antigravity and postural/trunk muscles)	2-3 days/week	1-2 sets of 8-15 reps	To moderate volitional fatigue, rest 2 min between sets	Increase resistance as tolerated 2-5% once she can perform 15 reps.
Flexibility (anterior chest, hip flexors, plantarflexors)	Daily	2 reps, hold 60 s each	Perform slowly so as not to elicit spasticity/clonus	Increase ROM as tolerated.
Neuromuscular Progressive balance activities (perform standing in corner with chair in front for protection)	2-3 days/week	5-10 min	Should provide sufficient challenge to cause occasional loss of balance	Increase difficulty by sensory manipulation; decrease base of support ; increase speed/amplitude of movement.
Functional Walking with cane with guarding by husband	Daily trials	As tolerated	As tolerated	Increase distance, speed as able.
Warm-up and cool-down	Before and after each session	2-3 min	RPE 9-10/20	Increase time to 5-10 min as total exercise time increases.

sides of the body and difficulty controlling the left upper extremity due to tremors. The client practiced balance exercises on land using sport skills including ball throwing, catching, and kicking. He also practiced sport mobility skills such as lunges, as well as walking in varying directions. Finally, a Euroglide was used to allow the client to work on balance and strengthening with weight shifts.

For home exercises, the client used a pool and weight room at his apartment complex. He also performed push-ups and purchased an exercise ball for strengthening and balance activities at home.

Exercise considerations: During the six months of exercise, fatigue was a significant issue, initially limiting his abilities and affecting his attitude. Disinhibition in his post-TBI personality created challenges that had to be addressed using a behavior modification approach. A system was set up that used three warnings prior to termination of exercise and rewards of special fun activities for good effort. This proved successful in keeping the client motivated and compliant.

Results: With regard to gait, the client progressed to walking while pushing his wheelchair from behind and finally to walking over smooth and uneven surfaces without any assistive devices or orthoses. He has progressed to being able to walk functional community distances, including walking the entire length of a shopping mall. His endurance has improved to allow such extended periods of gait with two brief rest periods, resulting in minimal fatigue afterward. At this point, he is not yet able to run. He is able to ascend and descend stairs independently using a handrail but continues to prefer to use the elevator at school due to crowded and distracting settings. He walks independently at all times at school, including traveling between classes. In icy conditions and outside of school, he is given contact guard assistance. Loss of balance is infrequent, and he is able to regain balance without assistance 95% of the time.

Follow-up

He is not yet riding a bike or skateboarding but has started roller skating at a rink. He has been able to complete two loops around the rink with three people giving contact guard assistance or with one person and the support of a short wall. His goal is to decrease the support required and increase distance in roller skating.

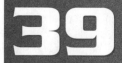

Spinal Cord Disabilities

Paraplegia and Tetraplegia

Stephen F. Figoni, PhD, RKT, FACSM

OVERVIEW OF THE PATHOPHYSIOLOGY

Spinal cord disabilities frequently result in paraplegia or tetraplegia, with segmental neuromuscular, autonomic, and physiologic impairment of the legs, arms, trunk or more than one of these. The majority of individuals with spinal cord disabilities acquire their disability during adolescence or early-middle adulthood from traumatic injuries to the spinal cord. Most traumatic spinal cord injuries (SCIs) result from motor vehicle accidents and falls, with fewer caused by sports (e.g., diving), violence, infection or tumor of the spinal cord, or surgical complications. Fewer traumatic SCIs occur during childhood and old age from these types of causes. In the United States, the incidence of new traumatic SCI is about 32 per million population, producing 8000 new SCIs per year and approximately 75,000 total SCI survivors in any given year.

Additionally, about 1 of every 1,000 live births in the United States results in spina bifida (SB), the congenital developmental form of spinal cord disability. Therefore, about 4,000 infants are born with this condition each year. Spina bifida is a defect due to neural tube abnormalities that usually becomes evident during prenatal sonogram or at birth. The pathogenesis of SB involves incomplete development and closure of the vertebral arch and results in spinal cord damage; usually of the myelomeningocele type affecting the lumbosacral neural segments and causing low-level paraplegia. Congenital and acquired or traumatic spinal cord disability can result in the same sensorimotor, autonomic, physiological, and locomotor impairments. However, in adolescents and adults with SB, secondary conditions tend to accumulate across the entire life span. Therefore, one needs to be aware of complicated medical and psychosocial histories that frequently include hydrocephalus, implanted cerebral shunts, multiple orthopedic and plastic surgeries, skin ulceration, tendinitis, gastrointestinal disorders, obesity, impaired mobility, latex allergy, learning disability, low self-esteem, depression, social immaturity, and hygiene and sexual issues.

Spinal cord disability from any etiology results in impairment or loss of sensorimotor and other functions in the trunk or extremities (or both) caused by damage to the neural elements within the spinal canal. Injury to the cervical segments (C1-C8) or the highest thoracic segment (T1) causes tetraplegia (formerly termed quadriplegia), with impairment of the arms, trunk, legs, and pelvic organs (bladder, bowels, and sexual organs). Injury to thoracic segments T2 to T12 causes paraplegia, with impairment to the trunk, legs, pelvic organs, or some combination of these. Injury to the lumbar or sacral segments of the cauda equina (L1-L5, S1-S4) results in impairment to the legs or pelvic organs or both. The neurological level and completeness of injury determine the degree of impairment.

Physiological impairment may include extensive muscular paralysis and sympathetic nervous system impairment. These impairments frequently result in two major exercise-related problems:

- Reduced ability to voluntarily perform large muscle group aerobic exercise (i.e., without electrical stimulation of paralyzed muscles)
- Inability to stimulate the cardiovascular system to support higher rates of aerobic metabolism

Therefore, catecholamine production by the adrenal medullae, skeletal muscle venous pump, and thermoregulation may be impaired, restricting exercise cardiac output to subnormal levels. Common secondary complications during exercise, especially in individuals with tetraplegia, may include limited positive cardiac chronotropic and inotropic states, excessive venous pooling, orthostatic and exercise hypotension, exercise intolerance, autonomic dysreflexia (a syndrome resulting from mass activation of autonomic reflexes causing extreme hypertension [>200/110 mmHg], headache, bradycardia, flushing, gooseflesh, unusual sweating, shivering, and nasal congestion).

EFFECTS ON THE EXERCISE RESPONSE

In persons with paraplegia, the primary pathologic effects are usually limited to paralysis of the lower body, precluding exercise modes such as walking, running, and voluntary leg cycling. Therefore, the upper body must be used for all voluntary activities of daily living and exercise: arm cranking, wheelchair propulsion, or ambulation with orthotic devices and crutches. The proportionally smaller active upper body muscle mass typically restricts peak values of power output, oxygen consumption ($\dot{V}O_2$), and cardiac output to approximately one-half of those expected for maximal leg exercise in individuals without SCI.

In persons with tetraplegia, the pathologic effects are more extensive than with paraplegia. The active upper body muscle mass is partially paralyzed, and the sympathetic nervous system may be completely separated from control by the brain. Upper body power output and $\dot{V}O_2$, as well as cardiac output, are typically reduced to approximately one-half to one-third of the levels seen in individuals with paraplegia. Furthermore, strenuous exercise may not be tolerated because of orthostatic and exercise hypotension, which may produce dizziness, nausea, and other symptoms. Peak heart rates for individuals with tetraplegia typically do not exceed 120 contractions per minute.

EFFECTS OF EXERCISE TRAINING

Arm exercise training adaptations are believed to be primarily peripheral (muscular), and may include increased muscular strength and endurance of the arm musculature in the exercise modes used. These may result in 10% to 20% improvements in peak power output and peak oxygen consumption ($\dot{V}O_{2peak}$), as well as enhanced sense of well-being. Central cardiovascular adaptations to exercise training, such as increased maximal stroke volume or cardiac output, have not yet been documented.

MANAGEMENT AND MEDICATIONS

Management of individuals with paraplegia or tetraplegia is complex because of the multitude of associated complications, which include the following:

- Skin. Individuals with spinal cord disability should avoid sitting for long periods without pressure relief; avoid abrasion or bumping of bony weight-bearing areas of the hips, especially ischial tuberosities, sacrum, and coccyx; and sit on a cushion.

- Bones. Those working with spinal cord disability patients should avoid dropping during transfers or allowing the person to fall (e.g., from a wheelchair or exercise equipment). These individuals have an increased risk for fractures secondary to osteoporosis.

- Stabilization. If trunk control and balance are impaired, sufficient strapping and seat belts should be used during upright exercise.

- Handgrip or foot placement. The hands or feet of individuals with weak or absent handgrip or impaired foot control should be secured to ergometer and exercise equipment handles or pedals with elastic bandages, gloves with Velcro straps, toe clips, tape, and the like.

■ Bladder. People should empty their bladder or leg bag just before exercise testing to avoid bladder overdistension or overfilling of the leg bag during exercise, as this may induce autonomic dysreflexia (with hypertension) in persons with paraplegia above T6 or those with tetraplegia.

■ Bowels. A regular bowel maintenance program is useful to avoid autonomic dysreflexic symptoms in individuals with tetraplegia or prevent accidental bowel movement during exercise.

■ Illness. Exercise should be postponed if the person is ill (e.g., bladder infection, pressure ulcer, cold, flu, allergy, unusual spasticity, autonomic dysreflexia, constipation).

■ Hypotension. If resting blood pressure before the test is below 80/50 mmHg, the individual should wear elastic support stockings and an abdominal binder, or both, to elevate resting blood pressure. Exercise should be avoided within 3 h of eating a large meal because food intake may induce hypotension. Regularly monitor blood pressure and symptoms of hypotension (e.g., dizziness, lightheadedness, nausea, pallor, cyanosis, extreme or sudden weakness, mental confusion, visual disturbances, inability to respond to questions or instructions).

■ Hypertension. Autonomic dysreflexia is possible in persons with paraplegia above T6 or with tetraplegia. Preventive measures include proper bowel and bladder management. Monitor blood pressure regularly, and check for dysreflexic signs and symptoms. Discourage "boosting" (i.e., induction of autonomic dysreflexia to improve exercise tolerance).

■ Pain. Discontinue arm exercise that aggravates chronic shoulder joint pain. Overuse syndromes are common in people who use their arms to transfer themselves into and out of and propel wheelchairs.

■ Orthopedic. Bone or joint swelling, discomfort, or deformity may indicate fracture or sprain. Do not aggravate painful chronic shoulder overuse syndromes as these may involve rotator cuff injury or impingement syndrome, requiring medical management.

Allow the person to take normal prescription medications. However, be aware of medications or drugs that induce either hypotension (e.g., Ditropan [oxybutynin chloride], Dibenzyline [phenoxybenzamine hydrochloride]) or diuresis (e.g., alcohol, diuretics).

RECOMMENDATIONS FOR EXERCISE TESTING

Exercise testing an individual with a spinal cord disability should take into account the following recommendations (see table 39.1):

■ For clinical cardiovascular exercise testing, consult a medical or allied health professional with specific training in exercise testing of persons with paraplegia or tetraplegia. Utilize any reproducible exercise mode that is not contraindicated, such as arm or leg cycle ergometry or both (with or without electrical stimulation of paralyzed muscles), wheelchair ergometry, and rowing.

■ Consider functional mobility testing with timed wheeling or walking (6 to 12 min) or a custom-designed mobility obstacle course that includes potential environmental barriers such as ramps, stairs, curbs, doorways, soft or uneven surfaces, and turns and involves transfers, lifting, carrying, and manipulation of objects on shelves.

■ Adapt the exercise equipment as needed, and provide for special requirements in terms of trunk stabilization (straps), securing of hands on crank handles (holding gloves), skin protection (seat cushion and padding), prevention of bladder overdistension (i.e., emptying of bladder or use of urinary collection device immediately before test), and vascular support to help maintain blood pressure and improve exercise tolerance (elastic stockings and abdominal binder).

■ Use an environmentally controlled thermoneutral or cool laboratory or clinic to compensate for impaired thermoregulation.

■ Design a discontinuous incremental testing protocol that allows monitoring of heart rate, blood pressure, rating of perceived exertion, symptoms, and exercise tolerance at each stage. Power output increments may range from 5 to 20 W depending on exercise mode, level and completeness of paraplegia or tetraplegia, and activity and training status.

■ Expect peak power outputs to range from 0 to 50 W for persons with tetraplegia and from 50 to 120 W for those with paraplegia. Treat postexercise hypotension and exhaustion with recumbency, leg elevation, rest, and fluid ingestion.

TABLE 39.1

Spinal Cord Injury: Exercise Testing

Methods	Measures	Endpoints*	Comments
Aerobic			
Arm ergometer Wheelchair ergometer Wheelchair treadmill Wheeling on track or treadmill	■ Peak HR, METs, or $\dot{V}O_{2peak}$	■ Serious dysrhythmia ■ >2 mm ST-segment depression/elevation ■ Ischemic threshold ■ T-wave inversion with significant ST change ■ SBP >250 mmHg or DBP >115 mmHg	■ Adjust incremental power levels to subject's capacity. ■ Peak HR will be low (110-130 contractions/min) in tetraplegia (above T1) due to sympathetic impairment. ■ Persons with tetraplegia will need gloves or hand wrappings. ■ Give rest periods between stages (i.e., stop exercise). ■ Watch for hypertension from autonomic dysreflexia or hypotension caused by orthostasis and exertion. ■ Indicates basic exercise tolerance and effort.
	■ BP ■ RPE (6-20)		
Flexibility			
Goniometry Stretching tests	Flexibility of shoulders, elbow, wrist, hip, and knee		Helpful in preventing contractures and injury.

*Measurements of particular significance; do not always indicate test termination.

RECOMMENDATIONS FOR EXERCISE PROGRAMMING

Exercise training can provide a variety of health-related benefits for the individual with a spinal cord disability. The following recommendations should be considered in the development of an exercise program (see table 39.2).

■ Cardiopulmonary training modes may include arm cranking, wheelchair ergometry, wheelchair propulsion on treadmill or rollers, and free-wheeling; swimming; vigorous sports such as wheelchair basketball, quad rugby, and racing; arm-powered cycling; vigorous activities of daily living such as ambulation with crutches and braces; seated aerobic exercises; and electrically stimulated leg cycle exercise (ESLCE) or ESLCE combined with arm cranking.

■ To prevent upper extremity overuse syndromes, (1) vary exercise modes from week to week; (2) strengthen muscles of the upper back and posterior shoulder, especially external shoulder rotators; and (3) stretch muscles of anterior shoulder and chest.

■ Use an environmentally controlled, thermo-neutral gym, laboratory, or clinic for persons with tetraplegia. Individuals with thermoregulatory abilities can exercise outdoors if provisions are made for extreme conditions. Because of complications with autonomic dysreflexia, an unfortunate common practice of spinal cord injured athletes, emptying the bladder or urinary collection device immediately before exercise may prevent dysreflexic symptoms during exercise. The person should drink plenty of fluids after exercise.

■ The greater the exercising muscle mass, the greater the expected improvements in all

TABLE 39.2

Spinal Cord Injury: Exercise Programming

Modes	Goals	Intensity/Frequency/Duration	Time to goal
Aerobic Arm ergometer Wheelchair ergometer Wheelchair treadmill Free wheeling Arm cycling Seated aerobics Swimming Wheelchair sports Electrically stimulated leg cycle ergometry, with/without arm ergometry	■ Increase active muscle mass and strength ■ Maximize overall strength for functional independence ■ Improve efficiency of manual wheelchair propulsion	■ 40-90% $\dot{V}O_2R$ ■ 3-5 days/week ■ 20-60 min/session	4-6 months
Strength Weight machines or dumbbells Wrist weights	■ Increase active muscle mass and strength ■ Maximize overall strength for functional independence ■ Improve efficiency of manual wheelchair propulsion	■ 2-3 sets of 8-12 reps ■ 2-4 days/week	4-6 months
Flexibility Stretching	Avoid joint contracture	Before aerobic or strength activities	4-6 months

physiologic and performance parameters. Arm training will probably induce training effects in the arm muscles only; combined arm and leg exercise may induce both muscular and cardiopulmonary training effects.

■ Remember such training principles as specificity, overload, progression, and regularity.

SPECIAL CONSIDERATIONS

There are many special considerations in persons with SCIs.

■ Depression is common among people with paraplegia or tetraplegia. Be supportive and set realistic goals.

■ Cognitive impairment and learning disability are common among individuals with SB.

■ Expect small but progressive improvements in fitness (<5% per week). Progress may be interrupted periodically due to chronic secondary health conditions.

■ Always supervise individuals with tetraplegia. If they are not exercising in their own wheelchair, two assistants may be needed for manual transfer of large individuals to and from exercise equipment. Monitor blood pressure and symptoms regularly during exposure to orthostatic or exercise stress. Hypotension is common and may necessitate the use of support stockings and abdominal binder. To achieve good program adherence, provide supportive structure and motivation for those who need it.

- Follow the precautions outlined earlier (see "Management and Medications") concerning skin, bones, stabilization, handgrip, bladder, bowels, illness, hypotension, hypertension, pain, orthopedic complications, and medications. If necessary, hypotensive individuals should use supine posture and wear support stockings and abdominal binder to help maintain blood pressure. Avoid contacting persons with SB with latex products (e.g., coating on equipment, stretch bands, latex gloves).

- Consult the physician and appropriate allied health personnel to answer specific questions concerning medical complications to which the person may be susceptible.

- For individuals with tetraplegia and high-level paraplegia, exercise should take place only in thermally neutral environments, such as a laboratory or clinic with air conditioning to control temperature and humidity.

- In many conditions, little research is available to support specific guidelines. Thus, for some conditions the exercise professional may want to make some innovative recommendations.

- Osteoporosis may exist in leg bones; contractures may be present.

- Persons with tetraplegia will usually display bradycardia and have peak heart rate limited to approximately 120 contractions per minute. They do not adapt acutely to stressors such as heat or cold (e.g., blood shunting, shivering, and sweating may be profoundly impaired or abolished) or to exercise because of sympathetic dysfunction, including vasomotor paralysis, cardiac sympathetic blockade, and adrenal denervation. Orthostatic and exercise hypotension is common; individuals with quadriplegia are also at risk for deep venous thrombosis leading to pulmonary embolism.

- Depending on level of injury, forced expiration can be limited or absent.

- Skeletal muscle paralysis depends on the level and completeness of injury, with upper motor neuron injury producing spastic paralysis and lower motor neuron injury producing flaccid paralysis. Spastic paralyzed muscles can be electrically stimulated to produce movements for functional or therapeutic purposes; flaccid paralyzed muscles do not respond to electrical stimulation techniques. Paralyzed leg muscles are also aggravated by venous pooling secondary to loss of the venous muscle pump.

- Sensory loss depends on level and completeness of injury according to dermatome maps. Insensate weight-bearing areas are at risk for pressure ulceration and need periodic pressure relief.

- In some settings, electrically stimulated muscle contractions can recruit sufficient muscle mass to significantly increase $\dot{V}O_{2peak}$.

- $\dot{V}O_{2peak}$ depends on total active muscle mass.

- Voluntary anal sphincter control is often lost along with abdominal muscle denervation, necessitating a special bowel care program. Be sure that the bladder is empty prior to exercise.

- Keep the exercise environment thermally neutral.

Suggested Web Sites

American Spinal Injury Association. www.asia-spinal-injury.org

Christopher and Dana Reeve Foundation Paralysis Resource Center. www.paralysis.org

National Spinal Cord Injury Association. www.spinal-cord.org

Paralyzed Veterans of America. www.pvamagazines.com

Spinal Cord Injury Information Pages. www.sci-info-pages.com

Wheelchair Sports, USA. www.wsusa.org

CASE STUDY

Spinal Cord Injury

A 55-year-old male was in a car accident 25 years prior to evaluation and sustained a thoracic SCI resulting in incomplete T7 paraplegia. The muscle strength of his upper extremities and upper thorax was normal; but his abdominal muscles, other trunk musculature, and lower extremities were paralyzed. He had marked spasticity in the hip and knee flexors and ankle plantarflexors. He had gained 50 lb (22.7 kg) over the previous 15 years. He lived independently without assistance, but transferred independently with great difficulty using a sliding board. He pushed a manual wheelchair independently in the community and drove an adapted sedan.

S: "My shoulders hurt and my arms get tired, and I get short of breath pushing my wheelchair up inclines."

O: Vitals

Height: 5 ft 9 in. (1.75 m)
Weight: 220 lb (99.8 kg)
BMI: 32.6 kg/m^2
Supine HR: 75 contractions/min
Supine BP: 150/85 mmHg
Upright HR: 85 contractions/min
Upright BP: 140/95 mmHg
Medications: Baclofen, Dulcolax, Lipitor, lisinopril, metformin, glyburide

Labs

Fasting blood glucose: 200 gm/dl
HbA1c: 7.0%
Total cholesterol: 250 mg/dl
LDL: 150 mg/dl
Triglycerides: 200 mg/dl
HDL: 30 mg/dl

Late middle-aged, obese, paraplegic male
Triceps skinfold: 25 mm
Standard 4 m (13 ft) ramp test (12:1 slope): 15 s
6 min wheel test (dense-carpeted surface): 600 m (0.4 miles)

Graded exercise test (arm crank)

Peak power: 80 W
Peak HR: 150 contractions/min
Termination secondary to arm muscle fatigue and dyspnea (central RPE 9/10, peripheral RPE 10/10)
ECG: Normal at rest, 2 mmHg ST depression in 4 leads during peak exercise

Pain

Bilateral shoulder: 6/10 pain during wheelchair locomotion on flat ground; 8/10 during transfers

A: 1. Bilateral shoulder rotator cuff tears without impingement syndrome
2. Upper extremity deconditioning secondary to shoulder pain
3. Obesity
4. Type 2 diabetes mellitus
5. Dyslipidemia
6. Hypertension
7. Possible coronary artery disease

P: 1. Consult physical therapist about shoulder pain.
2. Increase physical activity to improve metabolic control of blood glucose, blood lipids, and hypertension.
3. Dietary counseling is necessary.

Mode	Frequency	Duration	Intensity	Progression
Aerobic (arm ergometer)	3 days/week	To fatigue forward and backward	1 day: 25 W 2 days: five 1 min intervals at 35 W	Increase as tolerated to 30-60 min/session. Advance to supervised swimming 2 days/week.
Strength (rickshaw, lat pulldowns, rowing, incline bench press)	2 days/week	2 sets of 10 reps	80% 1RM	Increase weight. Reassess every 2 weeks.
Flexibility (anterior chest, hip flexors, plantarflexors)	3 days/week	20 s/stretch	Maintain stretch below discomfort point	Progress as tolerated up to 20 min for contracted muscles.
Neuromuscular	3 days/week			
Warm-up and cool-down	Before and after each session	10-15 min	Light	

4. Consult cardiology to evaluate possible myocardial ischemia.
5. Reevaluate effectiveness of medications for diabetes, hypertension, and dyslipidemia.

Exercise Program Goals: Phase I (month 1)

1. Increase daily physical activity by 25%. Find activities that do not aggravate shoulder pain. Consider aquatics, seated aerobics, and therapeutic exercises.

2. Pain-free ADLs using everyday wheelchair.
3. Physical therapy: Increase strength, endurance, and overall muscle balance of shoulder and upper back.

Exercise Program Goals: Phase II (months 2-12)

1. Exercise at home and in an accessible fitness facility/clinic 5 days/wk.
2. Lose 20 kg (44 lb) of fat weight.
3. Repeat graded exercise test after 12 months.

40

Muscular Dystrophy

Mark A. Tarnopolsky, MD, PhD

OVERVIEW OF THE PATHOPHYSIOLOGY

Muscular dystrophies (MDs) are a group of more than 30 genetic diseases characterized by progressive muscle weakness, defects in muscle proteins, and eventual death of muscle cells and tissue resulting in degeneration of the skeletal muscles. Depending on which type of MD an individual has, symptoms can be mild and progress slowly or may progress rapidly and produce severe muscle weakness, functional disability, and loss of the ability to walk. Although there are currently no specific treatments to stop or reverse any form of MD, recent strides made in understanding the genetic bases and cellular consequences (necrosis or apoptosis of muscle cells or both) of MD are encouraging and hopefully leading researchers toward effective treatments and a cure for MD someday. This chapter focuses on the most common MDs, including the dystrophinopathies (Becker MD [BMD] and Duchenne MD [DMD]), facioscapulohumeral (FSHD), limb girdle (LGMD), myotonic (MD), and Emery-Driefuss (EDMD), and excludes myopathies (e.g., channelopathy, metabolic, endocrine, congenital, and inflammatory) and congenital MD.

Complete and partial MDs (DMD and BMD, respectively) are caused by an X-linked recessive genetic disorder that results in a deficiency of the dystrophin protein, which links contractile proteins to the sarcolemma. Duchenne MD is the most common form of childhood MD and primarily affects boys (~1 in 3500 live male births). Symptoms include proximal muscle weakness beginning at 3 to 4 years of age, calf muscle hypertrophy, and a very high plasma creatine kinase (CK) activity. Duchenne MD progresses to involve distal muscles, at which time ambulation becomes more difficult. By the age of 10, most children with DMD use wheelchairs exclusively and will eventually develop scoliosis. Some children with DMD will also have cognitive developmental delays. The course of BMD is less aggressive, with most children remaining ambulatory beyond the age of 12. Severe respiratory and cardiac problems are common in children with DMD and BMD by the time they reach early adulthood.

The limb girdle MDs are broadly divided into autosomal recessive disorder (carrier parents have a 25% risk of an affected child) and autosomal dominant (an affected parent has a 50% chance of passing the disease on to offspring). The autosomal recessive form of LGMD has an earlier onset and a more rapid progression, often as severe as that seen in DMD. The LGMDs are usually caused by mutations in genes encoding for cytoskeletal proteins (e.g., sarcoglycans), although other proteins such as calpain 3 can also be involved. Individuals with LGMD are also at high risk for cardiac and respiratory problems as they age.

Facioscapulohumeral dystrophy is an autosomal dominant condition that is named after the muscles that are most affected. Recent discoveries show that the genetic cause of FSHD is related to a deletion in chromosome 4 in a noncoding region. The majority of individuals with FSHD will notice some facial weakness and periscapular weakness by the late teens, which will slowly progress to involve the biceps, tibialis anterior, and thigh muscles. Most people with FSHD remain ambulatory well into their 50s and 60s; however, there are rare cases of a more severe phenotype with infantile onset, cognitive delays, and hearing loss.

Emery-Dreifuss MD is usually an X-linked recessive disorder, although some forms are autosomal dominant. The X-linked form of EDMD is caused by a mutation in the emerin gene, while the autosomal dominant form is caused by a mutation in the lamin A/C gene. Both the lamin A/C and emerin genes are involved in the nuclear envelope and are critical for skeletal muscle satellite cell differentiation. The emerin form of MD is characterized by the development of elbow, Achilles tendon, and cervical spine contractures, followed by atrophy and weakness of the upper arms and peroneal muscles. The lamin A/C form of MD usually results in less severe proximal weakness of both the arms and legs with less contracture development. Both forms of EDMD are often associated with cardiac conduction blocks and atrial paralysis.

Myotonic MD is the most common form of adult-onset MD. It is an autosomal dominant disorder caused by a mutation (trinucleotide [CTG] expansion) in the untranslated region of the myotonin kinase gene. The size of the CTG expansion is reasonably well correlated with the severity of the phenotype. For the most common intermediate-severity form, slow progressive atrophy, weakness, and myotonia affect distal muscles with onset in the teens. In more severe cases, children can present with a congenital form with severe life-threatening weakness and cognitive delays, while in milder cases the disease may go unnoticed aside from premature cataracts. In addition to muscle-related problems, these individuals may have balding, cataracts, swallowing problems, cardiac conduction block, gastrointestinal dysmotility, and diabetes. Relatively recently, a second form of myotonic dystrophy has been recognized and characterized at the genetic level, leading to the designation of the more "classical" form already described as myotonic dystrophy type 1 (DM1) and the newer form as myotonic dystrophy type 2 (DM2). DM2 is caused by a tetra-nucleotide (CCTG) repeat in the zinc finger 9 gene, and shares most of the features of DM1 except for proximal muscle involvement, absence of a congenital form, no cognitive impairment, and often associated muscle pain.

EFFECTS ON THE EXERCISE RESPONSE

Isometric and isokinetic strength may be within normal limits early in the course of a dystrophy. For example, children with DMD often have normal strength until age 3 to 4, when progressive proximal weakness begins. It is also important to understand the underlying disease process and patterns of weakness. For example, clients with FSHD may have completely normal handgrip strength and yet be unable to raise their arms above their head. Expectedly, knee extension strength is more affected in limb girdle and dystrophinopathies as compared with DMD. The loss of isometric and isokinetic strength parallels the loss of functional capacities. Individuals without a structural cardiomyopathy usually have a normal heart rate, ventilation, and rating of perceived exertion at a given relative exercise intensity of cycling; however, the loss of strength renders the absolute values higher than those in age-matched controls. Alterations in gait pattern (e.g., waddling, high stepping, and excessive lordosis) can lead to an abnormally high oxygen cost per unit of work (speed) on a treadmill. For this reason, a cycle ergometer, and in severe cases, a reclining ergometer is most helpful in assessment and in exercise prescription. The use of orthotics can reduce the oxygen cost of ambulation, and testing the client with and without an orthosis may be beneficial.

EFFECTS OF EXERCISE TRAINING

Several prospective studies have examined the effect of resistance exercise on muscle strength in clients with dystrophinopathies. In general, from the results of five studies on more than 100 DMD clients, one can state that there is no evidence that exercise induces a more rapid decline in strength (i.e., overuse). Overall, about half of the participants experienced mild improvements in strength and activities of daily living with moderate resistance exercise and stretching (usually three times a week). In the more slowly progressive dystrophies (e.g., LGMD, FSHD, myotonic), several studies have used more traditional weight training programs (≤80% of 1-repetition maximum [1RM]) and shown increases in strength and functional capacity. In general, muscles with mild to moderate weakness are those that are most likely to show improvements. These muscles are weaker than antigravity strength and are likely to show improvement with exercise.

MANAGEMENT AND MEDICATIONS

In spite of substantial advances in the understanding of the molecular bases for the dystrophies, there is currently no cure. As a result, management is focused upon the maintenance of function through exercise, orthoses, medication, and in some cases surgery. Therapeutic exercise is focused on the prevention of contractures (stretching), attenuating (and in some cases maintaining or even temporarily increasing) strength (strength training), and maintaining cardiovascular health (aerobic exercise). Aerobic exercise is important in preventing body fat accumulation and reducing cardiovascular risk factors in dystrophies in which survival into adulthood is possible. Because most of the dystrophies primarily affect the proximal muscles, the main orthotic device that has been used is the knee-ankle-foot orthosis, which may prolong independent ambulation. In myotonic MD, where the weakness is distal, an ankle-foot orthosis is particularly helpful.

The main surgeries considered in clients with dystrophies are for release of contractures (e.g., ankles, adductors) and correction of scoliosis. It is very important for therapeutic exercise to be continued as much as possible during the perioperative period to prevent deconditioning. A traumatic fracture can be the precipitating factor halting independent ambulation. The only medications that have been consistently shown to attenuate strength loss in clients with dystrophinopathies are corticosteroids. Overall, these result in about a 4% to 6% increase in strength that can delay degeneration beyond critical levels of function. Corticosteroids are associated with a loss of bone mass, attenuation in linear growth, increased body fat, insulin resistance, cataracts, and increased blood pressure. Given that children with DMD have low bone mass even before they begin to take corticosteroids, it is important to measure bone mass prior to starting corticosteroids and to provide prophylaxis (calcium and vitamin D; in severe cases, bisphosphonates). Several studies have shown that creatine monohydrate supplementation (~0.1 g/kg per day) can increase muscle strength and lean body mass, and a Cochrane review has supported these independent findings.

RECOMMENDATIONS FOR EXERCISE TESTING

Important qualitative and quantitative information is obtained from exercise testing of an individual with MD. Clinicians should consider the following recommendations when completing these evaluations (see table 40.1). The primary focus of exercise programming is on gaining muscle strength and muscular endurance. Therefore, testing is designed to guide such programming. Muscular power and peak aerobic power are of secondary importance, especially from a day-to-day clinical perspective.

- Manual muscle testing (i.e., 5-point Medical Research Counsel scale) is often used in a clinical setting; however, a very large decline in strength can go undetected before the grade changes.

TABLE 40.1

Muscular Dystrophy: Exercise Testing

Methods	Measures	Endpoints*	Comments
Aerobic			
Cycle (ramp protocol 5 W/2 min; staged protocol 5-10 W/min)	▪ 12 lead ECG, HR	▪ Serious dysrhythmias ▪ >2 mm ST-segment depression or elevation ▪ Ischemia ▪ T-wave inversion with significant ST change ▪ Chest pain	12-lead initially for DMD, BMD, EDMD, or any patient over age 40.
	▪ BP	▪ SBP >250 mmHg or DBP >115 mmHg ▪ Hypotensive response	
	▪ RPE (6-20)	▪ Volitional fatigue	

Methods	Measures	Endpoints*	Comments
Muscular endurance and power Wingate test Isokinetic fatigue test	▪ Peak and mean power ▪ Mean power in first 5 and last 5 contractions	▪ 30 s or voluntary termination ▪ 50 contractions	Not possible in moderate to severe cases.
Strength Grip strength Knee extension Weight machine Spirometry	▪ Isokinetic torque at 30 and 180 rad/s ▪ Isometric ▪ Peak strength ▪ FVC, FEV$_1$	▪ Peak strength ▪ Peak value ▪ Best RM ▪ Best of 3 attempts	▪ 3 measurements. ▪ 2 min rest between speeds. ▪ Measure 1 proximal + 1 distal muscle in upper and lower extremities.
Flexibility Goniometry	ROM	Maximal range (3 attempts)	Ankle, knee, and hip are important.
Neuromuscular Gait/balance analysis	▪ Foot drop ▪ Trendelenburg gait ▪ Antalgic gait		Sophisticated equipment is required to semiquantitate.
Functional capacity Lifestyle-specific tests: ▪ Put on a T-shirt ▪ 4-stair climb ▪ Square (1 in.^{2} [2.54 cm^2]) cut art ▪ Supine to stand ▪ Walk/run 20 in. (50.8 cm)	▪ Time ▪ Time up and down ▪ Time to cut square (from standard 4 ft^2 [1.2 m^2] paper) ▪ Time to get up (feet together) ▪ Time from tape		▪ Indicate with/without handrail. ▪ Use plastic (children's) scissors. ▪ Use wheelchair if not ambulatory.

*Measurements of particular significance; do not always indicate test termination.

- Objective testing should include handgrip dynamometry and a handheld dynamometer at a minimum.
- Ideally, an isokinetic dynamometer (0°/s is isometric) should be used to follow individuals at least every 12 months (or more frequently for more rapidly progressive dystrophies).
- Objective testing should be used before any therapeutic trial (e.g., drugs, surgery).
- Pulmonary function testing should be a part of the battery of standard tests available to the clinician (minimum of FVC and FEV$_1$).
- In symptom-limited maximal graded exercise testing, heart rate, blood pressure, electrocardiogram (ECG), and rating of perceived exertion should be recorded.
- It is important to modify the testing and adapt the device to the individual.
- Body composition should be measured and followed using bioelectric impedance, dual-energy X-ray absorptiometry (DEXA) scan, or air displacement. These data can be used to provide dietary advice to maintain an acceptable percentage of body fat and to follow lean

mass. It is important that the same method be used longitudinally for each person because intertest variance is high. Ideally, the same person should perform each test to minimize intertester variability.

RECOMMENDATIONS FOR EXERCISE PROGRAMMING

The primary focus of exercise for individuals with MD is on gaining muscle strength and endurance while paying close attention to flexibility to aid in the prevention of contractures (see table 40.2).

- Provide manageable short-term goals to each individual and follow up closely in the initial stages of the program to ensure safety and encourage compliance.
- With weight training, start at a low percentage (~50%) of individual 1RM and with more than 10 repetitions. Gradually increase the percentage of 1RM as tolerated over a period of weeks to months. (This is a function of individual preference; however, some clients can eventually tolerate up to 75% of 1RM, three sets of 10-12 repetitions.) It is important to allow for at least 48 h of rest for a given muscle group

(e.g., Monday, Wednesday, Friday schedule). It is important to tell the client to "listen to your body" and to decrease the intensity if mild myalgias do not disappear after 36 to 48 h or if muscles cramp during activity. In addition, any myoglobinuria (red, brownish, tea colored) must be immediately reported to the clinician and no exercise completed until this is sorted out. Pigmenturia, prolonged myalgias, or a subjective loss of strength should be reported to the attending clinician, and the client should be evaluated.

- When muscles are weaker than antigravity strength, formal weights are essentially useless and the goal becomes to exercise through the available range of motion, and then to regain full range against gravity and to prevent contractures.
- For children, it is important to make the activities as game-like as possible.
- Stretching, to prevent contractures and to maintain overall flexibility, should be performed daily.
- Any client with dystrophy should exercise with a partner, drink plenty of fluids, and avoid strenuous exercise in conditions of high heat and humidity.

TABLE 40.2

Muscular Dystrophy: Exercise Programming

Modes	Goals	Intensity/Frequency/Duration	Time to goal
Aerobic Cycling Walking/treadmill Elliptical trainer Rowing Arm ergometry	- Maintain/increase aerobic capacity - Decrease cardiac risk factors	- 4-6 days/week - 50-80% HRR - 20-40 min/session - Until fatigue (goal: ≥20 min)	
Flexibility Stretching	- Increase ROM - Prevent contractures	- Daily - Hold for 20 s/stretch	4-12 weeks
Functional Activity-specific task (i.e., wheelchair propulsion)	Maintain and enhance proficiency in ADLs	Daily as tolerated	

SPECIAL CONSIDERATIONS

Knowledge of the characteristics of the specific dystrophy is very important in order to adapt the exercise testing and prescription to the individual. Cardiac involvement is the most significant ancillary factor to consider in exercise prescription. Cardiomyopathy can be seen in DMD, BMD, and some forms of LGMD and EDMD and can limit exercise capacity via a central pumping limitation (decreased oxygen delivery). Cardiac conduction defects (e.g., Atrio-ventricular blocks) can be seen with EDMD and myotonic MD. These may also limit oxygen delivery through incomplete filling of the atria or dropped contractions. An ECG and an echocardiogram should be performed on all DMD, BMD, EDMD, and LGMD clients with a cardiology consult before exercise prescription or testing.

Contractures are another important factor to consider in exercise prescription, for these may severely limit the ability to use certain testing or training devices. Exercise and range of motion are the mainstays of therapy in contracture treatment. Lack of motivation to exercise is a significant issue, particularly in individuals with myotonic MD and some more severely affected children with DMD.

Safety issues are important. For example, individuals with myotonic MD often find that they have more myotonia in the cold; hence, they should avoid swimming in cold water. Myotonia can also be a significant disability in sports that require a rapid relaxation of the hand (e.g., throwing sports). Recent evidence has shown that individuals with DMD (and likely many other types of dystrophy) have low bone mineral content. Dual-energy X-ray absorptiometry scanning for individuals with MD who wish to participate in contact sports may also be a consideration. If the bone mineral content is low, interventions can range from bisphosphonates and avoidance of all contact sports (severe) to recommending calcium supplements and follow-up (mild). Cataracts can limit the ability of clients with myotonic dystrophy to perform sports that require hand–eye coordination. A stationary cycle and cataract removal are possible suggestions for such a client.

Prednisone and deflazacort (corticosteroids) are often used in children with DMD and in some with BMD. These drugs cause an increase in fat mass and reduce bone mineral content. With obesity, it may be appropriate to initiate exercise using weight-supported activities. Any child on prednisone should be followed yearly with a DEXA scan, and all should be taking supplemental calcium and vitamin D. Exercise is the most potent modality to attenuate the negative effects of corticosteroids on muscle and bone and should be encouraged for all individuals on these drugs. Finally, there has been the suggestion that individuals with dystrophies are more likely to have malignant hyperthermia, which is a rare life-threatening condition caused by a drastic and uncontrollable increase in body temperature that eventually leads to circulatory collapse and death if untreated. Although true malignant hyperthermia (autosomal dominant genetic channelopathy) is not likely to be more prevalent in the dystrophy population per se than in other groups, the underlying muscle destruction could lead to an abnormally high release of myoglobin into the urine with resultant renal failure.

A high percentage of individuals with MD do not meet the daily required dietary intake for energy, for protein, and for a large number of vitamins and minerals as well. Given that many with MD do not expend much energy, a low energy intake is the likely cause of their inability to meet U.S. and Canadian dietary guidelines. Ideally, a dietary assessment by a nutritionist with dietary advice is recommended; however, from a practical perspective, most individuals with MD do not consume enough energy to meet the vitamin and mineral recommendations, and a multivitamin is often required.

It is important to consider several issues when working with an individual with dystrophy. Among these are safety, exercise intensity, mode of exercise, and psychological aspects.

Safety

Some dystrophies are associated with cardiomyopathy (e.g., dystrophinopathies, some types of LGMD) and others with conduction block (e.g., EDMD, myotonic MD). A diagnostic exercise stress test should be performed before the beginning of an exercise program. Some individuals may require other cardiac diagnostic procedures such as an echocardiogram and a cardiology consult before starting.

Even in the face of a conduction block and cardiomyopathy, the design of an exercise program is possible using well-established guidelines for individuals with primary cardiac problems. Plasma CK activity can fluctuate even without an antecedent trigger, so there is no point in following the activity of this marker. However, establishing a baseline plasma CK value is warranted. This may take several determinations until a mean value can be established and will also provide day-to-day variance in the measure. If an individual loses strength more rapidly than expected, check the plasma CK; and if it is more than 2 standard deviations (SDs) above the individual's mean, decrease the exercise intensity and review for other factors that may have contributed to this rise. Individuals with dark urine (tea colored or foamy, indicative of myoglobinuria) should notify their physician and cease physical activity until evaluated. Finally, bone mass may already be low in someone with dystrophy, and the mode of activity should be modified if bone mass is critically low.

Ergometry

Ergometers should be adaptable for arm cranking as well as cycling. The ergometer should be capable of functioning at very low work rates (≤5 W). In addition, the work rate increments should be capable of increasing in 1 to 2 W increments. A reclining cycle ergometer is sometimes required for individuals with poor balance or weakness to the degree that upright cycle ergometry would be dangerous.

Psychological Aspects

Participation in physical activity is important for all individuals with MD, because this is one of the few forms of activity in which an afflicted individual can feel a sense of control and self-direction. Physical activity allows a sense of self-determination and control over a disorder that often takes away one's independence. Daytime somnolence is a particular factor in myotonic MD that may be correlated with reduced motivation. Providing follow-up and support is important, particularly in the initial stages of the program, to enhance compliance and success.

Suggested Web Sites

National Center on Physical Activity and Disability. www.ncpad.org

Neuromuscular Disease Center. www.neuro.wustl.edu/neuromuscular

---

CASE STUDY

Limb Girdle Muscular Dystrophy

A 45-year-old male was diagnosed with autosomal dominant LGMD 10 years earlier, after he had noted difficulty running around the bases in a baseball league. He stopped all activities because he was told that exercise would make his disease worse. Since then, he had gained 25 lb (11 kg) and developed increasing difficulty climbing up the 10 steps to his bedroom (initially he had been fatigued when doing this; then his legs became heavy). He needed to use his arms to pull himself up the stairs. He also had osteoarthritis in the knees, but was otherwise healthy and did not smoke.

S: "I'm afraid I'll have to sell my house and move to a single-floor dwelling."

O: Vitals

Height: 5 ft 7 in. (1.7 m)
Weight: 198 lb (89.9 kg)
BMI: 31.1 kg/m²
Normal mental status, cranial nerves, reflex and sensory exam
Motor exam: Shoulder abductors 4/5; hip flexors 3/5; neck extension 4/5
More distal muscles graded at >4+/5
Routine blood tests (CBC, electrolytes, creatinine, BUN, and liver function): Normal
Serum CK: 430 U/L (normal: <230 U/L)
Spirometry: Normal

Grip strength: Right 35 kg (77 lb); left 32 kg (70.5 lb) (normal)
Isometric knee extension: Right 5 kg (11 lb); left 4 kg (8.8 lb) (>2 SD below lower limit of normal)

A: 1. LGMD limiting ADLs (stair climbing)
   2. Obesity
   3. Osteoarthritis (knees)

P: 1. Increase strength in the limb and knee extensors.
   2. Prescribe dietary counseling for weight loss.

Exercise Program Goals

1. Ability to ascend stairs
2. Increased knee extensor strength
3. Weight loss

Follow-Up

The client developed some knee pain when he first increased to 70% of 1RM; however, this resolved with 1 week of decreasing to 60% and taking an occasional acetaminophen. After 12 weeks, he could climb stairs without using his arms. His isometric knee extension strength improved to (right) 8 kg (17.6 lb) and (left) 7 kg (15.4 lb) by dynamometry. Grip strength and weight were unchanged, but he decreased to 25% body fat.

Mode	Frequency	Duration	Intensity	Progression
Aerobic (cycling)	3 days/week	8 min/session	THR (>120 contractions/min)	Increase to 15-20 min at HR >140 contractions/min as tolerated.
Strength (isometric knee extensions)	3 days/week	1 set of 12 reps	40% 1RM	Increase to 3 sets of 12 reps at 70% of 1RM.
Flexibility (all major muscle groups)	Daily	20-60 s/stretch	Maintain stretch below discomfort point	
Warm-up and cool-down	Before and after each session	10-15 min	RPE <10/20	

Epilepsy

Karl Otto Nakken, MD, PhD

OVERVIEW OF THE PATHOPHYSIOLOGY

Epilepsy is a common chronic neurological disorder characterized by recurrent unprovoked seizures due to brief, excessive discharges of electrical activity in the brain. An estimated 2.7 million Americans have epilepsy. Epilepsy afflicts all ages, but especially young children and the elderly. Approximately 10% of Americans will experience at least one seizure sometime during their lifetime, and about 3% of the population will have had a diagnosis of epilepsy by age 80. Epilepsy is also slightly more common in males than in females. Epilepsy can be caused by a number of factors, including genetic, congenital, and developmental factors among children and tumors, head trauma, central nervous system infections, injury, and stroke in adults. However, in 60% to 70% of individuals with epilepsy, the cause is of unknown origin. A diagnosis of epilepsy may not necessarily be a lifetime condition; some forms of epilepsy are limited to particular stages of childhood or events such as pregnancy. There is no cure per se, but epilepsy can usually be controlled with medication. In rare circumstances, surgery may be considered for uncontrollable seizures that do not respond to medication. Like any other chronic disease, epilepsy can often severely affect an individual's physical and mental health, including interfering with normal daily activities.

Seizures are temporary alterations in brain functions due to an abnormal electrical discharge within a select group of brain cells. For an electric discharge to create a seizure, a large number of cells abnormally linked together have to fire simultaneously, causing "an electrical brainstorm." The communication between nerve cells is delicately balanced by factors that can cause rapid increases (excitation) or decreases (inhibition) in electrical activity within these cells. In seizure disorders, the underlying abnormality may be either or both of the following: (a) loss of or damage to cells that inhibit excitatory cells or limit the spread of electrical discharges, or (b) an imbalance between excitatory (e.g., glutamate) and inhibitory (e.g., gamma-aminobutyric acid [GABA]) neurotransmitters, leading to increased excitability. Several diseases and injuries that affect the gray matter of the brain can lead to such an imbalance.

There are two main categories of seizures: those that are localized within a particular area of the brain, called partial seizures, and those that are distributed throughout the brain, called generalized seizures. Partial seizures involve an electrical disturbance to a specific area of just one cerebral hemisphere, and are the most common type of seizure experienced by individuals with epilepsy.

Acknowledgment
The editors wish to acknowledge the previous author of this chapter, Lorraine E. Bloomquist, EdD, FACSM.

Partial seizures are further subdivided into simple partial seizures, in which consciousness is retained, and complex partial seizures, in which consciousness is impaired or lost. Partial seizures can be caused by congenital dysplasia, hypoxia, trauma, infections, mass lesions, or stroke that may selectively damage specific areas of the brain, such as the hippocampus. Partial seizures can evolve into generalized seizures that affect both cerebral hemispheres from the beginning of the seizure and result in loss of consciousness, either briefly or for a longer period of time. In generalized seizures, genetic factors that regulate the production of neurotransmitters or neuronal membrane components appear to play a critical role.

Epileptic seizures increase the risk of trauma and fractures, dislocations, burns, and aspiration pneumonia. However, the consequences of epilepsy are numerous and extend far beyond seizures; just a few of the complicating factors in epilepsy are adverse drug effects; psychosocial problems due to social stigma; isolation; anxiety; depression; and restriction on education, transportation, and vocation. Most individuals with epilepsy are of normal intelligence, but there are also considerable neurological, cognitive, or psychiatric comorbidities or problems in this group.

An accurate diagnosis of seizure type and epilepsy syndrome is critical to achieving successful treatment. In addition to a thorough seizure history and neurological examination, individuals should have a neurophysiological and neuroimaging evaluation, including a standard electroencephalogram (EEG). Sometimes a prolonged video EEG recording obtained after sleep deprivation, magnetic resonance imaging (MRI), single-photon emission computed tomography (SPECT), and positron emission tomography (PET) may be useful in diagnosing epilepsy and helpful in identifying what region of the brain has been affected or helpful in the classification of the type of epileptic syndrome. A physical examination including blood tests should be done to rule out systemic disorders that can cause seizures (e.g., hypotension, diabetes, liver or kidney disease, hyperthyreosis, electrolyte deviations, alcohol abstinence). The diagnosis of epilepsy requires documenting the presence of recurrent, unprovoked seizures of cerebral origin.

Among the epilepsies are several syndromes characterized by age at seizure onset, seizure type, EEG findings, neurological status, response to treatment, and prognosis.

All kinds of paroxysmal occurring symptoms, with or without preserved consciousness, may be of epileptic origin. If seizures arise in a limited area of the brain, the initial ictal symptom reflects the function of that area. The ictal symptoms may have predominantly motor, sensory, autonomic, or psychic features. Epileptic seizures are classified according to their clinical features (semiology) and pattern seen in EEG. As already noted, they are divided into two main types: generalized and partial (focal) seizures.

Generalized Seizures

- **Absences.** Brief episodes (2-15 s) of staring with impairment of awareness and responsiveness. These seizures begin usually between 4 and 14 years and often resolve at the age of 18. The children are usually of normal intelligence.

- **Atonic seizures.** Brief episodes (<15 s) of sudden loss of muscle tone that causes the head to nod or the person to fall. These seizures start in childhood.

- **Tonic seizures.** Sudden bilateral stiffening of the body, including arms and legs. These seizures last less than 20 s and occur most commonly during sleep.

- **Myoclonic seizures.** Ultrashort jerks of a muscle or a group of muscles; most often bilateral jerks of the neck, shoulders, and upper arms. These seizures are seen in a variety of epilepsy syndromes.

- **Tonic-clonic seizures.** These major convulsions are the seizure type most people associate with epilepsy. The seizures begin with loss of consciousness and include a tonic phase (stiffening), a sudden cry, a fall, and a subsequent clonic phase consisting of jerking of the upper and lower limbs. Average duration is 1 to 2 min. Other signs include drooling, tongue biting, and bladder or bowel incontinence. The person may sleep or be confused after the seizure.

Partial Seizures

- **Simple partial.** In these seizures, the patient is alert and able to respond to questions and afterward remember what happened during the seizure. Such seizures may precede complex partial or secondary generalized tonic-clonic seizures. Dependent on the localization of the seizure onset, the attacks may have a diversity of symptoms, which can make diagnosis challenging; and vague symptoms may go unnoticed.

- **Complex partial.** In these commonly occurring seizures, staring is accompanied by impaired consciousness and recall. Semiautomatic movements, named automatisms, occur most often and involve mouth and face (lip smacking, chewing); upper limbs (fumbling, picking); vocal apparatus (grunts, repetition of words or phrases). They can also include more complex acts like walking, running, or undressing. Average duration is 30 to 120 s. Postictal confusion is common and usually lasts for less than 15 min.

EFFECTS ON THE EXERCISE RESPONSE

Individuals with epilepsy can participate in almost all sports and physical activities, provided they do so using common sense and some restrictions when indicated. The critical factor in recommending and planning exercise programs for individuals with epilepsy is seizure control. The primary concern is that the individual could risk bodily harm if a seizure should occur, especially in light of the type of activity he or she is participating in. Thus, the risk of exercise depends on the type of seizure and type of activity.

Advising people with epilepsy concerning physical exercise takes into consideration three categories:

- Sports with no restrictions
- Sports with restrictions (safety precautions, e.g., helmet when bicycling or horseback riding, life jacket in boats)
- Sports that are prohibited (e.g., rock or rope climbing, hang gliding, parachuting, unsupervised swimming, diving, and motor sports)

The risk of having a seizure during exercise is usually smaller than during the postexercise relaxation period. Physical exercise reduces the occurrence of epileptiform discharges in EEG and does not change the serum levels of the antiepileptic drugs to a clinically important extent. In 30% to 40% of the population with epilepsy, regular physical training yields a moderate seizure-protecting effect. However, in approximately 10%, strenuous exercise may act as a seizure precipitant. Among those prone to exercise-induced seizures, there seems to be a preponderance of patients with poor physical fitness and symptomatic epilepsies, that is, an underlying morphological brain lesion.

The underlying mechanisms of interaction between epilepsy and physical exercise are mainly unknown. The influence of exercise on the seizure threshold may be direct or indirect and may be both psychological and physiological. A uniform brain activation by increased attention and a stream of afferent impulses from receptors in muscle and tendon spindles, increased levels of beta-endorphins and catecholamines, a low-grade metabolic acidosis, stress reduction, and increased well-being may all contribute to an increased seizure threshold. A widespread misconception is that an exercise-induced increase in ventilation can provoke seizures.

EFFECTS OF EXERCISE TRAINING

Many individuals with epilepsy are overprotected and lead isolated and sedentary lives. Thus, they tend to be physically unfit and to avoid sport participation. However, studies have shown that people with epilepsy can achieve the same physiological and psychological benefits from regular physical exercise that apparently healthy individuals do.

MANAGEMENT AND MEDICATIONS

Individuals with epilepsy are an extremely heterogenous group of patients, especially with respect to how they respond and adapt to exercise. Information on seizure type(s), frequency and pattern, auras, known precipitants, medication, additional comorbidities, and past experiences with exercise should all be taken into consideration before an individual with epilepsy is allowed to participate in sport or other physical activities. Avoidance of seizure-precipitating factors like stress, sleep deprivation, alcohol, and irregular drug and food intake is important. The type of activity selected should take into account the individual's preferences and should occur in a safe and pleasant atmosphere. All personnel should be informed regarding the risk of a seizure and be trained and educated in how to respond if a seizure should occur.

Tonic-Clonic Seizures

General and immediate first aid procedures for tonic-clonic seizures include the following:

- Keep calm, and do not attempt resuscitation.
- Try to break a fall to prevent the head from being struck.
- Place the individual on his or her back and put a protecting towel or jacket under the head.
- Clear the area.

- Loosen the individual's tie, belt, and collar.
- Place the person's head to the side or roll the person onto the side to drain saliva.
- Do not put anything in the individual's mouth, and keep your hands away from the teeth.
- Do not administer liquids.
- If the seizure lasts longer than 3 min, if a second seizure begins soon after the first has ceased, or if the seizure occurs in water (danger of water aspiration), call 911 immediately.
- Look for medical identification (e.g., medic alert ID).
- Observe that the individual is breathing.
- Stay with the individual until you are sure that he or she is self-supporting.

Absence or Complex Partial Seizures

The following are first aid procedures for individuals with absence or complex partial seizures:

- Do not touch, but observe the individual's movement.
- Keep the person away from the pool side, the top of stairs, or anywhere a fall is possible.
- Remove harmful objects.
- Speak quietly and in a friendly manner.
- Stay with the individual until full consciousness returns.

If necessary, arrange for safe transportation and follow-up evaluation by medical staff after a seizure.

Treatment Options

Antiepileptic drugs (AEDs), various kinds of epilepsy surgery, vagal nerve stimulation, ketogenic diets, avoidance of seizure precipitants, and addressing psychosocial problems are the most commonly used therapies for epilepsy. Commonly used epilepsy drugs include the following:

- Luminal (phenobarbital): A barbiturate and the most widely used anticonvulsant worldwide. Side effects include sedation, hypnosis, dizziness, nystagmus, and ataxia.
- Dilantin (phenytoin): The first modern anticonvulsant drug produced. Side effects include clumsiness, insomnia, motor twitching, nausea, rash, gum overgrowth, hairiness, and thickening of features.

- Tegretol (carbamazepine): Used in the treatment of all types of partial seizures and in treatment of generalized tonic-clonic (grand mal) seizures. Tegretol is usually described as a first-line treatment. Side effects include drowsiness, headache, dizziness, blurred vision, difficulty in thinking, diarrhea, double vision, nausea, and vomiting.
- Depakene or Depakote (valproic acid): Useful in treating absence seizure (petit mal), myoclonic epilepsy, and primary generalized epilepsy (grand mal). Side effects include a decrease in appetite, nausea, and vomiting when starting on the drug. Depakote is the same drug as Depakene but made differently to avoid this problem. Dizziness, tremor, imbalance, and sedation may occur especially when valproic acid is used in conjunction with other drugs.
- Lamictal (lamotrigine): Used as add-on therapy for partial seizures (with or without secondary generalization) in adults and for partial and generalized seizures associated with the Lennox-Gastaut syndrome in children. Side effects include double vision (diplopia), drowsiness, dizziness, ataxia, headache, nausea and vomiting, and rash.
- Klonopin (clonazepam): Belongs to a family of drugs called benzodiazepines. Klonopin may be prescribed for a variety of seizure types and syndromes, including absence seizures, myoclonic, atonic (drop attacks), and Lennox-Gastaut syndrome. It is most often used as an add-on drug to other antiepileptic drugs. Side effects include drowsiness, slurred speech, double vision, dizziness, behavioral changes, depression, and worsening of tonic-clonic seizures.
- Neurontin (gabapentin): Typically prescribed as add-on therapy for partial seizures with or without secondary generalization (spread to become a grand mal seizure). Side effects include sedation, fatigue, dizziness, and unsteadiness.
- Keppra (levetiracetam): Used as an add-on therapy for partial seizures in adults. Side effects include sleepiness, unsteadiness, infection, behavior disturbance, and dizziness.
- Trileptal (oxcarbazepine): Related to Tegretol, TegretolXR, Carbatrol, and Epitol (carbamazepine). Trileptal was developed in an effort to combine the effectiveness of these related drugs with fewer side effects and drug interactions. It is used as single-drug therapy (monotherapy) and as add-on therapy (adjunctive) in adults and children 4 years of age and older with partial seizures. Side effects include fatigue, headache, dizziness, sleepiness, unsteadiness, nausea, vomiting, and double vision.

■ Topamax (topiramate): Used as an add-on medication for adults and children (2 to 16 years old) with partial seizures with or without secondary generalization or primary generalized tonic-clonic seizures, and for seizures associated with the Lennox-Gastaut syndrome. Side effects include difficulty with concentration, speech and language problems, cognitive slowing, drowsiness, dizziness, tingling of distal extremities and face, unsteadiness, and fatigue.

Drugs used in the treatment of epilepsy have different mechanisms of action, potential for pharmacokinetic interactions, and effect and side effect profiles. Most adverse effects are related to the target organ (the brain), for example somnolence, ataxia, tremor, dizziness, nausea, vomiting, increased or decreased appetite, and concentration and coordination difficulties. Rash, elevated liver enzymes, and hormonal changes may also be seen. Drug levels in serum and side effects need to be monitored. Most side effects tend to subside early after drug initiation, and many persons experience no side effects at all.

RECOMMENDATIONS FOR EXERCISE TESTING

When seizures are controlled, standard exercise testing can be used (see table 41.1). As strenuous exercise may precipitate seizures in unfit individuals, personnel should be alert, especially during and immediately after maximal testing. The exercise professional should be aware that certain medications (e.g., phenobarbital, Dilantin, Depakote) may cause side effects including lethargy, loss of coordination, tremors, weight changes, and inattention.

RECOMMENDATIONS FOR EXERCISE PROGRAMMING

With few exceptions, regular physical activity is recognized as beneficial to people including those with epilepsy. Several studies have shown that exercise training in individuals with epilepsy improves functional capacity and confers psychological and social benefits as well. Exercise does not seem to

TABLE 41.1

Epilepsy: Exercise Testing

Methods	Measures	Endpoints*	Comments
Aerobic Cycle (ramp protocol 17 W/min; staged protocol 25 W/3 min stage) Treadmill (1-2 METs/stage)	■ 12-lead ECG, HR	■ Serious dysrhythmias ■ >2 mm ST-segment depression or elevation ■ Ischemia ■ T-wave inversion with significant ST change ■ SBP >250 mmHg or DBP >115 mmHg ■ Volitional fatigue	Testing and screening may be warranted if risk factors/symptoms of CAD are present (see chapter 6 exercise testing table).
	■ BP		
	■ RPE (6-20)		
Muscular endurance 6 and 12 min walks	Distance	Time	Useful for measurement of improvement throughout conditioning program.
Strength Free weights Weight machines	1RM or MVC		

*Measurements of particular significance; do not always indicate test termination.

influence the average frequency of seizures or the serum concentrations of antiepileptic drugs to a clinically important degree. If seizures are controlled, persons with epilepsy are encouraged to participate in most athletic activities (see table 41.2), including collision and contact sports. It is important that the individual with epilepsy feel normal; this reinforces a positive self-image. Individual sports may be preferred above team activities. As training adaptations occur, for example weight loss or gain (as might result from such sports as cross country running or weight training), the dose of medications may need to be adjusted. Several factors that can influence or provoke seizures (and can possibly occur during sports or exercise) have been postulated, including fatigue, stress of competition, hypoxia, hypothermia, and hypoglycemia; however, no studies to date have shown conclusively that sport participation provokes seizures. While regular physical activity is beneficial to the individual with epilepsy, participation in certain sporting activities (e.g., scuba diving, rock climbing, boxing and other combative sports) is contraindicated.

Evidence-Based Guidelines

Glauser T, Ben-Menachem E, Bourgeois B, et al. ILAE treatment guidelines: Evidence-based analysis of antiepileptic drug efficacy and effectiveness as initial monotherapy for epileptic seizures and syndromes. Epilepsia. 2006 Jul;47(7):1091-1093.

Karceski S, Morrell M, Carpenter D. The expert consensus guideline series: Treatment of epilepsy. Epilepsy Behav. 2001;2(6).

Scherer A. New guidelines on the treatment of epilepsy with the new antiepileptic drugs from the Epilepsy Foundation. Epilepsy Behav. 2004;5(4):433-434.

Suggested Web Sites

Epilepsy Foundation of America. www.efa.org

Epilepsy Foundation of Northeast Ohio. www.efneo.org

University of Maryland Medicine. www.marylandepilepsy.com

TABLE 41.2

Epilepsy: Exercise Programming

Modes	Goals	Intensity/Frequency/Duration	Time to goal
Aerobic Large muscle activities	Increase $\dot{V}O_{2peak}$, work rate, and endurance	▪ 60-90% peak work rate ▪ 3-5 days/week ▪ 20-40 min/session ▪ Progressively increase intensity and duration	4-6 months
Strength Isotonic or isokinetic exercises	▪ Improve general fitness ▪ Prevent muscle atrophy	Low resistance, high reps to start	

CASE STUDY

Epilepsy

A 60-year-old man was a successful teacher when he developed epilepsy. He had several episodes with reduced consciousness; these also occurred while he was operating a vehicle. Sometimes he felt tingling on the right side of his face. Occasionally he would babble incoherently for several seconds. He had no known head injury. An EEG clearly showed epileptiform discharges in the left temporal lobe. Cerebral MRI was normal. Dilantin and Tegretol both caused a rash, but Depakote controlled his seizures. He wanted an exercise program to help control his weight and improve his fitness.

S: "I want to get in better shape."

O: Vitals

BP: 130/80 mmHg
HR: 80 contractions/min
Respirations: 14 breaths/min
Elderly male in no distress
Neurological exam: Slight tremor, mild ataxia, otherwise normal

Lungs and heart sounds: Normal
Normal peripheral pulses, no edema
ECG: Normal
Medications: Valproic acid

Graded exercise test (Bruce protocol)

Exercise tolerance: 5 METs
Peak HR: 150 contractions/min
No significant ST changes or dysrhythmias

A: 1. Complex partial seizures, etiology unknown
    2. Deconditioning

P: 1. Monitor blood levels, liver function tests, and side effects.
    2. Initiate a walking program.

Exercise Program Goals

1. Increase functional capacity
2. Reinforce lifestyle changes/medical management

Mode	Frequency	Duration	Intensity	Progression
Aerobic	3 days/week	20 min	THR (55-70% HR_{max}) RPE 11-14/20	Increase to 30 min at 60-70% HR_{max}. RPE 12-14/20 after 12 weeks.
Strength (all major muscle groups)	3 days/week	1 set of ≤10 reps	50-70% of 1RM	Increase to 2 sets of 10-12 reps after 12 weeks.
Flexibility (all major muscle groups)	3 days/week	20 s/stretch	Maintain stretch below discomfort point	Increase ROM as tolerated.
Warm-up and cool-down	Before and after each session	10-15 min	RPE <10/20	

Multiple Sclerosis

Kurt Jackson, PhD, PT, GCS ■ Janet A. Mulcare, PhD, FACSM

OVERVIEW OF THE PATHOPHYSIOLOGY

Multiple sclerosis (MS) is thought to be an auto-immune disease that damages the insulating myelin of the central nervous system. These inflammatory "attacks" occur randomly and vary widely in severity, frequency, and duration. The loss of myelin, the fatty material that insulates nerves, adversely affects rapid, smooth conduction along the neural pathways in the central nervous system and subsequently interferes with smooth, rapid, coordinated movement. Most patients are first diagnosed with the disease between the ages of 16 and 60 years with a peak at age 30. Multiple sclerosis is more common in women than men by a ratio of 2 or 3 to 1. The course of MS is unpredictable and can range from benign to rapidly progressing.

EFFECTS ON THE EXERCISE RESPONSE

Depending on the level and nature of impairment associated with the disease, individuals may experience a variety of symptoms that may directly affect their responses to a single exercise session. These symptoms may include the following:

- Spasticity
- Incoordination
- Impaired balance
- Fatigue
- Muscle weakness, paresis (partial paralysis), and paralysis
- Sensory loss and numbness
- Cardiovascular dysautonomia (dysfunction of the autonomic nervous system causing possible problems with cardioacceleration and reduction in blood pressure response)
- Tremor
- Heat sensitivity

EFFECTS OF EXERCISE TRAINING

Exercise training has no effect on the prognosis or progression of MS. However, exercise may improve short-term physical fitness and functional performance (e.g., strength, endurance, aerobic fitness, fatigability, and mobility).

For example, results from a recent meta-analysis show that exercise training is associated with small improvements in walking mobility among individuals with multiple sclerosis, with the greatest benefits resulting from supervised exercise training programs. In addition, a four-week aerobic training program consisting of five 30-minute sessions per week of bicycle ergometer exercise (individualized for exercise intensity) significantly improved aerobic threshold, health perception, increased levels of activity, and there was a tendency towards a reduction in general fatigue in individuals with MS. Furthermore, an eight-week progressive resistance training program significantly increased lower body strength, improved ambulation, and decreased self-reported fatigue in patients with MS.

MANAGEMENT AND MEDICATIONS

Several medications (disease-modifying agents) are now commonly prescribed to persons immediately following diagnosis of the disease. Clinical trials have shown a reduction in both the number and severity of exacerbations with these drugs. Often individuals with MS are also prescribed various medications to manage the assorted symptoms associated with the disease. The following are drugs that are commonly prescribed for persons with MS, along with common side effects that may alter exercise response, tolerance, or both.

Disease-Modifying Agents

- Interferon beta-1a (Avonex, Rebif): flu-like symptoms, injection site irritation
- Interferon beta-1b (Betaseron): flu-like symptoms, injection site irritation
- Glatiramer acetate (Copaxone): injection site irritation
- Mitoxantrone (Novantrone): fever or chill, swelling of legs, cough or shortness of breath
- Natalizumab (Tysabri): fatigue, joint pain, depression

Symptom Management

- Amantadine, modafinil (Provigil): May reduce fatigue.
- Baclofen (Lioresal), tizanidine (Zanaflex): May cause muscle weakness and fatigue.
- Amitriptyline (Elavil), fluoxetine (Prozac): May cause muscle weakness.
- Prednisone: May cause muscle weakness, reduced sweating, hypertension, diabetes, osteoporosis.

RECOMMENDATIONS FOR EXERCISE TESTING

Common symptoms that affect ambulation (e.g., lower extremity sensory decrement or loss, foot drop due to tibialis anterior weakness, balance difficulty, muscle spasticity, ankle clonus) often make treadmill testing impractical for this population. Therefore, the preferred mode of clinical exercise testing is either upright or recumbent leg cycle ergometry (see table 42.1). If a combination arm-leg ergometer is available, the increase in activated muscle mass may improve test results by eliciting greater cardiopulmonary stress. In both types of ergometry, toe clips and heel straps are recommended to ensure foot stability and counteract spasticity, tremor, and weakness in the lower extremities. When using the combination ergometer, arm and leg movements are mechanically linked to reduce the need for motor coordination. Individuals who are more severely impaired with significant lower extremity paresis or paralysis may use arm cranking as a viable alternative to leg cycling. However, the primary problem associated with arm cranking is that arm muscle fatigue occurs before a true cardiopulmonary maximum is elicited. The following are other recommendations for performing exercise testing with those who have MS.

- Morning is usually the optimal time to test.
- Use a continuous or discontinuous protocol of 3 to 5 min stages.
- Begin with a warm-up of unloaded pedaling or cranking.
- Use a fan for cooling.
- Increase the work rate for each stage by approximately 12 to 25 W and 8 to 12 W for legs and arms, respectively.
- Monitor heart rate and blood pressure.
- Use a category–ratio RPE scale to estimate stress level.
- Typical test termination criteria are volitional fatigue, achievement of maximal heart rate, or decrease or plateau in oxygen consumption ($\dot{V}O_2$) with increasing work rate.

Research has shown that $\dot{V}O_{2peak}$ varies greatly among individuals with MS and is to some extent related to the individual's lower extremity impairment. Because very few data are available that can be reported by gender, age, and impairment level, it is difficult to provide standard values as guidelines. In the absence of cardiovascular dysautonomia or severe muscle paresis, research has shown that most individuals with MS are able to reach 85% to 90% of their age-predicted maximal heart rate.

TABLE 42.1

Multiple Sclerosis: Exercise Testing

Methods	Measures	Endpoints*	Comments
Aerobic Schwinn Air-Dyne Recumbent cycle (17 W/min) Recumbent stepper Ramp protocol (12-25 W/3 min stage) Discontinuous protocol (3-5 min/stage) 6 and 12 min walk tests	■ Expired gases ■ HR ■ Rate–pressure product ■ RPE (6-20) ■ BP ■ Distance walked	■ $\dot{V}O_{2peak}$, METs ■ HR_{peak} ■ Volitional fatigue ■ SBP >250 mmHg or DBP >115 mmHg ■ Hypotensive response	■ $\dot{V}O_{2peak}$, METs, and RPE are often best for exercise prescription because of possible cardiovascular dysautonomia. ■ Attenuated BP response may occur.
Strength Isokinetics 10RM Manual muscle testing 30 s sit to stand test	■ Torque, power ■ 10RM weight ■ MMT grade ■ Number of sit to stands	Volitional fatigue	■ Isokinetics are reliable in persons with MS. ■ MMT least reliable and responsive to change. ■ Sit to stands are a functional measure of LE strength, power, and muscular endurance.
Flexibility Goniometry Sit and reach	■ Joint angles ■ Distance reached	Maximum ROM	Focus on ankle dorsiflexion, hip extension, finger/wrist extension, and two-joint muscles.
Neuromuscular Gait analysis Balance Tone Fatigue	■ Gait speed, distance ■ Berg Balance Scale ■ Ashworth Scale ■ Modified Fatigue Impact Scale	NA	Numerous functional scales are appropriate.

*Measurements of particular significance; do not always indicate test termination.

RECOMMENDATIONS FOR EXERCISE PROGRAMMING

Exercise prescription for individuals with MS should focus on maintenance, and when possible, on improvement of joint flexibility, muscular strength, balance, and cardiopulmonary endurance. Exercise professionals should be aware of the following when prescribing exercise programs for people with MS:

- Fatigue can reduce exercise tolerance.
- Impaired balance may affect the choice of exercise mode.
- Heat intolerance may affect intensity, duration, mode, and environmental demands.
- Spasticity may require special foot strapping.
- Sensory loss may preclude upright activities, such as walking or running.
- Muscle paresis can reduce exercise intensity and duration.

Despite these factors, most persons with mild to moderate disability can realize benefits of exercise training similar to those for persons without MS. People with more severe disability are less likely to demonstrate marked improvement with the use of traditional exercise methods.

Because fatigue is a common complaint, any intervention that can increase energy by improving efficiency should be incorporated into a well-balanced exercise program. This might include activities related to the areas already mentioned as well as activities that focus on weight control or reduction (see table 42.2). Finding exercise activities that have combined effects can help to improve exercise efficiency and reduce fatigue. For example, standing hip abduction with resistance can improve hip strength as well as single-leg balance.

SPECIAL CONSIDERATIONS

When working with an individual who has MS, exercise personnel need to keep in mind possible psychological dimensions as well as the variability of progression of the disease itself. There are also considerations relating to safety and the exercise environment. Many individuals with MS have some level of cognitive deficit that will affect their understanding of testing and training instructions. They may also have memory loss sufficient to require written instructions to supplement verbal cues. These individuals may require additional time for information processing as well as multiple forms of information presentation to ensure understanding.

The symptoms of MS commonly recur, resulting in progressive impairment. In some people, this progression is slow and may take years, while in others the disease may progress significantly within weeks or months. Exercise professionals should be aware of the various symptoms experienced by persons with this disease and should recognize the effects that such symptoms may have on exercise performance. The exercise professional should also be sensitive to daily variation in symptoms that can be influenced by changes in medications, sleep disorders, and increases in environmental or circadian temperature. Daily training expectations should be flexible to accommodate these factors. Personnel should be knowledgeable regarding transfers, lift-

TABLE 42.2

Multiple Sclerosis: Exercise Programming

Modes	Goals	Intensity/Frequency/ Duration	Time to goal
Aerobic Cycling Walking Swimming	Increase/maintain cardiovascular function	■ 60-85% HR_{peak} ■ 50-70% $\dot{V}O_{2peak}$ ■ 3-5 days/week ■ 30 min/session	4-6 months
Strength Weight machines Free weights Isokinetics Resistance bands	Increase strength, power, and functional performance	■ 2-3 days/week ■ 1-2 sets ■ 8-15 repetitions ■ 50-70% MVC	4-6 months
Flexibility Stretching	Increase/maintain ROM and manage spasticity	■ Perform daily. ■ Hold minimum of 30-60 s for 2 repetitions. ■ Contracture may require prolonged stretch >20 min.	Ongoing

ing, and assistance techniques for individuals with physical disabilities.

If clients experience an exacerbation, they should not be encouraged to exercise until the disease status returns to full remission, meaning that the symptoms manifested during the exacerbation have diminished or disappeared. Once it is determined that the person is in remission, a new baseline of exercise performance should be established and goals should be adjusted. For the client whose disease is progressing slowly, increased impairment may be very subtle, and distinct improvement may not be as obvious. In these cases, the goal of the exercise program may be simply to slow any further physical deterioration and optimize remaining function.

Some persons with MS have either attenuated or absent sudomotor (sweating) responses. This impairment can further compound the already heightened sensitivity to increases in internal and external temperature that appear to adversely affect many individuals with MS. Therefore, even for moderate-intensity aerobic exercise, room temperature should be kept neutral (72° to 76° F [~20° to 22° C]). Fans should be provided upon request. Persons with MS should be encouraged to drink water before, during, and after each exercise session. For moderate-intensity aquatic exercise, water temperature between 89° and 91° F (~28° and 29° C) is sufficiently comfortable and offers significant heat-dissipating potential. There is some evidence that precooling prior to aerobic exercise may have a beneficial effect on performance. In contrast, surface cooling during submaximal exercise does not appear to increase exercise time.

Urinary incontinence, as well as urgency and frequency, is common. Because of this concern, some individuals self-limit fluid intake. Education on the importance of adequate hydration with an increase in activity level may be needed. Proximity and accessibility of rest rooms is another important consideration.

The general lack of uniformity among research protocols in this area and the variability in aerobic exercise capacity among persons with MS make it difficult to develop absolute standards for comparison. Therefore, expected outcomes from training in this group are often less evident than they would usually be. Preliminary data show that after a six-month program of moderate aerobic exercise, people with MS may show an average aerobic fitness gain of 30%; however, the variability among individuals is extremely high (i.e., 2% to 54%). Evidence shows that as impairment increases, the magnitude of improvement in training response will be less and the length of time needed to observe improvements will be longer.

Evidence-Based Guidelines

Multiple sclerosis. National clinical guideline for diagnosis and management in primary and secondary care. National Collaborating Centre for Chronic Conditions. London, UK: National Institute for Clinical Excellence (NICE); 2004. p. 197.

Suggested Web Sites

National Center on Physical Activity and Disability. www.ncpad.org

National Multiple Sclerosis Society. www.nmss.org

CASE STUDY

Multiple Sclerosis

The client was a 51-year-old female with a 14-year history of relapsing-remitting MS. She was currently using Betaseron for her disease management and was taking Baclofen for her spasticity. She had no other significant past medical history. The patient was referred to a community-based wellness program for persons with chronic neurological disorders.

S: *"I would like to be able to walk farther with just a cane. I also want to feel more confident that I won't fall."*

O: Vitals

Height: 5 ft 5 in. (1.65 m)
Weight: 108 lb (49 kg)
BMI: 18.5 kg/m²
HR: 80 contractions/min
BP: 100/81 mmHg
ROM: WNL except for end-range tightness in left hip extension, ankle dorsiflexion, and shoulder external rotation

(continued)

Mode	Frequency	Duration	Intensity	Progression
Aerobic Recumbent stepper (NuStep), walking on indoor track lightly touching rail	3-5 days/week	7-10 min	• THR (60-75% HR_{max}) • RPE 11-13/20	• Increase to 30 min at 65-80% HRmax. • RPE 12-14/20. • Increase walking speed/distance.
Strength (focus on antigravity and postural/trunk muscles)	2-3 days/week	1-2 sets of 8-15 reps	To moderate volitional fatigue; rest 2 min between sets	Increase resistance as tolerated 2-5% once she can perform 15 reps.
Flexibility (anterior chest, hip flexors, plantarflexors)	Daily	2 reps, hold 60 s each	Perform slowly so as not to elicit spasticity/clonus	Increase ROM as tolerated.
Neuromuscular Progressive balance activities (perform standing in corner with chair in front for protection)	2-3 days/week	5-10 min	Should provide sufficient challenge to cause occasional loss of balance	Increase difficulty by sensory manipulation, decrease base of support, increase speed/amplitude of movement.
Functional Walking with cane with guarding by husband	Daily trials	As tolerated	As tolerated	Increase distance, speed as able.
Warm-up and cool-down	Before and after each session	2-3 min	RPE 9-10/20	Increase time to 5-10 min as total exercise time increases.

Strength: 4/5 in left upper extremity, 3+/5 in left lower extremity, 5/5 in right upper and lower extremity

Sensation: Moderate impairment of proprioception in left lower extremity

Tone: Moderate increase in extensor tone on left with 2-3 beat ankle clonus

Motor control: Moderate truncal and left-sided ataxia

Balance: 32/56 on the Berg Balance Scale, high fall risk

Gait: Ambulates household distances with 4-wheel walker

Functional tests

6 min walk test: 392 ft (119 m) with 4-wheel walker, HR 108 contractions/min

Five-repetition sit-to-stand test: 14 s

A: Client demonstrates poor functional endurance for walking as well as balance and coordination deficits which make her a high fall risk.

P: Instruct client in a comprehensive exercise program to improve functional endurance, antigravity muscle strength, and postural control.

Exercise Program Goals

1. Increase gait to community distances with use of walker or cane
2. Improve balance and postural control
3. Improve long-term health and wellness

Polio and Post-Polio Syndrome

Thomas J. Birk, PhD, MPT, FACSM

OVERVIEW OF THE PATHOPHYSIOLOGY

Poliomyelitis (polio) is a highly infectious viral disease that attacks the nervous system, causing inflammation of the motor neurons and total paralysis. Until vaccines became widely available in the late 1950s, polio was a debilitating childhood disease that crippled thousands of children in the United States every year. Polio has been eliminated in the United States and throughout most of the world, with the exception of several developing countries that remain polio endemic. Despite the possibility of paralysis and even death, most people exposed to the polio virus don't develop any symptoms or permanent damage. The remaining forms of polio are classified based on the severity of their symptoms:

Abortive Polio

Abortive polio does not involve the central nervous system and is considered a minor illness, occurring mainly in young children. Symptoms are described as flu-like, including a slight fever, headache, sore throat, vomiting, constipation, and diarrhea. Full recovery typically occurs in 24 to 72 h with no permanent side effects.

Nonparalytic Aseptic Meningitis

Approximately 8% to 10% of polio infections affect the outer covering (meninges) of the brain. Signs and symptoms last from two to 10 days and include symptoms similar to those of abortive polio, in addition to pain or stiffness in the back, neck, arms, or legs; muscle spasms or tenderness; and sensitivity to light. Recovery is complete.

Paralytic Polio

Less than 1% of those infected with the poliovirus develop paralysis. Paralysis appears in one to 10 days following symptoms that include loss of reflexes; severe muscle aches; and muscle spasms in the arms, legs, or back with paralysis worsening over time. Paralysis is likely permanent if muscle weakness or paralysis lasts a year or more, but muscle strength eventually returns in the majority of people.

Up to 40 years after contracting acute poliomyelitis during peak epidemic periods, at least one-fourth of the affected population have developed symptoms similar to those of the initial onset of the disease. Common symptoms include general fatigue and exhaustion with minimal activity, weakness, and muscle and joint pain. Other symptoms are sleep disorders and intolerance of cold. The collection of these symptoms is termed post-polio syndrome (PPS). Post-polio syndrome is more prevalent and intense in the muscles of the lower extremities (LE). Paramount to the diagnosis are new and increasing pain and weakness. New pain and weakness coupled with positive electromyography (EMG) and nerve conducting velocity findings facilitates greater diagnostic accuracy. The muscle weakness associated with PPS is secondary to chronic overload and eventual loss of motor units through the aging process. When a critical level of less than 50% of the original total number of motor units is reached, symptoms of fatigue, weakness, and pain become apparent. Other factors contributing to weakness, fatigue, and pain include excessive body fat (overloading already weakened leg muscles) and repetitive physical tasks (overloading a smaller muscle mass).

EFFECTS ON THE EXERCISE RESPONSE

The majority of individuals with PPS whose LE have been affected will have altered acute responses to exercise. Post-polio patients can be expected to exhibit significantly diminished leg strength and aerobic capacity when compared to asymptomatic post-polio individuals of similar age. These changes associated with PPS appear secondary to a loss of motor units whereby fewer motor units can be activated to generate muscle tension, resulting in diminished strength and endurance. Thus, an additional burden is placed on the remaining motor units, which can hasten the onset of fatigue. Aerobic power is diminished in many individuals with PPS and appears to be related to muscle weakness and deconditioning. A lack of LE muscle strength also limits walking speed. An everyday walking speed for someone with PPS imposes considerably greater cardiovascular stress than in apparently healthy adults and only somewhat less than in someone with congestive heart failure. Labile exercise blood pressures also pose potential risks that should be initially monitored. Secondary to premature peripheral fatigue, maximal heart rates are usually 20 to 30 contractions per minute lower than what would be expected for asymptomatic post-polio individuals of similar age. Concurrently, maximal oxygen consumption ($\dot{V}O_{2max}$) is typically up to 20% lower than would be seen in similarly aged counterparts.

EFFECTS OF EXERCISE TRAINING

Although there are few well-controlled prospective studies, the literature suggests that LE strength and aerobic capacity can be significantly increased in persons with PPS. The relative improvements in aerobic capacity have equaled those for asymptomatic post-polio persons of similar age. However, complications of prolonged high-intensity exercise were joint edema, possible deformity, and general muscle discomfort. Consequently, the best results were achieved at moderate intensities. Documented beneficial changes in stable PPS include the following:

- Increases of 15% to 20% in aerobic capacity with moderate-intensity exercise after at least eight weeks of training
- Increases in quadricep and hamstring muscle strength after at least six weeks of moderate to hard resistive training
- A tendency of warm water exercises of moderate intensity and duration to reduce pain and increase cardiovascular conditioning

Only some individuals with PPS exhibit a marked reduction in elbow flexor strength in response to upper extremity (UE) exercise training. However, diminished strength adaptations after 12 weeks are seen with moderate isometric hand exercise training. Studies evaluating UE adaptations suggest that each limb should be evaluated separately.

MANAGEMENT AND MEDICATIONS

Primary means of managing and treating PPS have included energy conservation, bracing and splinting, and medication. Strength and moderate-intensity aerobic exercise training have been used as adjunctive therapy. The performance of exercise testing and training in the morning of relatively nonstressful days is advised in order to avoid physical overstressing and effort overextending. To avoid excessive fatigue, encourage the use of a wheelchair or scooter if long periods of standing or walking are anticipated or planned. The following are some guidelines for bracing and splinting.

- Support the joint around which muscles have significantly weakened and when abnormal structural problems indicate excessive "wear and tear."

- Fitting and braces and splints should allow for sufficient range of motion during exercise.
- Braces and splints increase muscular efficiency during activities of daily living, not during exercise.
- Fasten one or more limbs to ergometer pedals or handles when necessary.

Medications for pain, chronic fatigue, and sleep disorders are commonly prescribed for individuals with PPS. Nonsteroidal anti-inflammatory drugs and muscle relaxants have been used to reduce symptoms of peripheral pain. Tricyclic antidepressants, such as Elavil, may increase heart rate and decrease blood pressure during rest and exercise. Electrocardiogram abnormalities have included false positive and false negative exercise test results, as well as possible T-wave changes and dysrhythmias, especially in persons with a cardiac history. Exercise may help to alleviate some of the prevalent anticholinergic side effects, such as constipation and lethargy. The therapeutic effect of these medications may be delayed by two to four weeks after the beginning of therapy. Additional medication changes include the following:

- Tricyclic antidepressants (Elavil) can negatively affect motivation.
- Antidepressants (e.g., Elavil, Pamelor, Sinequan, Prozac, Zoloft) inhibit neurotransmitters (i.e., serotonin, norepinephrine), thus decreasing anxiety and improving sleep.
- Bromocriptine mesylate, a postsynaptic dopamine receptor agonist, inhibited early morning fatigue in one study but has not been used with exercise.
- Pyridostigmine, an anticholinesterase drug, has shown some beneficial effects on quadriceps strength and subsequent walking; but the positive functional changes were found only in those with normal-sized motor units or less severe symptoms of PPS.

RECOMMENDATIONS FOR EXERCISE TESTING

Exercise testing of persons with PPS should incorporate the following principles:

- Optimally utilize available muscle mass.
- Avoid use of a painful or recently weakened limb during an exercise test.
- Use equipment that does not require complex motor coordination.
- Use submaximal exercise tests.
- Ideally use a four-limb ergometer (e.g., Schwinn Air-Dyne with foot straps or pegs [or both] for resting inactive or nonfunctional limbs
- Consider use of discontinuous protocols in readily fatigued individuals.

Four-limb ergometry is preferred, but for persons with severe lower limb involvement, an arm crank ergometer is recommended (see table 43.1). Four-limb ergometry activates the greatest possible

TABLE 43.1

Polio and Post-Polio Syndromes: Exercise Testing

Methods	Measures	Endpoints*	Comments
Aerobic			
Schwinn Air-Dyne	■ V̇O$_{2peak}$, physical work capacity	■ Serious dysrhythmias	■ Use only if diagnosed CAD or related symptoms are present.
Arm ergometer (or any upper/lower limb ergometer)		■ >2 mm ST-segment depression/elevation	
	■ 12-lead ECG, maximal HR	■ Ischemic threshold	■ Calculate efficiency index.
		■ T-wave inversion with significant ST changes	■ Estimates functional capacity and predicts type or amounts of ADLs and occupational tasks possible.
	■ BP	■ SBP >250 mmHg or DBP >115 mmHg	
	■ RPE 6-20	■ Volitional fatigue	
	■ METs		

(continued)

TABLE 43.1 *(continued)*

Methods	Measures	Endpoints*	Comments
Endurance 6 and 12 min walk 1-mile (1.6K) walk	▪ Distance ▪ Time	Note time, distance, symptoms at rest stops	▪ Can be adapted. ▪ 1-mile (1.6K) walk may be too long in some cases.
Strength Weight machines Dynamometers	▪ Submaximal endurance of stable and unstable limbs ▪ Maximal voluntary contraction	Fatigue	▪ Dynamometer: hip and knee flexion/extension and ankle dorsi- and plantarflexion should be measured; no more than a 6 s effort at 45° angle. ▪ Monitor and document changes caused by intervention or neuromuscular changes.
Flexibility Sit and reach Goniometry	▪ Reach distance ▪ Angle at full flexion/extension	▪ Full ROM ▪ Full ROM	▪ Sit and reach measures middle and lower back flexibility, which is important for static and dynamic balance. ▪ Goniometry measures specific joint active and passive ranges.
Neuromuscular Gait and balance analyses EMG/Nerve conduction studies	 ▪ Conduction velocities ▪ Action potential waveforms		▪ Gait and balance analyses are useful in determining static and dynamic balance and locomotion if ambulatory. ▪ Nerve conduction studies, along with EMG, are useful in diagnosis and prognosis of stable motor units and their available readiness.
Functional Sit to stand Lifting	▪ Balance and symmetry ▪ Balance, symmetry, and safety in techniques	▪ 10 reps completed; extensive use of arms; fatigue ▪ Potentially poor technique; fatigue	Use for ADLs and occupational tasks.

*Measurements of particular significance; do not always indicate test termination.

muscle mass, and if necessary the use of a painful or recently weakened limb or muscle group can be minimized while the other limbs are still allowed to exercise. Because it increases the active muscle mass, use of a four-limb ergometer presents a greater challenge for the cardiopulmonary system. The four-limb ergometer should include a cycling mechanism for the legs and either a cycling or push-pull mechanism for the arms. Work rate should be measurable, accurate, and repeatable.

The testing protocol should deviate from standard procedures by using a submaximal intensity over an increased period of time. Although some persons with PPS can be maximally tested, excessive residual fatigue and possible further reduction of motor units could result from excessive maximal testing. A submaximal intensity eliciting at least a "somewhat hard" rating of perceived exertion (RPE), performed continuously for at least 6 min, facilitates an accurate estimation of aerobic fitness while minimizing possible motor unit damage. Terminating the test at a "hard" RPE (15/20) should enable the tester to challenge the cardiopulmonary system to reach 85% of age-predicted maximum heart rate. If 85% is not reached and coronary artery disease is not suspected, an additional stage of higher intensity can be used and should not unduly debilitate the subject unless new and increasing peripheral pain and weakness were present prior to testing.

Research on validity and reliability for an effort-limited treadmill walk test in persons with PPS has shown that individuals tend to walk at their self-determined speed for as long as it takes to reach an RPE of 15 or "hard" or a pain intensity level of 7/10. The distance achieved using this protocol is similar to that with the "get up and go" test. The distance walked on the treadmill also correlates with pain during activities of daily living (ADLs).

Exercise MET (metabolic equivalent) values may range from 2 to 9 METs, depending on the limitation of skeletal muscle. Heart rate responses to acute maximal exercise may range from 120 contractions per minute (for elderly persons using only the arms) to 175 to 180 (for middle-aged persons using all four limbs). Both exercise systolic and diastolic blood pressures are generally similar to those observed for post-polio persons without PPS. Blood lactate concentration responses may range from 2 to 8 mmol/L during exercise testing. Ventilatory responses during exercise are approximately 10% to 20% lower than those observed in asymptomatic post-polio persons of similar age. Ratings of perceived exertion tend to focus on the peripheral component reflecting peripheral muscular fatigue.

Consequently, the most limiting factors appear to be peripheral fatigue and pain, as opposed to central cues such as dyspnea. Premature muscle fatigue and low $\dot{V}O_{2max}$ explain the lower maximal ventilation. Peak external power outputs during four-limb ergometry range from 15 to 200 W.

Exercise testing considerations may include utilization of stirrups, straps, or both for pedals and use of straps, gloves, or both for hands on the handlebars or arm crank handles. These adaptations will secure weakened limbs to equipment, thus providing more efficient application of force and protection of impaired limbs. Discontinuous protocols are advised for individuals with chronically weakened muscles because this facilitates higher central physiological responses while delaying fatigue of exercising muscles.

RECOMMENDATIONS FOR EXERCISE PROGRAMMING

The primary purpose of an exercise program for persons with PPS is similar to that for their asymptomatic counterparts: to prevent premature onset of hypokinetic diseases and maintain adequate muscle strength and endurance for occupational and leisure pursuits. However, individuals without PPS can usually perform a wider range of intensities and durations without long-lasting residual complications; the person with PPS usually has a narrower range of acceptable exercise intensities. If persons with PPS overestimate their maximum intensity, they may risk premature acceleration of motor unit loss. The following principles of aerobic exercise prescription are based on symptoms and history. Recent symptoms of pain and weakness warrant a preparticipation medical exam and neuromuscular evaluation (see table 43.2 for specific programming suggestions).

Exercise recommendations for individuals with PPS include the following:

- Involve as much stable musculature as possible.
- Include four-limb ergometry, therapeutic aquatics, and other non-weight-bearing activities.
- Conventional weight-bearing activities such as walking and running may be appropriate for some individuals with less involvement and without a history of muscle atrophy.
- An exercise intensity of 60% to 70% of peak oxygen consumption ($\dot{V}O_{2peak}$) or moderate-to-somewhat hard RPEs is recommended if there are no new symptoms or signs of weakness.

TABLE 43.2

Polio and Post-Polio Syndromes: Exercise Programming

Modes	Goals	Intensity/Frequency/Duration	Time to goal
Aerobic Schwinn Air-Dyne Arm ergometer	■ Increase cardiovascular condition ■ Increase endurance of stable limbs and maintain unstable limbs ■ Increase efficiency of ADLs and ambulation	■ 40-70% $\dot{V}O_{2peak}$ or peak HR ■ 3 days/week ■ 20-30 min/session (performed in intervals initially for sedentary clients)	■ Indeterminate. ■ Increase, if tolerated, to 40 min continuous exercise.
Strength Isotonic exercises Isometric exercises	■ Increase strength of stable limbs and maintain unstable limbs ■ Increase efficiency of ADLs and ambulation	■ 3 sets of 10-15 reps ■ 2-4 days/week ■ 3 sets of 6 s ■ 3 sets of 6 contractions at 67% of 1RM every 20° of ROM of stable musculature/joints ■ 3 days/week	
Flexibility Stretching (passive)	■ Increase ROM (if deficient) ■ Prevent contractures	■ Perform with both stable (unless painful) and unstable (mild intensity) musculature/joints ■ 5-7 days/week	

- An intensity of less than 50% of $\dot{V}O_{2peak}$ is recommended if there has been a recent change in weakness or symptoms.

- Clients who have severe atrophic polio and have recent weakness should not exercise.

- A frequency of three sessions a week is recommended.

- Performing exercise on alternate days is optimal to attain beneficial physiological changes without overtaxing the reduced number of motor units.

Determining the optimal exercise frequency for individuals with PPS should be based on the client's degree of deconditioning and symptoms:

- If the client is severely deconditioned or has been sedentary for more than one year, and has not had new weakness or symptoms, an initial total exercise duration of up to 20 min per session in 2 to 4 min intervals is recommended.

- If weakness and symptoms are recent, a total duration of 15 min per session, divided into 3 min intervals, is recommended.

- Clients who exercise irregularly should exercise for less than 25 min per session and divide the session into 5 min intervals or less.

- If the client regularly participates in exercise, 30 to 40 min of continuous activity is appropriate.

Routine exercise is appropriate in most cases of PPS. Furthermore, some individuals without recent weakness or symptoms but with a history of ventilator use or of four-limb involvement should have a thorough preparticipation medical examination and should be supervised for two months to ensure safety. Any questions about exercise prescription should be directed to a physician and appropriately trained health professional. Increased fatigue, weakness, or pain in a particular area should alert the individual to decrease intensity or duration of exercise or both. If symptoms continue for more than two weeks and are exacerbated by exercise, then exercise should be terminated, and appropriate medical follow-up is suggested.

SPECIAL CONSIDERATIONS

Most sedentary individuals with PPS are encouraged to consult a physician or appropriately trained health professional before beginning an exercise program. These professionals can supervise and monitor responses to exercise over a two-month period. This will facilitate beneficial physical and psychological tolerance to exercise. Depression has a higher incidence in persons with PPS than in the asymptomatic post-polio population. Appropriate supervision should help the individual with PPS with not only the physical but also the mental and emotional obstacles to beginning and continuing an exercise program.

Following an initial two-month period of supervision and perhaps follow-up, individuals with PPS should be able to self-monitor and adjust their exercise program. However, performing a submaximal evaluation every three to six months is recommended in order to compare exercise responses and to ensure fitness improvement and maintenance. If questions or concerns arise, an appropriately trained health professional should be consulted. The individual's own physician and an American College of Sports Medicine–certified rehabilitation therapist would be appropriate.

Other special considerations are as follows:

- Weakness and pain may be present in the lower limbs of patients with braces or orthotic appliances.
- Full or partial loss of sensation, as well as fasciculations and paresthesia, may be present in lower limbs.
- Spasms and fasciculations (involuntary twitching of muscle fibers) indicate a need to decrease work period and increase recovery period.
- Progressive sudden fatigue indicates overly high intensity.
- Clients may lack motivation or compliance secondary to clinical depression.
- Rest periods during the day may be necessary in the initial stages of the exercise program.

Evidence-Based Guidelines

Halstead LS. Managing post-polio: A guide to living and aging well with post-polio syndrome. 2nd ed. Washington, DC: ABI Professional; 2006.

Kling C, Persson A, Gardulf A. The health-related quality of life of patients suffering from the late effects of polio (post-polio). J Adv Nurs. 2000;32(1):164.

March of Dimes. Post-polio syndrome: Identifying best practices in diagnosis & care. 2001. Available from www.marchofdimes.com/files/PPSreport.pdf.

Maynard, FM, Headley JL, eds. Handbook on the late effects of poliomyelitis: For physicians and survivors. 2nd ed. St. Louis: Post-Polio Health International; 1999.

National Institute of Neurological Disorders and Stroke. Post-polio syndrome fact sheet. 2005. Available from www.ninds.nih.gov/disorders/post_polio/detail_post_polio.htm.

Post-Polio Health International. A statement about exercise for survivors of polio. 2003. Available from www.post-polio.org/ipn/pnn19-2A.html#sta.

CASE STUDY

Post-Polio Syndrome

A 52-year-old man was diagnosed with paralytic polio at age 8. He had not used assistive devices, but was considering an orthotic or device of some type to prevent left "foot drop" and "stubbing his toe." He complained of increased left lower leg fatigue with moderate walking distances (up to 150 ft [46 m]). He gained almost 10 lb (4.5 kg) over the prior six months, secondary to not being able to walk as far without increasing left lower leg fatigue and pain. He had taken over-the-counter nonsteroidal anti-inflammatory drugs for lower extremity pain (7/10 worst, 3/10 best) and fatigue. He was attempting to walk at least three times a week for up to 30 min. He was employed as a salesman and lived with his wife.

(continued)

S: "My left front lower leg gets weak and painful after just a little bit of walking, and then I can't pick up my foot."

O: Vitals

Height: 5 ft 11 in. (1.80 m)
Weight: 168 lb (76.3 kg)
BMI: 21.2 kg/m²
Resting HR: 75 contractions/min (standing)
Resting BP: 126/82 mmHg (standing)
Nonobese middle-aged male, pleasant, upbeat affect
Stands in slight lumbar hyperextension with mild anterior pelvic tilt and slight hip flexion bilaterally
More than 50% of body weight on right side while standing without an assistive device, appliance, or orthotic
Left lower extremity: Knee mildly hyperextended
Moderate atrophy left mid-anterior lower leg to ankle, with diminished muscle tone
Sensation diminished to light touch, vibration, sharp-dull, and temperature
Reflexes absent in left lower leg: Achilles and knee extensor
EMG: Significant motor unit amplitude and duration with increased fasciculations (on anterior left lower leg, tibialis anterior)
Passive flexibility: Grossly normal

Active flexibility

L hip flexion: 95°
L hip extension: 20°
L knee extension: 0°
L knee flexion: 100°
L dorsiflexion: −1°
L plantarflexion: 36°
Balance: Moderate perturbation results in hip strategy particularly on left LE
Sit and reach: 6 in. (15.5 cm)
Sit to stand: 6 reps in 45 s before fatigue
Gait:
Initially right step decrease with moderate lack of left dorsi and plantarflexion
After approximately 150 ft (46 m), severe lack of left dorsiflexion with poor plantarflexion resulting in significantly decreased right step
Trunk flexion increased beyond 10° from the vertical after 150 ft
Pelvic rotation moderately excessive on left
Minimal left hip extension/flexion after approximately 150 ft
Significant decrease in left knee flexion/extension and heel plant/toe-off
Step and stride length reduced by over 75% on right after 150 ft

Strength

Left lower extremity: Grossly 3+/5 (3 reps)
Left lower extremity: Hip flexion/extension/abduction/adduction: Grossly 3+/5 (3 reps)
Knee (flexion/extension): Grossly 3 to 3+/5 (3 reps)
Ankle (plantarflexion/dorsiflexion): Grossly 2+/5 (3 reps)
Right lower extremity: Grossly 4/5 (3 reps), all movements
Aerobic: Estimated max 7 METs

A: 1. Decreased active range of motion for dorsiflexion in foot drop
2. Significantly weakened left dorsiflexors (tibialis anterior, extensor digitorum, hallucis extensors, and peroneus tertius)
3. Weakened left hip and knee
4. Gait/walking intolerance and poor mechanics
5. "Less than fair" standing balance

P: 1. Fit for left ankle-foot orthosis (AFO): Fabricate from carbon fiber with an oil damper resistance (small shock absorber with hydraulic resistance) to not totally stop plantarflexion.
2. Prescribe an exercise/rehabilitation program, particularly for left lower extremity and lower leg/ankle.
3. Prescribe a gait and dynamic stand balance program.

Exercise Program Goals

1. Perform gait with AFO
2. Increase left leg strength, particularly dorsiflexors
3. Increase active ROM (AROM) for dorsiflexion of left foot
4. Decrease left lower leg pain to less than 2/10 while walking greater than 150 ft
5. Increase aerobic capacity
6. Increase dynamic stand balance

Follow-Up

The client's aerobic capacity increased 20% in 8 weeks without further exacerbation of left lower leg symptoms. His left dorsiflexors increased by 12% in muscle strength and 15% in AROM after 8 weeks. The left hip and knee increased approximately 10% in muscle strength. His gait/walking improved to 300 ft (91 m) before there was an increase in pain beyond 3/10, and decreased dorsiflexion AROM, without the use of the AFO. With the AFO, he was able to walk over 1000 ft (305 m) before there was notice of pain. Dynamic stand balance improved to "fair plus" without the AFO and was similar with it after 8 weeks of training.

Mode	Frequency	Duration	Intensity	Progression
Aerobic (Schwinn Air-Dyne)	3 days/week	25 min/session (initially)	5 min/interval; 60-80% of HRR	Increase by 5 min every 3 weeks.
Strength (lower extremities)	Daily	Left: 6 reps at 40% of 1RM Right: 6 reps at 70% of 1RM	Left: 40% of 1RM Right: 70% of 1RM (use multiangle or 60% of MVC)	Reassess every 2 weeks and increase weight if appropriate.
Flexibility	5 days/week	60 s/stretch		
Neuromuscular				
Warm-up and cool-down	Before and after each session	5-10 min	RPE <10/20	

44

Amyotrophic Lateral Sclerosis

Vanina Dal Bello-Haas, PhD, PT ■ Lisa Stroud Krivickas, MD

OVERVIEW OF THE PATHOPHYSIOLOGY

Amyotrophic lateral sclerosis (ALS) is the most common type of adult-onset motor neuron disease. The primary characteristic of this idiopathic, progressive, and eventually fatal disease is degeneration of the lower (LMN) and upper motor neurons (UMN). Symptoms of ALS with LMN involvement include muscle weakness and atrophy, muscle cramps, hyporeflexia, and fasciculations, whereas UMN involvement results in spasticity, hyperreflexia, and loss of dexterity. The average age at diagnosis is 55 years, but onset can occur at any time from the teenage years to older adulthood. Amyotrophic lateral sclerosis is a terminal illness, with approximately 50% of individuals surviving for up to three years following diagnosis, 20% for up to five years, and 10% for up to 10 years.

Amyotrophic lateral sclerosis progresses at a steady rate without any periods of remission. The rate of progression is highly variable; some individuals lose strength very rapidly, while in others the disease progresses so slowly that they remain at a high functional capacity for many years. The primary cause of death in ALS is respiratory failure due to inadequate ventilation secondary to respiratory muscle weakness. Factors that indicate a better prognosis include a younger age of onset, age of limb involvement, and a slower progression of symptoms prior to diagnosis.

Approximately 90% to 95% of individuals diagnosed with ALS have sporadic ALS, meaning that there is no apparent cause. Factors involved in the pathogenesis of ALS include oxidative stress, neuroinflammation, microglial cell activation, mitochondrial dysfunction, abnormal protein aggregation, and abnormalities of axonal transport. Another potential cause of ALS is glutamate toxicity (excitotoxicity). Excitotoxicity is caused by glutamate receptors that become overactivated and allow large amounts of calcium ions to enter the cell. Excess intracellular calcium stimulates various enzymatic activities that result in damage to cell structures. Glutamate toxicity is likely due to a defective protein that interferes with normal aerobic energy metabolism. An antiglutamate drug, riluzole, has recently shown some therapeutic benefit in the treatment of ALS.

Acknowledgment
The editors wish to acknowledge the previous author of this chapter, Karen Lo Nau White, PhD, TP, FACSM.

Approximately 10% of ALS is due to the familial form of ALS, which is nearly always transmitted in an autosomal dominant pattern. Despite a considerable amount of ongoing research, there are currently no pharmacologic therapies that reverse or halt ALS.

Major factors contributing to disability in individuals with ALS include muscle weakness, spasticity, lack of motor control, and progressive respiratory failure. Weakness can occur in any skeletal muscle with the exception of the extraocular and sphincter muscles, which are generally spared. Initial signs and symptoms of weakness are typically asymmetric and focal, occurring in the distal upper or lower extremity, trunk, or bulbar muscles. Individuals presenting with initial symptoms in the bulbar region (e.g., difficulty speaking, chewing, and swallowing) may not have significant extremity weakness until later in the progression of the disease. Other people have significant extremity weakness but develop bulbar weakness much later.

During the early stages of ALS, denervated muscle fibers become reinnervated by neighboring motor units, which helps to maintain muscle strength and may be a key element in the preservation of function among individuals with slow progression. One characteristic of the immature neuromuscular junction of the newly reinnervated muscle fiber is that it can experience transmission failure, contributing to increased transient muscle fatigue, with no permanent damage to the motor neuron. However, there is a theoretical concern that extreme exercise or overexertion may hasten motor neuron death. Many physicians have been extremely cautious about prescribing exercise for people with ALS, yet there is no clear evidence that overuse weakness occurs in this population.

EFFECTS ON THE EXERCISE RESPONSE

Typical limiting factors for ALS include the individual's muscular strength, endurance, and degree of fatigue. Muscle fatigue also occurs before the cardiovascular system reaches maximal capacity during exercise. Individuals with early ALS may still be functioning at near-normal levels and be able to reach their maximal aerobic capacity, although this near-normal functioning level is the rare exception. Individuals with pulmonary impairments may find that ventilation is their limiting factor, and for this reason dyspnea should be monitored closely. People with spasticity may not be able to exercise at speeds

fast enough to elicit a cardiovascular response due to poor coordination. Muscle weakness, joint laxity, and poor coordination and balance make many modes of exercise testing unsafe or impractical.

Allied health professionals should also be aware that over a third of individuals with ALS have been found to have cognitive and behavioral changes, and a very small percentage develop frontotemporal dementia (ALS-FTD) or parkinsonism-dementia complex (PDC). People with ALS-FTD show signs and symptoms of frontal and temporal lobe dysfunction (e.g., cognitive decline; executive functioning impairments; difficulties with planning, organization, and concept abstraction; and personality and behavior changes); those with ALS-PDC show additional signs of parkinsonism (i.e., bradykinesia, rigidity, tremor) related to neuronal degeneration in the substantia nigra. Individuals with ALS but without FTD have been reported to have a wide variety of cognitive impairments (especially difficulties with verbal fluency and language comprehension). Thus cognitive impairments or impairments related to ALS-FTD or ALS-PDC may limit people's ability to participate in exercise testing or an exercise training program.

EFFECTS OF EXERCISE TRAINING

Muscle weakness and atrophy associated with ALS result from disuse and may be minimized with exercise training. Incorporating regularly practiced exercise will strengthen healthy muscle fibers and possibly mildly improve affected muscles. Studies of single ALS muscle fibers have shown that the contractile properties of the remaining muscle fibers are normal and that muscle fiber hypertrophy occurs, possibly to compensate for lost fibers. If healthy muscle fibers remain trainable, this may permit an individual with ALS to maintain strength and function for a longer period of time. Strengthening the muscles of respiration should likewise optimize the functional ability of intact fibers and prolong the time before pulmonary impairments become severely restrictive. Improving or maintaining aerobic capacity may have positive benefits on functional ability by maximizing the efficiency of innervated muscle fibers, and may improve psychological well-being, appetite, and sleep. Amyotrophic lateral sclerosis cannot be reversed, and people eventually lose functional capacity despite their best efforts. Maintaining joint range of motion (ROM) and muscle length will also help prevent contractures and minimize pain, and will make it easier for caregivers to provide assistance for individuals with ALS who can no longer take care of themselves.

MANAGEMENT AND MEDICATIONS

The drug riluzole is the only medication currently approved by the Food and Drug Administration for ALS. Riluzole has been shown to prolong survival by two to three months, without improving functional status. Optimal management of nutrition and respiratory function has been shown to prolong life to a greater extent than any pharmacologic therapies to date. Additional medical management of ALS focuses on controlling secondary symptoms. Medications are available to decrease muscle spasticity (e.g., Lioresal, tizanidine, and diazepam), sialorrhea (e.g., tricyclic antidepressants, scopolamine transdermal patch, glycopyrrolate, botulinum toxin injections), pseudobulbar affect (e.g., amitriptyline, paroxetine, combination of dextromethorphan and quinidine), anxiety, depression, and pain. Any dose of symptomatic treatments must be titrated carefully to avoid potential side effects. Medications prescribed to reduce spasticity can also increase weakness, sedation, and dizziness, while antidepressant agents can cause hypotension and sedation.

Other therapeutic interventions may include the following:

- A recommendation for orthotics, adaptive equipment, assistive devices, and other environmental modifications
- Nutritional supplementation and placement of a feeding tube for those with dysphagia or malnutrition
- Augmentative communication devices for those with dysarthria
- Noninvasive positive pressure ventilation for respiratory muscle weakness
- Emotional support and counseling for the individual and the family
- Home health personnel to assist with caregiving
- A discussion with the patient and appropriate caregivers regarding issues related to end of life (e.g., hospice, use of a ventilator, taking a patient off a ventilator, the use of lifesaving techniques)

RECOMMENDATIONS FOR EXERCISE TESTING

Safety is a key consideration when exercise testing individuals with ALS. Due to variability in presentation (e.g., unilateral vs. bilateral, upper limb vs. lower limb and may or may not include bulbar weakness), the mode selected should maximize safety and function based on individual needs. Equipment may have to be modified to increase support. For severely affected individuals, assessing ability to complete functional tasks may be more useful than traditional exercise testing. Functional assessment is one of the primary tools for monitoring ALS progression (see table 44.1). The ALS Functional Rating Scale is commonly used to assess disease progression. Results from exercise testing can be highly variable, depending on the stage of ALS, extent of involvement, and rate of progression (from near normal to severely compromised). Before starting a test, the individual should be asked about his or her daily activities so that an estimate of functional capacity and an appropriate exercise test protocol can be developed.

RECOMMENDATIONS FOR EXERCISE PROGRAMMING

Goals of an exercise training program for individuals with ALS include the following:

- Maximizing functional capacity of the innervated muscle fibers
- Preventing or minimizing the effects of disuse atrophy
- Preventing limitations in ROM and muscle length
- Maximizing aerobic capacity, endurance, and functional level for as long as possible

Individuals with ALS will become weaker and more functionally limited despite any type or amount of exercise. This fact must be understood and accepted by both the health professional and the patient. Modest improvements may occur at the onset of an exercise training program, but severity and number of impairments will increase and overall function will inevitably decrease over time. Because ALS is progressive, the overall goal of an exercise training program is to maintain a higher functional level and quality of life than the individual would have otherwise. Specific goals must

TABLE 44.1

Amyotrophic Lateral Sclerosis: Exercise Testing

Methods	Measures	Endpoints	Comments
Aerobic Recumbent cycle Arm or all-extremity ergometer	■ HR ■ RPE ■ BP ■ METs ■ $\dot{V}_E$	■ Fatigue ■ Signs of overwork	■ Useful in determining exercise prescription. ■ Can be used to screen for hypertension. ■ Can be used to estimate functional capacity and predict the types and amounts of ADLs possible. ■ Useful in indicating whether dyspnea will be a limiting factor in exercise performance. ■ Maximal testing is not appropriate for most; submaximal or functional tests are sufficient.
Endurance If ambulatory, 6 min walk test	Distance or time	■ Time (or distance) ■ Fatigue ■ Signs of overwork	May have to adjust distance trials based on individual.
Strength Weight machines Dynamometers	■ Number of repetitions ■ Maximal voluntary contraction		■ Expect strength to decrease as the disease progresses. ■ Spasticity may influence results.
Flexibility Goniometry	ROM		
Neuromuscular Gait analysis Balance analysis			Used to determine safety and need for assistive devices.
Functional capacity Sit to stand ADLs Performance-based tests	■ Amount of assistance needed ■ Time to complete activities	■ Fatigue ■ Signs of overwork	Used to determine safety, the need for assistive devices, adaptive equipment, and compensatory interventions.

be continuously modified to adapt to individual changes. Exercise training programs must be at a level that will minimize disuse atrophy but be cautious enough to avoid fatigue and overwork, as both may be detrimental to individuals with ALS (see table 44.2). Once exercise becomes so tiring or is so difficult that it prevents someone from completing daily activities, it is no longer appropriate.

SPECIAL CONSIDERATIONS

Because research evidence for exercise training is limited with this population, goals should be practical, exercise intensity and duration should be low to moderate, rest periods should be frequent, expectations should be realistic, and careful monitoring is essential. Strengthening exercises should

TABLE 44.2

Amyotrophic Lateral Sclerosis: Exercise Programming

Modes	Goals*	Intensity/Frequency/Duration	Time to goal
Aerobic			
Recumbent cycling Walking (limited) Pool exercises Swimming	Increase/maintain work capacity and endurance	■ 50-80% peak HR** ■ 11-13/20 RPE ■ 3 sessions/week ■ Up to 30 min/day in 10 min sessions if necessary ■ As tolerated, without excessive fatigue	4-6 months
Strength			
Dynamic exercises (weight machines, modified cuff weights, Theraband) Static exercises Active ROM exercises	■ Increase or maintain strength of uninvolved limbs ■ Increase or maintain strength of involved limbs if they have greater than grade 3 muscle strength ■ Increase or maintain trunk strength ■ Increase or maintain ability to perform ADLs and ambulation	■ Low to moderate intensity ■ Low to moderate load ■ 1 or 2 sets of 8-12 reps ■ Perform on nonaerobic training days ■ Reduce resistance and reps as weakness progresses	4-6 months
Flexibility			
Stretching Active and passive ROM exercises	■ Prevent contractures ■ Increase/maintain ROM	■ Daily ■ 1 to 2 sessions/day	Ongoing
Functional performance			
	■ Increase or maintain ability to perform ADLs ■ More beneficial when a "traditional" exercise program is no longer possible	As tolerated, without excessive fatigue	

*Due to the progressive nature of the disease, goals need to change as the disease progresses.

**80% peak HR is recommended for individuals in the early stages of ALS.

target muscles that are stronger than grade 3/5 on the Medical Research Council strength scale (i.e., the muscle should be strong enough to move the joint fully against gravity and at least be able to hold the joint against minimal resistance). Exercise training is not appropriate for all individuals with ALS, and eventually there will come a point with all ALS patients when the disease limits any potential benefits of exercise training. Individuals most likely to benefit from an exercise program are those in the early stages of ALS and with a slower rate of disease progression. Ideally, exercise programs should be managed in conjunction with a trained health care professional who is knowledgeable about the nature of ALS.

The following are other considerations:

- The risk of injury is present due to flaccid limbs (e.g., catch, bump), joint discomfort (especially in shoulders), laxity (extreme caution needed), or stiffness. Constant vigilance is necessary because of muscle weakness and poor balance (support trunk to maximize safety). Straps or wraps may be necessary to keep feet and hands secured. Treadmills can be especially unsafe for people with muscle weakness and poor balance.

- Pulmonary function (restrictive in nature) is decreased secondary to respiratory muscle weakness and decreased vital capacity, inspiratory and expiratory pressures, and reserve volumes. Supine positions can increase respiratory symptoms. Pulmonary function testing should be part of standard testing (e.g., measuring forced vital capacity [FVC]).

- Clients may be emotionally labile (pseudobulbar affect), depressed, or anxious. Psychological symptoms need to be aggressively managed. Increased frustration and decreased motivation may result from lack of improvement despite effort.

- Clients may have difficulty chewing and swallowing if bulbar area is affected. Presence of a feeding tube may affect exercise capacity immediately after insertion.

- Cognitive impairments or ALS-FTD may limit the individual's ability to participate in an exercise training program. Although FTD differs from Alzheimer's disease in that FTD is not primarily a memory problem, exercise prescription for the client exhibiting these cognitive impairments can be modified from the exercise recommendations for Alzheimer's patients (see chapter 48).

Evidence-Based Guidelines

Andersen PM, Borasio GD, Dengler R, et al. EFNS Task Force on Diagnosis and Management of Amyotrophic Lateral Sclerosis: Guidelines for diagnosing and clinical care of patients and relatives. Eur J Neurol. 2005;12(12):921-938.

Piepers S, van den Berg L. Evidence-based care in amyotrophic lateral sclerosis. Lancet Neurol. 2006;5(2):105-106.

Suggested Web Sites

Amyotrophic Lateral Sclerosis Association. www.alsa. org

National Center on Physical Activity and Disability. www.ncpad.org/disability/fact_sheet.php?sheet=141

CASE STUDY

Amyotrophic Lateral Sclerosis

A 44-year-old female noticed increasing difficulty playing sports because of right foot slapping, as well as difficulty doing up the snaps on her son's pajamas. She was diagnosed with ALS. Over a period of 11 months postdiagnosis, the upper limb weakness progressed from hand to shoulder, affecting the left side only. Although she was no longer able to pinch with her left hand, she was able to move her left elbow and shoulder through range against gravity, without resistance. She was unable to dorsiflex her right ankle at all. At the time of presentation, she was wearing an AFO on the right foot.

S: "I would like to stay as active as possible."

O: Vitals

Height 5 ft 4 in. (1.63 m)
Weight: 122.0 lb (55.4 kg)
Resting HR: 72 contractions/min
BP: 126/78 mmHg
Visible muscle wasting in all extremities distally
Fasciculations in the lower extremities and left upper extremity
Maximal isometric strength:
Hip flexion: Right 44.0 lb (20 kg); left 52.8 lb (24 kg)
Knee extension: Right 74.4 lb (34 kg); left 83.6 lb (38 kg)
Ankle dorsiflexion: Right 0 lb (0 kg); left 33 lb (15 kg)
Shoulder flexion: Right 48.4 lb (22 kg); left 35.2 lb (16 kg)
Elbow flexion: Right 79.2 lb (36 kg); left 61.6 lb (28 kg)
Grip strength: Right 42.5 lb (19.3 kg); left 12.5 lb (5.7 kg)

Recumbent cycle test (discontinuous protocol, feet strapped to pedals):
Peak output: 60 W
$\dot{V}O_{2peak}$: 32.5 ml · kg^{-1} · min^{-1}
Peak HR: 132 contractions/min at RPE 15/20 (approximately 75% of age-adjusted maximum HR)

A: 1. ALS progressing slowly
   2. Ambulatory, but weakness in lower extremities
   3. Light to moderate resistance training appropriate for most muscle groups

P: 1. Formulate a low- to moderate-intensity exercise program based on client's interest.
   2. Maintain flexibility.

Exercise Program Goals

1. Maintain endurance
2. Maintain strength
3. Maintain ROM

Follow-up

Seven months later, the client developed a left drop foot and increasing weakness in the right lower extremity. She was advised to use a wheelchair for long-distance mobility. She is no longer able to move her left upper limb through a full ROM on her own and is noticing some mild to moderate weakness in the right upper limb. Intervention focus changed to compensatory strategies. Exercise program was limited to daily active and passive ROM exercises.

Mode	Frequency	Duration	Intensity	Progression*
Aerobic Swimming	3 days/week	As tolerated	Self-selected	As tolerated
Strength	3 days/week Nonaerobic days	1-2 sets of 8-12 reps	Low to moderate	As tolerated
Flexibility Passive, right foot Active, other joints All major muscle groups	Daily	20 s/stretch 3 reps for each stretch	Maintain stretch below discomfort point	
Neuromuscular	Individualized			
Functional	Individualized			
Warm-up and cool-down	Before and after each session	10 min		

*Client to record exercise and activities in a daily log and note signs and symptoms. Although some improvement may be made initially, expect decrease or reversal as disease progresses, which will require readjustment to exercise program.

45

Cerebral Palsy

James J. Laskin, PT, PhD

OVERVIEW OF THE PATHOPHYSIOLOGY

Cerebral palsy (CP) consists of a group of permanent yet nonprogressive physical disabilities that appear early in life, usually in infancy or early childhood. Cerebral palsy is characterized by limited ability to move and maintain balance and posture due to abnormal development or damage in one or more areas of the brain that control muscle tone and spinal reflexes. The subsequent changes in muscle tone and spinal reflexes depend on the location and extent of the injury within the brain. Motor disorders associated with CP can also lead to disturbances in sensation, perception, cognition, communication, and behavior. The exact medical classification of CP depends on the type of muscle tone and the injury site (see table 45.1).

In the United States, CP is one of the most common congenital disorders of childhood, affecting approximately two to four neonates per 1,000 live births. The type of brain anomaly associated with CP has two common etiologies:

1. Failure of the brain to develop properly:
   - Occurrence within the first or second trimester (or both) of embryonic development
   - Disruption of the normal developmental process, which may be caused by genetic disorder, chromosomal abnormality, or faulty blood supply

2. Neurological disorder:
   - Injury to brain before, during, or after birth
   - Lack of oxygen, bleeding in brain, toxic injury or poisoning, head trauma, metabolic disorder, or infection of nervous system

The Cerebral Palsy-International Sport and Recreation Association (CP-ISRA) has developed a classification system based on an individual's "function." The CP-ISRA system is intended for use with those diagnosed with CP as well as individuals with other conditions characterized by nonprogressive brain lesions (e.g., stroke, traumatic brain injury, and tumor). Many Paralympic sports (e.g., swimming and track and field) have moved to a functional classification system to match an athlete's disabilities with sport-specific abilities. Within the context of CP and exercise, however, the CP-ISRA system allows for the grouping of individuals of similar "abilities," including the following groups:

- CP1: Severe spastic or athetoid tetraplegia. The person is unable to propel a manual wheelchair independently and has nonfunctional lower extremities, very poor to no trunk stability, and severely decreased function in the upper extremity.

- CP2: Moderate to severe spastic or athetoid tetraplegia. The person is able to propel a manual wheelchair slowly and inefficiently, and has differential function abilities between upper and lower extremities and fair static trunk stability.

TABLE 45.1

Medical Classification of Cerebral Palsy

Category	Site of injury	Presentation
Pyramidal	Cortical system	Spastic, hyperreflexia, "clasp knife" hypertonia, prone to contractures
Extrapyramidal	Basal ganglia and cerebellum	Athetosis, ataxia, "lead pipe" rigidity chorea
Mixed	Combination of above	Combination of above

Based on P.A. DeLuca, 1996, "The musculoskeletal management of children with cerebral palsy," *Pediatric Clinics of North American* 43(5): 1135-1150.

■ CP3: Moderate spastic tetraplegia or severe spastic hemiplegia. The person is able to propel a manual wheelchair independently; may be able to ambulate with assistance; and has moderate spasticity on the lower extremities, fair dynamic trunk stability, and moderate limitations to function in the dominant arm.

■ CP4: Moderate to severe spastic diplegia. The person ambulates with aids over short distances and has moderate to severe involvement of the lower extremities, good dynamic trunk stability, and minimal to near-normal function of the upper extremities at rest.

■ CP5: Moderate spastic diplegia. The person ambulates well with assistive devices, has minimal to moderate spasticity in one or both lower extremities, and is able to run.

■ CP6: Moderate athetosis or ataxia. The person ambulates without assistive devices and has poor static and good dynamic trunk stability, good upper extremity range and strength, and poor throwing and grasp and release; lower extremity function improves from walking to running or cycling.

■ CP7: True ambulatory hemiplegia. The person has mildly to moderately affected upper extremity and minimally to mildly affected lower extremity.

■ CP8: Minimally affected diplegia, hemiplegia, athetosis, or monoplegia.

Given the overwhelming challenges that many individuals with CP face with activities of daily living, it is no surprise that the level of physical fitness is very low in this population. Particularly for the wheelchair user, the risk for secondary conditions related to physical inactivity such as obesity, type 2 diabetes, hypertension, and cardiovascular disease is greater than that of their able-bodied peers.

EFFECTS ON THE EXERCISE RESPONSE

Specific research examining the exercise responses in individuals with CP is limited. Historically, individuals with CP have not typically participated in physical fitness programs, structured or unstructured; but when they do undergo physiological assessment, they often achieve higher than expected exercise response values. However, studies examining the cardiovascular and metabolic responses to exercise have shown that individuals with CP tend to have higher heart rates, blood pressure, and lactate concentrations for a given submaximal work rate than their able-bodied peers.

Individuals with CP tend to have slightly lower peak physiological responses (10-20%) than able-bodied controls. Reduced mechanical efficiency, due to the added energy required to overcome muscle tonus in spastic CP has also been reported . Physical work capacity has been reported to be as much as 50% lower than that of able-bodied subjects. Low fitness levels in individuals with CP are likely the result of poor exercise habits, difficulty performing skilled movements, contralateral and ipsilateral muscle imbalances, and often poor functional strength. Fatigue and stress are also factors that have a negative impact on the exercise performance. In addition, individuals with CP commonly report a transient increase in spasticity and incoordination after a strenuous exercise session.

EFFECTS OF EXERCISE TRAINING

Given the nature of this physical disability, there is no reason to expect that individuals with CP cannot benefit from a regular program focusing on muscular strength, flexibility, aerobic endurance, or some combination of these. Because the risk for cardiovascular disease and stroke is greater in the sedentary physically disabled population than in able-bodied counterparts, it is imperative to collect a comprehensive medical and health history in people with CP before they engage in any form of regular physical activity.

A small but growing body of literature indicates that individuals with CP do respond and adapt to training. There is also documented anecdotal evidence in this population of improvement in sense of wellness, body image, and capacity to perform activities of daily living, as well as a lessening of severity of symptoms such as spasticity and athetosis. In addition, athletes with CP and their coaches consistently report improvements in peak oxygen uptake, higher ventilatory threshold, increased work rate at a given submaximal heart rate, increased range of motion, improved coordination and skill of movements, and increased strength and muscular endurance, as well as skeletal muscle hypertrophy. An additional benefit that many individuals with CP report is an overall attenuation in spasticity with participation in a long-term exercise program. The benefit of decreased muscle tone allows for improved function and a decreased use of antispasmodic medications. Collectively, these anecdotal reports are supported by the performances of numerous athletes at national and international competitions.

MANAGEMENT AND MEDICATIONS

As with any client, one should perform appropriate physical screening to rule out any contraindications or precautions before initiating an exercise program. Before a physical fitness assessment is selected or the exercise prescription is developed, the individual's specific needs, goals, and limitations must be addressed. The Use of the CP-ISRA classification system allows the health professional gain insight into the type and modes of exercise that should be used, as well as any special considerations that will help maximize the individual's performance. One must note that the symptoms of spasticity and athetosis increase with stress and fatigue.

Medications may be a confounding factor for exercise testing or exercise programming. Antiseizure medications are commonly prescribed for individuals with CP because seizure or seizure tendencies are present in 60% or more of them. Three commonly used drugs to control seizures are phenobarbital, phenytoin, and carbamazepine.

Some antiseizure medications have a depressant effect on the central nervous system, thus possibly blunting the physiologic responses to exercise. Carbamazepine has the fewest side effects, which may include mental confusion or irritability, dizziness, nausea, weight loss, and sensitivity to sunburn. It is also important to note that, in some instances, the paradoxical effect of hyperactivity may be a result of these medications.

Antispasmodics and muscle relaxants are two other classes of medications frequently prescribed to individuals with CP. Antispasmodic medications decrease muscle tone, which enables the individual to perform physical activities with greater ease. However, a serious side effect of these drugs is drowsiness and lethargy. These medications act systemically; therefore, an already low-tone trunk may be compromised in its ability to act as a base of support, thus further limiting extremity function. Increasingly, these medications (specifically baclofen) are now being delivered directly via an intrathecal pump. The pump is implanted subcutaneously and does not pose any concern for exercise or exercise testing. However, during the period of time when the dosage is being titrated to maximize the effectiveness of the intervention, the clinician may see marked decreases in muscle tone with corresponding decreased coordination and weakness.

RECOMMENDATIONS FOR EXERCISE TESTING

Limited research is available to substantiate testing protocols, principles, and techniques for the CP population. The commonly used modalities to test individuals with CP include leg cycle ergometry, Schwinn Air-Dyne ergometry, wheelchair ergometry, and the treadmill. Wheelchair ergometry is the preferred mode of testing the cardiorespiratory fitness of nonambulatory individuals with CP. For persons who are able to ambulate but who have lower extremity joint contractures, lower extremity or lumbar pain, or poor balance, or those who are at high risk for falls, the use of a body support system in conjunction with a treadmill would be a prudent option. The treadmill alone will give the optimal response for ambulatory individuals with adequate balance and coordination (see table 45.2).

The selection of testing methods is dependent on the abilities of the client. The selection of the test protocol should complement an individual's physical capacities and should be easily tolerated. For those in a wheelchair, wheelchair ergometry or arm crank ergometry provides the best outcomes. The use of

TABLE 45.2

Cerebral Palsy: Exercise Testing

Methods	Measures	Endpoints*	Comments
Aerobic Ambulatory: ■ Treadmill ■ Cycle ergometer ■ Schwinn Air-Dyne ■ NuStep** Wheelchair user: ■ Wheelchair ergometer ■ Arm crank ergometer ■ NuStep ■ Recumbent bike	■ ECG, HR ■ BP ■ RPE (6-20) ■ $\dot{V}O_{2max}$	■ Serious dysrhythmia ■ >2 mm ST-segment depression/elevation ■ Ischemic threshold ■ T-wave inversion with significant ST change ■ SBP >250 mmHg or DBP >115 mmHg ■ Volitional fatigue	■ Use exercise methods that are reciprocal and cadences that are relatively slow if spasticity is a concern. ■ Record current medications/dosages; any change in medication usage may confound test–retest data.
Endurance Using the methods listed above: ■ 6 and 12 min walk/push ■ 1-mile (1.6K) walk/push ■ Multistage submaximal protocols	■ Distance ■ HR ■ RPE (6-20)	Note vitals, time, distance, symptoms at rest stops	■ Same concerns as listed for aerobic methods. ■ The specific measure or endpoint or both may have to be individualized.
Strength Free weights Weight machines Hydraulic resistance	■ 8RM ■ 25RM ■ Number of reps in 1 min	Maximum ROM	■ Same concerns as listed for aerobic methods. ■ Ensure that client moves through the entire available ROM. ■ To minimize the effects of spasticity, use a slow cadence; a metronome may help keep the client at the right prescribed pace.
Flexibility Goniometry	Joint angles at full flexion/extension	■ Pain ■ Increased spasticity	ROM may be limited due to spasticity, athetosis, or contractures.
Neuromuscular ■ Gait ■ Balance			These are useful measurements because CP may affect motor regions or pathways in the CNS, which could influence the exercise prescription.

*Measurements of particular significance; do not always indicate test termination.

**Allows for combined upper and lower extremity activity.

personal wheelchairs increases comfort with and tolerance of testing during wheelchair ergometry if such accommodations are available. An orientation and practice time should be allowed in order to ensure that exercise test termination results from cardiorespiratory and muscular limitations and not the condition itself. Leg cycle ergometry, Schwinn Air-Dyne ergometry, or the treadmill may be the testing method elected for ambulatory individuals with CP. Balance and coordination are also a concern with ambulatory CP and should be taken into consideration in the choice of the testing method. Persons with CP may be unable to perform leg cycle ergometry because of inadequate hip flexion caused by excessive spasticity, fixed deformities, or both. Practice time should also be allowed when the feet are strapped to the pedals during leg cycle or Schwinn Air-Dyne ergometry. The primary objectives of exercise testing are

- to identify challenges and barriers to engagement in regular physical activity,
- to uncover risk for secondary conditions,
- to determine functional capacity and limitations to exercise programming, and
- to determine appropriate intensity range for cardiovascular and muscular strength and endurance exercise training.

Medication and special considerations for exercise testing include the following:

- Antiseizure medications (including phenobarbital, phenytoin, and carbamazepine) and antispasmodic medications may decrease aerobic capacity and results from other tests because of a decrease in attention span, motivation, or both.
- Concomitant cognitive, visual, hearing, and speech and swallowing difficulties may be present.
- Do not assume decreased cognitive ability on the basis of the presence of drooling or the quality of verbal skills.
- Use testing modalities that are reciprocal and cadences that are relatively slow if spasticity is a concern.
- Record current medications and dosages; any change in medication usage may confound test–retest data.
- Strap the hands or feet to the pedals during arm and leg cycle ergometry, respectively.
- Use of gloves for wheelchair exercise testing is recommended.

- Uninterrupted supervision and spotting during testing are required.
- Those with significant involvement present with mouths that have developed with a very acute angle of the mandible, making a satisfactory seal with a standard mouthpiece difficult.
- Posttest fatigue may result in a significant increase in spasticity, causing a marked decrease in function.

RECOMMENDATIONS FOR EXERCISE PROGRAMMING

The progressive goal of all exercise training is to improve health and increase daily functional activities. As with exercise testing, research pertaining to exercise prescription for individuals with CP is limited. Because of the nature and variability in presentation of CP, the practitioner will need to implement exercise programs using creative adaptations. The average individual with CP will benefit the most from a balanced program of muscular strength, flexibility, and aerobic endurance. The practitioner must take into consideration the individual's abilities, interests, and personal goals. Specific exercises should be designed such that the individual can be independent. Progression should be gradual and should increase at the individual's own rate and in accordance with the principle of specific adaptations to imposed demands (see table 45.3). The special considerations listed in the section on exercise testing are equally applicable to exercise programming. The primary goals of exercise programming are to identify and mediate the barriers to participation and to determine an exercise regimen that complements the individual's interests and abilities and enhances quality of life. These goals are achieved with an exercise program that

- is performed at moderate intensities respecting spasticity, limited range of motion, and pain;
- preferably entails daily participation; and
- allows for adequate rest between sets and sessions.

Suggested Web Sites

Cerebral Palsy International Sports and Recreation Association. www.cpisra.org/

National Center on Physical Activity and Disability. www.ncpad.org/

United Cerebral Palsy. www.ucp.org/

TABLE 45.3

Cerebral Palsy: Exercise Programming

Modes	Goals	Intensity/Frequency/Duration	Time to goal
Aerobic Ambulatory: ■ Schwinn Air-Dyne ■ Any upper and lower limb ergometer Wheelchair: ■ Arm ergometer	Increase aerobic capacity and endurance	■ 40-85% $\dot{V}O_2R$ ■ 3-5 days/week ■ 20-40 min/session ■ Emphasize duration over intensity	Variable
Endurance Ambulatory: ■ 6 to 15 min walks Wheelchair: ■ 6 to 15 min pushes	Improve distance covered	1-2 sessions/week	Variable
Strength Free weights or weight machines	Improve muscle strength of involved and uninvolved muscle groups	■ 3 sets of 8-12 reps ■ 2 days/week ■ Resistance as tolerated	Variable
Flexibility Stretching (involved and uninvolved joints)	Improve ROM directly related to capacity for ADLs	Before and after aerobic and endurance exercise	Variable

CASE STUDY

Cerebral Palsy

A 46-year-old woman was not currently participating in any form of regular physical activity. She worked full-time as a grant writer for a progressive university research institute. The university had just opened a new recreation facility that was not only accessible but also had equipment specifically designed for individuals with impaired mobility. These developments inspired her to investigate beginning an exercise program. Her mobility limitations were related to her spastic tetraplegia, resulting from trauma at birth. As a child she underwent rigorous physical therapy, and was relatively active throughout high school as a competent manual wheelchair user. Fifteen years earlier she decided to use a power chair for work only, but had not used her manual chair for the past 10 years. She

felt that her spasticity had become much worse, and over the previous few years she had less energy and found it more difficult to perform routine activities of daily living. She was able to ambulate short distances at home and in the office, but recently even these short walks left her short of breath. She also felt that the increased spasticity and lack of mobility had caused significant joint pain in her hips and knees. She reported having gained over 25 lb (11.3 kg) during the previous three years. She was a nonsmoker and did not drink alcohol regularly. Currently she was on no prescription medications, taking Aleve or Tylenol as needed. She had no chronic cardiovascular diseases such as hypertension or diabetes, but did have a very strong family history of diabetes.

S: *"I think I'm getting worse and I would really like to try starting an exercise program, but I need help and guidance."*

O: Vitals

HR: 85 contractions/min
BP: 110/90 mmHg
Middle aged female, moderately overweight
Knees and hips without inflammation or effusion
Mobility via power wheelchair
Able to stand unsupported and walk 3 m without assistance
Mild to moderate spasticity in bilateral upper extremities
Moderate to severe spasticity in bilateral lower extremities
Full functional active and passive ROM in upper extremities but must move very slowly to avoid triggering moderate spasticity
Significantly reduced passive and active lower extremity ROM:
Knee flexion contracture: Right 10°; left 13°
Hip flexion contracture: Right 12°; left 20°
Dorsiflexion bilateral ankles: 0°
Upper extremity strength: Normal
Lower extremity strength: Limited from spasticity
Submaximal aerobic test (modified 3-stage NuStep recumbent stepper):

Work rate setting 1 (65 steps/min): 95 contractions/min
Work rate setting 2 (65 steps/min): 116 contractions/min
Work rate setting 3 (65 steps/min): 122 contractions/min
8RM strength test:
Chest press: 65 lb (29.5 kg)
Seated row: 55 lb (24.9 kg)
Seated abdominal curl: 45 lb (20.4 kg)
Lat pulldown: 75 lb (34 kg)
Medications: Aleve and Tylenol prn

A: 1. Cerebral palsy with spastic tetraplegia
   2. Easily fatigable

P: 1. Prescribe a weight loss diet.
   2. Initiate an exercise program.
   3. Utilize an unweighting system to take 5-10% of body weight while treadmill walking.
      - Improve efficiency of gait.
      - Increase duration of ambulation.
      - Ensure safety—minimize risk of falls.
   4. Encourage use of manual wheelchair.

Exercise Program Goals

1. Improved aerobic capacity, overall strength, and flexibility
2. Weight loss
3. Use of manual wheelchair at home and socially

Mode	Frequency	Duration	Intensity	Progression
Aerobic Recumbent stepper (Nu-Step	3-5 days/week	Two or three 10 min sessions	Work rate of 65 steps/min	Increase to 45 min over 4-8 weeks.
Strength (focus on antigravity and postural/trunk muscles)	3-5 days/week	2 sets of 8-12 reps, resistance as tolerated	To fatigue	Progress as tolerated to total exercise time of 60-90 min.
Flexibility (anterior chest, hip flexors, plantarflexors)	3-5 days/week	60 s/stretch	Maintain stretch below discomfort point	Progress as tolerated up to 20 min for contracted muscles.
Warm-up and cool-down	Before and after each session	5-10 min		

46

Parkinson's Disease

Elizabeth J. Protas, PhD, PT, FACSM ■ Rhonda K. Stanley, PhD, PT
Joseph Jankovic, MD

OVERVIEW OF THE PATHOPHYSIOLOGY

Parkinson's disease (PD) is a chronic, progressive neurologic disorder involving the division of the nervous system that regulates muscle reflexes, the extrapyramidal system. Parkinson's disease is believed to be caused by a reduction in the neurotransmitter dopamine, which is produced in the substantia nigra, a component of the basal ganglia. In PD, the dopaminergic cells that produce dopamine deteriorate and eventually die off. The loss of dopamine within the brain results in the symptoms of PD, which include resting tremor, bradykinesia (slow movements), rigidity, and gait and postural abnormalities. Symptoms of PD do not occur until there is greater than 80% loss of dopaminergic cells.

The term parkinsonism refers to the collective symptoms of PD, namely tremor, rigidity, bradykinesia, and postural instability. Idiopathic PD is the most common form of parkinsonism and usually occurs in individuals over the age of 50. It is found slightly more frequently in men than in women and may be less prevalent in African blacks and Asians. Parkinson's disease is believed to afflict an estimated 1.5 million U.S. adults, and this figure will likely continue to rise as the U.S. adult population continues to advance in age. There is no known cause of PD; however, both genetics and environment (e.g., exposure to toxins) are thought to be factors. Other contributing factors may include aging, autoimmune responses, and mitochondrial dysfunction.

The severity of an individual's PD can be simply classified as early, moderate, or advanced.

- Early disease: The individual has been newly diagnosed with PD, with only minor symptoms of tremor or stiffness.
- Moderate disease: The individual begins to experience limited movement, with mild to moderate tremor.
- Advanced disease: The individual begins to experience significant limitations in activity, regardless of treatment or medication.

Severity of PD can be categorized based on a more comprehensive assessment that can then be used to guide treatment and prognosis. For example, a malignant clinical course of PD identifies those persons with PD who have had symptoms evident for less than one year but whose disability has progressed rapidly, and their prognosis is poor.

Parkinson's disease can be classified according to

- Age at onset (<40 [juvenile]; between 40 and 70; >70)
- Clinical symptom (tremor predominant, akinetic-rigidity predominant, postural instability–gait difficulty predominant)

- Mental status (dementia present/absent)
- Clinical course (benign, progressive, malignant)
- Disability (Hoehn and Yahr stage 1.0-5.0)

The Hoehn and Yahr scale is used to describe how the symptoms of PD progress. The scale is divided into stages from 0 to 5 relative to the level of disability.

- Stage 1: Symptoms on one side of the body only
- Stage 2: Symptoms on both sides of the body, no impairment of balance
- Stage 3: Balance impairment, mild to moderate disease, physically independent
- Stage 4: Severe disability, but still able to walk or stand unassisted
- Stage 5: Wheelchair bound or bedridden unless assisted

The motor symptoms that occur with PD affect many aspects of movement. Tremors can be evident both at rest and with action. Rigidity often begins in the neck and shoulders and spreads to the trunk and extremities, making movement difficult. The ability to move fingers, hands, arms, or legs rapidly is drastically reduced (bradykinesia), and motor control to rise from a chair is lessened. Standing posture is characterized by increased kyphosis and flexed knees and elbows, as well as adducted shoulders. Gait is described as slow and shuffling, with shortened festinating steps (short, fast, rigid, shuffling gait), decreased arm swing, and difficulty initiating a step (start hesitation). Postural righting reflexes are compromised and eventually lost (an individual with a Hoehn and Yahr disability level stage of 3 is unable to recover balance on a pull test). Falls can become a recurring problem. Episodes of decreased movement or freezing become more frequent during walking. Passage through doorways or narrowed spaces becomes more difficult. Activities of daily living can be affected by minute, illegible handwriting (micrographia), the inability to cut food or handle utensils, difficulty swallowing food, difficulty turning in bed and rising from bed, and the need for assistance with dressing and bathing. Individuals with PD have problems with both the volume and the understandability of their speech. Communication disorders are exacerbated by a loss of facial expression (hypomimia). The motor symptoms contribute to the impairment displayed by individuals with PD.

EFFECTS ON THE EXERCISE RESPONSE

Considerable variability exists among individuals with PD, which makes it difficult to detail the exercise responses in this population. Symptoms may fluctuate from hour to hour, day to day, and week to week, regardless of the precision of the exercise intervention strategy. Autonomic nervous system dysfunction is common; this can cause problems with thermal regulation during exercise as well as altered heart rate and blood pressure responses during exercise. Movement disorders and muscular rigidity decrease exercise efficiency, resulting in higher heart rate and oxygen consumption responses during submaximal exercise. Walking may be severely impaired in this population, but other activities such as stair climbing may be easily accomplished. It is common for individuals with PD to freeze and hesitate, which makes certain activities more difficult than others. During single sessions of exercise, significant loss of upright posture (increasing kyphosis) can occur as well.

EFFECTS OF EXERCISE TRAINING

Exercise training in individuals with PD can have significantly varied outcomes because of the complexity and progressive nature of the disease, as well as the effects of medications. Research has demonstrated numerous benefits of exercise for individuals in all stages of PD, even though many of these benefits may be short-lived, especially as the disease progresses. Exercise has not been shown to halt or reverse the symptoms, but will help most people with PD improve their quality of life and ability to perform activities of daily living. Documented benefits of exercise for individuals with PD include improvements in the following:

- Motor performance
- Trunk rotation
- Hand–eye coordination
- Stability and balance during walking
- Nonmotor symptoms
- Muscle volume and strength

The Michael J. Fox Foundation has recently funded a number of clinical trials on exercise and PD that will hopefully provide more information on this subject in the near future. Exercise has also recently been shown to reduce the overall risk of developing PD in men by as much as 60% if they exercise vigorously beginning early into adulthood.

MANAGEMENT AND MEDICATIONS

Pharmacologic intervention is the most successful way of treating many of the symptoms of PD. Drug therapy in PD is primarily aimed at correcting or preventing neurochemical imbalances in relation to reduced dopamine production by lowering epinephrine and norepinephrine levels and raising acetylcholine levels in the brain. The following are the most common antiparkinsonian medications:

- Dopaminergics (e.g., levodopa, levodopa/carbidopa, amantadine, pergolide, bromocriptine, pramipexole, ropinirole)
- Anticholinergics (e.g., benztropine, trihexyphenidyl).
- Monoamine oxidase type B (MAO-B) inhibitors (e.g., deprenyl, selegiline)

Most PD medications have both peripheral and central side effects. The most common side effects are gastrointestinal distress, confusion, delusional states, hallucination, insomnia, and changes in mental activity. Long-term use of drug therapies, particularly dopaminergics and MAO-B inhibitors, can result in movement disorders (e.g., dyskinesias), dystonias, and clinical fluctuations of motor disability. More than 50% of all individuals with PD treated for more than five years with drug therapies have reduced responses to the drugs and display clinical fluctuation of motor disability.

Most people with PD take multiple medications to alleviate their symptoms. It is quite common for an attending neurologist to proceed by trial and error in an effort to determine the combination and dosage of drugs that work best. A key medication for PD is levodopa, a metabolic precursor to dopamine that can pass through the blood–brain barrier. In the brain, levodopa is metabolized into dopamine and increases the amount of dopamine available in the basal ganglia. Levodopa is also metabolized in peripheral muscle, which can lessen the amount of drug that can enter the brain's circulation. Carbidopa is combined with levodopa in the drug Sinemet to reduce the peripheral metabolism of levodopa and increase the amount of the drug that passes through the blood–brain barrier. How exercise conditioning affects the peripheral metabolism of levodopa is not yet known.

An important point to stress regarding drug therapy in the medical management of individuals with PD is that the effectiveness of the drugs declines over time, and the variability of individual responses to the drugs make understanding of the influences on drug absorption, metabolism, and effectiveness critical. Reduced absorption of medications may be affected by strenuous exercise, concomitant use of anticholinergic drugs, autonomic dysfunction, recent food intake, amount of protein in the diet, iron supplementation, and level of aerobic fitness.

There are a number of special considerations regarding antiparkinsonian medications and exercise testing.

- Levodopa/carbidopa can produce exercise bradycardia and transient peak-dose tachycardia and dyskinesia.
- Pramipexole, ropinirole, and pergolide may lower blood pressure and exacerbate dyskinesia.
- Selegiline is associated with dyskinesia and produces mood elevation.
- Medication plasma level may influence exercise performance.
- Whenever possible, people should be tested at peak dose, usually 45 min to 1 h after medication has been taken.
- Some individuals who fluctuate clinically may demonstrate a brief, intense peak-dose tachycardia.
- Some people may have intense and severe dyskinesias at peak dose.
- Some medications are associated with cardiac dysrhythmias.
- Caution should be used in testing an individual who has had a recent change in medications because the impact may be unpredictable.
- A single exercise session may increase, decrease, or not affect the time to peak dose-response.
- Individuals who fluctuate clinically should be tested both on and off medications to establish performance ranges.

Many of these concerns regarding possible medication effects during exercise testing are equally applicable to exercise training; however, several additional considerations should be noted.

- Some people display an impaired chronotropic response to aerobic exercise, making it difficult to reach target heart rates.

- Heart rate responses to a given exercise activity may vary greatly from day to day, depending on the medication plasma level.

- Heart rates should be carefully observed during aerobic exercise for evidence of this variability.

- Exercise outcomes may be dependent upon consistently exercising at the same time after the last medication dose.

- Observe for changes in parkinsonian symptoms during exercise training that might be related to changes in drug absorption or metabolism (e.g., increases or decreases in dyskinesias, bradykinesia, dystonias, freezing, and tremor).

- Noting the time to peak-dose onset may be useful in following an individual's medication response to exercise training.

- Recent evidence suggests that sympathetic denervation of the heart may occur early in the disease and affect exercise responses.

RECOMMENDATIONS FOR EXERCISE TESTING

Individuals with PD who have balance deficits or freezing episodes should not be tested on treadmills without the use of a safety support harness or careful guarding. An appropriate cycle ergometer protocol may be selected if harness support is not available. If metabolic gases are to be collected, the use of a breathing mask is recommended, as individuals with PD may have difficulty maintaining a seal around a mouthpiece.

There is some evidence that people in stages 1 and 2 on the Hoehn and Yahr scale have aerobic capacities comparable to those of healthy individuals, with greater variability and lower capacities anticipated for stages 3 and 4. Individuals with PD are in an age group that is at high risk for latent cardiovascular disease, and as such should be carefully screened for coronary artery disease risk factors and any signs or symptoms. Most individuals with PD can ride a bike ergometer or perform arm crank ergometry even if they are in an "off" period and unable to walk without assistance. Nonroutine motor behaviors are often easily accomplished with ergometry (see table 46.1).

RECOMMENDATIONS FOR EXERCISE PROGRAMMING

Parkinson's disease is a complex disorder that is often difficult to evaluate. Complicating the exercise prescription may be direct, indirect, and composite effects of PD. Direct effects are those that occur directly as a result of PD, for example, tremor and rigidity. Indirect effects, such as aerobic deconditioning or loss of range of motion from inactivity, occur along with the disease. Composite effects may be a combination of the direct central nervous system changes and compensatory musculoskeletal symptoms, such as changes in axial mobility and balance problems. Exercise interventions could have a minimal effect on the symptoms resulting directly from the disease process, but appropriately designed interventions may alter the indirect or composite effects of musculoskeletal and cardiopulmonary changes or both (see table 46.2). Parkinson's disease can interfere with motor planning and motor memory; thus repeated demonstrations along with written and visual cues are needed to ensure adherence. In some instances, supervision may be necessary for participation in an exercise intervention.

Evidence-Based Guidelines

Pahwa R, et al. Practice parameter: Treatment of Parkinson disease with motor fluctuations and dyskinesia (an evidence-based review). Report of the Quality Standards Subcommittee of the American Academy of Neurology. Neurology. 2006;66:983-995.

Suchowersky O, et al. Practice parameter: Diagnosis and prognosis of new onset Parkinson disease (an evidence-based review). Report of the Quality Standards Subcommittee of the American Academy of Neurology. Neurology. 2006;66:968-974.

Suchowersky O, et al. Practice parameter: Neuroprotective strategies and alternative therapies for Parkinson disease (an evidence-based review). Report of the Quality Standards Subcommittee of the American Academy of Neurology. Neurology. 2006;66:976-982.

Suggested Web Site

Medline Plus. www.nlm.nih.gov/medlineplus/parkinsonsdisease.html

TABLE 46.1

Parkinson's Disease: Exercise Testing

Methods	Measures	Endpoints*	Comments
Aerobic			
Leg or arm ergometer	■ 12-lead ECG, HR	■ Serious dysrhythmias ■ >2 mm ST-segment depression or elevation ■ Ischemic threshold ■ T-wave inversion with significant ST change	■ Prevalence of dysrhythmias is high. ■ Use HR response to determine impact of medications. ■ Autonomic dysfunction is common.
	■ BP	■ SBP >250 mmHg or DBP >115 mmHg ■ Hypotensive response ■ Volitional fatigue	
	■ $\dot{V}O_{2max}$ ■ METs ■ RPE (6-20)		
Endurance			
6 and 12 min walk	Distance	Note vitals, symptoms, time, distance at rest stops	Aerobic training may improve walking velocity.
Strength			
Weight machines	Maximal voluntary contraction		Use with electromyography to determine strength deficits.
Flexibility			
Goniometry	Joint angles at full extension/flexion		Especially important to measure ROM of neck, trunk, shoulders, hip, and knees.
Neuromuscular			
Gait and balance analysis Reaction time Balance Gait	■ Pull test, 360° turn, functional turn ■ Timed walk, velocity, cadence, step length	Level of difficulty	■ Use gait analysis if functional gait training and/or motor intervention is necessary. ■ Classify disability level and define existing balance deficits. ■ Reaction time is important to determine whether driving competence is questionable.
Functional			
Sit and stand Mobility	Time		Multiple attempts in the sit and stand may suggest quadriceps weakness and/or poor motor control. Weight training should specifically target quadriceps.

*Measurements of particular significance; do not always indicate test termination.

TABLE 46.2

Parkinson's Disease: Exercise Programming

Modes	Goals	Intensity/Frequency/Duration	Time to goal
Aerobic Leg and arm ergometry Rowing	Maintain or improve work capacity	▪ 60-80% peak HR ▪ 3 days/week ▪ ≤60 min/session	3 months
Endurance Short walking sessions (20-30 min; supervised)	Increase work capacity	▪ Speed dependent on individual ▪ 4-6 sessions/day	
Strength Weight machines Closed kinetic chain activities	Maintain strength of arms, shoulders, legs, and hips	▪ Use light weights ▪ 1 set of 8-12 reps ▪ 3 sessions/week	
Flexibility Stretching	Increase/maintain ROM and manage spasticity	1-3 sessions/week	
Functional ADLs Postural changes	Maintain capacity to perform as many ADLs as possible		

CASE STUDY

Parkinson's Disease

A 62-year-old woman had bilateral total knee replacements and was referred to physical therapy for knee rehabilitation after the surgery. The program included strengthening of the knee and hip muscles, gait training, ROM exercises, general exercise for endurance, and pain reduction. After completing the rehabilitation program, however, she still had difficulty walking. She showed shortened step lengths and was referred to a neurologist, who made a diagnosis of idiopathic Parkinson's disease. Antiparkinsonian medications were prescribed, and she was referred to physical therapy. She had difficulty in performing activities of daily living (e.g., bathing, grooming, rising from a chair and bed, turning over in bed) and complained of getting tired easily. She also lacked confidence in making conversation and had a fear of choking.

S: *"I'm afraid of freezing and falling."*

O: Vitals

Elderly woman in no distress; masked facies and neck flexed with stooped shoulders; cranial nerves intact; slurred speech; poor finger-to-nose and heel-to-shin coordination. Romberg's sign: positive; slight flexion of knees while standing; reduced ROM in neck, shoulders, trunk, hips, knees, and ankles; normal strength; festinating gait with reduced arm swing.

Gait study: Slow, shortened steps, narrowed base of support and instability (festinating gait)

50 ft (15.2 m) walk time: 16 s

(continued)

Gait velocity: 0.73 m/s

Step length: Left 36.6 cm (14.4 in.); right 38.4 cm (15.1 in.)

Pull test: Unable to recover balance (Hoehn and Yahr stage 3.0)

360° turn: 6.7 s

Functional reach: 8.5 in. (21.6 cm)

A: 1. Status postbilateral knee replacement surgery
   2. Parkinson's disease
      - Gait and balance impairment
      - Difficulty in transfers (turning in bed, getting up)

- Decreased flexibility
- Decreased endurance
- Impaired orofacial functions

P: 1. Prescribe Sinemet/anticholinergic medication.
   2. Initiate a physical rehabilitation program.

Exercise Program Goals

1. Ambulate with confidence
2. Improve balance
3. Self-sufficiency with transfers
4. Improve endurance

Mode	Frequency	Duration	Intensity	Progression
Aerobic (walking, swimming[a])	3 days/week	30 min	Self-selected	As tolerated
Strength (resistance[b])	2 days/week	3 sets	Hold for 10 s each	As tolerated
Flexibility (stretching[c])	1 day/week	20 s/stretch 30 min total	3 reps, hold for 10 s each	
Neuromuscular (gait and balance,[d] orofacial[e])	1 day/week 2 day/week	15-20 min	3 reps, hold for 10 s each	
Functional (transfer exercises[f])	1 day/week	15-20 min	3 reps, hold for 10 s each	
Warm-up and cool-down	Before and after each session			

[a]Perform during peak drug response.

[b]Resistance exercises include shoulder shrug, shoulder squeeze, trunk twist, hip bridge, straight-leg raise, leg kick, toe/heel raise, standing against the wall, and wall push-up.

[c]Stretching exercises include head turns and tilts, chin tuck, arm stretch, wrist circles, finger/thumb circles, back extension, hamstring stretch, bringing knees to chest, hip roll, calf stretch, and ankle circles.

[d]Gait training requires an attentional strategy—for example, reminding about taking larger steps and walking with alternate arm swing, or using visual or auditory cues to improve step length. Balance training includes tandem walking, sideways walking, backward walking, standing on one limb, alternate standing on toes and heels, and turning the head and looking over the shoulders while standing.

[e]Orofacial exercises include chin tucks in and out, eyebrow lifts, deep breathing, sticking the tongue out and in, saying "u-k-r" loudly, lip presses, whistling, circling the tongue inside the lips, long blowing through the mouth, big smiles, face squeezes, and cheek stretches.

[f]Transfer training includes bed turns (sequential trunk rolling and pushing up) and getting up (leaning forward, shifting weight, and standing up quickly).

PART VIII

Cognitive, Psychological, and Sensory Disorders

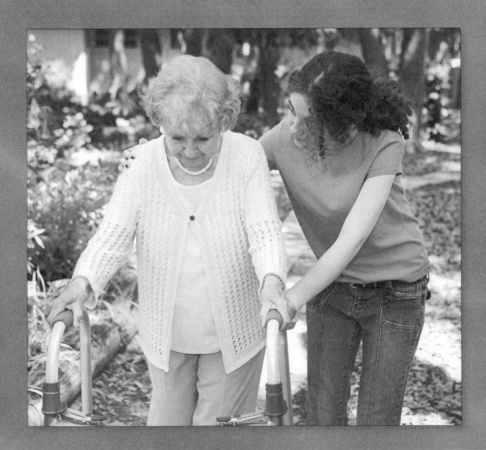

Intellectual Disabilities

Patricia Fegan, PhD

OVERVIEW OF THE PATHOPHYSIOLOGY

Intellectual disability (ID) is a common developmental disorder, affecting an estimated 7.5 million U.S. citizens, and is a lifelong chronic condition. Factors attributable to this condition affect the structure or function of the developing brain, or both, with symptoms ranging from mild to severe. Individuals with ID tend to be sedentary and rarely participate in exercise programs, which puts them at significant risk for numerous chronic health conditions. Determinants of exercise participation for individuals with ID include personal characteristics (age, level of adaptive behavior, and health status), perceived benefits, socio-emotional barriers, and access barriers to exercising. No longer referred to as mentally retarded, individuals with ID are experiencing greater social inclusion and acceptance in society.

Individuals are considered to have an ID if they meet all three of the following criteria:

- Significant limitation in intellectual functioning (IQ below 70-75).
- Significant limitations in two or more adaptive skills—the basic conceptual, social, and practical skills one needs for everyday life
- Incidence of the ID before age 18

There are over 400 potential causes of ID, including genetic and nutritional disorders, birth or childhood trauma, infectious diseases and poisons as in fetal alcohol syndrome, maternal drug use, and ingestion of leaded substances. Other causes include poverty, malnutrition, severe stimulus deprivation, and lack of educational supports that promote intellectual development and adaptive skills learning. While normal probability estimates indicate that 3% or 7.5 million U.S. citizens have an ID, the actual number of individuals receiving services through the educational or social service systems because of ID is often 1% to 2%. This discrepancy arises because most people with ID have very mild forms of the disability, do not require or use any special services, and therefore are not identified.

Many systems exist for classifying ID. The World Health Organization and the American Psychiatric Association use intelligence test scores to determine the level of severity of ID. Presently, the American Association on Intellectual and Developmental Disabilities (AAIDD) proposes a five-level classification system ranging from none to intermittent, limited, extensive, and pervasive disability. The classification system is based on the relationship between the individual's functioning and the environment and the supports necessary to maximize the individual's functioning. The intensity of needed support for

Acknowledgment

The editors wish to acknowledge the previous author of this chapter, Bo Fernhall, PhD, FACSM.

an individual within a specific subclassification is as follows:

- Intermittent: Short-term support is on an "as needed" basis.
- Limited: Episodic, longer-term low-intensity support is needed.
- Extensive: Daily support is needed in some environments.
- Pervasive: Constant high-intensity support is needed across all environments.

Assessing the support required for an individual with an ID and developing the individualized support plan include four steps:

- Step 1: Identify relevant support areas: Human development, teaching and education, home living, community living, employment, health and safety, behavioral, social and protection, and advocacy.

- Step 2: Identify relevant support activities for support areas: The AAIDD has identified numerous support activities for each of the nine support areas mentioned in step 1.

- Step 3: Evaluate the level or intensity of support needs: One system used for this purpose is the Supports Intensity Scale (SIS), which evaluates practical support requirements of a person with an ID through a positive and thorough interview process. This system provides a summary of the frequency, daily support time, or type of support (or some combination of these) for each relevant support activity and can be found at the SIS Web site (see "Suggested Web Sites").

- Step 4: Write the individualized supports plan to reflect the individual: An individualized profile is written based on the information from steps 1 through 3. This profile guides the planning team in developing an individualized supports plan (ISP).

Ninety percent of all people with ID require either no support, intermittent support, or limited support. The remaining 10% have a greater incidence of coexisting conditions usually requiring extensive or pervasive support. These coexisting conditions include autism, seizure disorders, cerebral palsy, and sensory deficits. An important note is that the level of support one needs is not uniform across all life activities. For example, some people may need only limited support in self-care but extensive support in a vocational setting.

Individuals with ID frequently react inappropriately to social and emotional situations due to misinterpretation of the situation rather than to a lack of appropriate responses. Additionally, they are often ill prepared to handle the many social and emotional situations they encounter because of difficulties generalizing information or learning from past experiences. However, people with ID can learn to act appropriately and function well in social settings.

The motor abilities and skills of people with ID are typically delayed, but early intervention is effective in offsetting the gap between this population and those without ID. Motor skill development delays are also exacerbated by a lack of movement experiences, as well as physical disabilities, obesity, and other co-occurring conditions (e.g., hearing loss, visual impairments) that are often observed in this population. Overweight and obesity are common conditions among individuals with ID, posing problems with body mechanics, postural deviations, and balance and increasing risk for other diseases. Thus, physical activity performed on uneven surfaces or requiring rapid changes of direction can cause anxiety and pose greater risk of injury.

The most recognizable (although not the most prevalent) genetic condition associated with ID is Down syndrome (Ds). In the United States, about 5000 children are born with Ds each year. Among the more than 80 clinical characteristics associated with Ds, those that affect physical performance include poor muscle tone; short neck, legs, fingers, and arms in relation to torso; broad hands and feet; perceptual difficulties; poor balance, vision, and audition; immature respiratory and cardiovascular systems; and obesity.

Individuals with Ds also tend to be hypotonic (i.e., have abnormally low muscle tone), particularly in the flexor muscles, and have lax ligaments that permit greater than normal body flexibility. Weak ligaments and muscles also predispose these individuals to sprains and strains. Approximately 10% to 20% of those with Ds have atlantoaxial instability between vertebrae C1 and C2, which increases the risk for spinal cord compression and injury.

Many people with Ds also have comorbidities. Approximately 40% have heart defects such as atrioventricular and ventricular septal defects, many of which are repaired during infancy. In addition, about 20% of individuals with ID (which includes the Ds sub-population) are classified as obese, with a strong inverse relationship between IQ and adiposity. Other conditions such as hypothyroidism, visual defects, hearing loss, digestive problems, and respiratory problems are common among those with Ds. Adults with Ds age more rapidly than others, and the incidence of Alzheimer's disease is three to five times greater than in those without Ds.

EFFECTS ON THE EXERCISE RESPONSE

Individuals with ID who require extensive or pervasive supports have not for the most part participated in studies involving conventional exercise testing and training. On average, individuals with ID, irrespective of age, tend to have lower maximal heart rates and peak oxygen consumption ($\dot{V}O_{2peak}$) levels than their nondisabled peers. Those with ID but without Ds achieve maximal heart rates 8% to 20% lower than the nondisabled population. Although these lower $\dot{V}O_{2peak}$ values (e.g., ranging from 25 to 41 ml $\cdot$ kg^{-1} $\cdot$ min^{-1} and 25 to 35 $\cdot$ kg^{-1} $\cdot$ min^{-1} in children and young adults, respectively) are shown in the majority of research, there is wide interindividual variability. Some persons within this population can achieve average or above-average levels of cardiovascular fitness. Recent studies suggest that a sedentary lifestyle, lack of motivation during an exercise test, lower peak ventilation (peak $\dot{V}_E$), and possible chronotropic incompetence are factors that may be partially responsible for the reduced maximal heart rates and $\dot{V}O_{2peak}$ values in individuals with ID (without Ds).

Persons with Ds appear to be unable to achieve the same level of cardiorespiratory fitness as those with ID who do not have Ds. Individuals with Ds typically have peak heart rates approximately 30 to 35 contractions per minute lower and $\dot{V}O_{2peak}$ levels 30% to 35% lower than their intellectually disabled peers without Ds. Age does not appear to affect $\dot{V}O_{2peak}$ in individuals with Ds; average values for both children and young adults are within the range of 18 to 25 ml $\cdot$ kg^{-1} $\cdot$ min^{-1}. Chronotropic incompetence has been identified as a physiologic condition in most individuals with Ds and therefore is likely responsible for these significantly lower heart rates. Recent data suggest that people with Ds display an altered hormonal profile at rest and during exercise compared to those without ID. At rest, individuals with Ds showed significantly higher levels of circulating catecholamines, insulin, and leptin but lower levels of testosterone and cortisol than nondisabled persons. During submaximal exercise, catecholamine and cortisol levels fail to increase, whereas insulin concentrations are significantly higher in the Ds group compared to controls. This altered endocrine profile is partially responsible for the low cardiovascular fitness. Other anatomical and physiological anomalies associated with Ds that may further limit cardiorespiratory capacity include pulmonary hypoplasia, a reduced peak $\dot{V}_E$, skeletal muscle hypotonia, a high prevalence of circulatory abnormalities and heart defects (e.g., a narrowed aorta), and small nasal and oral cavities. In addition to a reduced aerobic capacity, muscle strength in individuals with ID (with or without Ds) is typically 30% to 50% lower than what would be expected of their nondisabled counterparts and may be a further limiting factor in aerobic capacity.

EFFECTS OF EXERCISE TRAINING

For the most part, exercise training is beneficial for people with ID. However, the majority of exercise training studies on cardiovascular and skeletal muscle adaptations in the ID population have received criticism because of small sample sizes, failure to assess study outcomes utilizing validated test protocols for this population, or the lack of control groups. Nonetheless, findings on exercise training adaptations for individuals with ID are consistent throughout the literature. Some studies demonstrate that individuals with ID (without Ds) can significantly improve $\dot{V}O_{2peak}$ (by 16%) following 16 weeks of Air-Dyne cycling. Improvements in $\dot{V}O_{2peak}$ of 10% to 20% are expected for persons without Ds. Other potential endurance training outcomes for persons with ID but without Ds include

- increased maximum work rate,
- increased time to exhaustion, and
- improved peak $\dot{V}_E$.

The exact mechanisms surrounding the improved functional capacity in individuals with ID are not completely described; however, individuals with ID but not Ds exhibit adaptations such as improvements in stroke volume, cardiac output, and muscle metabolism. At the same time, strength training appears to yield expected improvements in muscular strength and endurance, typically ranging from 20% to 50% when standard resistance training recommendations for the general population have been followed.

Because persons with Ds have some alterations in body structures (e.g., heart defects), their ability to respond to exercise training with improved fitness may be altered or attenuated. Few studies have examined the effect of exercise training in people with Ds; but a recent meta-analysis showed that participating in aerobic exercise for 10 to 16 weeks improved performance (i.e., time to exhaustion), increased maximal work rate, and increased peak $\dot{V}_E$. However, endurance exercise training had no impact on $\dot{V}O_{2peak}$ or body weight. Interestingly, when endurance exercise training is combined with light, progressive resistance training, significant improvements in $\dot{V}O_{2peak}$ have been observed, suggesting that a combined program of resistance and aerobic exercise training may have a larger impact on cardiovascular fitness than aerobic exercise alone in people with Ds. Furthermore, a strong correlation has been demonstrated between $\dot{V}O_{2peak}$ and leg strength in people with Ds.

The inability of endurance exercise training to significantly reduce body weight is in accordance with findings from the literature on non-ID populations. Investigations of people without intellectual impairments show that a combination of exercise and caloric restriction is more effective in achieving weight loss than exercise training alone. Thus, promoting healthy food choices combined with exercise training to achieve healthy living is recommended in the ID population.

MANAGEMENT AND MEDICATIONS

While exercise has no effect on one's intelligence quotient, many adapted behaviors such as practical skills are influenced by regular exercise training. In addition, exercise training plays an important role in helping individuals with ID live independently, sustain their own health, and be gainfully employed. Employment opportunities often include jobs that demand manual labor skills and the stamina to sustain those skills over long periods of time. Therefore, the health and fitness of persons with ID have significant economic and social consequences.

Because the rate of secondary disabilities and other health problems among people with ID is high, these individuals are more likely than others to be taking a variety of medications.

- Anticonvulsive medications (for seizure disorders), antidepressant medications, and stimulants (for hyperactivity disorders) may negatively affect motor performance; alter heart rate; and cause irritability, lethargy, fatigue, headaches, blurred vision, dizziness, drowsiness, mood swings, or general malaise. These effects may influence the individual's level of concentration, motivation, and ability to understand instructions.

- Antianxiety medications can affect the autonomic nervous system, producing blurred vision, contraction of the pupils, decreased sweating, salivation, and dizziness.

- Cardiac medications such as beta-blockers may further blunt exercise heart rate responses.

- Thyroxine replacement therapy (for hypothyroidism) can produce palpitations, chest pain, muscle cramps, and sweating until the correct dosage is achieved.

RECOMMENDATIONS FOR EXERCISE TESTING

Assessing cardiorespiratory fitness levels in individuals with ID can target those in need of intervention and provide a starting point to set goals for exercise prescription. Because obesity, congenital heart defects, pulmonary abnormalities (heart defects and pulmonary problems are more common in those with Ds), atlantoaxial instability (in those with Ds), physical inactivity, and low endurance capacities are prevalent in persons with ID, risk factor screening prior to exercise testing is recommended. Making note of current medications (e.g., those that may affect exercise performance) and comorbidities is also indicated prior to exercise testing.

Testing Aerobic Function

Measurement of $\dot{V}O_{2max}$ during a maximal aerobic exercise test is currently considered the gold standard of assessing cardiovascular fitness. However, individuals with ID may have difficulty with this type of assessment due to problems with task comprehension, motivation, attention deficits, physical disabilities, and motor delays. Thus meeting the criteria for $\dot{V}O_{2max}$ is difficult, and $\dot{V}O_{2peak}$ is typically used as an alternate fitness measure. To facilitate optimal performance outcomes, practice sessions should be scheduled prior to the actual exercise test to familiarize the individual with the protocol, environment, and staff. In addition, this familiarization time can be used to determine the person's capability to perform the test protocol or exercise activity, adjust the protocol to ensure validity of test results and safety, or select an alternate activity if necessary. Individuals with ID may require substantial modifications to test protocols. Assessments using typical health-related physical fitness tests of those who need extensive or pervasive supports may not be possible; therefore, task analysis or measurement of physical activity may be preferred in this group. To help ensure valid testing, the following recommendations should be followed:

- Select a measurement activity that the individual is capable of performing.

- Ensure appropriate testing attire.
- Provide ample warm-up and cool-down activities particularly when large range of motion, strenuous effort, and aerobic activities are involved.
- Provide adequate time for test familiarization and practice testing (one to three familiarization sessions may be necessary depending on the individual). Once the person is able to perform the initial test stages without undue stress and behavioral problems, he or she is deemed ready to undergo the actual exercise test.
- Adhere to all safety precautions; ensure that participants do not fall or fear falling.
- Tailor the protocol to the individual.
- Provide a positive testing environment with frequent positive reinforcement.
- Demonstrate the task while giving short action-word instructions.
- Ask the client to repeat instructions to ensure that they understand.

Exercise test protocol selection is based on individual ability. Treadmill protocols are typically low level, involve a constant speed, and increase the gradient every 1 or 2 min. Speed can be increased toward the end of the test in order to elicit a maximal response as long as grade is not increased at the same time. If ambulatory limitations or poor coordination precludes the use of the treadmill, other modes of exercise should be selected (e.g., the Schwinn Air-Dyne and cycle ergometer have been validated for exercise testing in this population). See table 47.1. Maximal exercise testing is not always appropriate or feasible; submaximal field-based testing is an acceptable alternative.

Commonly used field tests designed to assess cardiorespiratory fitness include step testing, bicycle ergometry, and running and walking tests. However, few of these have been validated on individuals with ID. Because persons with ID may not be physically capable of performing certain modes of activity, to the exercise professional should use a field test validated for this population.

The following are field tests currently validated for use in children with ID:

- The 1-mile Rockport Walk Fitness Test (RWFT)
- The 20 m shuttle run
- The 16 m shuttle run
- The 600 yard run/walk

Reliable and valid field tests for adults with ID include the following:

- The 1-mile RWFT
- The 1.5-mile run/walk

TABLE 47.1

Intellectual Disabilities: Exercise Testing

Methods	Measures	Endpoints*	Comments
Aerobic			
Schwinn Air-Dyne or cycle ergometer (25 W/2 min stage)	• HR		• Peak HR is usually lower than age predicted.
Treadmill (Naughton, Balke protocols; speed 2-0.5 mph)	• BP	• SBP >250 mmHg or DBP >115 mmHg	
Field tests (adults):	• $\dot{V}O_{2peak}$		• $\dot{V}O_{2peak}$ is usually lower than age/gender predicted.
• 1-mile RWFT (1.6K)	• METs	• Volitional fatigue	
• 1.5-mile (2.4K) run/walk	• RPE		
Field tests (children):		• Distance	• A pacer will assist the individual during field tests.
• 20 m PACER	• Completed laps	• Inability to complete laps in required time	
• 16 m PACER	• Time		
• 600 yd walk/run			• More individuals will walk rather than run.
• 1-mile RWFT			

(continued)

TABLE 47.1 *(continued)*

Methods	Measures	Endpoints*	Comments
Strength—upper body			
Isokinetic tests	▪ Time	▪ Completion of 3 trials	
Isometric push-up	▪ Repetitions	▪ Correct position no longer held	
Bench press (weight machines)	▪ Weight lifted	▪ Volitional fatigue	▪ Ensure that there are 1-2 spotters for bench press.
Handgrip dynamometer	▪ Kilograms		▪ Free weight use necessitates appropriate supervision.
Extended arm hang	▪ Time	▪ Fingers leave bar	
Flexed arm hang	▪ Time	▪ Chin contacts or drops below the bar	
Strength—trunk			
Trunk lift	▪ Joint angles	▪ 12 in./30 cm	▪ Beware of excessive arching of the back.
Curl-up	▪ Repetitions	▪ Curl exceeds 3 s or 75 curls are reached	▪ Curl not counted if feet come off floor.
Modified curl-up	▪ Repetitions		
Flexibility			
Shoulder stretch	▪ Degree of stretch	▪ Does not count if fingers touch	▪ Proceed with caution for persons with Ds.
Modified Apley test	▪ Achieve 0-3 points	▪ One trial each leg	▪ Requires sturdy table.
Modified Thomas test	▪ Achieve 0-3 points		
Back-saver sit and reach	▪ Degree of stretch (inches or centimeters)	▪ Complete four attempts	▪ Requires flex-tester box.
Target stretch test	▪ Achieve 0-2 points	▪ Hold position for 1-2 s	▪ Requires goniometer.

Testing for Muscular Strength

Both isokinetic and isometric strength testing protocols have been validated in individuals with ID. Performing an aerobic warm-up and at least one practice isokinetic trial prior to isokinetic strength testing is recommended. The following are typical procedures for isokinetic strength testing:

- The client performs at 60° or 90°/s.
- Two trials of six repetitions are used.

- The highest isokinetic contraction is considered the peak torque.

Isometric strength is evaluated by various modes including handgrip dynamometry, push-ups, curl-ups, arm hangs from a bar, trunk lifts, and bench press (see table 47.1). When using bench press testing, the evaluator must take extra care in monitoring the client. Caution is advised with the use of free weights in individuals with ID. Proper supervision in a weight room is recommended.

Testing Flexibility

Various tests are suitable for examining flexibility in ID individuals (see table 47.1). However, due to joint laxity, one must take care when testing flexibility in people with Ds.

RECOMMENDATIONS FOR EXERCISE PROGRAMMING

Because of a high incidence of sedentary lifestyle, obesity, and very low exercise capacity, prescreen all individuals with ID is advised before starting an exercise training program in order to identify any existing conditions that may affect the exercise response or the safety of exercise. Individuals with atlantoaxial instability should not engage in exercises with strong neck flexion or extension. This would exclude participation in activities such as gymnastics and diving.

During the early stages of exercise training, the main focus is to promote daily physical activity, which may necessitate varying the exercise intensity to encourage regular participation. Once activity is habitual, emphasis moves to increasing exercise duration and intensity (refer to table 47.2).

Motivating people with ID to perform to the best of their ability is often a challenge. A number of strategies can help to enhance motivation:

- Considering individual preferences when prescribing exercise will make the difference in whether the client truly engages in an activity or just goes through the motions, and will likely improve adherence.

- Activities should be selected according to the individual's chronological age and modified to accommodate the person's functional abilities and mental age. Because clients with ID have difficulty applying past experience and previously learned information to new tasks,

TABLE 47.2

Intellectual Disabilities: Exercise Programming

Modes	Goals	Intensity/Frequency/ Duration	Time to goal
Aerobic Walk, walk/jog Schwinn Air-Dyne Swim Aerobics (or other exercise to music) Cycle	▪ Weight control or loss ▪ Improve cardiovascular fitness ▪ Improve work capacity	▪ 60-80% $\dot{V}O_{2peak}$ ▪ 60-80% peak HR ▪ 3-7 days/week ▪ 20-60 min/session	4-6 months
Strength Weight machines Isometrics Exercise/resistance bands Caution about the use of free weights	Increase strength of large muscle groups	▪ 70-80% of 1RM ▪ 3 sets of 8-12 reps ▪ 1-2 min rest between sets ▪ Monitor closely to prevent injury	10-12 weeks
Flexibility Passive stretching Active-assisted stretching Active stretching	▪ Improve ROM of selected joints ▪ Improve flexibility about a joint	▪ Hold stretch to a position of mild discomfort ▪ 3-5 days/week ▪ 3-5 reps not to exceed 30 s each ▪ Monitor closely to prevent injury	▪ 10-12 weeks ▪ Not recommended for individuals with Ds

the progression from familiar to unfamiliar must occur gradually and must be strongly reinforced.

- Because verbalization is more abstract, demonstration or modeling, physical prompting, or manipulation of body parts should accompany verbal instructions. Verbal instructions should be precise, short, and simple and should use action words—for example, words like "walk," "run," or "hop" instead of "go."

- The use of picture cards as reminders of how to do the activity, as well as visual tracking of progress is beneficial.

- Physical activity skills are better taught in environments where they are used than in an artificial laboratory setting.

- Proper technique in all activities and skills should be reinforced.

- Behavior management principles such as cueing, reinforcing, and correcting should enhance success.

- Day-to-day consistency in structure, behavior, and expectations helps promote learning.

- If an individual with ID can acquire some of the skills needed to participate in an activity, the parts of the activity that he or she cannot perform are accommodated through physical assistance or adaptations of equipment. Peer tutors often provide the physical assistance, whereas modified equipment and rule changes can allow individuals with ID to participate in an inclusive setting.

- Generally, exercise session time should be reduced because most individuals with ID are not motivated to work through the discomfort of a long, intense exercise session.

- Make the activity fun. Most people with ID are more motivated to work hard if they enjoy the activity. Music is often a great motivator. Use of testing or training equipment (i.e., treadmill, ergometer) as the power source for a favorite movie, television show, or music has proven successful.

- Use simple movement patterns and demonstrate the task numerous times.

- External pacers are also helpful in maintaining exercise intensity, as individuals with ID have particular difficulty with understanding the concept of exercise intensity.

- Encourage regular exercise as a way to enhance participation and success in organized sport programs such as Special Olympics.

Persons with ID do not appear to differ from the general population in their response to resistance exercise training. Therefore, standard exercise guidelines are used for prescribing resistance training in this population (see table 47.2). In most cases, people with ID should start with weight machines or bands and, if appropriate, progress to free weights. In general, keep the number of repetitions or trials per set low while using low to moderate weights. If the individual has hypotonicity, provide longer rest periods between activities and decrease the number of repetitions per set.

SPECIAL CONSIDERATIONS

Although many of the organizational and instructional methods used in exercise programming for nondisabled individuals are applicable to those with ID, careful planning and organization of the exercise program are needed. Emphasis on frequency, intensity, and duration is appropriate; but because intensity is particularly difficult for this population to understand, the use of external pacers is recommended.

Numerous medical problems associated with Ds will necessitate medical clearance prior to engagement in any exercise program. Again, careful planning of the exercise program is imperative. As with any program that includes aerobic and resistance training activities, progression is an important consideration. Gradual changes in exercise programming should be introduced and monitored; additional caution is warranted for muscle hypotonia and lax ligaments, which often cause postural and orthopedic impairments such as lordosis, dislocated hips, kyphosis, flat pronated feet, forward head, and total body slump. Exercises and physical activities that cause hyperflexion are contraindicated because they place undue stress on the body and contribute to hernias, dislocations, and strains or sprains. Muscle strengthening exercises that stabilize joints are encouraged. Poor balance, eyesight, and hearing in some people with Ds will necessitate adapted equipment and instructional strategies typically used with persons who have sensory impairments.

Evidence-Based Guidelines

Grey IM, Hastings RP. Evidence-based practices in intellectual disability and behaviour disorders. Curr Opin Psychiatry. 2005;18:469-475.

World Health Organization. Atlas: Global resources for persons with intellectual disabilities. World Health Organization 2007. 103 p.

Suggested Web Sites

American Association on Intellectual and Developmental Disabilities. www.aaidd.org

American Psychiatric Association. www.psych.org

American Psychological Association. www.apa.org

National Center on Physical Activity and Disability. www.ncpad.org

National Down Syndrome Society. www.ndss.org

Special Olympics, Inc. www.specialolympics.org

Supports Intensity Scale Web site. www.siswebsite.org/

CASE STUDY

Intellectual Disabilities

A 35-year-old female with Ds experienced significant weight gain and was recently diagnosed with type 2 diabetes. Having been selected to compete in cycling at the Special Olympics World Summer Games, she wanted to be able to perform her best. She had an intellectual disability but lived in her own home with intermittent supports from family and friends in most domains. She worked in the laundry of a special school and volunteered at a summer camp. She was a nonsmoker and had trained with Special Olympics in swimming and cycling since the age of 8 years.

S: *"I want to win a medal at the Special Olympics World Summer Games."*

O: Vitals

Height: 4 ft 10 in. (1.47 m)
Weight: 183 lb (83.01 kg)
BMI: 38.41 kg/m^2
HR: 71 contractions/min
BP: 106/70 mmHg
Body composition: Triceps + subscapular skinfold: 41 mm
Resting metabolic rate: 1260 kcal/day
Graded exercise test: Stopped at 3.0 mph and a grade of 12% because of fatigue and shortness of breath
Peak HR: 147 contractions/min
$\dot{V}O_{2peak}$: 22.4 ml · kg^{-1} · min^{-1}
Peak ventilation: 60 L/min
Respiratory exchange ratio: 1:14
Medications: Riomet (1 tsp prior to meal)

Strength tests

Handgrip: 26.8 kg
Trunk lift: 23 cm

A: 1. Ds; minimal verbalization; very determined; controls own diabetes
   2. Mildly abnormal aortic valve of uncertain pathology
   3. Requires endocarditis prophylaxis
   4. Low aerobic capacity, peak HR
   5. Weak upper and lower extremities
   6. Severe obesity, normal metabolic status

P: 1. Prescribe aerobic exercise, alternating walking, cycling, and swimming.
   2. Improve muscle strength using exercise bands and isometric weights.
   3. Decrease body weight and relative body fat using exercise and diet.
   4. Prescribe diabetic diet counseling.

Exercise Program Goals

1. Improve cycling times in the 500 m, 1K, and 5K
2. Increase muscle strength and endurance
3. Improve cardiovascular fitness
4. Weight loss to 135 lb (61 kg)

Mode	Frequency	Duration	Intensity	Progression
Aerobic (walk, swim, cycle)	6-7 days/week	20-30 min	As tolerated	Increase to 45 min over 3-6 weeks; 60 min over 6-12 weeks.
Strength (circuit weight training, exercise bands)	2-3 days/week	1-2 sets of 8-12 reps	60% of 1RM	Gradually increase to 80% of 1RM after 2 weeks. Increase to 2-3 sets after 2-6 weeks. Increase to 3-4 sets after 6-9 weeks.
Flexibility				
Warm-up and cool-down	Before and after each session	10-15 min		

48

Alzheimer's Disease

James H. Rimmer, PhD ■ Donald L. Smith, MS, RCEP

OVERVIEW OF THE PATHOPHYSIOLOGY

Alzheimer's disease (AD) is a chronic progressive and eventually fatal brain disorder that affects more than 5.1 million Americans, with an annual cost of treatment estimated at $100 billion. By the year 2050, it is estimated that 13.2 million people in the United States will suffer from Alzheimer's. Alzheimer's disease is also the most common cause of dementia and the seventh leading cause of death in the United States. Although the etiology of AD is still being investigated, current accepted theories include reduced biosynthesis of the neurotransmitter acetylcholine, neural protein anomalies, and a genetic predisposition among likely causes of AD. Alzheimer's disease is a devastating condition that destroys brain cells, causing problems with memory, thinking, and behavior that lead to disability and decreased quality of life among older adults. After the age of 65, the percentage of those affected with AD doubles with every decade of life, with the highest prevalence occurring in those 85 or older. There is still no known cure for AD, but efforts aimed at preventing and controlling the effects of Alzheimer's have become a national health care priority, especially in light of the rapid changes in aging demographics of the U.S. population.

The pathophysiology of AD begins in the entorhinal cortex and proceeds to the hippocampus, an important structure in memory formation. As the hippocampal neurons degenerate, short-term memory begins to falter; and as the disease spreads to other regions of the brain, particularly the cerebral cortex, functions such as language and reason are affected. In the regions of the brain attacked by AD, nerve cells or neurons degenerate, losing their connections or synapses with other neurons, leading to the eventual death of some neurons. Atrophy of the cerebral cortex results in intellectual impairment, which progresses from increasing loss of memory to total disability. This deterioration is manifested in the brains of individuals with AD at autopsy (a definite diagnosis of AD is still possible only when an autopsy reveals the hallmark features of the disease).

The pathological features of AD include amyloid plaques, neurofibrillary tangles, and synaptic and neuronal cell death. Granulovacuolar degeneration in the hippocampus and amyloid deposition in blood vessels are also common during histological examination, but are not required for a diagnosis of AD. Overwhelming evidence has confirmed that tangles occur in dying nerve cells following the accumulation of beta-amyloid proteins. These sticky tangles are the twisted, abnormal, pretzel-like filaments that form inside the nerve cells as they die. Beta-amyloids "gum up" the space between the nerve cells, are toxic to nerve cells, and interfere with the normal function of the brain. Formation of tangles is the result of neuronal breakdown and is the end-stage event resulting from the accumulation of the beta-amyloid fibrils over time. One can compare Alzheimer's to heart disease, where reducing cholesterol levels aids in prevention and treatment.

As in heart disease, the cholesterol equivalent present in AD is beta-amyloid, which must be lowered to reduce the progression of neurofibrillary tangles that exacerbate the disease over time.

Despite the great increase in research on AD, the diagnosis before death remains elusive. At present, there is no universally accepted set of criteria for a pathologic diagnosis. The disease was first recognized in 1907 by the German psychiatrist Alois Alzheimer. From 1907 to 1983, diagnosis was based solely on exclusion criteria, meaning that other conditions such as brain tumors, strokes, infections, head trauma, and other potential etiologies had to be ruled out before a person was diagnosed as having AD. These differential diagnoses are typically eliminated via magnetic resonance imaging scanning or screening. Alzheimer's disease is also characterized by the presence of dementia of insidious onset and a progressive deteriorating course. In 1984, the National Institute for Neurological and Communicative Disorders and Stroke and the Alzheimer's Disease and Related Disorders Association (NINCDS-ADRDA) task force formalized the definition and structured the disease into three categories: definite, probable, and possible AD.

In definite AD, diagnosis is confirmed at autopsy by histopathologic findings of neurofibrillary plaques and tangles. In probable AD, dementia is established clinically and confirmed by neuropsychological tests (cognitive loss accompanied by memory loss). In possible AD, the major clinical sign is unusual losses of memory. Other symptoms include deterioration of language and perception, judgment problems that compromise the person's ability to carry out activities of daily living (ADLs), and behavioral problems such as agitation and paranoia. Alzheimer's disease is progressive and degenerative. Experts in this field have documented common patterns of symptom progression that occur in many individuals with AD and have developed several models for understanding AD. The Phase Model divides AD into three phases that include characteristic indicators of the disease:

- Phase I: Forgetfulness, about where items are placed, appointments, and names, for example, as well as anxiety associated with the forgetting
- Phase II: Confusion and intellectual impairment, including problems with short-term memory, concentration, and orientation
- Phase III: Increased delusions, agitation, loss of basic abilities, and incontinence

The clinical director of the New York University School of Medicine's Silberstein Aging and Dementia Research Center developed the Staging Model, which divides AD into seven stages. Each stage corresponds to classic symptoms of AD, including the following:

- Stage 1: No impairment. Individuals experience no memory problems and none are evident to a health care professional during a medical interview.
- Stage 2: Very mild cognitive impairment. Individuals are aware that they are having memory lapses, such as misplacing of personal items and forgetting of names. No obvious deficits are noticed by friends, family, or coworkers or during a medical interview.
- Stage 3: Mild cognitive decline (early-stage AD). Others begin to notice deficiencies in the person's recall of familiar words and names, retention of information after reading a passage, and ability to plan and organize. These deficiencies may be measurable in clinical testing or during a detailed medical interview.
- Stage 4: Moderate cognitive decline (mild or early-stage AD). Clear-cut deficiencies are evident from medical assessment in the areas of recalling recent events, performing mathematical tasks, performing complex tasks (e.g., managing finances), and recollecting one's own history; and the person may appear withdrawn in socially or mentally challenging situations.
- Stage 5: Moderately severe cognitive decline (moderate or midstage AD). Major gaps in memory emerge, such as recalling the date, the day of the week, or the current season. The individual may require assistance with certain ADLs; however, people with stage 5 AD usually have no difficulty feeding themselves or with incontinence.
- Stage 6: Severe cognitive decline (moderately severe or midstage AD). Memory continues to decline; significant personality changes may emerge; people may require assistance with ADLs (e.g., dressing themselves), experience disruption to circadian rhythms, experience incontinence, and tend to wander.
- Stage 7: Very severe cognitive decline (severe or late-stage AD). Individuals lose the ability to respond to their environment, to speak, and ultimately to control movement.

Although the life expectancy among persons with the disease varies, early mortality is seen among those who develop AD early in life and in men. However, persons with AD can often live for several years with the condition, dying eventually from pneumonia or other diseases. The duration of AD from time of diagnosis to death can be 20 years or more, with an average length of four to eight years. Former U.S. President Ronald Reagan had AD for a decade from 1994 to 2004. At the present time, there is no cure, and for the most part treatment has been limited. Nonetheless, the future care of AD appears promising, and investigators are getting closer to finding new medications that can slow the progression. With the baby boomers preparing for retirement starting in 2010, there is a sense of urgency about better understanding the causes of AD and developing better treatments for dealing with the condition in a substantially larger group of older adults. As technology and medicine continue to advance the human life span beyond age 85, AD will receive more focus among researchers, funding agencies, and health care providers.

MANAGEMENT AND MEDICATIONS

The primary goal of AD treatment is to improve memory and cognition and to delay the progression of disease. Currently five drugs are approved by the Food and Drug Administration for the treatment of AD: acetylcholinesterase inhibitors donepezil, rivastigmine, galantamine, and tacrine, and the N-methyl-D-aspartate receptor antagonist memanatine. The acetylcholinesterase inhibitors help raise acetylcholine levels in the brain which may help compensate for the loss of functioning brain cells in people with AD. Of the four acetylcholinesterase inhibitors, tacrine is less likely to be prescribed due to possible side effects (e.g., possible liver damage). Memantine, used to treat moderate to severe AD, appears to regulate glutamate activity, a chemical involved in information processing, storage, and retrieval.

In addition to prescribed medication, the antioxidants vitamin E and selegiline have been shown to help slow the progression of AD. A variety of other drugs used to treat psychiatric symptoms associated with dementia, including antidepressants, hypnotics, and neuroleptics, have been employed in the management of AD. These drugs help to control depression, psychotic behavior, agitation, aggression, and sleep disturbances, which are often symptoms associated with AD. As a result of the older age of onset, many clients with Alzheimer's are also on other medications to control hypertension, arthritis, heart disease, Parkinson's disease, and other conditions. A wide variety of medications are commonly encountered with clients who have Alzheimer's; see the relevant chapters and the appendix.

EFFECTS ON THE EXERCISE RESPONSE AND EXERCISE TRAINING

The number of scientific studies on the effects of exercise training on persons with AD is limited. Very often the discussion of exercise and AD is based largely on the vast amount of literature on exercise in older adults or adults with certain health conditions (i.e., arthritis, Parkinson's, etc.). Practically speaking, it would seem appropriate to suggest then that older adults with AD can gain many, if not all, of the benefits that older adults without AD achieve, such as improved mobility, fitness, and quality of life. In the limited number of clinical investigations on exercise and AD, exercise has resulted in

- substantial gains in physical fitness and mood, maintenance of function in multiple language measures, and a slower than typical decline in mental status after a year of exercise;
- significant improvement on four cognitive measures after three months of aerobic exercise; and
- improved health and decreased levels of depression following exercise training.

And in cases of more severe dementia, exercise has been shown to reduce the frequency of unwanted behaviors such as wandering, pulling at clothing, making repetitive noises, swearing, and aggressive acts, as well as to improve communication and social participation. The benefits and risks associated with exercise and AD vary considerably, based on the age of onset, comorbidities, stage of disease, and the client's current age and health status.

RECOMMENDATIONS FOR EXERCISE TESTING

Because of the effect of AD on mental capacity, laboratory tests, including those involving treadmills and bike ergometers, may be difficult or impossible to obtain or may be unreliable, especially during the mid to late stages of the disease. Many individuals with AD have a high level of agitation or impaired cognition and therefore do not tolerate lengthy testing sessions. Thus, exercise testing may be best suited for those with early-stage Alzheimer's. When exercise testing is recommended for a client with AD, several practice sessions should be conducted prior to the actual test. If the client becomes agitated or confused, the test should be stopped and scheduled for another day, or another test modality should be selected. Additionally, all testing should be conducted in the morning because most people with AD function better during the early hours of the day. Because of the age of this population, patients should be carefully screened for other chronic conditions, such as coronary artery disease or hypertension, as well as their individual symptoms of AD (see table 48.1).

RECOMMENDATIONS FOR EXERCISE PROGRAMMING

Exercise training for individuals with AD has three major considerations:

- to minimize problems arising from the declining physical and mental health of the participant
- to recognize behavioral changes that may cause the client to become agitated with the exercise program or the exercise setting*to support caregivers' willingness to continue bringing the person to the exercise program as the disease progresses

Thus, a low-intensity program at the client's usual ADL levels is recommended. For this level of involvement, exercise testing is unnecessary.

TABLE 48.1

Alzheimer's Disease: Exercise Testing

Methods	Measures	Endpoints*	Comments
Aerobic Cycle (ramp protocol 10 W/ min; staged protocol 25 W/3 min stage) Treadmill (1 MET/3 min stage)		■ Use ACSM test termination criteria ■ Serious dysrhythmias ■ >2 mm ST-segment depression or elevation ■ Ischemic threshold ■ T-wave inversion with significant ST change	Note time, distance, symptoms at rest stops.
Strength Use machines whenever possible to avoid injury.	10RM weight		When no equipment is available, perform certain timed exercises such as sit to stand and wall push-ups.
Flexibility Upper arms and legs	■ Apley test for the upper arms and shoulders ■ Modified sit and reach for the lower legs (from a seated position)		

*May be applicable only to individuals in the early stages of Alzheimer's.

During the early stages of AD, most clients should be able to participate in some form of physical activity. One of the most common problems associated with exercise programming for adults with AD is memory loss. Clients may forget to come to the exercise session or may find that they have forgotten how to perform certain activities. Depression is also quite common during the early stage of the disease and may result in the client's withdrawal from the program. The cornerstones of an exercise program for this population are consistency, patience, and enjoyment. The exercise leader must constantly provide verbal encouragement and support to maintain the client's interest in the program. During the early stages of exercise training, simple repetitive exercises like walking, riding a stationary bike, or lifting a certain amount of weight on various exercise machines will be easier than more complex routines (see table 48.2).

Precautions

- In the early stages of the condition, participation is extremely important in terms of establishing some sort of regular routine that the client can sustain for as long as possible.

- Emotional instability or outbursts may affect the exercise program in the later stages.

- Low-intensity exercise should be the main focus, involving activities that the person enjoys and can successfully perform.

- Constant supervision during physical activity is necessary during the mid to later stages of Alzheimer's.

The middle stage of AD presents a different set of challenges for the exercise leader. As the disease progresses, the program should become more simple and the leader should consider what reasonable criteria should be used to terminate the program. One of the major concerns during later stages of AD involves behavior. Because agitation is one of the hallmark symptoms of the disease, it is not unusual for a client to become resistant to continuing the exercise program. A client with good exercise adherence during the early stage may suddenly decide to drop out. Memory loss during this stage is more pronounced than earlier, and the client may need verbal or physical guidance in maintaining the exercise routine.

Extreme outbursts of anger and physical aggression can occur during this stage. Often such behavior will last for only a few minutes and the client will immediately forget that the incident occurred. The exercise leader must remember that this is a symptom of the disease and therefore should not take such outbursts personally. He or she must work through the agitation with the support of the caregiver, who may or may not be present during the exercise session. For some caregivers, the brief period away from their loved one is much desired. However, if the individual has a high level of agitation, it may be necessary to have the caregiver present to work through certain behaviors. In some cases, the caregiver may be in the facility and "on call" but wouldn't necessarily have to be in the same room. Sometimes music can help the person relax during the exercise session provided that it is not too loud and has a sound that is appealing to the participant.

TABLE 48.2

Alzheimer's Disease: Exercise Programming

Modes	Goals	Intensity/Frequency/Duration	Time to goal
Aerobic			
Enjoyable activities involving large muscle groups Familiar activities Determine RPE 10-15/20 (in clients with adequate comprehension)	▪ Increase functional health (i.e., maintaining ability to perform various activities and instrumental activities of daily living) ▪ Increase endurance necessary for community ambulation	▪ Monitor HR or RPE ▪ 40-60 min/session (may be broken up into smaller 15-20 min activities)	▪ Emphasize enjoyment rather than performance improvements. ▪ Increase duration by adding daily activities that require exercise (e.g., walking to the mail box or gardening).

During the advanced and final stage of the disease, the client will require constant supervision and physical assistance. Language skills will be greatly diminished and language comprehension extremely limited. The exercise program must be guided on an individual basis. Incontinence and limited mobility are common. Range of motion and strength exercises will be the major focus during this stage.

SPECIAL CONSIDERATIONS

People with AD commonly have a higher level of restlessness or agitation at the end of the day, which experts have labeled "sundowning." This increased state of agitation, activity, and negative behaviors is associated with high levels of fatigue and tiredness later in the day. Therefore the exercise program should be scheduled for an earlier time in the day, preferably in the morning, when the client's agitation level is usually at its lowest and mental cognition is at its highest.

If the client is exercising at home with a family member, a daily walk may be the optimal way to establish a structured routine. However, if the client refuses to exercise at home, attending a day care program once or twice a week may be better. As the disease progresses, walking may be the only exercise the individual is capable of carrying out; and once ambulation is no longer a possibility, because of either the inability to walk or the risk of wandering, maintenance of range of motion becomes crucial.

The hallmark exercise program is one that keeps the client active at various times during the day (e.g., 10 min exercise routines), poses a low risk of injury from falls, and has a strong behavioral component (e.g., effective reinforcement strategies).

When developing the training program be sure to consider the following elements:

Strength Training: Therabands

- Strengthen postural muscles.
- Focus on areas of weakness (i.e., quadriceps, hip extensors).
- Use 10 to 12 reps or less as tolerated.

Aerobic Training: Walking and Chair Aerobic Exercises

- Emphasize enjoyment.
- Maintain function.

Flexibility Training

- Stretch postural muscle groups.
- Focus on exercises that can be done on a raised platform (i.e., mat table) or chair; getting down or up from the floor will be difficult.

Evidence-Based Guidelines

California workgroup on guidelines for Alzheimer's disease management. Guidelines for Alzheimer's disease management: Final report. Los Angeles. 2002. Available from www.alzla.org/medical/FinalReport2002.pdf.

Doody RS, Stevens JC, Beck C, et al. Practice parameter: Management of dementia (an evidence-based review). Report of the Quality Standards Subcommittee of the American Academy of Neurology. Neurology. 2001;56(9):1154-1166.

Eccles M, Clarke J, Livingstone M, et al. North of England evidence based guidelines development project: Guideline for the primary care management of dementia. BMJ. 1998;317(7161):802.

Suggested Web Sites

Alzheimer's Association. www.alz.org/

National Association of Social Workers. www.helpstartshere.org/Default.aspx?PageID=1238

National Center on Physical Activity and Disability. www.ncpad.org

National Institute on Aging, National Institutes of Health. www.nia.nih.gov/alzheimers

CASE STUDY

Alzheimer's Disease

An active, healthy-appearing 78-year-old male learned that he might have Alzheimer's disease, which upset him. He had two years of unusual memory loss, including not remembering the bases he had been stationed at or the proud duties he had completed during his 31-year military career. He became so disoriented that walking only a few blocks home would take a few hours. These occurrences were becoming more frequent; and his language and perception were deteriorating, making it difficult to read and communicate. Depression soon followed, and he began having loud outbursts. Tests ruled out the possibility of brain tumors, stroke, infection, or trauma. He tried taking a cholinesterase inhibitor to improve his memory and function but experienced the side effects of nausea, vomiting, and anorexia. Over the preceding year he had lost 15 lb (7 kg), become considerably weaker, and had difficulty performing basic ADLs such as household tasks and carrying groceries. He had started using a cane to prevent falls and was referred to an exercise program to increase strength and improve balance.

S: "My doctor says I might have Alzheimer's and need exercise to help prevent falls and increase my strength."

O: Vitals

Height: 5 ft 10 in. (1.78 m)
Weight: 160 lb (72.73 kg)
BMI: 23.0 kg/m^2

Anxious; ambulates with cane
Musculoskeletal exam: Poor performance on certain strength measures
6 min walk: Estimated $\dot{V}O_{2max}$ 13 ml · kg^{-1} · min^{-1} (poor)
Sit and reach: 12.5 in. (31.75 cm) (poor)
Functional performance: Failed to lift 5 lb (2.27 kg) weight higher than shoulder
Timed stand: 1 leg, 20 s; 1 leg with cane, 58 s

A: 1. Possible Alzheimer's
   2. Generalized weakness/sarcopenia
   3. Recent falls; unclear if balance deficit or secondary to weakness
   4. Cardiorespiratory deconditioning

P: 1. Initiate a daily exercise program
   2. Follow up with testing every 6 mo
   3. Arrange counseling with registered dietitian

Exercise Program Goals

1. Maintain functional independence
2. Improve strength and balance
3. Promote regular physical activity participation most days of the week
4. Set specific number of steps/day and provide client with simple pedometer to monitor daily activity

Mode	Frequency	Duration	Intensity	Progression
Aerobic	4-5 sessions/week	20 min	RPE 10-14	Add 5 min to activity as tolerated.
Strength (all major muscle groups)	3 sessions/week	1-3 sets of 10-12 reps		Use light hand weights, add weight as needed.
Flexibility (all major muscle groups)	3 sessions/week	20 s		Increase ROM as tolerated.
Warm-up and cool-down	Before and after each session	5 min	RPE 6-7	

Mental Illness

Gary S. Skrinar, PhD, FACSM ■ Dori S. Hutchinson, ScD

OVERVIEW OF THE PATHOPHYSIOLOGY

An estimated one in four U.S. adults aged 18 and over suffers from a diagnosable mental illness. Mental illness is a major public health problem, yet is often undiagnosed and undertreated. Mental illness refers collectively to any one of 300 different diagnosable mental disorders characterized by disturbances in a person's thoughts, emotions, or behavior. Mental disorders represent clinically significant behavioral or psychological patterns in individuals that are typically associated with distress, disability, or increased risk of suffering. Mental illness can affect a person's cognitive, behavioral, and social functioning. In severe cases, it is characterized by significant functional impairment resulting in an inability to carry out normal daily life tasks, possible hospitalization, and often a need for psychotropic medication. Mental illness is the leading cause of disability and a significant contributor to loss in the U.S. economy. In recent years the cost of not treating mental illness has far exceeded the direct costs of treatment, as the U.S. economy loses an estimated $113 billion a year due to untreated and mistreated mental illness while an estimated $55 billion is spent on treatment and support.

An estimated 4.9% of the U.S. population have a serious mental illness, including an estimated 14 million adults with diagnosed depression, bipolar disorder, or schizophrenia. Serious mental illness often has a devastating impact on people's lives.

Those who suffer from mental illness often lose their valued roles as students, employees, and citizens due to the disabling effects of the illness and the treatment itself. Many of the medications prescribed to reduce the symptoms of mental illness can cause serious adverse health effects, including metabolic syndrome, diabetes, dyslipidemia, obesity, and osteoporosis. High morbidity and mortality rates in the United States are largely due to preventable health conditions that are strongly associated with physical activity levels. The level of physical activity is a powerful contributor to the disability experience and recovery efforts of people who live with a serious mental illness and federal mandates are pressuring health care systems to provide interventions that will increase physical activity in persons with serious mental illness as a critical lifestyle practice.

EFFECTS ON THE EXERCISE RESPONSE

Specifically diagnosed mental illness (e.g., depression, schizophrenia, personality disorders) does not alter the exercise response to a single exercise session (i.e., exercise testing) unless concurrent pharmacological therapy plays a dual role (i.e., propranolol minimizes social phobia but also influences cardiovascular function). In addition, it is common for persons with psychiatric disabilities to be diagnosed with a secondary medical condition (e.g., metabolic syndrome, diabetes, hypertension) that could have a primary or concurrent effect on the exercise response. When one is planning single or multiple bouts of exercise for individuals with mental illness, one must consider the primary diagnosed mental illness and current medications as well as comorbidities that could influence the safety and efficacy of exercise.

EFFECTS OF EXERCISE TRAINING

Exercise programming has been safely and successfully conducted with individuals who have severe psychiatric disabilities. Changes in fitness, performance time, and body composition are important and can be expected in this population if standard components of exercise prescription are followed. Programs that include supervision by both exercise and psychiatric rehabilitation personnel are preferred. Concomitant positive changes in the psychological profile may include the following:

- Improved mood
- Improved self-concept
- Improved work behavior
- Decreased depression and anxiety
- Improved social networks

The majority of studies reviewed indicate that exercise has an antidepressive effect and is recommended for inclusion in both inpatient and outpatient treatment programs. A number of studies have substantiated the benefits of exercise in the treatment of depression, and in many cases better treatment outcomes with a variety of mental disorders. Emotional and physical fitness are central to people's ability to control their lives, and exercise is a key component of creating options in living, learning, and working, Further research is needed to clarify all the potential benefits in relation to all types of mental disorders, including the role of exercise in preventing mental illness.

MANAGEMENT AND MEDICATIONS

Because individuals with severe psychiatric disabilities are usually taking some type of psychiatric medication (e.g., antianxiety, antidepressant, antipsychotic), consider reviewing the client's current medications prior to any exercise. The following lists the most common drugs and psychiatric medications used in treating mental illness.

- Antipsychotic medications: Antipsychotics are used to treat severe cases of mental illness such as schizophrenia. These medications include clozapine (Clozaril), olanzapine (Zyprexa), and many others. Side effects include weight gain, sedation, nausea, and vomiting.

- Antidepressant medications: Antidepressants help improve symptoms of depression such as sadness, hopelessness, lack of energy, difficulty concentrating, and lack of interest in activities. Antidepressant medications include citalopram (Celexa), paroxetine (Paxil, Paxil CR), and many others. Side effects include insomnia, weight gain, and dizziness.

- Antianxiety medications: These are used to treat anxiety and panic disorders. Antianxiety medications include alprazolam (Xanax), lorazepam (Ativan), and many others. Side effects include drowsiness, potentiation of alcohol effects, and withdrawal.

Some medications prescribed for mental illness have the same action when prescribed for other disabilities but are utilized for different purposes. For example, the beta-blocker propranolol is commonly prescribed for individuals with cardiovascular disease to help reduce the oxygen requirement of the heart at rest and during exercise, thereby reducing the signs and symptoms of angina. Propranolol is also prescribed to reduce social phobias in individuals with anxiety disorders. When prescribed for mental disorders, beta-blockers reduce the amount of nervous system stimulation and consequently the anxiety associated with social situations. Thus, propranolol has the same cardiovascular effect when prescribed for social phobias as it does when prescribed for heart disease. Possible side effects may occur when psychopharmacologic medications are taken in combination with other medications. Complications from use of alcohol or nicotine in combination with psychopharmacologic medications increase the risk of adverse drug–drug interactions in mentally ill individuals and should be continually reviewed.

RECOMMENDATIONS FOR EXERCISE TESTING

When exercise testing is indicated, both field and laboratory evaluations should be preceded by extensive orientation to the exercise testing facilities, mode of exercise, and personnel. The psychological and emotional status of individuals with psychiatric disabilities varies from day to day and is frequently influenced by the type of medications prescribed. Psychological status may affect people's motivation and ability to perform exercise protocols that depend on volitional maximal efforts. Individuals with psychiatric disorders can be uncomfortable or unaccustomed to treadmill testing, probably as a result of the effects of medication (e.g., fatigue, dehydration, depression, sedentary lifestyle). Gait disturbances associated with tardive dyskinesia, a possible side effect of antipsychotic medications, and anxiety responses associated with certain diagnoses can affect the safety and efficacy of testing in this population. Thus bike ergometers offer a less intimidating and more dependable mode of testing for this group. The recommendation is to consider this mode of testing whenever possible to reduce the anxiety associated with treadmill testing, which may increase a person's sense of vulnerability and lack of control. Measuring gas exchange during exercise testing is rarely if ever indicated, particularly in light of the level of anxiety that is often present.

Special considerations for exercise testing and training include the following:

- Allowing time for the individual to practice the test or mode of exercise

- Familiarizing the client with staff and surroundings

- Understanding that anxiety disorders, social phobias, and lack of motivation are commonly caused by emotional conditions, medication, or both

- Using cycle testing in clients with drug-induced side effects

- Emphasizing low to moderate intensity and enjoyment of participation

The following are medications that may affect the exercise response:

- Beta-blockers: Attenuation of HR response

- Proxilin: Possible increase in blood pressure

- Nefazodone: Infrequent tachycardia, hypertension, ventricular extrasystoles, and angina pectoris

- Antipsychotic medication: Possible gait disturbances in relation to tardive dyskinesia, and often dehydration

- Antidepressants: Insomnia, weight gain, and dizziness

- Antianxiety medication: Drowsiness, potentiation of alcohol effects, and withdrawal

Mental Illness: Exercise Testing and Programming

For testing and programming methodologies, see guidelines for the general population in *ACSM's Guidelines for Exercise Testing and Prescription, Eighth Edition*. If the client has a specific medical problem, see the corresponding chapter in this book (e.g., if the patient has a history of MI, see chapter 6 of this text for tables on exercise testing and programming).

RECOMMENDATIONS FOR EXERCISE PROGRAMMING

In most cases, a good starting point when developing the exercise prescription for individuals with mental illness is to follow standard American College of Sports Medicine protocols for working with apparently healthy individuals, unless comorbidities are present. Because maximal values are infrequently achieved during initial testing, a more conservative approach is recommended in the choice of the exercise intensity level. Exercise programs involving walking or running, as well as group dynamic movement activities at low to moderate intensity (50-65% of maximum heart rate) lasting from 20 to 60 min, have been shown to be safe and effective in this population. Because physical inactivity, high body fat, and low self-esteem are common in those with serious mental illness, the recommendation is to use a structured, supervised program initially to reinforce the elements of exercise programming and exercise education.

Evidence-Based Guidelines

Evidence based practice: Listed by the Implementing Evidence-Based Practices for Severe Mental Illness Project. Implementing dialectical behavioral therapy. Psychiatr Serv. 2002;53(2):171-178.

Evidence based practice: Mental health: A report of the surgeon general. Rockville, MD: U.S. Department of Health and Human Services, Substance Abuse and Mental Health Services Administration, Center for Mental Health Services, National Institutes of Health, National Institute of Mental Health; 1999. p. 286-287.

Torrey W, Drake RE, Dixon L, Burns B, et al. Implementing evidence-based practices for persons with severe mental illnesses. Psychiatr Serv. 2001;52(1):45-52.

Suggested Web Sites

American Psychological Association. www.apa.org

Bazelton Center for Mental Health Law. www.bazelon.org

Boston University, Education, Center for Psychiatric Rehab. www.bu.edu/cpr

National Alliance of Mental Illness. www.nami.org

National Association of State Mental Health Program Directors. www.nasmhpd.org

National Mental Health Association. www.nmha.org

American Psychiatric Association. www.psych.org

Substance Abuse and Mental Health Law. www.samhsa.gov

CASE STUDY

Mental Illness—Schizophrenia

A 47-year-old male with a 27-year history of a schizophrenia diagnosis, substance abuse in remission, and a more recent history of type 2 diabetes, high blood pressure, and obesity enrolled in a supported healthy lifestyle program for persons with serious mental illness. His immediate goal was to improve his cardiovascular fitness, stabilize his blood sugars, and lose some of the weight that had accumulated over recent years due to the atypical antipsychotic medications he had been prescribed to ameliorate his symptoms. While on these medications, he had gained considerable weight (50 lb [19 kg]), a very common side effect of this type of treatment, and developed type 2 diabetes and hypertension. He had tried unsuccessfully to increase his physical activity levels on his own and had referred himself to the healthy lifestyle program with the support of his physician and psychiatrist. The achievement of these health goals was critical to his long-term goal of returning to work as a computer technician with increased functional health.

S: *"I have been able to manage my mental illness, but the side effects of my treatment have significantly decreased my physical health. As a result, I have very little stamina, feel poorly, and cannot work."*

O: Vitals

Height 5 ft 10 in. (1.78 m)
Weight 248 lb (112.7 kg)
BMI: 35.6 kg/m²
HR: 74 contractions/min
BP: 150/95 mmHg
Abdominal circumference: 44 in. (1 m)
Obese, 47-year-old man, normal appearance
Well-managed schizophrenia (SCI-PANSS)
Poor glucose management as indicated by FPG (T2DM >125)
Medications: Zyprexa

A: 1. Schizophrenia disorder NOS (not otherwise specified)
   2. Substance abuse disorder
   3. Type 2 diabetes, obesity, hypertension

P: 1. Continue medical and psychiatric treatment.
   2. Initiate a therapeutic lifestyle program including moderate, daily physical exercise and nutritional plan to support rehabilitation goals.

Exercise Program Goals

1. Sustain a moderate exercise program
2. Improve self-esteem and reduce anxiety
3. Weight loss

Mode	Frequency	Duration	Intensity	Progression
Aerobic	≥ 4 days/wk	20-30 min/session	RPE 11-14/20	P Limit to 30 min/session
Strength (all major muscle groups)	2 days/wk	1 set of 8-12 reps	50-70% of 1RM	Increase gradually to 2 sets
Flexibility (all major muscle groups)	5 days/wk	20-60 s/stretch	Maintain stretch below discomfort point	
Warm-Up/Cool-down	Before and after each session	5-10 min each session		

50

Stress and Anxiety Disorders

Gregory A. Hand, PhD, FACSM ■ Jason R. Jaggers, MS
Wesley D. Dudgeon, PhD

OVERVIEW OF THE PATHOPHYSIOLOGY

Despite its prevalence and the profound influence that stress has on our physical and mental health, on the economy, and on the quality and quantity of life, there is no consensus regarding its definition. Stress is difficult to define and measure because the experience is highly subjective with respect to the types of stimuli that produce it and the symptoms that follow. The most recognized definition of stress was conceived by Hans Selye over 70 years ago, who stated that stress or the stress syndrome is "the non-specific response of the body to any demand for change." Selye theorized that the body goes through three predictable stages—alarm reaction, adaptation, and exhaustion—when confronted with a stressor (anything that causes stress). The term used to describe these stages was the general adaptation syndrome (GAS). Selye's definition is widely accepted today, due in part to its simplicity and its characterization of stressors as "non-specific," referring to the endless possibilities of psychological and physiological stressors. Contemporary opinions tend to view stress as more than just a matter of environmental stressors and instead to focus on how well individuals feel they can cope with various environmental stressors. For example, according to

one of the more contemporary definitions, "Stress is a condition or feeling experienced when a person perceives that demands exceed the personal and social resources the individual is able to mobilize." Despite the many uncertainties with respect to our understanding of what stress is or is not, there is little disagreement that stress is a serious, prevalent, and menacing problem in the United States and that the persistent and ever-increasing number of new stressors today is detrimental to our health, to the economy, and to our relationships and the quality and quantity of life.

In contrast to the lack of agreement on the definition of stress, there is more of a consensus about how the body responds to stress (regardless of how stress is defined), especially in terms of physiological responses and adaptations. In this context, stress has been defined as the physiological changes resulting from a stressor. Physiological changes occur rapidly once a stressor is registered. For example, activation of the sympathetic nervous system is almost instantaneous, followed moments later by activation of the hypothalamic-pituitary-adrenal (HPA) axis. This response is the same whether an individual is running from a perceived threat or sitting in heavy traffic that will make him or her late for a business meeting. These automatic physiological responses to stress have been fine-tuned throughout the course of human evolution in response to the myriad physical challenges to survival. Modern-day stress has more to do with emotional threats than with physical threats; but unfortunately, our bodies still react with the prehistoric "fight-or-flight" responses that are now not only unnecessary but potentially damaging and deadly. Recent advances in the study of stress have focused on the associated central neural pathways, including the hypothalamus, limbic system, frontal cortex, and brainstem loci. These regions of the brain are critical for numerous high-level functions such as memory, cognition, emotion, and reward and are all altered by stressful stimulation.

While the stress response is similar among individuals, what is perceived as stressful varies tremendously. Interpreting and responding to stressful stimulation depend on the individual's appraisal of the stressor. The factors that determine the response include inherent characteristics such as genetic predisposition and physiological limitations, as well as environmental factors such as the context of the situation and previous experiences. Often a research subject reports a very low level of perceived stress while a blood sample shows a high level of stress hormone release. In any case, chronic stimulation of the physiological stress response has been shown to either cause or exacerbate a number of physiological and psychological diseases and disorders, including cardiovascular disease, immunosuppression, and major depressive and anxiety disorders.

Perceived stress can elicit a greater pathological response that includes extreme worry or apprehension, occurring frequently without any real threat. This condition, termed "anxiety," encompasses a group of disorders that are similar but each have distinct specific behavioral characteristics. These include phobias, obsessive-compulsive disorder, posttraumatic stress disorder, panic disorder, and generalized anxiety disorder (GAD). Anxiety can be subdivided into transient feelings that are typically evoked by an acute event or perceived threat (state anxiety) and personality characteristics that determine how prone an individual is to perceiving events as threatening (trait anxiety). The anxiety that is experienced as a normal response to actual events is distinguishable from clinical anxiety disorders. For example, criteria that distinguish GAD are (1) the experience of excessive anxiety on more days than not for at least six months, (2) difficulty in controlling worry, and (3) an association with three or more of six symptoms (restlessness, fatigue, lack of concentration, irritability, muscle tension, sleep disturbances).

The etiologies of anxiety disorders are still unclear. Numerous neurobiological pathways are potential components involved with anxiety. Most notably, the central norepinephrine and serotonergic systems have both been implicated in anxiety disorders. From a cognitive perspective, subjects who suffer from anxiety disorders typically exhibit a heightened inclination toward recalling information that includes a real or perceived threat. However, anxiety disorders are poorly understood, and there is a dearth of information regarding biological markers for anxiety. Therefore, establishing an exercise-associated anxiolytic effect has been very difficult and is based almost entirely on self-reported anxiety levels.

EFFECTS ON THE EXERCISE RESPONSE

The physiological adjustments during a graded exercise stress test are typically not altered by heightened stress levels or anxiety disorders. In extreme cases of chronic stress or anxiety, there is a potential for abnormal neuroendocrine responses at moderate- and high-intensity test stages. These abnormal responses usually are manifested as a reduced time on the treadmill or bike and reduced peak oxygen consumption. As in other clinical populations, concurrent pharmacological interventions may negatively affect the exercise response. Therefore a thorough medical history and listing of current medications are critically important prior to a graded exercise stress test.

EFFECTS OF EXERCISE TRAINING

Exercise training has various positive effects on stress and anxiety levels, while overtraining can have negative ramifications.

Stress

Most studies using human or animal subjects have shown that exercise training reduces the intensity or the number of symptoms associated with stress. Most of these studies have focused on large muscle, rhythmic exercise and have used physiological measures of stress, self-reported perceived stress, or both. For example, human studies have shown enhanced mood following acute exercise in both clinical and nonclinical subject pools. These studies indicate that an exercise session of 20 to 30 min is optimal for an anxiolytic effect, with longer sessions showing significant diminishing returns. Animal and human studies indicate that cardiovascular fitness is associated with a reduced heart rate and blood pressure response to a perceived stressor. In addition, electromyographic studies in human subjects demonstrate a reduced level of muscle tension in the head and upper and low body in resting individuals following aerobic exercise. Aerobic exercise programs lasting several months appear to optimally reduce chronic stress symptoms as reported by study participants.

Anxiety

Numerous studies indicate a significant decrease in state anxiety observed approximately 30 min following a 20 to 30 min session of moderate to intense aerobic exercise. A number of those studies showed a slightly heightened level of anxiety immediately following the exercise session. In clinical populations, reports indicate a small to moderate exercise-induced anxiolytic effect regardless of exercise intensity. The anxiolytic effect of exercise training has been compared experimentally to that of a number of other therapeutic interventions, including various forms of meditation, distraction therapies, and pharmacological interventions. It appears that acute sessions of aerobic exercise are as effective as meditation or antianxiety drugs in reducing an individual's level of anxiety. Further, the effects of exercise last longer than therapies involving distraction from the stimulus. While an exercise session of at least 20 min seems to be necessary for exercise-induced anxiolytic effects, exercise intensity may not be a critical factor. Few studies have addressed the effects of resistance exercise training, but those that have done so show either no anxiolytic effect or an effect at moderate-intensity training.

Negative Responses to Exercise Training

While many investigations have demonstrated a beneficial effect of exercise training in persons with high stress and anxiety levels, it is important to be cognizant of studies showing disturbed mood states associated with overtraining (chronically pushing beyond the healthy physical and psychological limits of exercise training). Overtraining is usually characterized by decreased performance and fatigue, depression, heightened levels of anxiety, decreased libido, and loss of appetite. In more extreme cases, overtraining syndrome is associated with generalized immunosuppression resulting from abnormal endocrine function. It is critical for all individuals, especially those with high levels of stress and anxiety to have a realistic view of healthy physical activities in terms of both exercise mode and intensity.

MANAGEMENT AND MEDICATIONS

Management of stress and anxiety disorders can be addressed through psychotherapy and behavioral therapy or pharmacological intervention or some combination of these. Psychotherapy takes a variety of forms, but all are designed to help people recognize stress and anxiety and develop new ways to cope with problems. Often, biofeedback or some other form of self-examination is included in therapy sessions in an attempt to train the individual to control stress and anxiety. Anxiolytic drugs are designed to correct chemical imbalances in the brain. A number of categories of medicines are used in the treatment of stress or anxiety disorders, including the following:

■ Azaspirones/Buspirone: For the treatment of GAD, medications in this class are partial agonists for serotonin receptors and work by helping to regulate the antidepressant and antianxiety effects of serotonin. These drugs are non-habit forming and are tolerated well, usually without serious side effects.

■ Benzodiazepines: This drug class is the most commonly prescribed for anxiety disorders and includes several drugs, all of which are central nervous system depressants. They work as sedatives through reducing the individual's state of arousal. They are fast acting as compared to drugs in some other classes, but can be very habit forming and evoke withdrawal symptoms when discontinued.

■ Beta-blockers: Known mainly for their use in regulating blood pressure and heart function, beta-blockers can also be used to control certain stress or anxiety symptoms such as sweating, heart palpitations, and muscle tremors.

■ Tricyclics (TCA): These groups of drugs are best known for treatment of depression but are also effective in controlling panic attacks. They work through increasing the amount of serotonin, norepinephrine, and to a lesser degree dopamine in the brain. Beneficial effects are not noticeable for two to four weeks. These drugs also elicit significant side effects, such as weight gain, lethargy, and dizziness.

■ Monoamine oxidase inhibitors (MOIs): This category of medications, which prevents the metabolism and breakdown of several neurochemicals, is used for a number of disorders including panic disorder, posttraumatic stress disorder (PTSD), and social phobias. They are typically used in more severe cases or when other treatments are ineffective, as MOIs require certain food restrictions and interact negatively with a number of other drugs.

■ Serotonin reuptake inhibitors: This drug class includes selective serotonin reuptake inhibitors (SSRIs) and serotonin-norepinephrine reuptake inhibitors (SNRIs). They normalize neurochemical levels in the brain by increasing the amount of serotonin or norepinephrine. These drugs are relatively new and are widely used for stress and anxiety disorders as well as depression.

Typical drug treatment regimens initially use less potent and less habit-forming medications and move through more potent drugs as the level of drug effectiveness is established. Some of these drug categories have significant side effects that can impair an individual's capacity and desire to be physically active. It is recommended that the individual participate in a monitored exercise program, at least until drug–activity interactions can be established. As with some other clinical populations, there is little information regarding the interaction of medications and exercise training.

RECOMMENDATIONS FOR EXERCISE TESTING

The process of exercise testing an individual in treatment for stress or anxiety disorders does not differ from the procedures used for testing in the apparently healthy population. In assessing the individual's current level of fitness, tone must remember that a number of drug classes used for treatment of this population can reduce functional capacity, induce dizziness or inhibit motor function, or reduce the desire to perform at a high level of exertion.

In the context of the broad array of tests for cardiovascular fitness, including maximal and submaximal tests, there is no reason to think that the majority of this population would respond differently than a healthy population of the same age.

Therefore one would expect that, other than for individuals with medication-associated side effects, maximal stress tests could be used. As with other clinical populations, a modified Bruce protocol, which starts at a lower speed than the standard Bruce protocol but can still be used as a maximal test, would be appropriate. Further, because of potential effects of the condition or drugs (or both) on balance and concentration, a cycle ergometer test may be appropriate.

Assessment of muscular fitness should include endurance and flexibility as well as muscular strength. There is no evidence to indicate that people with stress or anxiety disorders will demonstrate a significant reduction in muscular fitness, although they are generally characterized as untrained and deconditioned. As the population is also typically unfamiliar with resistance training, a 3RM (3-repetition maximum), 6RM, or 10RM may be used in lieu of the standard 1RM test to predict muscular strength. As with any untrained or deconditioned group, it may be necessary to test muscular strength on multiple occasions. Muscular endurance can be safely tested in this population using the YMCA bench press test, which has men press an 80 lb (36 kg) load and women press a 35 lb (16 kg) load 30 times per minute, with the rating of muscular endurance based on the number of repetitions completed.

Stress or Anxiety Disorder: Exercise Testing and Programming

For testing and programming methodologies, see guidelines for the general population in *ACSM's Guidelines for Exercise Testing and Prescription, Eighth Edition*. If the client has a specific medical problem, see the corresponding chapter in this book (e.g., if the patient has a history of MI, see chapter 6 and testing and programming tables).

RECOMMENDATIONS FOR EXERCISE PROGRAMMING

Individuals presenting with stress or anxiety disorders should be evaluated for a range of physical functioning, including functional aerobic capacity, muscular strength, body composition, and flexibility. In addition, neuromuscular function should be assessed, as these conditions and a number of medications prescribed for them can affect perception, alertness, and coordination. These effects should be documented, as they can affect all components of the exercise prescription.

- The goal for persons with stress or anxiety disorders is to meet the American College of Sports Medicine (ACSM) recommendations for aerobic and resistance exercise. However, a number of condition- and medication-related side effects may necessitate a reduction in expectations over the short term, and perhaps reduce rates of progression over the long term.

- Much of this population will be unfamiliar with resistance training. Aerobic exercise has been used as the predominant therapeutic modality for stress and anxiety disorders, and exercise training as an affective therapeutic modality for stress. Therefore, resistance programming most likely could take a secondary role to aerobic activities for these individuals. The resistance training program should adhere to the ACSM guidelines for exercise testing and prescription for safe exercise training. A beneficial rule of thumb for resistance training progression is the 2+2 method, according to which the exercise resistance is increased when the participant is able to complete two repetitions above the number originally prescribed after two consecutive exercise sessions.

SPECIAL CONSIDERATIONS

Participants with stress or anxiety disorders should be monitored for general physical and emotional health, with particular attention given to novices during the introductory period. Those unaccustomed to activity are particularly prone to injury due to condition- and medication-related side effects and are at increased risk for withdrawal from an activity program. The exercise supervisor should emphasize the importance of reporting increased feelings of tiredness or exhaustion, shortness of breath or chest discomfort, heart palpitations, any unusual emotional swings, or increased effort in performing everyday activities. Further, exercise staff members should be trained in and required to follow universal precaution practices. Monitoring the medical regimen of the exercise participant is important, as changes in prescription medications may affect overall functional capacity. In addition, the exercise supervisor should emphasize the importance of reporting anything about the exercise setting (e.g., a particular mode of exercise) that makes a client anxious.

Evidence-Based Guidelines

Baldwin DS, Anderson IM, Nutt DJ, et al. Evidence-based guidelines for the pharmacological treatment of anxiety disorders: Recommendations from the British Association for Psychopharmacology. J Psychopharmacol. 2005;19(6):567-596.

Mclean PD, Woody SR. Anxiety disorders in adults: An evidence-based approach to psychological treatment. New York: Oxford University Press; 2001. p. xvi, 369.

Nejad L, Volny K. Treating stress and anxiety: A practitioner's guide to evidence-based approaches. Bancyfelin, UK: Crown House; 2008.

Suggested Web Sites

American Institute of Stress. www.stress.org

American Psychological Association. www.apa.org

Mayo Clinic. www.mayoclinic.org

National Institute of Mental Health, National Institutes of Health. www.nimh.nih.gov/health/index.shtml

CASE STUDY

Stress and Anxiety Disorder

A 37-year-old Caucasian male was recently prescribed a 10 mg dosage of the serotonin reuptake inhibitor Zoloft. He was having trouble falling asleep and often laid awake worrying about many "what ifs" in his life. His work began to suffer because he became easily distracted from important assignments due to constant worry about job security and supporting his family. He also began to worry about his health as he approached 40; he knew that he should exercise but said, "I've been so busy at work that I don't have the time and am too exhausted after leaving the office."

S: *"I'm worried about my health and want to get in shape but am just too busy and tired all the time."*

O: Vitals

Height: 6 ft 1 in. (1.85 m)
Weight: 192 lb (87.1 kg)
BMI: 25.3 kg/m²
HR: 88 contractions/min
BP: 144/96 mmHg
Central adiposity; waist circumference 38 in (96.5 cm)

(continued)

Labs

Fasting glucose: 92 mg/dl
Total cholesterol: 195 mg/dl
Triglyceride: 148 mg/dl

Graded exercise test (modified Bruce protocol)

Peak work rate: 4.2 mph (6.8 km/h) @ 16% grade
Total treadmill time: 11.25 min
Test termination from volitional exhaustion
Peak RPE: 19 out of 20
Peak HR: 180 contractions/min
Peak BP: 200/98 mmHg
$\dot{V}O_{2peak}$: 43 ml · kg^{-1} · min^{-1}
ECG: Sinus rhythm at rest and throughout exercise and recovery
No dysrhythmias observed or reported
No report of chest discomfort
Body composition: 27.3% fat (DEXA)
Bone density: 1.2 g/cm^2
Medications: Zoloft

A: 1. Sedentary
   2. Stage 1 hypertension
   3. Overweight

P: 1. Begin a combined moderate-intensity aerobic and resistance training regimen in an attempt to reduce anxiety and fatigue while also increasing overall health and quality of life.

2. After 6-8 weeks, monitor performance and body composition outcomes, assess subjective progress, and update the regimen as needed.

Exercise Program Goals

1. Short-term goals (1-2 mo):
   - Attend majority (~90%) of exercise sessions.
   - Walk/jog for 30 min at a moderate intensity 3-5 days a week. This may be done in multiple sessions lasting a minimum of 10 min throughout the day.
   - Increase muscular strength on all exercises.
   - Increase lean tissue mass.
   - Decrease fat mass.
   - Reduce anxiety.
2. Long-term goals (6 mo):
   - Walk/jog for 60 min at a moderate-intensity 3-5 days a week.
   - Increase muscular strength.
   - Increase lean tissue mass.
   - Decrease fat mass.
   - Reduce anxiety.
   - Improve subjective QOL.

Mode	Frequency	Duration	Intensity	Progression
Aerobic Walking/Jogging Cycling	3-5 days/wk	20-30 min	50% to 85% of APHR$_{max}$	Increasing frequency, duration, intensity
Strength (8-10 separate exercises targeting major muscle groups)	2 days/wk	1 set of 8-12 reps. per exercise	Resistance set at ~60-85% of max	Frequency and reps. remain constant, increasing resistance based on the 2+2 method
Flexibility (Static stretching for major upper and lower body muscles)	Following each session	Hold stretch for 15-30 sec	Stretch to point of tightness, avoid discomfort	ROM will increase over time
Warm-Up/Cool-down	Before and after each session	5-10 min	30-45% APHR$_{max}$	Low-intensity, large muscle activity

APHR$_{max}$ – Age Predicted Maximum Heart Rate, ROM – Range of Motion, RM – Repetition Maximum, Reps. – Repetitions

Deaf and Hard of Hearing

M. Kathleen Ellis, PhD ■ Tracy Karasinski, MSW

OVERVIEW OF THE PATHOPHYSIOLOGY

An estimated 31.5 million U.S. citizens have some form of hearing loss, including an estimated 738,000 with hearing loss at the severe to profound level. Individuals who are deaf and hard of hearing can generally participate in all forms of physical activities independently, with a small percentage requiring some minor adaptations. Hearing loss is a generic term that applies to people who are hard of hearing or deaf. The following are two common terms used to characterize people with hearing loss:

- Hard of hearing: A mild to severe level of hearing loss in which individuals who have some range of useful hearing and intentionally use it for the purpose of communication, usually with the assistance of an auditory device.

- Deaf: A severe to profound level of hearing loss in which a person is unable to use residual hearing for processing information or communicative purposes, even with the use of amplification devices. People who are deaf may or may not use sign language as their primary mode of communication.

The four different types of hearing loss include conductive, sensorineural, mixed, and central hearing loss. A conductive hearing loss is one in which sound cannot effectively pass through the outer or middle ear in order to reach the inner ear. Conductive hearing losses can sometimes be medically or surgically corrected. The following are causes of this type of hearing loss:

- Loss of the outer ear structure due to injury, disease, or birth defect

- Buildup of impacted wax or infection of the external ear structure

- Blockages within the middle ear Eustachian tubes caused by infections or diseases

- Otitis media, most commonly caused by infection, affecting the middle ear structure

- Otosclerosis, progressive deafness of unknown etiology, caused by formation of spongy bone, especially around the oval window, resulting in stiffening of stapes and preventing proper vibration

Sensorineural hearing loss (also known as nerve deafness) is the most common type of hearing loss and occurs when the outer and middle ear is intact

Acknowledgment
The editors wish to acknowledge the previous author of this chapter, Lorraine E. Colson Bloomquist, EdD, FACSM.

but the inner ear structures, the cochlea and the delicate hair cells and associated nerves have deteriorated. The cochlea is the region where sensory receptors convert sound waves into neural impulses that are transmitted to the brain for interpretation. Most individuals who are classified as deaf or hard of hearing have a sensorineural hearing loss. Individuals with sensorineural hearing loss may also demonstrate issues with balance, especially younger children and those with Ménière's disease. Balance is typically affected because of the location of the vestibular apparatus within the inner ear. Most sensorineural hearing losses are caused by

- idiopathic (unknown) factors (~50% of cases);
- hereditary and genetic factors (60 different types have been identified);
- illnesses such as meningitis, mumps, scarlet fever, encephalitis, and measles;
- maternal illnesses during pregnancy (e.g., herpes viruses, measles, toxoplasmosis);
- head trauma affecting the hearing mechanism or any ear structure;
- prematurity; and
- aging and excessive noise exposure such as that from noisy work environments, city life, machinery, rock concerts, and listening to loud music through earphones (as a group, these conditions are the most common causes of hearing deterioration over time).

Mixed hearing losses include a combination of conductive and sensorineural hearing losses and involve multiple ear structures. This type of hearing loss is common among senior citizens.

The fourth type of hearing loss, central hearing loss, involves the central nervous system's nuclei or the associated nerves and is caused by damage or impairment to this area in the pathways leading to the brain or within the brain. Central hearing loss is not common and is sometimes classified as a sensorineural hearing loss.

In many cases, individuals with hearing loss could gain some assistance through the use of a hearing aid, which is the most common assistive device used to treat hearing loss. However, only approximately 20% of those who could benefit from using a hearing aid actually do so. In its simplest form, a hearing aid is a device that is worn in the ear and amplifies sound. Hearing aid technology has advanced considerably in recent years; today's hearing aids are very sophisticated and often tailored to an individual's particular hearing loss.

Many digital hearing aids are programmable and can be adjusted by the user for maximal benefit in a particular listening environment, such as a noisy restaurant or a quiet office, or when the person is on the telephone. While hearing aids often offer tremendous benefit to persons with hearing loss, it is important to note that they do not correct or restore normal hearing. Rather, they are designed to provide amplification so that the person can make the best of use residual hearing. The following are the positions in which the most common types of hearing aids are worn:

- Behind the ear (BTE)
- In the ear (ITE)
- In the canal (ITC)
- Completely in the canal (CIC)
- On the chest or body (in special cases worn by young children and persons with multiple or more severe disabilities)

In addition to hearing aids, there are more than 200 kinds of assistive devices that amplify sounds, convert auditory cues to light or vibration systems, or do both. For example, persons with hearing loss may use a listening system in classrooms, auditoriums, or gyms. The listening system, consisting of a transmitter and a receiver, uses FM radio frequencies or infrared signals to relay speech from a microphone (worn by the speaker) directly to the person wearing the receiver. This helps to combat the background noise, distance, and echo that can interfere with clear speech understanding. Other devices include visual warning devices such as fire alarms or smoke detectors, visual or tactile alarm clocks, door signals, and baby monitors.

A relatively recent development for persons with profound hearing loss is the surgical insertion of a cochlear implant. Unlike hearing aids, which amplify sound in order to be detected by damaged sensory cells within the ear structure, a cochlear implant bypasses the nonfunctioning hair cells in the cochlea and directly stimulates the auditory nerve. Approximately a quarter of a million children and adults have a hearing loss severe enough to benefit from a cochlear implant; and nearly 60,000 people worldwide have received cochlear implants, with the United States representing almost half that number. While as yet an expensive treatment (approximately $30,000-$50,000) that requires lengthy postoperative speech and sound therapies, cochlear implantation can improve the lives of people with profound hearing loss.

Cochlear implants are often recommended for those whose hearing loss is too severe to benefit from hearing aids. A cochlear implant consists of two basic parts, an internal device that is surgically placed in the inner ear and an external sound processor. The external processor may resemble a hearing aid and is typically worn behind the ear, or in the case of many young children, on the body. The sound processor captures sound, which is converted into digital signals that are transmitted to the implanted electrodes in the cochlea. These digital signals stimulate the auditory nerve, which sends the information to the brain for interpretation into meaningful sound.

EFFECTS ON THE EXERCISE RESPONSE

Hearing loss generally does not alter the exercise response to any form of physical activity. As there are no physical restrictions directly associated with hearing loss that would lead to concerns during participation, most individuals can participate at a high intensity of exercise or sport without any special considerations. The majority of research in this area has shown that people with hearing loss do not differ significantly from others with respect to exercise. However, deaf individuals, both children and adults, have been reported to have a higher incidence of overweight and obesity than their hearing counterparts.

In assessing fitness and implementing exercise programs for individuals with hearing loss, special consideration should be given to those with sensorineural hearing loss, because some may also exhibit deficiencies in dynamic balance and spatial orientation. These deficiencies may in turn affect their cardiorespiratory efficiency in exercises or activities requiring high levels of balance. Attention should be given when conducting an exercise test using protocols such as those involving the treadmill or step tests. The increased cardiorespiratory efficiency required to compensate for balance and spatial awareness deficiencies while exercising on these modalities may negatively affect the client's test results. Furthermore, these protocols place the individual at an increased risk of falling.

The extent of exercise familiarity, as well as the ability for full involvement including communication and understanding, is an important consideration when those with hearing loss undertake exercise and physical activities. An individual with a profound hearing loss may not be able to hear music at an acceptable level for participation; however, he or she may feel the vibrations either through the floor or by holding a vibration-transmitting object such as a balloon while completing movements. Many people with more severe to profound hearing losses also have difficulty with spoken communication, leading to fewer social opportunities, lower self-concept, decreased self-esteem, lack of self-confidence, and isolation. Early-onset hearing loss, primarily before the age of 4 years, may also lead to difficulty with language acquisition and the development of reading skills; if no assistance is provided, this may significantly affect academic achievement and lead to frustration associated with not understanding both the spoken and written language.

EFFECTS OF EXERCISE TRAINING

Regular exercise in individuals with hearing loss produces the same positive physiological, psychological, and skill benefits as for individuals with no hearing loss. Additional benefits may include the following:

- More opportunities to improve socialization skills in group activities
- Practice of movement skills leading to improvements in balance and spatial orientation
- Increased communication proficiency among group leaders and group members
- Improved self-image, confidence, and self-concept and reduced social isolation

An important consideration in work with individuals who have hearing loss is to document all currently prescribed medications, whether related to hearing loss or a comorbidity. While medications are not typically prescribed to treat hearing loss per se, one must note other medical conditions and treatments (e.g., coronary artery disease) and consider specific prescriptions when testing and developing an exercise program. In some cases, people with temporary hearing loss caused by infections or fluids in their ears are prescribed medications. Children with hearing loss may take medications (e.g., Ritalin) for hyperactivity. Possible side effects of these medications need to be considered, including the following:

- Loss of appetite
- Abdominal pain
- Weight loss or gain, especially if corticosteroids are prescribed to suppress inflammation
- Insomnia

- Tachycardia
- Long-term effects that may have implications for the cardiovascular system and normal growth and development

RECOMMENDATIONS FOR EXERCISE TESTING

If an individual with a hearing loss does not have signs or symptoms of other comorbidities or balance or spatial orientation deficiencies, exercise testing can follow standard protocols. When someone with a hearing loss has a balance or spatial orientation deficiency, care should be taken to ensure his or her safety during testing on protocols requiring balance, and testing protocols with lower balance or orientation requirements should perhaps be substituted in order to ensure accurate results. When signs or symptoms of other primary disease are present, however, exercise testing should follow recommended procedures for that particular disorder.

Additional considerations for individuals with hearing loss may include the following:

- Presenting all instructions in writing, in picture form, via signing, or on a video
- Allowing the person to describe or demonstrate the test protocol before the test begins
- Giving visual or tactile reinforcement to increase motivation
- Taking precautionary measures to prevent the individual from tripping or falling, especially someone who has demonstrated balance or spatial orientation deficiencies

Deaf and Hard of Hearing: Exercise Testing and Programming

For testing and programming methodologies, see guidelines for the general population in *ACSM's Guidelines for Exercise Testing and Prescription, Eighth Edition*. If the client has a specific medical problem, see the corresponding chapter in this book (e.g., if the patient has a history of asthma, see chapter 19 and testing and programming tables).

RECOMMENDATIONS FOR EXERCISE PROGRAMMING

People with hearing loss can generally participate in all types of physical activity. Exercise prescription procedures should follow American College of

Sports Medicine (ACSM) guidelines for the apparently healthy individual.

SPECIAL CONSIDERATIONS

An important special consideration for individuals who are deaf or hard of hearing is to ensure effective communication during exercise testing and training sessions. While individuals with hearing losses may use a variety of communication strategies, those who are hard of hearing typically rely on hearing aids and other assistive listening devices in order to maximize use of residual hearing, whereas many deaf individuals use a spectrum of modalities ranging from verbal communication to manual sign language systems to a combination of the two. Manual sign language systems include American Sign Language (ASL), Conceptually Accurate Signed English (CASE), Signed Essential English (SEE), finger spelling, and gestures. In some cases, use of interpreters may be necessary to facilitate communication and provide access to medical and exercise services and programs. Certified oral interpreters are professionals who silently mouth the words of the person speaking to be directly speech read by the deaf person Cued speed interpreters use the same strategies as oral interpreters with the addition of hand signals, which serve as cues for specific speech sounds. Other sign language interpreters specialize in one or more of the various sign language systems.

Caution is warranted when one is speaking directly to an individual with a hearing loss, as even the best, most experienced speech readers are able to pick up only approximately 30% of spoken language. One of the reasons is that the sounds for many words are formed in the throat or the back of the mouth, making it impossible to see how they are produced and to interpret them. Only words that are formed by the lips and tongue are produced in a way that is visible; however, not all these are readable because sounds can be silent (e.g., *s/f*) and different letters can look similar on a speaker's lips (e.g., *s/t/p*). Therefore, ensuring understanding of critical concepts and communication is imperative, and understanding should never be assumed. If difficulty in communication persists, use visual means such as paper and pencil or black- or whiteboards specifically for this purpose. The goal is effective communication, no matter how it is achieved.

Multiple strategies can be used to enhance the prospects of effective communication. Possibly the most important detail to be aware of is the communication preference of the individual and incorporate that into the exercise program. The following are some additional strategies that can enhance communication effectiveness:

- Always face the person so that he or she can see your face, lips, eyes, and body.
- Maintain eye contact and speak directly to the person, not to the interpreter if one is present (think of the interpreter as if he or she were invisible).
- Demonstrate exactly what is required from start to finish, as many people who are deaf or hard of hearing are very visual learners.
- Use as many visual cues and concrete examples as possible.

Exercise and medical professionals who work with individuals with a hearing loss may need to also consider the following recommendations and guidelines for exercise testing and training:

- Be aware that some individuals with hearing loss may exhibit below-average fitness levels or balance and orientation skills.
- The speaker should stay near the individual and maintain eye contact to enable speech reading.
- The speaker should use facial expressions, body language, gestures, and common signs or cues such as thumbs up or down to communicate emotions and meanings.
- The speaker should avoid chewing gum or food, covering the mouth, or having an untrimmed mustache, as each of these hinders clear view of the lips and mouth and affects speech reading.
- The speaker should use normal enunciation and loudness regardless of whether the person is deaf or hard of hearing or uses a hearing aid, cochlear implant, or no assistive listening device.
- Visual and tactile cues should be used to enhance understanding; this includes having a black- or whiteboard available to use when necessary.
- A demonstration of the routine or activity is helpful and could be done in person or via a video demonstration.
- If an individual's speech is unclear or difficult to understand, the listener should not pretend that he or she understands but rather ask for clarification.

- Avoid loud, constant background noise, as such sounds may cause headaches (from echoes and vibrations), prevent hearing aid users from attending to a speaker, or reduce the effective use of hearing aids.
- Unnecessary or extra physical or visual movements in the area behind the speaker (called "visual noise") should be avoided.
- The individual should be oriented to all aspects of the facility and environment, with special attention to emergency aspects such as exits and fire evacuation procedures.
- People should be taught to be visually aware and observant of their surroundings, especially when they are near moving vehicles or in other potentially dangerous situations (e.g., where others are cycling, jogging, skating, or cross country racing).
- Facilities should be equipped with strobe or visual fire alarms or other alerting devices or strategies. Alerting devices or strategies include use of the buddy or tapping system, very loud sounds (as with a bullhorn), vibrations, colorful flags, or flashing lights.
- Normal speech enunciation and volume should be used for speaking to an individual who has a hearing aid or cochlear implant.
- Some basic cue or feedback signs, for words such as "ready," "start," "faster," "ok," "stop," or whatever words are necessary for activity, should be established.
- A videotape of the test or activity, as well as demonstration, should be shown before the activity is to begin. Instructions should also be in written form.
- Hearing aids and external cochlear implant devices should be removed before participation in activities involving contact and in water activities.
- Removal of hearing aids during contact sports, self-defense activities, aquatics, and gymnastics should be suggested.
- External cochlear implant apparatus should be removed before participation in activities like aquatics and in situations in which electrostatic discharge (ESD) is likely. Electrostatic discharge is commonly associated with plastic equipment and apparatus, such as plastic mats, ball pits, and bats and may damage the "maps" in the electrodes implanted in the individual's cochlea.

- It is important for individuals with tympanic membrane tubes to prevent water entry into the ear canal. Swimmers should wear personal earplugs covered by a water cap and should swim only under the advice of a physician.

- People who wear a hearing aid or use a cochlear implant should take care to avoid injuries or damage when engaging in head-impact sports (e.g., soccer).

- If a balance or spatial orientation deficiency is evident, one should be cautious about involving the person in activities requiring these skills, such as activities using the balance beam, springboard diving, or bicycling.

- Activities and facilities must comply with the Americans with Disabilities Act.

- Exercise professionals should familiarize themselves with the support devices and resources (e.g., amplified phones, sound wizards, interpreters) available for health care providers.

- An activity or testing routine should remain consistent to allow individuals to become adjusted to expectations.

The following are medications commonly used by persons with hearing loss:

- Ritalin: Children taking this hyperactivity drug may experience such side effects as tachycardia, weight loss, abdominal pain, loss of appetite, or difficulty sleeping.

- Antibiotics: Children or adults taking this class of medications for conditions such as ear infections and ear inflammation may experience side effects like diarrhea, nausea, vomiting, sensitivity to sun, weakness or fatigue, and loss of appetite.

Evidence-Based Guidelines

Rosenfeld R. An evidence-based approach to otitis media. Pediatr Clin North Am. 1996;43(6):1165-1181.

Suggested Web Sites

Americans with Disabilities Act. www.ada.gov/

Deaf Linx. www.deaflinx.com/

National Institute on Deafness and Other Hearing Disorders. www.nidcd.nih.gov/health/hearing/hearingaid.asp

Sign language browser. www.commtechlab.msu.edu/sites/aslweb/

CASE STUDY

Deaf or Hard of Hearing

A 14-year-old athlete attended public school with an educational placement of 70% inclusive setting and 30% within a self-contained deaf education classroom. His hearing loss was classified as congenital profound bilateral sensorineural hearing loss. Due to the level of hearing loss, he was unable to hear high-pitched tones like the sound of a whistle or to understand speech at normal communicative levels. While he understood some communication through speech reading, his primary communication modality was sign language. Because of his exceptional athletic skills, he participated with many of his hearing peers in various sporting events, including basketball, baseball, football, and track. In addition, he participated in local recreation soccer and hockey leagues as these sports were not offered through the school he attended. In fact, he participated in an all-state travel hockey team and played the position of forward. Practice for travel hockey was year-round and occurred on most mornings for 2 h. In general physical education classes, he compared favorably to other high school males on the President's Physical Fitness Test. He worked well with his teammates and reacted quickly to facial expressions, body language and movements, and common gestures used in various sports. Over the years,

team sports had helped to develop his skills in leadership, interdependence, communication, and teamwork. Because he had a high level of skill and could compete with his peers in all activities, sports were his main recreational activity.

S: "I want to become a better, more competitive hockey player."

O: Vitals

Neurological examination intact, except cranial nerve VIII, profound hearing loss

A: Profound, bilateral sensorineural hearing loss; otherwise typical athlete

P: 1. Encourage participation in USA hockey developmental program to enhance skill performance.
2. Notify coach to use black-/whiteboard, visual signals, directions, and demonstrations, interpreter during practices, and to inform officials to use visual signals during competitions.

Exercise Program Goal

Play hockey for Team USA in Deaf Olympics

Mode	Hockey-Specific Exercises	Progression
Lower Body Exercises	Squats, lunges, plyometrics Incorporate multi-muscle exercises by changing the squat to a squat/overhead press, etc. Plyometrics could include box jumps, one leg forward/back/side, etc Stretch for specific muscle groups after each segment	2-3 days per week start Start with body weight only and add weights gradually Warning: never go to muscle failure with young individuals
Upper Body Exercises	Pushups, rows, DB shoulder exercises, core Planks, situps and rotational chops for core Stretch for specific muscle groups after each segment	2-3 days per week to start Start with body weight push-ups, medium weight rows (machine and dumbbell) Progress by adding weight and decreasing rest
Endurance	Lunges to end of hall, 10 push-ups, 10 squat jumps, lunge back, 20 sit-ups, plank for one minute, rest for one minute Lunge to end of hall, 10 bicep curl/ overhead press, 10 box jumps, lunge back, plank for one minute, rest for one minute	2-3 days per week to start Increase repetitions on intervals gradually
Flexibility	Stretch all major muscle groups before, during and after workouts	Daily, on and off days, in and out of season
Intensity	Train harder in the off-season Reduce intensity during in-season, couple with practices	
Warm-up/Cool-down	Before and after each session	

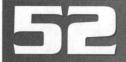

Visual Impairment

Larry J. Leverenz, PhD, ATC

OVERVIEW OF THE PATHOPHYSIOLOGY

Visual impairment (VI) is vision loss that represents a significant limitation of visual ability resulting from disease, trauma, or a congenital or degenerative condition that cannot be corrected by conventional means, including refractive correction, medication, or surgery. Legal blindness is vision of 20/200 or less with the best correction (while one is wearing glasses). Legal blindness is the ability to see at 20 ft (6.1 m) what the normal eye sees at 200 ft or 61 m (i.e., ≤1/10 of normal vision), termed blind due to lack of visual acuity. Blind by visual field means having a visual field of less than 10 ft of central vision or having tunnel vision (e.g., retinitis pigmentosa). Total blindness is lack of visual perception or the inability to recognize a strong light shone directly into the eye, sometimes termed "no light perception."

In approximately 95% of individuals who are considered blind, there is some residual vision that can be used to allow the person to participate in normal daily activities. Visual impairment is the second least common disability in childhood (next to deaf-blind). Visual impairment is more prevalent with advancing age. Approximately 500,000 persons in the United States are classified as legally blind.

In younger populations, causes of VI are attributed to birth defects, including congenital cataracts and optic nerve disease. Another, uncommon cause of VI in children is retinopathy of prematurity (excessive oxygen in incubators), although there are many individuals aged 18 and older with this condition as well. Tumors, injuries, and infectious diseases are possible but less common causes of VI. In persons who are elderly, diabetes, macular degeneration, glaucoma, and cataracts are leading the leading causes of VI. Visual impairment may also occur concomitantly in people with cerebral palsy and mental retardation.

EFFECTS ON THE EXERCISE RESPONSE

Visual impairment generally does not alter the exercise response to a single exercise session. However, some individuals may have associated poor balance, forward head posture, low cardiovascular fitness, obesity, lack of confidence, timidity, self-stimulatory behaviors such as rocking, and fewer social skills than others; any one these conditions could affect the exercise response irrespective of the person's degree of VI. Verbal cues are essential during testing. Loss of visual field—that is, peripheral vision—may affect mobility.

Acknowledgment
The editors wish to acknowledge the previous author of this chapter, Lorraine E. Colson Bloomquist, EdD, FACSM.

EFFECTS OF EXERCISE TRAINING

Individuals with a VI can participate in many vigorous physical activities with some adaptations. In fact, regular exercise in individuals with VI produces the same positive physiological and psychological benefits as in individuals without a disability. Additional benefits include the following:

- Greater opportunities to improve socialization skills
- Practice and improvement in balance skills, which may be low
- Improvement in self-image, confidence, and spatial orientation
- Improvement in cardiovascular fitness
- Decrease in obesity

Depending on the degree of VI, the primary treatment is corrective lenses or eyeglasses. Eyeglasses, though, may not correct VI completely. Individuals who are visually impaired frequently wear glasses to correct acuity problems associated with nearsightedness or farsightedness, but eyeglasses are not the norm in this population. Glasses do not correct vision above the 20/200 level (i.e., some people wear glasses, but this does not correct vision to normal, especially sunglasses for light sensitivity when one is outside).

One encouraging note is that there are numerous highly trained world-class blind athletes. A number of organizations specializing in competitive sport participation (e.g., United States Association of Blind Athletes) for men and women with varying degrees of VI sponsor local, state, regional, national, and international competitions. Blind and VI athletes frequently participate in sporting events that include many of the typical Olympic sports of track and field, swimming, and Nordic and alpine skiing, to mention just a few.

MANAGEMENT AND MEDICATIONS

There are no commonly prescribed medications for apparently healthy adults with VI. The only possible common scenario involves people with glaucoma who may need to use eye drops before or following exercise. If an individual with VI has other primary problems (e.g., coronary artery disease or diabetes), one should note and consider specific medications for those problems when testing and training (see chapters 6, 7, 8, and 24).

RECOMMENDATIONS FOR EXERCISE TESTING

Providing that an individual with a VI does not have any signs or symptoms of other primary conditions, standard exercise testing protocols can be used. When signs or symptoms of other primary diseases are present, exercise testing should follow recommended procedures for the particular disorder (see the table on exercise testing and programming for persons with VI).

The exercise professional may need to follow certain additional guidelines for a person with a VI:

- Have all instructions described verbally or on audio tape.
- Allow the person to describe or demonstrate the test protocol before the test begins.
- Give tactile and verbal reinforcement to motivate the participant.
- Allow the person to stand close to the tester to use residual vision, or to lightly touch handrails or the tester when necessary.

The following are special considerations for exercise testing and training:

- Be aware that clients may have lower than average fitness levels.
- Balance may be poor, so the client may need to use handrails for occasional support.
- Play an audio tape describing the test, activity, or sport. Ask the client to repeat the instructions verbally before beginning.
- Manually and verbally orient the client to all testing and training facilities and equipment.
- Use verbal cues for reinforcement.
- Pair the client with a partner for running and other activities.
- Avoid jumping or other high-impact activities if the client has had a detached retina, has high myopia, or has had a cataract surgically removed (aphakia).
- Keep the facility clear of clutter.

RECOMMENDATIONS FOR EXERCISE PROGRAMMING

Individuals with VI can generally participate in all types of physical activity, one should understand that blind by loss of field leads to greater difficulty in mobility than blind by acuity. The exercise prescription procedure is the same as for individuals without VI, though it may be advisable to consider the following special precautions:

- Manually or verbally orient the person to facilities.
- Keep instructions in large print or Braille or use a strong magnifying glass.
- Play an audio tape describing the routine or activity.
- Ensure that eyeglasses are securely held to the face.
- Allow the person to run or exercise with a partner.
- Have the person run with a short tether to a partner or while holding a partner's upper arm.
- Give regular tactile and verbal cues and feedback to prevent boredom.
- Avoid tracking activities such as handball and tennis.
- Consider offering goal ball, a specialized team sport in which all are blindfolded and a large bell ball is used.
- Most individual sports, such as swimming, weight training, dance, track and field, golf, and aerobics, are appropriate.
- Ensure that people with aphakia (absence of natural lens of eye that occurs when a cataract has been surgically removed), detached retina, or high myopia do not engage in high-impact activities such as jumping.
- Orient the person to all aspects of the facility with special attention to exits, use of the pool, and fire evacuation procedures.
- Keep areas clear of clutter for safe movement.
- Keep doors either closed or wide open.

- Keep equipment in the same place at all times so that individuals can memorize locations.
- Paint or tape (use white) floors or walls where changes occur (e.g., stairs, ramp, pool edge, locker room entrance and exit and lockers themselves).
- Keep areas well lit (e.g., stairs, pool, and equipment).
- A handrail or grab bar can be installed for accessing equipment.
- Keep a sound source, radio, or tape recorder at one end of the room or at the shallow end of the pool for direction orientation.

Visual Impairment: Exercise Testing and Programming

For testing and programming methodologies, see guidelines for the general population in *ACSM's Guidelines for Exercise Testing and Prescription, Eighth Edition*. If the client has a specific medical problem, see the corresponding chapter in this book (e.g., if the patient has a history of MI, see chapter 6 and testing and programming tables).

Suggested Web Sites

American Association for Physical Activity and Recreation. www.aahperd.org/aapar

American Association of Adapted Sports Programs. www.aaasp.org

American Foundation for the Blind. www.afb.org

Association of Services for the Blind and Visually Impaired. www.asb.org

Helen Keller National Center for the Deaf/Blind. www.helenkeller.org

International Blind Sports Association. www.ibsa.es

International Paralympic Committee. www.paralympic.org

The Lighthouse. www.lighthouse.org

National Beep Baseball Association. www.nbba.org

Palaestra: Forum of Sport, Physical Education & Recreation for Those with Disabilities. www.palaestra.com

PE Central, Adapted Physical Education page. www.pecentral.org/adapted/adaptedmenu.html

United States Association of Blind Athletes. www.usaba.org

CASE STUDY

Visual Impairment

35-year-old computer specialist wanted to increase his ~~r~~dic skiing skill and endurance. He had partial sight; that ~~~~he could see light and shapes, but the glare of the snow ~~~~de it almost impossible to see anything when skiing so he ~~~~ed with a guide. He and his guide needed to determine a ~~~~ning regimen that was compatible to both. He had excel- ~~~~t communication skills through working with his guide. ~~~~ had been skiing for three years and wanted to "step up" ~~~~program to enter some of the competitive events held ~~~~ally. When not skiing, he ran or rode a tandem bike with ~~~~wife. He considered himself in relatively good shape but ~~~~nted to increase his intensity to the competitive level. He ~~~~ no other health problems.

"I want to be competitive athletically for the first time ~~~~my life."

O: Vitals

35-year-old male, no known health problems
Detects light and shapes
Visual acuity: Left, 20/400; Right, 20/500
Graded exercise test (cycle ergometer, 25 W/3 min stage)
$\dot{V}O_{2max}$ (estimated): 42.4 ml $\cdot$ kg^{-1} $\cdot$ min^{-1}

A: 1. Severe visual impairments
    2. Average aerobic fitness and strength for age

P: 1. With assistance from ski coach, increase Nordic skiing skills.
    2. With assistance from exercise professional, increase aerobic fitness and strength.
    3. Compete in local skiing events, with the possibility of competing at some higher level.

~~M~~ode	Frequency	Duration	Intensity	Progression
~~A~~erobic ~~R~~ecumbent Stepper ~~(N~~uStep™), Walking ~~n~~ indoor track lightly ~~to~~uching rail.	6 days/wk			Per exercise professional (e.g., coach, personal trainer, health/fitness instructor)
~~St~~rength (focus on ~~an~~tigravity and postural/ ~~tr~~unk muscles)	2 days/wk			Per exercise professional (e.g., coach, personal trainer, health/fitness instructor)
~~Fl~~exibility (anterior chest, ~~hi~~p flexors, plantar ~~fl~~exors)	3-7 days/wk			Per exercise professional (e.g., coach, personal trainer, health/fitness instructor
~~W~~arm-Up/Cool-down	Before and after each session			Per exercise professional (e.g., coach, personal trainer, health/fitness instructor

Appendix

Common Medications

ß-Blockers

Use or condition: Hypertension, angina, arrhythmias including supraventricular tachycardia, increasing AV block to slow ventricular response in atrial fibrillation, acute myocardial infarction, migraine headache, anxiety; mandatory as part of therapy for HF due to systolic dysfunction

Drug name	Brand name†
Acebutolol**	Sectral**
Atenolol	Tenormin
Betaxolol	Kerlone
Bisoprolol	Zebeta
Esmolol	Brevibloc
Metoprolol	Lopressor SR, Toprol XL
Nadolol	Corgard
Penbutolol**	Levatol**
Pindolol**	Visken**
Propranolol	Inderal
Sotalol	Betapace
Timolol	Blocadren

**ß-Blockers with intrinsic sympathomimetic activity.

ß-Blockers in Combination With Diuretics

Use or condition: Hypertension, diuretic, glaucoma

Drug name	Brand name†
Atenolol, chlorthalidone	Tenoretic
Bendroflumethiazide, nadolol	Corzide
Bisoprolol, hydrochlorothiazide	Ziac
Metoprolol, hydrochlorothiazide	Lopressor HCT
Propranolol, hydrochlorothiazide	Inderide
Timolol, hydrochlorothiazide	Timolide

α- and ß-Adrenergic Blocking Agents

Use or condition: Hypertension, chronic heart failure, angina

Drug name	Brand name†
Carvedilol	Coreg
Labetalol	Normodyne, Trandate

α1-Adrenergic Blocking Agents

Use or condition: Hypertension, enlarged prostate

Drug name	Brand name†
Doxazosin	Cardura
Tamsulosin	Flomax
Prazosin	Minipress
Hytrin	Terazosin

Central α2-Agonists and Other Centrally Acting Drugs

Use or condition: Hypertension

Drug name	Brand name†
Clonidine	Catapres, Catapres-TTS patch
Guanfacine	Tenex
Methyldopa	Aldomet
Reserpine	Serpasil

Central α2-Agonists in Combination With Diuretics

Use or condition: Hypertension

Drug name	Brand name†
Methyldopa + hydrochlorothiazide	Aldoril
Reserpine + chlorothiazide	Diupres
Reserpine + hydrochlorothiazide	Hydropres

Adapted, by permission, from ACSM, 2009, *ACSM's guidelines to exercise testing and prescription*, 8th ed. (Philadelphia, PA: Lippincott, Williams, and Wilkins).

Nitrates and Nitroglycerin

Use or condition: Angina, vasodilator in chronic HF

Drug name	Brand name†
Amyl nitrite	Amyl Nitrite
Isosorbide mononitrate	Ismo, Imdur, Monoket
Isosorbide dinitrate	Dilatrate, Isordil, Sorbitrate
Nitroglycerin, sublingual	Nitrostat, NitroQuick
Nitroglycerin, translingual	Nitrolingual
Nitroglycerin, transmucosal	Nitrogard
Nitroglycerin, sustained release	Nitrong, Nitrocine, Nitroglyn, Nitro-Bid
Nitroglycerin, transdermal	Minitran, Nitro-Dur, Transderm-Nitro, Deponit, Nitrodisc, Nitro-Derm
Nitroglycerin, topical	Nitro-Bid, Nitrol

Calcium Channel Blockers (Nondihydropyridines)

Use or condition: Angina, hypertension, increasing AV block to slow ventricular response in atrial fibrillation, paroxysmal supraventricular tachycardia, headache

Drug name	Brand name†
Diltiazem extended release	Cardizem CD, Cardizem LA, Dilacor XR, Tiazac
Verapamil immediate release	Calan, Isoptin
Verapamil long acting	Calan SR, Isoptin SR
Verapamil COER-24	Covera HS, Verelan PM

Calcium Channel Blockers (Dihydropyridines)

Use or condition: Hypertension, angina, neurological deficits after subarachnoid hemorrhage

Drug name	Brand name†
Amlodipine	Norvasc
Felodipine	Plendil
Isradipine	DynaCirc CR
Nicardipine sustained release	Cardene SR
Nifedipine long acting	Adalat, Procardia XL
Nimodipine	Nimotop
Nisoldipine	Sular

Cardiac Glycosides

Use or condition: Chronic heart failure in the setting of dilated cardiomyopathy, increasing AV block to slow ventricular response with atrial fibrillation

Drug name	Brand name†
Digoxin	Lanoxin

Direct Peripheral Vasodilators

Use or condition: Hypertension, hair loss, vasodilation for heart failure

Drug name	Brand name†
Hydralazine	Apresoline
Minoxidil	Loniten

Angiotensin-Converting Enzyme (ACE) Inhibitors

Use or condition: Hypertension, coronary artery disease, chronic heart failure due to systolic dysfunction, diabetes, chronic kidney disease, heart attack, scleroderma, migraine

Drug name	Brand name†
Benazepril	Lotensin
Captopril	Capoten
Cilazapril*	Inhibace
Enalapril	Vasotec
Fosinopril	Monopril
Lisinopril	Zestril, Prinivil
Moexipril	Univasc
Perindopril	Aceon
Quinapril	Accupril
Ramipril	Altace
Trandolapril	Mavik

*Available only in Canada.

ACE Inhibitors in Combination With Diuretics

Use or condition: Hypertension, chronic heart failure

Drug name	Brand name†
Benazepril + hydrocholorthiazide	Lotensin
Captopril + hydrocholorthiazide	Capozide
Enalapril + hydrocholorthiazide	Vaseretic
Lisinopril + hydrocholorthiazide	Prinzide, Zestoretic
Moexipril + hydrocholorthiazide	Uniretic
Quinapril + hydrocholorthiazide	Accuretic

ACE Inhibitors in Combination With Calcium Channel Blockers

Use or condition: Hypertension, chronic heart failure, angina

Drug name	Brand name†
Benazepril + amlodipine	Lotrel
Enalapril + felodipine	Lexxel
Trandolapril + verapamil	Tarka

Angiotensin II Receptor Antagonists

Use or condition: Hypertension

Drug name	Brand name†
Candesartan	Atacand
Eprosartan	Tevetan
Irbesartan	Avapro
Losartan	Cozaar
Olmesartan	Benicar
Telmisartan	Micardis
Valsartan	Diovan

Angiotensin II Receptor Antagonists in Combination With Diuretics

Use or condition: Hypertension, chronic heart failure, angina

Drug name	Brand name†
Candesartan + hydrochlorothiazide	Atacand HCT
Eprosartan + hydrochlorothiazide	Teveten HCT
Irbesartan + hydrochlorothiazide	Avalide
Losartan + hydrochlorothiazide	Hyzaar
Telmisartan + hydrochlorothiazide	Micardis HCT
Valsartan + hydrochlorothiazide	Diovan HCT

Diuretics

Use or condition: Edema, chronic heart failure, polycystic ovary syndrome, certain kidney disorders (i.e., kidney stones, diabetes insipidus, female hirsutism, osteoporosis)

Thiazides

Drug name	Brand name†
Chlorothiazide	Diuril
Hydrochlorothiazide (HCTZ)	Microzide, Hydrodiuril, Oretic
Indapamide	Lozol
Metolazone	Mykron, Zaroxolyn
Polythiazide	Renese

"Loop" Diuretics

Drug name	Brand name†
Bumetanide	Bumex
Ethacrynic acid	Edecrin
Furosemide	Lasix
Torsemide	Demadex

Potassium-Sparing Diuretics

Drug name	Brand name†
Amiloride	Midamor
Triamterene	Dyrenium

Aldosterone Receptor Blockers

Drug name	Brand name†
Eplerenone	Inspra
Spironolactone	Aldactone

Diuretic Combined With Diuretic

Drug name	Brand name†
Amiloride + hydrochlorothiazide	Moduretic
Triamterene + hydrochlorothiazide	Dyazide, Maxzide

Antiarrhythmic Agents

Use or condition: Specific for drug but include suppression of atrial fibrillation and maintenance of NSR, serious ventricular arrhythmias in certain clinical settings, increase in AV nodal block to slow ventricular response in atrial fibrillation

Drug name	Brand name†
Class IA	
Disopyramide	Norpace
Moricizine	Ethmozine
Procainamide	Pronestyl, Procan SR
Quinidine	Quinora, Quinidex, Quinaglute, Quinalan, Cardioquin
Class IB	
Lidocaine	Xylocaine, Xylocard
Mexiletine	Mexitil
Phenytoin	Dilantin
Tocainide	Tonocard
Class IC	
Flecainide	Tambocor
Propafenone	Rythmol
Class II	
ß-Blockers	Refer to appendix page \bb\
Class III	
Amiodarone	Cordarone, Pacerone
Bretylium	Bretylol
Sotalol	Betapace
Dofetilide	Tikosyn
Class IV	
Calcium channel blockers	Refer to appendix page 398

Antilipemic Agents

Use or condition: Elevated blood cholesterol, low-density lipoproteins, triglycerides, low high-density lipoproteins, and metabolic syndrome

Category	Drug name	Brand name†
A	Cholestyramine	Questran, Cholybar, Prevalite
A	Colesevelam	Welchol
A	Colestipol	Colestid
B	Clofibrate	Atromid
B	Fenofibrate	Tricor, Lofibra
B	Gemfibrozil	Lopid
C	Atorvastatin	Lipitor
C	Fluvastatin	Lescol
C	Lovastatin	Mevacor
C	Lovastatin + niacin	Advicor
C	Pravastatin	Pravachol
C	Rosuvastatin	Crestor
C	Simvastatin	Zocor
D	Atorvastatin + amlodipine	Caduet
E	Niacin	Niaspan, Nicobid, Slo-Niacin
F	Ezetimibe	Zetia
F	Ezetimibe + simvasatin	Vytorin

A = bile acid sequestrants; B = fibric acid sequestrants; C = HMG-CoA reductase inhibitors; D = HMG-CoA reductase inhibitors + calcium channel blocker; E = nicotinic acid, F = cholesterol absorption inhibitor.

Blood Modifiers (Anticoagulant or Antiplatelet)

Use or condition: To prevent blood clots, heart attack, stroke, intermittent claudication, or vascular death in patients with established peripheral arterial disease (PAD) or acute ST-segment elevation myocardial infarction; also used to reduce aching, tiredness, and cramps in hands and feet. Plavix is critical to maintain for one year after PCI for DES patency.

Drug name	Brand name†
Cilostazol	Pletal
Clopidogrel	Plavix
Dipyridamole	Persantine
Pentoxifylline	Trental
Ticlopidine	Ticlid
Warfarin	Coumadin

Respiratory Agents

Main drug classes for respiratory conditions include steroidal anti-inflammatory agents and bronchodilators.

Steroidal Anti-Inflammatory Agents

Use or condition: Allergy symptoms including sneezing, itching, and runny or stuffed nose; shrinking nasal polyps; various skin disorders; asthma

Drug name	Brand name†
Beclomethasone	Beclovent, QVAR
Budesonide	Pulmicort
Flunisolide	AeroBid
Fluticasone	Flovent
Fluticasone and salmeterol (ß2 receptor agonist)	Advair Diskus
Triamcinolone	Azmacort

Bronchodilators

Use or condition: Dilate the bronchi and bronchioles to decrease airway resistance and facilitate airflow. Bronchodilators include anticholinergics (acetylcholine receptor antagonists and anticholinergics with sympathomimetics), sympathomimetics (β2-Receptor Agonists), xanthine derivatives, leukotriene antagonists and formation inhibitors, and mast cell stabilizers.

Anticholinergics (Acetylcholine Receptor Antagonists)

Use or condition: To prevent wheezing, shortness of breath, and troubled breathing caused by asthma, chronic bronchitis, emphysema, and other lung diseases

Drug name	Brand name†
Ipratropium	Atrovent

Anticholinergics With Sympathomimetics (β2-Receptor Agonists)

Use or condition: Chronic obstructive pulmonary lung disease (COPD)

Drug name	Brand name†
Ipratropium and albuterol	Combivent

Sympathomimetics (β2-Receptor Agonists)

Use or condition: To prevent wheezing, shortness of breath, and troubled breathing caused by asthma, chronic bronchitis, emphysema, and other lung diseases

Drug name	Brand name†
Albuterol	Proventil, Ventolin
Metaproterenol	Alupent
Pirbuterol	Maxair
Salmeterol	Serevent
Salmeterol and fluticasone (steroid)	Advair
Terbutaline	Brethine

Xanthine Derivatives

Use or condition: To prevent wheezing, shortness of breath, and troubled breathing caused by asthma, chronic bronchitis, emphysema, and other lung diseases

Drug name	Brand name†
Theophylline	Theo-Dur, Uniphyl

Leukotriene Antagonists and Formation Inhibitors

Use or condition: To prevent wheezing, shortness of breath, and troubled breathing caused by asthma, chronic bronchitis, emphysema, and other lung diseases

Drug name	Brand name†
Montelukast	Singulair
Zafirlukast	Accolate
Zileuton	Zyflo

Mast Cell Stabilizers

Use or condition: To prevent wheezing, shortness of breath, and troubled breathing caused by asthma, chronic bronchitis, emphysema, and other lung diseases

Drug name	Brand name†
Cromolyn inhaled	Intal
Nedocromil	Tilade
Omalizumab	Xolair

Antidiabetic Agents

Use or condition: To control glucose levels. Antidiabetic agents include biguanides, glucosidase inhibitors, insulins, meglitinides, sulfonylureas, thiazolidinediones, and incretin mimetics.

Biguanides (Decrease Hepatic Glucose Production and Intestinal Glucose Absorption)

Use or condition: Type 2 or adult-onset diabetes

Drug name	Brand name†
Metformin	Glucophage, Riomet
Metformin and glyburide	Glucovance

Glucosidase Inhibitors (Inhibit Intestinal Glucose Absorption)

Use or condition: Type 2 or adult-onset diabetes

Drug name	Brand name†
Miglitol	Glyset

Insulins

Use or condition: Type 1, or sometimes type 2 or adult-onset diabetes

Rapid acting	Intermediate acting	Intermediate- and rapid-acting combination	Long acting
Humalog	Humulin L	Humalog Mix	Humulin U
Humulin R	Humulin N	Humalog 50/50	Lantus injection
Novolin R	Iletin II Lente	Humalog 70/30	Levemir
Iletin II R	Iletin II NPH	Novolin 70/30	
	Novolin L		
	Nivalin N		
Humalog	Humulin L	Humalog Mix	Humulin U

Meglitinides (Stimulate Pancreatic Islet Beta Cells)

Use or condition: Type 2 or adult-onset diabetes

Drug name	Brand name†
Nateglinide	Starlix
Repaglinide	Prandin, Gluconorm

Sulfonylureas (Stimulate Pancreatic Islet Beta Cells)

Use or condition: Type 2 or adult-onset diabetes

Drug name	Brand name†
Chlorpropamide*	Diabinese
Gliclazide	Diamicron
Glimepiride*	Amaryl
Glipizide*	Glucotrol
Glyburide	DiaBeta, Glynase, Micronase
Tolazamide*	Tolinase
Tolbutamide*	Orinase

*These drugs have been associated with increased cardiovascular mortality.

Thiazolidinediones (Increase Insulin Sensitivity)

Use or condition: Type 2 or adult-onset diabetes

Drug name	Brand name†
Pioglitazone	Actos
Rosiglitazone	Avandia

Incretin mimetics (Increase Insulin and Decrease Glucagon Secretion)

Use or condition: Type 2 diabetes

Drug name	Brand name†
Glucagon-like peptide 1	Byetta

Obesity Management

Main drug classes include appetite suppressants and lipase inhibitors.

Appetite Suppressants

Use or condition: Morbid obesity and metabolic syndrome

Drug name	Brand name†
Sibutramine	Meridia

Lipase Inhibitors

Use or condition: Morbid obesity and metabolic syndrome

Drug name	Brand name†
Orlistat	Xenical

†Represent selected brands; these are not necessarily all-inclusive.

Effects of Medications on Heart Rate, Blood Pressure, the Electrocardiogram (ECG), and Exercise Capacity

Medications	Heart rate	Blood pressure	ECG	Exercise capacity
I. ß-Blockers (including carvedilol and labetalol)	↓* (R and E)	↓ (R and E)	↓ HR* (R) ↓ ischemia† (E)	↑ in patients with angina; ↓ or ↔ in patients without angina
II. Nitrates	↑ (R) ↑ or ↔ (E)	↓ (R) ↓ or ↔ (E)	↑ HR (R) ↑ or ↔ HR (E) ↓ ischemia† (E)	↑ in patients with angina ↔ in patients without angina; ↑ or ↔ in patients with chronic heart failure (CHF)
III. Calcium channel blockers Amlodipine Felodipine Isradipine Nicardipine Nifedipine Nimodipine Nisoldipine Diltiazem Verapamil	↑ or ↔ (R and E) ↓ (R and E)	↓ (R and E)	↑ or ↔ HR (R and E) ↓ ischemia† (E) ↓ HR (R and E) ↓ ischemia† (E)	↑ in patients with angina; ↔ in patients without angina
IV. Digitalis	↓ in patients with atrial fibrillation and possibly CHF Not significantly altered in patients with sinus rhythm	↔ (R and E)	May produce nonspecific ST-T–wave changes (R) May produce ST-segment depression (E)	Improved only in patients with atrial fibrillation or in patients with CHF
V. Diuretics	↔ (R and E)	↔ or ↓ (R and E)	↔ or PVCs (R) May cause PVCs and "false positive" test results if hypokalemia occurs May cause PVCs if hypomagnesemia occurs (E)	↔, except possibly in patients with CHF

(continued)

Medications	Heart rate	Blood pressure	ECG	Exercise capacity
VI. Vasodilators, nonadrenergic	↑ or ↔ (R and E)	↓ (R and E)	↑ or ↔ HR (R and E)	↔, except ↑ or ↔ in patients with CHF
ACE inhibitors, and angiotensin II receptor blockers	↔ (R and E)	↓ (R and E)	↔ (R and E)	↔, except ↑ or ↔ in patients with CHF
α-Adrenergic blockers	↔ (R and E)	↓ (R and E)	↔ (R and E)	↔
Antiadrenergic agents without selective blockade	↓ or ↔ (R and E)	↓ (R and E)	↓ or ↔ HR (R and E)	↔
VII. Antiarrhythmic agents (all antiarrhythmic agents may cause new or worsened arrhythmias [proarrhythmic effect])				↔
Class I	↑ or ↔ (R and E)	↓ or ↔ (R) ↔ (E)	↑ or ↔ HR (R)	
Quinidine			May prolong QRS and QT intervals (R)	
Disopyramide			Quinidine may result in "false negative" test results (E)	↔
			May prolong QRS and QT intervals (R)	
Procainamide	↔ (R and E)	↔ (R and E)	May result in "false positive" test results (E)	↔
	↔ (R and E)	↔ (R and E)	↔ (R and E)	↔
Phenytoin				
Tocainide				
Mexiletine			May prolong QRS and QT intervals (R)	↔
Moricizine	↔ (R and E) ↓ (R)		↔ (E)	
Propafenone	↓ or ↔ (E)	↔ (R and E) ↔ (R and E)	↓ HR (R) ↓ or ↔ HR (E)	
Class II				
ß-Blockers (see I)				
Class III				
Amiodarone	↓ (R and E)	↔ (R and E)	↓ HR (R) ↔ (E)	↔
Sotalol				
Class IV				
Calcium channel blockers (see III)				

Medications	Heart rate	Blood pressure	ECG	Exercise capacity
VIII. Bronchodilators	↔ (R and E)	↔ (R and E)	↔ (R and E)	Bronchodilators ↑ exercise capacity in patients limited by bronchospasm
Anticholinergic agents Xanthine derivatives	↑ or ↔ (R and E)	↔	↑ or ↔ HR May produce PVCs (R and E)	
Sympathomimetic agents	↑ or ↔ (R and E)	↑, ↔, or ↓ (R and E)	↑ or ↔ HR (R and E)	↔
Cromolyn sodium	↔ (R and E)	↔ (R and E)	↔ (R and E)	↔
Steroidal anti-inflammatory agents	↔ (R and E)	↔ (R and E)	↔ (R and E)	↔
IX. Antilipemic agents	Clofibrate may provoke arrhythmias, angina in patients with prior myocardial infarction Nicotinic acid may ↓ BP All other hyperlipidemic agents have no effect on HR, BP, and ECG			↔
X. Psychotropic medications Minor tranquilizers	May ↓ HR and BP by controlling anxiety; no other effects			
Antidepressants	↑ or ↔ (R and E)	↓ or ↔ (R and E)	Variable (R)	
Major tranquilizers	↑ or ↔ (R and E)	↓ or ↔ (R and E)	Variable (R)	
Lithium	↔ (R and E)	↔ (R and E)	May result in T-wave changes and arrhythmias (R and E)	
XI. Nicotine	↑ or ↔ (R and E)	↑ (R and E)	↑ or ↔ HR May provoke ischemia, arrhythmias (R and E)	↔, except ↓ or ↔ in patients with angina
XII. Antihistamines	↔ (R and E)	↔ (R and E)	↔ (R and E)	↔
XIII. Cold medications with sympathomimetic agents	Effects similar to those described for sympathomimetic agents, although magnitude of effects is usually smaller			↔

(continued)

Medications	Heart rate	Blood pressure	ECG	Exercise capacity
XIV. Thyroid medications Only levothyroxine	↑ (R and E)	↑ (R and E)	↑ HR May provoke arrhythmias ↑ ischemia (R and E)	↔, unless angina worsened
XV. Alcohol	↔ (R and E)	Chronic use may have role in ↑ BP (R and E)	May provoke arrhythmias (R and E)	↔
XVI. Hypoglycemic agents Insulin and oral agents	↔ (R and E)	↔ (R and E)	↔ (R and E)	↔
XVII. Blood modifiers (anticoagulants and antiplatelets)	↔ (R and E)	↔ (R and E)	↔ (R and E)	↔ ↑ or ↔ in patients limited by intermittent claudication (for cilostazol only)
XVIII. Pentoxifylline	↔ (R and E)	↔ (R and E)	↔ (R and E)	↔ in patients limited by intermittent claudication
XIX. Anti-gout medications	↔ (R and E)	↔ (R and E)	↔ (R and E)	↔
XX. Caffeine	Variable effects depending on previous use Variable effects on exercise capacity May provoke arrhythmias			
XXI. Anorexiants/diet pills	↑ or ↔ (R and E)	↑ or ↔ (R and E)	↑ or ↔ HR (R and E)	Increased HR and BP common with norepinephrine reuptake inhibitors (e.g., sibutramine)

*ß-Blockers with intrinsic sympathomimetic activity lower resting HR only slightly.

†May prevent or delay myocardial ischemia (see text).

Abbreviations: PVCs = premature ventricular contractions; ↑ = increase; ↔ = no effect; ↓ = decrease; R = rest; E = exercise; HR = heart rate.

Suggested Readings

Chapter 1

Exercise Physiology

American College of Sports Medicine. ACSM's guidelines for exercise testing and prescription. 8th ed. Thompson WR, Gordon NF, Pescatello LS. Philadelphia: Lippincott Williams & Wilkins; 2008. 400 p.

American College of Sports Medicine. ACSM's resource manual for guidelines for exercise testing and prescription. 6th ed. Ehrman JK, ed. Philadelphia: Lippincott Williams & Wilkins; 2009. 896 p.

American College of Sports Medicine. ACSM's resources for clinical exercise physiology: Musculoskeletal, neuromuscular, neoplastic, immunologic, and hematologic conditions. Myers JN, Herbert WG, Humphrey R. Philadelphia: Lippincott Williams & Wilkins; 2002. 276 p.

Swain DP, Leutholtz BC. Exercise prescription: A case study approach to the ACSM guidelines. 2nd ed. Champaign, IL: Human Kinetics; 2007. 208 p.

Exercise in Chronic Disease and Disability

Frontera WR, Slovik DM, Dawson DM, eds. Exercise in rehabilitation medicine. 2nd ed. Champaign, IL: Human Kinetics; 2006. 464 p.

Sherrill C. Adapted physical activity, recreation, and sport: Cross-disciplinary and lifespan. 6th ed. Madison, WI: Brown & Benchmark; 2003. 736 p.

Skinner JS. Exercise testing and exercise prescription for special cases: Theoretical basis and clinical application. 3rd ed. Philadelphia: Lea & Febiger; 2005. 418 p.

Medicine

Fauci AS, Braunwald E, Kasper DL, Hauser SL, Longo DL, Jameson JL, Loscalzo J, eds. Harrison's principles of internal medicine. 17th ed. New York: McGraw-Hill; 2008. 2754 p.

Pharmacology

Kastrup E. Drug facts and comparisons. St. Louis: Facts and comparisons; 2008. 3120 p.

Chapter 2

American College of Sports Medicine. ACSM's guidelines for exercise testing and prescription. 8th ed. Thompson WR, Gordon NF, Pescatello LS. Philadelphia: Lippincott Williams & Wilkins; 2008. 400 p.

American College of Sports Medicine. ACSM's resource manual for guidelines for exercise testing and prescription. 6th ed. Ehrman JK, ed. Philadelphia: Lippincott Williams & Wilkins; 2009. 896 p.

Ehrman JK, Gordon PM, Visich PS, Keteyian SJ. Clinical exercise physiology. Champaign, IL: Human Kinetics; 2003. 619 p.

Gunn SN, Brooks AG, Withers RT, Gore CJ, Owen N, Booth ML, Bauman AE. Determining energy expenditure during some household and garden tasks. Med Sci Sports Exerc. 2002;34(5):896-902.

Guralnik JM, Ferrucci L, Pieper CF, et al. Lower extremity function and subsequent disability: Consistency across studies, predictive models, and value of gait speed alone compared with the short physical performance battery. J Gerontol, Series A, Biol Sci Med Sci. 2000;55:M221-223.

Jette AM, Jette DU, Ng J, Plotkin DJ, Bach MA. Are performance-based measures sufficiently reliable for use in multicenter trials? Musculoskeletal Impairment (MSI) study group. J Gerontol, Series A, Biol Sci Med Sci. 1999;54:M3-6.

Kastrup E. Drug facts and comparisons. St. Louis: Facts and Comparisons; 2008. 3120 p.

Rikli RE, Jones CJ. Development and validation of a functional fitness test for community-residing older adults. J Aging Phys Act. 1999;7:129-161.

Rikli RE, Jones CJ. Functional fitness normative scores for community-residing older adults, ages 60-94. J Aging Phys Act. 1999;7:162-181.

Stadnyk AN, Glezos JD. Drug-induced heat stroke. Can Med Assoc J. 1983;128(8):957-959.

Thompson PD, Franklin BA, Balady GJ, et al. Exercise and acute cardiovascular events: Placing the risks into perspective. A scientific statement from the American Heart Association Council on Nutrition, Physical Activity, and Metabolism and the Council on Clinical Cardiology. Circulation. 2007;115(17):2358-2368.

Chapter 3

American College of Sports Medicine. ACSM's guidelines for exercise testing and prescription. 8th ed. Philadelphia: Lippincott Williams & Wilkins; 2008. 400 p.

Andrade J, Ignaszewski A. Exercise and the heart: A review of the early studies, in memory of Dr R.S. Paffenbarger. BCMJ. 2007;49(10):540-546.

Blair SN, Kampert JB, Kohl HW III, et al. Influences of cardio-respiratory fitness and other precursors on cardiovascular disease and all-cause mortality in men and women. JAMA. 1996;276:205-210.

Blair SN, Kohl HW, Paffenbarger RS Jr., et al. Physical fitness and all-cause mortality. A prospective study of healthy men and women. JAMA. 1989;262:2395-2401.

Booth FW, Chakravarthy MV, Gordon SE, Spangenburg EE. Waging war on physical inactivity: Using modern molecular ammunition against an ancient enemy. J Appl Physiol. 2002;93(1):3-30.

Booth FW, Gordon SE, Carlson CJ, Hamilton MT. Waging war on modern chronic diseases: Primary prevention through exercise biology. J Appl Physiol. 2000;88(2):774-787.

Booth FW, Lees SJ. Fundamental questions about genes, inactivity, and chronic diseases. Physiol Genomics. 2007;28(2):146-157.

Church TS, Barlow CE, Earnest CP, et al. Associations between cardiorespiratory fitness and C-reactive protein in men. Arterioscler Thromb Vasc Biol. 2002;22(11):1869-1876.

Church TS, Earnest CP, Skinner JS, et al. Effects of different doses of physical activity on cardiorespiratory fitness among sedentary overweight or obese postmenopausal women with elevated blood pressure: A randomized controlled trial. JAMA. 2007;297(19):2081-2091.

Dishman RK, Washburn RA, Heath GW. Physical activity epidemiology. Champaign, IL: Human Kinetics; 2004. 496 p.

Durstine JL, Moore GE, LaMonte MJ, Franklin BA, eds. Pollock's textbook of cardiovascular disease and rehabilitation. Champaign, IL: Human Kinetics; 2008. 411 p.

Eckel RH, Grundy SM, Zimmet PZ. The metabolic syndrome. Lancet. 2005;365:1415-1428.

Hamilton MT, Hamilton DG, Zderic TW. Exercise physiology versus inactivity physiology: An essential concept for understanding lipoprotein lipase regulation. Exerc Sport Sci Rev. 2004;32(4):161-166.

Hamilton MT, Hamilton DG, Zderic TW. Role of low energy expenditure and sitting in obesity, metabolic syndrome, type 2 diabetes, and cardiovascular disease. Diabetes. 2007;56(11):2655-2667.

Haskell WL. J.B. Wolffe Memorial Lecture. Health consequences of physical activity: Understanding and challenges regarding dose-response. Med Sci Sports Exerc. 1994;26(6):649-660.

Haskell WL, Lee IM, Pate RR, et al. Physical activity and public health: Updated recommendation for adults from the American College of Sports Medicine and the American Heart Association. Circulation. 2007;116(9):1081-1093.

Haskell WL, Lee IM, Pate RR, et al. Physical activity and public health: Updated recommendation for adults from the American College of Sports Medicine and the American Heart Association. Med Sci Sports Exerc. 2007;39(8):1423-1434.

Hoffman C, Rice D, Sung HY. Persons with chronic conditions. Their prevalence and costs. JAMA. 1996;276(18):1473-1479.

Jakicic JM, Marcus BH, Gallagher KI, et al. Effect of duration and intensity on weight loss in overweight, sedentary women: A randomized trial. JAMA. 2003;290(10):1323-1330.

Kannel WB, Vasan RS, Keyes MJ, et al. Usefulness of the triglyceride-high-density lipoprotein versus the cholesterol-high-density lipoprotein ratio for predicting insulin resistance and cardiometabolic risk (from the Framingham Offspring Cohort). Am J Cardiol. 2008;101(4):497-501.

LaMonte MJ, Durstine JL, Yanowitz FG, et al. Cardiorespiratory fitness and C-reactive protein among a tri-ethnic sample of women. Circulation. 2002;106(4):403-406.

Lee CD, Blair SN, Jackson AS. Cardiorespiratory fitness, body composition, and all-cause and cardiovascular disease mortality in men. Am J Clin Nutr. 1999;69:373-380.

McTiernan A. Mechanisms linking physical activity with cancer. Nat Rev Cancer. 2008 Mar;8(3):205-211.

O'Donnell CJ, Elosua R. Cardiovascular risk factors. Insights from Framingham Heart Study. Rev Esp Cardiol. 2008;61(3):299-310.

Pecatello LS, Franklin BA, Fagard R, et al. American College of Sports Medicine position stand: Exercise and hypertension. Med Sci Sports Exerc. 2004;36(3):533-553.

Stampfer MJ, Hu FB, Manson JE, et al. Primary prevention for coronary artery disease in women through diet and exercise. N Engl J Med. 2000;343:16-22.

Thomas RJ, King M, Lui K, et al. AACVPR/ACC/AHA 2007 performance measures on cardiac rehabilitation for referral to and delivery of cardiac rehabilitation/secondary prevention services. J Am Coll Cardiol. 2007;50(14):1400-1433.

Wing RR, Jakicic J, Neiberg R, et al., Look Ahead Research Group. Fitness, fatness, and cardiovascular risk factors in type 2 diabetes: Look ahead study. Med Sci Sports Exerc. 2007;39(12):2107-2116.

Chapter 4

American College of Sports Medicine. ACSM's guidelines for exercise testing and prescription. 8th ed. Thompson WR, Gordon NF, Pescatello LS. Philadelphia: Lippincott Williams & Wilkins; 2008. 400 p.

American College of Sports Medicine. ACSM's resource manual for guidelines for exercise testing and prescription. 6th ed. Ehrman JK, ed. Philadelphia: Lippincott Williams & Wilkins; 2009. 896 p.

Durstine JL, Moore GE, LaMonte MJ, Franklin BA. Pollock's textbook of cardiovascular disease and rehabilitation. 1st ed. Champaign, IL: Human Kinetics; 2008. 411 p.

Ehrman JK, Gordon PM, Visich PS, Keteyian SJ. Clinical exercise physiology. 2nd ed. Champaign, IL: Human Kinetics; 2008. 690 p.

Frontera WR, Slovik DM, Dawson DM. Exercise in rehabilitation medicine. 2nd ed. Champaign, IL: Human Kinetics; 2006. 454 p.

Heyward VH. Advanced fitness assessment and exercise prescription. 5th ed. Champaign, IL: Human Kinetics; 2006. 425 p.

Skinner JS. Exercise testing and exercise prescription for special cases. Theoretical basis and clinical application. 3rd ed. Philadelphia: Lippincott Williams & Wilkins; 2005. 418 p.

Chapter 5

Armstrong N, van Mechelen W, eds. Paediatric exercise science and medicine. Oxford: Oxford University Press; 2000.

Bar-Or O. Pediatric sports medicine for the practitioner: From physiologic principles to clinical applications. New York: Springer-Verlag; 1983.

Bouchard C, Malina RM, Prusse L. Genetics of fitness and physical performance. Champaign, IL: Human Kinetics; 1997.

Canadian Society for Exercise Physiology. Measurement in pediatric exercise science. Docherty D, ed. Champaign, IL: Human Kinetics; 1996.

Dugan S. Exercise for preventing childhood obesity. Phys Med Rehabil Clin N Am. 2008;19:205-216.

Goldberg B, ed. Sports and exercise for children with chronic health conditions. Champaign, IL: Human Kinetics; 1995.

Malina RM, Bouchard C. Growth, maturation, and physical activity. Champaign, IL: Human Kinetics; 1991.

Maron BJ, Zipes DP. Thirty-sixth Bethesda Conference: Eligibility recommendations for competitive athletes with cardiovascular abnormalities. J Am Coll Cardiol. 2005;45:1313-1375.

Mitchell JH, Maron BJ, Epstein SE. Sixteenth Bethesda Conference: Cardiovascular abnormalities in the athlete: Recommendations regarding eligibility for competition. J Am Coll Cardiol. 1985;6:29-30.

Norman A-C, Drinkard B, McDuffie J, Ghorbani S, Yanoff L, Yanovski J. Influence of excess adiposity on exercise fitness and performance in overweight children and adolescents. Pediatrics. 2005;115:690-696.

Rowland TW. Developmental exercise physiology. Champaign, IL: Human Kinetics; 1996.

Rowland TW. Exercise and children's health. Champaign, IL: Human Kinetics; 1990.

Rowland TW, ed. Pediatric laboratory exercise testing: Clinical guidelines. Champaign, IL: Human Kinetics; 1993.

Swallen K, Reither E, Haas S, Meier A. Overweight, obesity and health related quality of life among adolescents: The National Longitudinal Study of Adolescent Health. Pediatrics. 2005;115:340-347.

Thompson D, Obarzanek E, Franko D, Barton B, Morrison J, Biro F, Daniels S, Striegel-Moore R. Childhood overweight and cardiovascular disease risk factors: The National Heart, Lung, and Blood Institute Growth and Health Study J Pediatr. 2007;150:18-25.

Tomassoni TL. Clinical Sciences Symposium: The role of exercise in the diagnosis and management of chronic disease in children and youth. Med Sci Sports Exerc. 1996;28(4):403-435.

Chapter 6

Ades PA, Savage PD, Brawner CA, Lyon CE, Ehrman JK, Bunn JY, Keteyian SJ. Aerobic capacity in patients entering cardiac rehabilitation. Circulation. 2006;113:2706-2712.

American College of Sports Medicine. ACSM's guidelines for exercise testing and prescription. 8th ed. Thompson WR, Gordon NF, Pescatello LS. Philadelphia: Lippincott Williams & Wilkins; 2008. 400 p.

Dominguez H, Torp-Pedersen C, Koeber L, et al. Prognostic value of exercise testing in a cohort of patients followed for 15 years after acute myocardial infarction. Eur Heart J. 2001;22:273-276.

Dutcher JR, Kahn J, Grines C, Franklin B. Comparison of left ventricular ejection fraction and exercise capacity as predictors of two- and five-year mortality following acute myocardial infarction. Am J Cardiol. 2007;99:436-441.

Franklin BA. Coronary revascularization and medical management of coronary artery disease: Changing paradigms and perceptions. Eur J Cardiovasc Prev Rehabil. 2006;13:669-673.

Franklin BA, Gordon NF. Contemporary diagnosis and management in cardiovascular exercise. 1st ed. Newtown, PA: Handbooks in Health Care; 2005.

Giannuzzi P, Tavazzi L, Temporelli PL, et al. Long-term physical training and left ventricular remodeling after anterior myocardial infarction: Results of the exercise in anterior myocardial infarction (EAMI) trial. J Am Coll Cardiol. 1993;1821-1829.

Hambrecht R, Niebauer J, Marburger C, et al. Various intensities of leisure time physical activity in patients with coronary artery disease: Effects on cardiorespiratory fitness and progression of coronary atherosclerotic lesions. J Am Coll Cardiol. 1993;22:468-477.

Hosokawa S, Hiasa Y, Takahashi T, Itoh S. Effect of regular exercise on coronary endothelial function in patients with recent myocardial infarction. Circulation. 2003;67:221-224.

Kendziorra K, Walther C, Foerster M, et al. Changes in myocardial perfusion due to physical exercise in patients with stable coronary artery disease. Eur J Nucl Med Mol Imaging. 2005;32:813-819.

Lee B-C, Chen S-Y, Hsu H-C, et al. Effect of cardiac rehabilitation on myocardial perfusion reserve in postinfarction patients. Am J Cardiol. 2008;101:1395-1402.

Leon AS, Franklin BA, Costa F, et al. Cardiac rehabilitation and secondary prevention of coronary heart disease. An American Heart Association scientific statement from the Council on Clinical Cardiology (Subcommittee on Exercise, Cardiac Rehabilitation, and Prevention) and the Council on Nutrition, Physical Activity, and Metabolism (Subcommittee on Physical Activity, in collaboration with the American Association of Cardiovascular and Pulmonary Rehabilitation). Circulation. 2005;111:369-376.

Mazzini MJ, Stevens GR, Whalen D, Ozonoff A, Balady GJ. Effect of an American Heart Association Get With the Guidelines program-based clinical pathway on referral and enrollment into cardiac rehabilitation after acute myocardial infarction. Am J Cardiol. 2008;101:1084-1087.

Senaratne MP, Smith G, Gulamhusein SS. Feasibility and safety of early exercise testing using the Bruce protocol after acute myocardial infarction. J Am Coll Cardiol. 2000;35:1212-1220.

Swain DP, Franklin BA. Is there a threshold intensity for aerobic training in cardiac patients? Med Sci Sports Exerc. 2002;34:1071-1075.

Taylor RS, Brown A, Ebrahim S, et al. Exercise-based rehabilitation for patients with coronary heart disease: Systematic review and meta-analysis of randomized controlled trials. Am J Med. 2004;116: 682-692.

Wenger NK. Current status of cardiac rehabilitation. J Am Coll Cardiol. 2008;51:1619-1631.

Williams MA, Haskell WL, Ades PL, et al. Resistance exercise in individuals with and without cardiovascular disease: 2007 update. A scientific statement from the American Heart Association Council on Clinical Cardiology and Council on Nutrition, Physical Activity, and Metabolism. Circulation. 2007;116:572-584.

Chapter 7

Adams J, Cline MJ, Hubbard M, McCullough T, Hartman J. A new paradigm for post-cardiac event resistance exercise guidelines. Am J Cardiol. 2006;97:281-286.

American Association of Cardiovascular and Pulmonary Rehabilitation. Guidelines for cardiac rehabilitation and secondary prevention programs. 4th ed. Champaign, IL: Human Kinetics; 2004.

American College of Sports Medicine. ACSM's guidelines for exercise testing and prescription. 8th ed. Thompson WR, Gordon NF, Pescatello LS. Philadelphia: Lippincott Williams & Wilkins; 2008. 400 p.

Boden WE, O'Rourke RA, Teo KK, et al. Optimal medical therapy with or without PCI for stable coronary disease. N Engl J Med. 2007;356:1503-1516.

Brubaker PH, Miller HS. Coronary artery revascularization. In: Durstine JL, Moore GE, LaMonte MJ, Franklin BA, eds. Pollock's textbook of cardiovascular disease and rehabilitation. Champaign, IL: Human Kinetics; 2008. p. 285-292.

Convertino VA. Effect of orthopedic stress on exercise performance after bed rest: Relation to inhospital rehabilitation. J Cardiac Rehabil. 1983;3:660-663.

Džavík V, Buller CE, Lamas GA, et al. Randomized trial of percutaneous coronary intervention for subacute infarct-related coronary artery occlusion to achieve long-term patency and improve ventricular function. The Total Occlusion Study of Canada (TOSCA)-2 Trial. Circulation. 2006;114:2449-2457.

Eisenberg MJ, Wou K, Nguyen H, et al. Use of stress testing early after coronary artery bypass graft surgery. Am J Cardiol. 2006;97:810-816.

Feuerstadt P, Chai A, Kligfield P. Submaximal effort tolerance as a predictor of all-cause mortality in patients undergoing cardiac rehabilitation. Clin Cardiol. 2007;30:234-238.

Franklin BA. Coronary revascularization and medical management of coronary artery disease: Changing paradigms and perceptions. Eur J Cardiovasc Prev Rehabil. 2006;13:669-673.

Hambrecht R, Walther C, Möbius-Winkler S, et al. Percutaneous coronary angioplasty compared with exercise training in patients with stable coronary artery disease. A randomized trial. Circulation. 2004;109:1371-1378.

Hannan EL, Wu C, Walford G, et al. Drug-eluting stents vs. coronary-artery bypass grafting in multivessel coronary disease. N Engl J Med. 2008;358:331-341.

Hochman JS, Lamas GA, Buller CE, et al. Coronary intervention for persistent occlusion after myocardial infarction. N Engl J Med. 2006;355:2395-2407.

Katritsis DG, Ioannidis JPA. Percutaneous coronary intervention versus conservative therapy in nonacute coronary artery disease. A meta-analysis. Circulation. 2005;111:2906-2912.

Kavanagh T, Hamm LF, Beyene J, et al. Usefulness of improvement in walking distance versus peak oxygen uptake in predicting prognosis after myocardial infarction and/or coronary artery bypass grafting in men. Am J Cardiol. 2008;101:1423-1427.

Sato S, Makita S, Majima M. Additional physical activity during cardiac rehabilitation leads to an improved heart rate recovery in male patients after coronary artery bypass grafting. Circulation. 2005;69:69-71.

Stewart KJ, Badenhop D, Brubaker PH, Keteyian SJ, King M. Cardiac rehabilitation following percutaneous revascularization, heart transplant, heart valve surgery, and for chronic heart failure. Chest. 2003;123:2104-2111.

Taylor RS, Brown A, Ebrahim S, et al. Exercise-based rehabilitation for patients with coronary heart disease: Systematic review and meta-analysis of randomized controlled trials. Am J Med. 2004;116:682-692.

Treat-Jocobson DJ, Lindquist R. Exercise, quality of life, and symptoms in men and women five to six years after coronary artery bypass graft surgery. Heart & Lung. 2007;36:387-397.

Tu JV, Pashos CL, Naylor CD, Chen E, Normand SL, Newhouse P, McNeil BJ. Use of cardiac procedures and outcomes in elderly patients with myocardial infarction in the United States and Canada. N Engl J Med. 1997;336:1500-1505.

Williams MA, Haskell WL, Ades PA, et al. Resistance exercise in individuals with and without cardiovascular disease: 2007 update. A scientific statement from the American Heart Association Council on Clinical Cardiology and Council on Nutrition, Physical Activity, and Metabolism. Circulation. 2007;116:572-584.

Wu S-K, Lin Y-W, Chen C-L, Tsai S-W. Cardiac rehabilitation vs. home exercise after coronary artery bypass graft surgery. A comparison of heart rate recovery. Am J Phys Med Rehabil. 2006;85:711-717.

Chapter 8

American Association of Cardiovascular and Pulmonary Rehabilitation. Guidelines for cardiac rehabilitation and secondary prevention programs. 4th ed. Champaign, IL: Human Kinetics; 2004.

American College of Sports Medicine. ACSM's guidelines for exercise testing and prescription. 8th ed. Thompson WR, Gordon NF, Pescatello LS. Philadelphia: Lippincott Williams & Wilkins; 2008. 400 p.

Anderson JL, Adams CD, Antman EM, et al. ACC/AHA 2007 guidelines for the management of patients with unstable angina/non–ST-elevation myocardial infarction—executive summary. J Am Coll Cardiol. 2007;50:652-726.

Anti-platelet therapy. Boston: Independent Drug Information Service (cited 2007 Dec 28). [Online]. Available from www.rxfacts.org.

Balady GJ, Williams MA, Ades PA, et al. Core Components of cardiac rehabilitation/secondary prevention programs: 2007 update. Circulation. 2007;115:2675-2682.

Chaitman BR. Exercise testing. In: Zipes D, Libby P, Bonow R, Braunwarld E, eds. Heart disease. 7th ed. Philadelphia: Saunders; 2005. p. 153-186.

Durstine JL, Moore GE, LaMonte MJ, Franklin BA, eds. Pollock's textbook of cardiovascular disease and rehabilitation. Champaign, IL: Human Kinetics; 2008. 411 p.

Fletcher GF, Mills WC, Taylor WC. Update on exercise stress testing. Am Fam Physician. 2006;74(10).1749-1754.

Froelicher V, Shetler K, Ashley E. Better decisions through science: Exercise testing scores. Prog Cardiovasc Dis. 2002;44:395-414.

Gibler WB, Cannon CP, Blomkalns AL, et al. Practical implementation of the guidelines for unstable angina/non–ST-segment elevation myocardial infarction in the emergency department. Circulation. 2005;111:2699-2710.

Kern MJ. Coronary blood flow and myocardial ischemia. In: Zipes D, Libby P, Bonow R, Braunwarld E, eds. Heart disease. 7th ed. Philadelphia: Saunders; 2005. p. 1103-1129.

King ML, Williams MA, Fletcher GF, et al. AHA/AACVPR scientific statement medical director responsibilities for outpatient cardiac rehabilitation/secondary prevention programs. Circulation. 2006;112:3354-3360.

Lee TH. Approach to the patient with chest pain. In: Zipes D, Libby P, Bonow R, Braunwarld E, eds. Heart disease. 7th ed. Philadelphia: Saunders; 2005. p. 1129-1140.

Lee TH. Chronic coronary artery disease. In: Zipes D, Libby P, Bonow R, Braunwarld E, eds. Heart disease. 7th ed. Philadelphia: Saunders; 2005. p. 1281-1355.

Morrow DA, Scirica BM, Karwatowska-Prokopczuk E, et al. Effects of ranolazine on recurrent cardiovascular events in patients with non–ST elevation acute coronary syndromes—the MERLIN-TIMI 36 Randomized Trial. JAMA. 2007;297:1775-1783.

Smith SC, Allen J, Blair SN, et al. AHA/ACC Guidelines for secondary prevention for patients with coronary and other atherosclerotic vascular disease: 2006 update. Circulation. 2006;113:2363-2372.

Chapter 9

Atwood JE, Myers J. Exercise hemodynamics of atrial fibrillation. In: Falk RH, Podrid PJ, eds. Atrial fibrillation: Mechanisms and management. Philadelphia: Lippincott-Raven; 1997. p. 219-239.

Atwood JE, Myers J, Sullivan M, et al. The effect of cardioversion on maximal exercise capacity in patients with chronic atrial fibrillation. Am Heart J. 1989;118:913-918.

Atwood JE, Myers J, Sullivan M, et al. Maximal exercise testing and gas exchange in patients with chronic atrial fibrillation. J Am Coll Cardiol. 1988;11:508-513.

Atwood JE, Myers JN, Tang XC, et al. Exercise capacity in atrial fibrillation: A substudy of the Sotalol-Amiodarone Atrial Fibrillation Efficacy Trial (SAFE-T). Am Heart J. 2007;153(4):566-572.

Lip GYH, Tse HF. Management of atrial fibrillation. Lancet. 2007;370:604-618.

Mertens DJ, Kavanagh T. Exercise training for patients with chronic atrial fibrillation. J Cardiopulm Rehabil. 1996;16:193-196.

Ueshima K, Myers J, Graettinger WF, et al. Exercise and morphologic comparison of chronic atrial fibrillation and normal sinus rhythm. Am Heart J. 1993;126:260-261.

Ueshima K, Myers J, Morris CK, et al. The effect of cardioversion on exercise capacity in patients with atrial fibrillation. Am Heart J. 1993;126:1021-1024.

Vanhees LD, Schepers J, Defoor S, et al. Exercise performance and training in cardiac patients with atrial fibrillation. J Cardiopulm Rehabil. 2000;20:346-352.

Watson T, Shanstila E, Lip GYH. Modern management of atrial fibrillation. Clin Med. 2007;7:28-34.

Wyse DE, Waldo AL, DiMarco JP, et al. A comparison of rate and rhythm control in patients with atrial fibrillation (the AFFIRM study). New Engl J Med. 2002;347:1825-1833.

Chapter 10

ACC/AHA/ESC 2006 guidelines for management of patients with ventricular arrhythmias and the prevention of sudden cardiac death. J Am Coll Cardiol. 2006;48:247-346.

ACC/AHA/NASPE 2002 guideline update for implantation of cardiac pacemakers and antiarrhythmia devices: Summary article: A report of the American College of Cardiology/ American Heart Association Task Force on Practice Guidelines (ACC/AHA/NASPE Committee to Update the 1998 Pacemaker Guidelines). Circulation. 2002;106:2145-2161.

Lampert R, Cannom D, Olshansky B. Safety of sports participation in patients with implantable cardioverter defibrillators: A survey of Heart Rhythm Society members. J Cardiovasc Electrophysiol. 2006;17(1):11-15.

Lampman RM, Knight, BP. Prescribing exercise training for patients with defibrillators. Am J Phys Med Rehabil. 2000;79(3):292-297.

Saksena S, Madan N. Management of the patient with an implantable cardioverter defibrillator in the third millennium. Circulation. 2002;106:2642-2646.

Vanheesa L, Kornaate M, Defoor J, et al. Effect of exercise training in patients with an implantable cardioverter defibrillator. Eur Heart J. 2004;25(13):1120-1126.

Chapter 11

Das P, Rimington H, Chambers J. Exercise testing to stratify risk in aortic stenosis. Eur Heart J. 2005;26(13):1309-1313.

Diagnosis and management of acute rheumatic fever and rheumatic heart disease in Australia: An evidence-based review. National Guidelines Clearinghouse, 2006 (cited 2008 Jan 10). [Online]. Available from www.guideline.gov/summary/summary.aspx?doc_id=10369.

Feigenbaum H. Echocardiography. 6th ed. Philadelphia: Lippincott Williams & Wilkins; 2005.

Gibbons R. ACC/AHA 2002 Guideline update for exercise testing: Summary article. A report of the American College of Cardiology/American Heart Association Task Force on Practice Guidelines (Committee to Update the 1997 Exercise Testing Guidelines). Circulation. 2002;106:1883.

Hirsh J, Guyatt G, Albers GW, Schünemann HJ. The Seventh ACCP Conference on Antithrombotic and Thrombolytic Therapy: Evidence-based guidelines. Chest. 2004;126:172S-173S.

Opie LH. Drugs for the heart. 6th ed. Philadelphia: Saunders; 2004.

Skinner JS. Exercise testing and exercise prescriptions for special cases: Theoretical basis and clinical application. 2nd ed. Media, PA: Lea & Febiger; 2004.

Vuyisile TN, Gardin JM, Skelton TN, Gottdiener JS, Scott CG, Enriquez-Sarano M. Burden of valvular heart diseases: A population-based study. Lancet. 2006;368(9540):1005-1011.

Zipes D, Libby P, Bonow R, Braunwarld E. Heart disease. 7th ed. Philadelphia: Saunders; 2005.

Chapter 12

Arena R, Myers J, Guazzi M. The clinical and research applications of aerobic capacity and ventilatory efficiency in heart failure: An evidence-based review. Heart Fail Rev. 2007 Nov 7 (e-pub).

Braith RW, Beck DT. Resistance exercise: Training adaptations and developing a safe exercise prescription. Heart Fail Rev. 2008;13:69-79.

Brubaker PH, Joo KC, Stewart K, Fray B, Moore B, Kitzman DW. Chronotropic incompetence and its contribution to exercise intolerance in older patients with diastolic versus systolic heart failure. J Cardiopulm Rehabil. 2006;26:86-89.

Dubach P, Myers J, Dziekan G, et al. Effect of exercise training on myocardial remodeling in patients with reduced left ventricular function after myocardial infarction: Application of magnetic resonance imaging. Circulation. 1997;95:2060-2067.

ExTraMATCH Collaborative. Exercise training meta-analysis of trials in patients with chronic heart failure. BMJ. 2004;328:189-192.

Feiereisen P, Delagardelle C, Vaillant M, Lasar Y, Beissel J. Is strength training the more efficient training modality in chronic heart failure? Med Sci Sports Exerc. 2007;39:1910-1917.

Gianuzzi P, Temporelli PL, Corra U, et al. Antiremodeling effect of long-term exercise training in patients with stable chronic heart failure: Results of the exercise in left ventricular dysfunction and chronic heart failure (ELVD-CHF) trial. Circulation. 2003;108:554-559.

Hambrecht R, Gielen S, Linke A, et al. Effects of exercise training on left ventricular function and peripheral resistance in patients with chronic heart failure: A randomized trial. JAMA. 2000;283:3095-3101.

Hunt SA, Abraham WT, Chin MH, et al. ACC/AHA 2005 guideline update for the diagnosis and management of chronic heart failure in the adult—summary article. J Am Coll Cardiol. 2005;46:1116-1143.

McElvie RS. Exercise training in patients with heart failure: Clinical outcomes, safety, and indications. Heart Fail Rev. 2007;13:3-11.

Myers J. Principles of exercise prescription for patients with chronic heart failure. Heart Fail Rev. 2008;13:61-68.

Myers J, Dziekan G, Goebbels U, et al. Influence of high-intensity exercise training on the ventilatory response to exercise in patients with reduced ventricular function. Med Sci Sports Exerc. 1999;31:929-937.

Piepoli MF, Flather M, Coats AJS. Overview of studies of exercise testing in chronic heart failure: The need for a prospective randomized multicenter European trial. Eur Heart J. 1998;19:830-841.

Pina IL, Apstein CS, Balady GD, et al. Exercise and heart failure: A statement from the American Heart Association Committee on Exercise, Rehabilitation and Prevention. Circulation. 2003;107:1210-1225.

Working Group on Cardiac Rehabilitation and Exercise Physiology and Working Group on Heart Failure of the European Society of Cardiology. Recommendations for exercise training in chronic heart failure patients. Eur Heart J. 2001;22:125-135.

Chapter 13

American Heart Association. 2007 heart and stroke statistical update. Dallas; 2007: American Heart Association.

Arena R, Myers J, Williams MA, Gulati M, Kligfield P, Balady GJ, et al. Assessment of functional capacity in clinical and research settings: A scientific statement from the American Heart Association Committee on Exercise, Rehabilitation, and Prevention of the Council on Clinical Cardiology and the Council on Cardiovascular Nursing. Circulation. 2007;116(3):329-343.

Bengel FM, Ueberfuhr P, Schiepel N, Nekolla SG, Reichart B, Schwaiger M. Effect of sympathetic reinnervation on cardiac performance after heart transplantation. N Engl J Med. 2001;345(10):731-738.

Braith RW, Edwards DG. Exercise following heart transplantation. Sports Med. 2000;30(3):171-192.

Fletcher GF, Balady GJ, Amsterdam EA, Chaitman B, Eckel R, Fleg J, et al. Exercise standards for testing and training: A statement for healthcare professionals from the American Heart Association. Circulation. 2001;104(14):1694-1740.

Kavanagh T. Exercise rehabilitation in cardiac transplantation patients: A comprehensive review. Eura Medicophys. 2005;41(1):67-74.

Kobashigawa JA, Leaf DA, Lee N, Gleeson MP, Liu H, Hamilton MA, et al. A controlled trial of exercise rehabilitation after heart transplantation. N Engl J Med. 1999;340(4):272-277.

Marconi C, Marzorati M. Exercise after heart transplantation. Eur J Appl Physiol. 2003;90(3-4):250-259.

Pierce GL, Magyari PM, Aranda JM Jr., Edwards DG, Hamlin SA, Hill JA, et al. Effect of heart transplantation on skeletal muscle metabolic enzyme reserve and fiber type in end-stage heart failure patients. Clin Transpl. 2007;21(1):94-100.

Pina IL, Apstein CS, Balady GJ, Belardinelli R, Chaitman BR, Duscha BD, et al. Exercise and heart failure: A statement from the American Heart Association Committee on Exercise, Rehabilitation, and Prevention. Circulation. 2003;107(8):1210-1225.

Schwaiblmair M, Scheidt WV, Uberfuhr P, Reichart B, Vogelmeier C. Lung function and cardiopulmonary exercise performance after heart transplantation: Influence of cardiac allograft vasculopathy. Chest. 1999;116(2):332-339.

Schwaiblmair M, von Scheidt W, Uberfuhr P, Ziegler S, Schwaiger M, Reichart B, et al. Functional significance of cardiac reinnervation in heart transplant recipients. J Heart Lung Transpl. 1999;18(9):838-845.

Stewart KJ, Badenhop D, Brubaker PH, Keteyian SJ, King M. Cardiac rehabilitation following percutaneous revascularization, heart transplant, heart valve surgery, and for chronic heart failure. Chest. 2003;123(6):2104-2111.

Taylor DO, Edwards LB, Boucek MM, Trulock EP, Aurora P, Christie J, et al. Registry of the International Society for Heart and Lung Transplantation: Twenty-fourth official adult heart transplant report—2007. J Heart Lung Transpl. 2007;26(8):769-781.

Williams MA, Haskell WL, Ades PA, Amsterdam EA, Bittner V, Franklin BA, et al. Resistance exercise in individuals with and without cardiovascular disease: 2007 update: A scientific statement from the American Heart Association Council on Clinical Cardiology and Council on Nutrition, Physical Activity, and Metabolism. Circulation. 2007;116(5):572-584.

Chapter 14

American College of Sports Medicine. ACSM's guidelines for exercise testing and prescription. 8th ed. Philadelphia: Lippincott Williams & Wilkins; 2008. 400 p.

American College of Sports Medicine. Position stand: Exercise and hypertension. Med Sci Sports Exerc. 2004;36:533-553.

Appel LJ, Brands MW, Daniels SR, et al. Dietary approaches to prevent and treat hypertension: A scientific statement from the American Heart Association. Circulation. 2006;47:296-308.

Chobanian AV, Bakris GL, Black HR, et al. The seventh report of the Joint National Committee on Prevention, Detection, Evaluation, and Treatment of High Blood Pressure. The JNC 7 report. JAMA. 2003;289:2560-2572.

Fields LE, Burt VL, Cutler JA, Hughes J, Roccella EJ, Sorlie P. The burden of adult hypertension in the United States 1999 to 2000: A rising tide. Hypertension. 2004;44:398-404.

Fletcher GF, Balady GJ, Amsterdam EA, et al. Exercise standards for testing and training: A statement for healthcare professionals from the American Heart Association. Circulation. 2001;104:1694-1740.

Franklin BF, Gordon NF. Contemporary diagnosis and management in cardiovascular exercise. Newtown, PA: Handbooks in Healthcare; 2005.

Gibbons RJ, Balady GJ, Bricker JT, et al. ACC/AHA 2002 guideline update for exercise testing; a report of the American College of Cardiology/American Heart Association Task

Force on Practice Guidelines; Committee on Exercise Testing. Circulation. 2002;106:1883-1892.

Gordon NF, Contractor A, Leighton RF. Resistance training for hypertension and stroke patients. In: Graves JE, Franklin BA, eds. Resistance training for health and rehabilitation. Champaign, IL: Human Kinetics; 2001.

Pickering TG, Hall JE, Appel LJ, et al. Recommendations for blood pressure measurement in humans and experimental animals: Part 1: Blood pressure measurement in humans. Hypertension. 2005;45:142-161.

Rosendorff C, Black HR, Cannon CP, et al. Treatment of hypertension in the prevention and management of ischemic heart disease: A scientific statement from the American Heart Association. Circulation. 2007;115:2761-2788.

Williams MA, Haskell WL, Ades PA, et al. Resistance exercise update in individuals with and without cardiovascular disease: 2007 update: A scientific statement from the American Heart Association. Circulation. 2007;116:572-584.

Chapter 15

Aboyans V, Criqui MH, Denenberg JO, et al. Risk factors for progression of peripheral arterial disease in large and small vessels. Circulation. 2006;113(22):2623-2629.

Ad Hoc Committee on Reporting Standards. Suggested standards for reports dealing with lower extremity ischemia. J Vasc Surg. 1986;4:80-94.

Dawson DL, Cutler BS, Hiatt WR, et al. A comparison of cilostazol and pentoxifylline for treating intermittent claudication. Am J Med. 2000;109:523-530.

Gardner AW, Katzel LI, Sorkin JD, et al. Exercise rehabilitation improves functional outcomes and peripheral circulation in patients with intermittent claudication: A randomized controlled trial. J Am Geriatr Soc. 2001;49:755-762.

Gardner AW, Montgomery PS, Flinn WR, et al. The effect of exercise intensity on the response to exercise rehabilitation in patients with intermittent claudication. J Vasc Surg. 2005;42:702-709.

Gardner AW, Skinner JS, Smith LK. Effects of handrail support on claudication and hemodynamic responses to single-stage and progressive treadmill protocols in peripheral vascular occlusive disease. Am J Cardiol. 1991;68:99-105.

Hirsch AT, Haskal ZJ, Hertzer NR, et al. ACC/AHA 2005 guidelines for the management of patients with peripheral arterial disease (lower extremity, renal, mesenteric, and abdominal aorta). J Am Coll Cardiol. 2006;47:1239-1312.

Izquierdo-Porrera AM, Gardner AW, Powell CC, Katzel LI. Effects of exercise rehabilitation on cardiovascular risk factors in older patients with peripheral arterial occlusive disease. J Vasc Surg. 2000;31:670-677.

Murabito JM, D'Agostino RB, Silbershatz H, et al. Intermittent claudication. A risk profile from the Framingham Heart Study. Circulation. 1997;96:44-49.

Norgren L, Hiatt WR, Dormandy JA, et al. Inter-society consensus for the management of peripheral arterial disease (TASC II). J Vasc Surg. 2007;45:suppl S:S5-S67.

Regensteiner JG, Hiatt WR. Exercise rehabilitation for patients with peripheral arterial disease. Exerc Sport Sci Rev. 1995;23:1-24.

Skinner JS, Strandness Jr. DE. Exercise and intermittent claudication: I. Effect of repetition and intensity of exercise. Circulation. 1967;36:23-29.

Treesak C, Kasemsup V, Treat-Jacobson D, et al. Cost-effectiveness of exercise training to improve claudication symptoms in patients with peripheral arterial disease. Vasc Med. 2004;9:279-285.

Womack CJ, Sieminski DJ, Katzel LI, et al. Improved walking economy in patients with peripheral arterial occlusive disease. Med Sci Sports Exerc. 1997;29:1286-1290.

Yao ST, Needham TN, Gourmoos C, et al. A comparative study of strain-gauge plethysmography and Doppler ultrasound in the assessment of occlusive arterial disease of the lower extremities. Surgery. 1972;71:4-9.

Chapter 16

Best PA, Tajik AJ, Gibbons RJ, Pellikka PA. The safety of treadmill exercise stress testing in patients with abdominal aortic aneurysms. Ann Int Med. 1998;139(8):628-631.

Braverman AC. Exercise and the Marfan syndrome. Med Sci Sports Exerc. 1998;30(10 suppl):S387-395.

Cheitlin MD, Douglas PS, Parmley WM. Task force 2: Acquired valvular heart disease. 26th Bethesda Conference: Recommendations for determining eligibility for competition in athletes with cardiovascular abnormalities. J Am Coll Cardiol. 1994;24(4):874-880.

Dalman RL, Tedesco MM, Myers J, Taylor CA. Abdominal aortic aneurysm disease: Mechanism, stratification, and treatment. Ann NY Acad Sci. 2006;1085:92-109.

DeRubertis BG, Trocciola S, Ryer EJ, et al. Abdominal aortic aneurysm in women: Prevalence, risk factors, and implications for screening. J Vasc Surg. 2007;46:630-635.

Egelhoff CJ, Budwig RS, Elger DF, et al. Model studies of the flow in abdominal aortic aneurysms during resting and exercise conditions. J Biomech. 1999;32:1319-1329.

Ellis CJ, Haywood GA, Monro JL. Spontaneous coronary artery dissection in a young woman resulting from an intense gymnasium "work-out." Int J Cardiol. 1994;47:193-194.

Fleming C, Whitlock EP, Beil TL, Lederle FA. Screening for abdominal aortic aneurysm: A best-evidence systematic review for the US Preventive Services Task Force. Ann Int Med. 2005;142:203-211.

Provenzale JM, Barboriak DP, Taveras JM. Exercise-related dissection of cranio-cervical arteries: CT, MR, and angiographic findings. J Comput Assist Tomogr. 1995;19(2):268-276.

Pyeritz RE, Francke U. Conference report: The second international symposium on the Marfan syndrome. Am J Med Genet. 1993;47:127-135.

Thomas MC, Walker RJ, Packer S. Running repairs: Renal artery dissection following extreme exertion. Nephrol Dial Transpl. 1999;14:1258-1259.

Chapter 17

Casaburi R, Burns MR, Porszasz J, et al. Physiologic benefits of exercise training in rehabilitation of severe COPD patients. Am J Respir Crit Care Med. 1997;155:1541-1551.

Casaburi R, Kakafka D, Cooper CB, et al. Improvement in exercise tolerance with the combination of tiotropium and pulmonary rehabilitation in patients with COPD. Chest. 2005;127:809-817.

Casaburi R, Patession A, Ioli F, et al. Reductions in exercise lactic acidosis and ventilation as a result of exercise training in patients with obstructive lung disease. Am Rev Respir Dis. 1991;143:9-18.

Celli BR, MacNee W. Standards for the diagnosis and treatment of patients with COPD: A summary of the ATS/ERS position paper. Eur Respir J. 2004;23:932-946.

Cooper CB. The connection between chronic obstructive pulmonary disease symptoms and hyperinflation and its impact on exercise and function. Am J Med. 2006;119(10A):S21-S31.

Cooper CB. Exercise in chronic pulmonary disease: Aerobic exercise prescription. Med Sci Sports Exerc. 2001;33(7 suppl):S671-679.

Cooper CB. Exercise in chronic pulmonary disease: Limitations and rehabilitation. Med Sci Sports Exerc. 2001;33(7 suppl):S643-646.

Cooper CB, Tashkin DP. Recent developments in inhaled therapy in stable chronic obstructive pulmonary disease. BMJ. 2005;330:640-644.

Global strategy for the diagnosis, management, and prevention of chronic obstructive pulmonary disease. NHLBI/WHO workshop summary, updated 2007. London: Global Initiative for Chronic Obstructive Lung Disease (GOLD); 2007 Dec.

Kesten S, Casaburi R, Kukafka D, Cooper CB. Improvement in self-reported exercise participation with the combination of tiotropium and rehabilitative exercise training in COPD patients. Int J Chron Obstruct Pulmon Dis. 2008;3:127-136

Myers J, Prakash M, Froelicher V, et al. Exercise capacity and mortality among men referred for exercise testing. N Engl J Med. 2002;346:793-801.

Ofir D, Laveneziana P, Webb KA, et al. Mechanisms of dyspnea during cycle exercise in symptomatic patients with GOLD stage I chronic obstructive pulmonary disease. Am J Respir Crit Care Med. 2008;177:622-629.

Pitta F, Troosters T, Spruit MA, et al. Characteristics of physical activities in daily life in chronic obstructive pulmonary disease. Am J Respir Crit Care Med. 2005;171:972-977.

Ries AL, Bauldoff GS, Carlin BW, et al. Pulmonary rehabilitation: Joint ACCP/AACVPR evidence-based clinical practice guidelines. Chest. 2007;131:4S-42S.

Storer TW. Exercise in chronic pulmonary disease: Resistance exercise prescription. Med Sci Sports Exerc. 2001;33:S680-692.

Chapter 18

ATS/ACCP statement on cardiopulmonary exercise testing. Am J Respir Crit Care Med. 2003;167:211-277.

Clinical exercise testing with reference to lung diseases: Indications, standardization and interpretation strategies. ERS Task Force on Standardization of Clinical Exercise Testing. European Respiratory Society. Eur Respir J. 1997;10:2662-2689.

Hsia CC. Cardiopulmonary limitations to exercise in restrictive lung disease. Med Sci Sports Exerc. 1999;31:S28-32.

Hsia CC. Coordinated adaptation of oxygen transport in cardiopulmonary disease. Circulation. 2001;104:963-969.

Marciniuk DD, Watts RE, Gallagher CG. Reproducibility of incremental maximal cycle ergometer testing in patients with restrictive lung disease. Thorax. 1993 Sep;48(9):894-898.

Sharma S. Restrictive lung disease. www.emedicine.com/MED/topic2012.htm.

West JB. Pulmonary pathophysiology—the essentials. 7th ed. Baltimore: Lippincott Williams & Wilkins; 2007.

Chapter 19

Anderson SD. How does exercise cause asthma attacks? Curr Opin Allergy Clin Immunol. 2006;6(1):37-42.

Borg GAV. Pyschophysical bases of perceived exertion. Med Sci Sports Exerc. 1982;14;377-381.

Celli BR, MacNee W, Agusti A, et al. ATS/ERS Task Force: Standards for the diagnosis and treatment of patients with COPD: A summary of the ATS/ERS position paper. Eur Respir J. 2004;23;932-946.

Centers for Disease Control and Prevention. National surveillance for asthma—United States, 1980-2004. MMWR. 2007;56:912-915.

Clark CJ, Cochrane LM. Physical activity and asthma. Curr Opin Pulm Med. 1999;5:68-75.

Clark CJ, Cochrane L, Mackay E. Low-intensity peripheral muscle conditioning improves exercise tolerance and breathlessness in COPD. Eur Respir J. 1996;9:2590-2596.

Global Initiative for Asthma Management and Prevention, NHLBI/WHO workshop report, U.S. Department of Health and Human Services. Bethesda, MD: National Institutes of Health; 1995. Pub. no. 95-3659.

Leff JA, Busse WW, Pearlman D, et al. Montelukast, a leukotriene-receptor antagonist, for the treatment of mild asthma and exercise-induced bronchoconstriction. N Engl J Med. 1998;339:147-152.

Morton AR, Fitch KD. Asthma. In: Skinner SJ, ed. Exercise testing and exercise prescription for special cases. 2nd ed. Philadelphia: Lea & Febiger; 1993.

National Heart, Lung, and Blood Institute, National Asthma Education and Prevention Program. Expert panel report 3: Guidelines for the diagnosis and management of asthma: Full report 2007. Bethesda, MD: NHLBI; 2007 Aug. Pub. no. 07-4051.

Nelson JA, Strauss L, Skowronski M, Ciufo R, Novak R, McFadden ER. Effect of long-term salmeterol treatment on exercise-induced asthma. N Engl J Med. 1998;339:1783-1786.

Rundell KW, Lemanske RF, Wilber RL. Exercise-induced asthma: Pathophysiology and treatment. Champaign, IL: Human Kinetics; 2002.

Storms WW. Asthma associated with exercise. Immunol Allergy Clin North Am. 2005;25(1):31-43.

Chapter 20

Cerny FJ, Pullano TP, Cropp GJ. Cardiorespiratory adaptations to exercise in cystic fibrosis. Amer Rev Respir Dis. 1982;126(2):217-220.

Cystic Fibrosis Foundation Patient Registry: Annual data report 2006. Available from www.cff.org/UploadedFiles/research/ClinicalResearch/2006%20Patient%20Registry%20Report.pdf.

Godfrey S. Exercise testing in children. Philadelphia: Saunders; 1974. p. 35.

Hodson M, Geddes D, Bush A. Cystic fibrosis. 3rd ed. London: A Hodder Arnold; 2007.

Klijn PH, Oudshoorn A, van der Ent CK, van der Net J, Kimpen JL, Helders PJ. Effects of anaerobic training in children with cystic fibrosis: A randomized controlled study. Chest. 2004;125(4):1299-1305.

Nixon, PA. Role of exercise in the diagnosis and management of pulmonary disease in children and youth. Med Sci Sports Exerc. 1996;28(4):414-420.

Nixon PA, Joswiak ML, Fricker FJ. A six-minute walk test for assessing exercise tolerance in severely ill children. J Pediatr. 1996;129:362-366.

Nixon PA, Orenstein DM, Curtis SE, Ross EA. Oxygen supplementation during exercise in cystic fibrosis. Am Rev Respir Dis. 1990;142(4):807-811.

Nixon PA, Orenstein DM, Kelsey SF, Doershuk CF. The prognostic value of exercise testing in patients with cystic fibrosis. New Engl J Med. 1992;327:1785-1788.

Orenstein DM, Henke KG, Costill DL, Doershuk CF, Lemon PJ, Stern RC. Exercise and heat stress in cystic fibrosis patients. Pediatr Res. 1983;17:267-269.

Orenstein DM, Nixon PA. Patients with cystic fibrosis. In: Franklin BA, Gordon S, Timmis CG, eds. Exercise in modern medicine. Baltimore: Williams & Wilkins; 1989. p. 204-214.

Orenstein DM, Noyes BE. Cystic fibrosis. In: Casaburi R, Petty TL, eds. Principles and practice of pulmonary rehabilitation. Philadelphia: Saunders; 1993. p. 439-458.

Schneiderman-Walker J, Pollock SL, Corey M, Wilkes DD, Canny GJ, Pedder L, Reisman JJ. A randomized controlled trial of a 3-year home exercise program in cystic fibrosis. J Pediatr. 2000;136:304-310.

Selvadurai HC, Blimkie CJ, Meyers N, Mellis CM, Cooper PJ, Van Asperen PP. Randomized controlled study of in-hospital exercise training programs in children with cystic fibrosis. Pediatr Pulmonol. 2002;33:194-200.

Serisier DJ, Coates AD, Bowler SD. Effect of albuterol on maximal exercise capacity in cystic fibrosis. Chest. 2007;131:1181-1187.

Chapter 21

Biring MS, Fournier M, Ross DJ, Lewis MI. Cellular adaptations of skeletal muscles to cyclosporin. J Appl Physiol. 1998; 84:1967-1975.

Division of Transplantation, Bureau of Health Resources Development. 2005 annual report of the US Scientific Registry for Transplant Recipients and the Organ Procurement and Transplantation Network—transplant data: 1995-2004. Rockville, MD: Health Resources and Services Administration, U.S. Department of Health and Human Services; 2005.

Garone S, Ross DJ. Bronchiolitis obliterans syndrome: Review of our knowledge and treatment strategies. Curr Opin Organ Transpl. 1999;4:254-263.

Grossman RF, Maurer JR. Pulmonary considerations in transplantation. Clinics Chest Med. 1990;11:2.

Hokanson JF, Mercier JG, Brooks GA. Cyclosporine A decreases rat skeletal muscle mitochondrial respiration in vitro. Am J Respir Crit Care Med. 1995;151:1848-1851.

Iber C, Simon P, Skatrud JB, et al. The Breuer-Hering reflex in humans: Effects of pulmonary denervation and hypocapnia. Am J Respir Crit Care Med. 1995;152:217-224.

Joint statement of the American Society for Transplant Physicians (ASTP)/American Thoracic Society (ATS)/European Respiratory Society (ERS)/International Society for Heart and Lung Transplantation (ISHLT). International guidelines for the selection of lung transplant candidates. Am J Respir Crit Care Med. 1998;158:335-339.

Miyoshi S, Trulock EP, Schaefers H-J, et al. Cardio-pulmonary exercise testing after single and double lung transplantation. Chest. 1990;97:1130-1136.

Ross DJ, Waters PF, Mohsenifar A, et al. Hemodynamic responses to exercise after lung transplantation. Chest. 1993;103:46-53.

Schwaiblmair M, von Scheidt W, Uberfuhr P, et al. Functional significance of cardiac reinnervation in heart transplant recipients. J Heart Lung Transpl. 1999;18(9):838-845.

Stiebellehner L, Quittan M, End A, et al. Aerobic endurance training program improves exercise performance in lung transplant recipients. Chest. 1998;113(4):906-912.

Trulock EP, Christie JD, Edwards LB, et al. Registry of the International Society for Heart and Lung Transplantation: Twenty-fourth official adult lung and heart-lung transplantation report—2007. J Heart Lung Transpl. 2007;26:782.

Chapter 22

Durstine JL, Grandjean PW, Davis PG, et al. The effects of exercise training on serum lipids and lipoproteins: A quantitative analysis. Sports Med. 2001;31(15):1033-1062.

Durstine JL, Thompson PD. Exercise in the treatment of lipid disorders. Cardiol Clin. 2001;19(3):471-488.

Fletcher B, Berra K, Ades P, et al. Managing abnormal blood lipids: A collaborative approach. Circulation. 2005;112:3184-3209.

Kelley GA, Kelley KS. Aerobic exercise and HDL2-C: A meta-analysis of randomized controlled trials. Atherosclerosis. 2006;184:207-215.

Kelley GA, Kelley KS. Aerobic exercise and lipids and lipoproteins in children and adolescents: A meta-analysis of randomized controlled trials. Atherosclerosis. 2007;191:447-453.

Kelley GA, Kelley KS, Franklin B. Aerobic exercise and lipids and lipoproteins in patients with cardiovascular disease: A meta-analysis of randomized controlled trials. J Cardiopulm Rehabil. 2006;26(3):131-139.

Kelley GA, Kelley KS, Tran ZV. Aerobic exercise and lipids and lipoproteins in women: A meta-analysis of randomized controlled trials. J Women's Health. 2004;13(10):1148-1164.

Kelley GA, Kelley KS, Tran ZV. Aerobic exercise, lipids and lipoproteins in overweight and obese adults: A meta-analysis of randomized controlled trials. Int J Obes. 2005;29(8):881-893.

Kraus WE, Houmard JA, Duscha BD, et al. Effects of the amount and intensity of exercise on plasma lipoproteins. N Engl J Med. 2002;347:1483-1492.

Kwiterovich PO Jr. The metabolic pathways of high-density lipoprotein, low-density lipoprotein, and triglycerides: A current review. Am J Cardiol. 2000;86(12A):5L-10L.

Shepherd J. Economics of lipid-lowering in primary prevention: Lessons from the West of Scotland Coronary Prevention Study. Am J Cardiol. 2001;87(5A):19B-22B.

Superko HR. Lipoprotein subclasses and atherosclerosis. Frontiers Biosci. 2001;1(6):D355-365.

Williams MA, Haskell WL, Ades PA, et al. Resistance exercise in individuals with and without cardiovascular disease: 2007 update: A scientific statement from the American Heart Association Council on Clinical Cardiology and Council on Nutrition, Physical Activity, and Metabolism. Circulation. 2007 Jul 31;116(5):572-584.

Chapter 23

Beyer N, Asdahl M, Strange B, et al. Improved physical performance after orthotopic liver transplantation. Liver Transpl Surg. 1999;5(4):301-209.

Diesel W, Noakes TD, Swanepoel C, Lambert M. Isokinetic muscle strength predicts maximum exercise tolerance in renal patients on chronic hemodialysis. Am J Kidney Dis. 1990;16:109-114.

Johansen K. Physical functioning and exercise capacity in patients on dialysis. Adv Ren Replace Ther. 1999;6(2):141-148.

Krasnoff JB. Liver disease, transplant, and exercise. Clin Exerc Physiol. 2001;3(1):27-34.

Krasnoff J, Painter PL. The physiologic consequences of inactivity and bed rest. Adv Ren Replace Ther. 1999;6(2):124-132.

Krasnoff JB, Vintro AQ, Ascher NL, Bass NM, Paul SM, Dodd MJ, Painter PL. A randomized trial of exercise and dietary counseling after liver transplantation. Am J Transpl. 2006 Aug;6(8):1896-1905.

Moore GE, Brinker KR, Stray-Gundersen J. Determinants of V̇O2 peak in patients with end-stage renal disease: On and off dialysis. Med Sci Sports Exerc. 1993;25:18-23.

Painter PL. Exercise after renal transplantation. Adv Ren Replace Ther. 1999;6(2):159-164.

Painter PL. Physical functioning in end-stage renal disease patients: Update 2005. Hemodial Int. 2005;9:218-235.

Painter PL, Carlson L, Carey S, Paul SM, Myll J. Physical functioning and health-related quality-of-life changes with exercise training in hemodialysis patients. Am J Kidney Dis. 2000;35(3):1-12.

Painter PL, Johansen KL. Improving physical functioning: Time to become a part of the routine care. Am J Kidney Dis. 2005;48:167-170.

Painter PL, Moore GE. The impact of rHu erythropoetin on exercise capacity in hemodialysis patients. Adv Ren Replace Ther. 1994;1(1):55-65.

Painter PL, Stewart AL, Carey S. Physical functioning: Definitions, measurement and expectations. Adv Ren Replace Ther. 1999;6(2):110-123.

Ritland S, Foss N, Skrede S. The effect of standardized work load on "liver tests" in patients with chronic active hepatitis. Scand J Gastroenterol. 1982;17:1013-1016.

Chapter 24

Albright A, Franz M, Hornsby G, Kriska A, Marrero D, Ullrich I, Verity LS. American College of Sports Medicine position stand. Exercise and type 2 diabetes. Med Sci Sports Exerc. 2000;32(7):1345-1360.

American Diabetes Association. Diagnosis and classification of diabetes mellitus. Diabetes Care. 2008;31(suppl 1):31:S55-S60.

American Diabetes Association. Nutrition recommendations and interventions for diabetes: A position statement of the American Diabetes Association. Diabetes Care. 2008;31(suppl 1):S61-S78.

American Diabetes Association. Physical activity/exercise and diabetes. Diabetes Care. 2004;27(suppl 1):S58-S62.

Buse JB, Ginsberg HN, Bakris GL, Clark NG, et al, American Heart Association, American Diabetes Association. Primary prevention of cardiovascular diseases in people with diabetes mellitus: A scientific statement from the American Heart Association and the American Diabetes Association. Circulation. 2007;115(1):114-126.

Centers for Disease Control and Prevention. National diabetes fact sheet: General information and national estimates on diabetes in the United States, 2005. Atlanta: U.S. Department of Health and Human Services, Centers for Disease Control and Prevention; 2005.

DCCT Research Group, The. The effect of intensive treatment of diabetes on the development and progression of long-term complications in insulin-dependent diabetes mellitus. N Engl J Med. 1993;329(14):977-986.

Nathan DM, Cleary PA, Backlund JY, Genuth SM, Lachin JM, Orchard TJ, Raskin P, Zinman B, Diabetes Control and Complications Trial/Epidemiology of Diabetes Interventions and Complications (DCCT/EDIC) Study Research Group. Intensive diabetes treatment and cardiovascular disease in patients with type 1 diabetes. N Engl J Med. 2005;353(25):2643-2653.

Orchard TJ, Temprosa M, Goldberg R, Haffner S, Ratner R, Marcovina S, Fowler S, Diabetes Prevention Program Research Group. The effect of metformin and intensive lifestyle intervention on the metabolic syndrome: The Diabetes Prevention Program randomized trial. Ann Int Med. 2005;142(8):611-619.

Schade DS, Valentine V. To pump or not to pump. Diabetes Care. 2002;25(11):2100-2102.

Chapter 25

American College of Sports Medicine position stand. Appropriate intervention strategies for weight loss and prevention of weight regain for adults. Med Sci Sports Exerc. 2001;33:2145-2156.

Aronne LJ. Classification of obesity and assessment of obesity-related health risks. Obesity Res. 2002;10 suppl 2 Dec:105S.

Atkinson RL, Walberg-Rankin J. Physical activity, fitness, and severe obesity. In: Bouchard C, Shephard RJ, Stephens T, eds. Physical activity, fitness, and health. Champaign, IL: Human Kinetics; 1994. p. 696-711.

Klein S, Allison DB, Heymsfield SB, et al. Waist circumference and cardiometabolic risk. A consensus statement from Shaping America's Health: Association for Weight Management and Obesity Prevention; NAASO, the Obesity Society; the American Society for Nutrition; and the American Diabetes Association. Diabetes Care. 2007;30:1647-1652.

Ogden CL, Carroll MD, Flegal KM. High body mass index for age among US children and adolescents, 2003-2006. JAMA. 2008;299(20):2401-2405.

Ogden CL, Carroll MD, McDowell MA, Flegal KM. Obesity among adults in the United States—no change since 2003–2004. NCHS data brief no 1. Hyattsville, MD: National Center for Health Statistics; 2007.

Sorace P, Lafontaine T. Lifestyle intervention: A priority for long-term success in bariatric patients. ACSM's Health & Fitness Journal. 2007;11:19-25.

Chapter 26

Abellan van Kan G, Rolland Y, Bergman H, et al. The IANA Task Force on frailty assessment of older people in clinical practice. J Nutr Health Aging. 2008;12(1):29-37.

Ahmed N, Mandel R, Fain MJ. Frailty: An emerging geriatric syndrome. Am J Med. 2007;120(9):748-753.

Bette RR, Bonder MBW. Functional performance in older adults. 2nd ed. Philadelphia (PA): Davis; 2001. 544 p.

Folstein MF, Forstein S, McHugh PR. Mini Mental State: A practical method for grading the cognitive state of patients for the clinician. J Psychiatr Res. 1975;12:189-198.

Fried LP, Darer J, Walston J. Frailty. In: Cassel CK, ed. Geriatric medicine: An evidence-based approach. New York (NY): Springer-Verlag; 2003. p. 1067-1076.

Heath JM, Stuart MR. Prescribing exercise for frail elders. J Am Board Fam Med. 2002;15(3):218-228.

Larson EB. Exercise, functional decline and frailty. J Am Geriatr Soc. 1991;39(6):635-636.

Laurie WF. The Cleveland experience: Functional status and services. Use, in multidimensional functional assessment: The OARS methodology. Durham, NC: Duke University Center for the Study of Aging and Human Development; 1978.

Mahoney FI, Barthel DW. Functional evaluation: The Barthel Index. Maryland State Med J. 1965;14:61-65.

Nelson ME, Rejeski WJ, Blair SN, Duncan PW, Judge JO, King AC, et al. Physical activity and public health in older adults: Recommendation from the American College of Sports Medicine and the American Heart Association. Circulation. 2007;116(9):1094-1105.

Singh MAF. Exercise and aging. Clinics Geriatric Med. 2004;20(2):201-221.

Singh MAF. Exercise to prevent and treat functional disability. Clinics Geriatric Med. 2002;18(3):431-462.

Skelton DA, Beyer N. Exercise and injury prevention in older people. Scand J Med Sci Sports. 2003;13(1):77-85.

Struck BD, Ross KM. Health promotion in older adults: Prescribing exercise for the frail and home bound. Geriatrics. 2006;61(5):22-27.

Topinková E. Aging, disability and frailty. Ann Nutr Metab. 2008;52(suppl 1):6-11.

Walston J, Hadley EC, Ferrucci L, et al. Research agenda for frailty in older adults: Toward a better understanding of physiology and etiology: Summary from the American Geriatrics Society/National Institute on Aging Research Conference on Frailty in Older Adults. J Am Geriatr Soc. 2006;54(6):991-1001.

Zubenko GS, Sunderland T. Geriatric psychopharmacology: Why does age matter? Harv Rev Psychiatry. 2000;7(6):311-333.

Chapter 27

Courneya K, Friedenreich C. Physical exercise and quality of life following cancer diagnosis: A literature review. Ann Behav Med. 2005;21:171-179.

Courneya KS, Mackey JR, Bell GJ, et al. Randomized controlled trial of exercise training in postmenopausal breast cancer survivors: Cardiopulmonary and quality of life outcomes. J Clin Oncol. 2003;21:1660-1668.

Demark-Wahnefried W, Hars V, Conaway MR, et al. Reduced rates of metabolism and decreased physical activity in breast cancer patients receiving adjuvant chemotherapy. Am J Clin Nutr. 1997;65:1495.

Demark-Wahnefried W, Pinto B, McGritz ER. Promoting health and physical function among cancer survivors: Potential for prevention and questions that remain. J Clin Oncol. 2006;24:5125-5131.

Doyle C, Kushi LH, Byers T, et al. Nutrition and physical activity during and after cancer treatment: An American Cancer Society guide for informed choices. 2006;56:323-353.

Galvao DA, Newton RU. Review of exercise intervention studies in cancer patients. J Clin Oncol. 2005;23:899-909.

Holmes MD, Chen WY, Feskanich D, et al. Physical activity and survival after breast cancer diagnosis. JAMA. 2005;293:2479-2486.

Knols R, Aaronson NK, Uebelhart D, et al. Physical exercise in cancer patients during and after medical treatment: A systematic review of randomized and controlled clinical trials. J Clin Oncol. 2005;23:3830-3842.

McKelly M, Campbell KL, Rowe BH, et al. Effects of exercise on breast cancer survivors: A systematic review and meta-analysis. CMAJ. 2006;175:34-41.

McTiernan A. Physical activity after cancer: Physiologic outcomes. Cancer Invest. 2004;22:68-81.

Meyerhardt JA, Giovannucci EL, Holmes MD, et al. Physical activity and survival after colorectal cancer diagnosis. J Clin Oncol. 2006;24:3527-3534.

Meyerhardt JA, Heseltine D, Niedzwiecki D, et al. Impact of physical activity on cancer recurrence and survival in patients with stage III colon cancer: Findings from CALGB 89803. J Clin Oncol. 2006;24:3535-3541.

Schmitz KS, Holtzman J, Courneya KS, et al. Controlled physical activity trials in cancer survivors: Systematic review and meta-analysis. Cancer Epidemiol Biomarkers Prev. 2005;14:1588-1595.

Schwartz AL. Physical activity after a cancer diagnosis: Psychosocial outcomes. Cancer Invest. 2004;22:82-92.

Schwartz AL, Winters K, Gallucci B. Exercise effects on bone mineral density in premenopausal and postmenopausal women with breast cancer receiving adjuvant chemotherapy. Oncol Nurs Forum. 2007;34:627-642.

Chapter 28

Bopp CM, Phillips KD, Fulk LJ, Hand GA. Clinical implications of therapeutic exercise in HIV/AIDS. J Assoc Nurs AIDS Care. 2003;14:73-78.

Bopp CM, Phillips KD, Sowell RL, Dudgeon WD, Hand GA. Physical activity and immunity in HIV-infected individuals. AIDS Care. 2004;16:387-393.

Dudgeon WD, Phillips KD, Bopp CM, Hand GA. Physiological and psychological effects of exercise interventions in HIV disease. AIDS Patient Care STDS. 2004;18:1-16.

Dudgeon WD, Phillips KD, Carson JA, Brewer RB, Durstine JL, Hand GA. Counteracting muscle wasting in HIV-infected individuals. HIV Med. 2006;7:299-310.

Fulk LJ, Kane BP, Phillips KD, Bopp CM, Hand GA. Depression in HIV-infected patients: Allopathic, complementary, and alternative treatments. J Psychosom Res. 2004;57:339-351.

Hand GA, Phillips KD, Dudgeon WD, Lyerly GW, Durstine JL, Burgess SE. Moderate intensity exercise training reverses functional aerobic impairment in HIV-infected individuals. AIDS Care. 2008;20:1066-1074, .

LaPerriere A, Antoni MH, Schneiderman N. Exercise intervention attenuates emotional distress and natural killer cell decrements following notification of positive serologic status for HIV-1. Biofeedback Self Regul. 1990;15:229-242.

LaPerriere A, Fletcher MA, Klimas N. Aerobic exercise training in an AIDS risk group. Int J Sports Med. 1991;12:53-57.

Roge BT, Calbet JA, Moller K, Ullum H, Hendel HW, Gerstoft J, Pedersen BK. Skeletal muscle mitochondrial function and exercise capacity in HIV-infected patients with lipodystrophy and elevated p-lactate levels. AIDS. 2002;16:973-982.

Schmitz HR, Layne JE, Humphrey R. Exercise and HIV infection. In: Myers JN, Herbert WG, Humphrey R, eds. ACSM's resources for clinical exercise physiology: Musculoskeletal, neuromuscular, neoplastic, immunologic, and hematologic conditions. Philadelphia: Lippincott Williams & Wilkins, 2002. p. 206-218.

Spence DW, Galantino MA, Mossberg KA, Zimmerman SO. Progressive resistance exercise: Effect on muscle function and anthropometry of a select AIDS population. Arch Phys Med Rehabil. 1990;71:644-648.

Ullum H, Palmø J, Halkjaer-Kustensen J, Diamant M, Klokker M, Kruuse A, LaPerriere A, Pedersen BK. The effect of acute exercise on lymphocyte subsets, natural killer cells, proliferative response, and cytokines in HIV seropositive persons. J Acquir Immune Defic Syndr. 1994;7:1122-1132.

Chapter 29

Beyer N, Asdahl M, Strange B, et al. Improved physical performance after orthotopic liver transplantation. Liver Transpl Surg. 1999;5(4):301-309.

Green GA, Moore G. Exercise and organ transplantation. J Back Musculoskel Rehabil. 1998;10:3-11.

Kempeneer GLG, Noakes TD, Van Zyl-Smit R, et al. Skeletal muscle limits the exercise tolerance of renal transplant recipients: Effects of a graded exercise program. Am J Kidney Dis. 1990;16:57-65.

Krasnoff JB. Liver disease, transplant, and exercise. Clin Exerc Physiol. 2001;3(1):27-34.

Krasnoff JB, Painter PL, Vintro AQ, et al. A randomized trial of exercise and dietary counseling after liver transplantation. Am J Transpl. 2006;6:1896-1905.

Painter PL. Exercise following organ transplantation: A critical part of the routine post transplant care. Ann Transpl. 2005;10:28-30.

Painter PL, Luetkemeier MJ, Moore GE, et al. 1997. Health-related fitness and quality of life in organ transplant recipients. Transplantation. 64:1795-1800.

Painter PL, Tomlanovich S, Hector L, et al. Cardiorespiratory fitness in pancreas-kidney transplant recipients. Transpl Proc. 1998;30:651-652.

Van den Ham EC, Kooman JP, Christiaans MH, et al. Relation between steroid dose, body composition and physical activity in renal transplant patients. Transplantation. 2000;69(8):1591-1598.

Chapter 30

Clapp L, et al. Acute effects of thirty minutes of light-intensity, intermittent exercise on patients with chronic fatigue syndrome. Phys Ther. 1999;79(8):749-756.

DeBecker PJ, Roeykens M, Reynders N, et al. Exercise capacity in chronic fatigue syndrome. Arch Int Med. 2000;160(21):3270-3277.

Edmonds M, McGuire H, Price J. Exercise therapy for chronic fatigue syndrome. Cochrane Database Syst Rev. 2004;CD003200.

Fukada K, Straus SE, Hickie I, et al. The chronic fatigue syndrome: A comprehensive approach to its definition and study. International Chronic Fatigue Study Group. Ann Int Med. 1994;121:953-959.

Fulcher KY, White PD. Strength and physiological response to exercise in patients with chronic fatigue syndrome. J Neurol Neurosurg Psychiatry. 2000;69(3):289.

LaManca JJ, Sisto SA. Chronic fatigue syndrome. In: Myers JN, Herbert WG, Humphrey R, eds. ACSM's resources for clinical exercise physiology: Musculoskeletal, neuromuscular, neoplastic, immunologic, and hematologic conditions. Phila-

delphia: Lippincott Williams & Wilkins; 2002. p. 219-232.

Ottenweller JE, Sisto SA, McCarty RC, et al. Hormonal responses to exercise in chronic fatigue syndrome. Neuropsychobiology. 2001;43(1):34-41.

Powell P, Bentall RP, Nye FJ, et al. Randomized controlled trial of patient education to encourage graded exercise in chronic fatigue syndrome. BMJ. 2001;322:387-390.

Reeves WC, Wagner D, Nisenbaum R, et al. Chronic fatigue syndrome—a clinically empirical approach to its definition and study. BMC Med. 2005;3:19.

Reid S, Chalder T, Cleare A, et al. Chronic fatigue syndrome. Clin Evidence. 2005;14:1366-1378.

Shepard RJ. Chronic fatigue syndrome. A brief review of functional disturbances and potential therapy. J Sports Med Phys Fit. 2005;45(3):381-392.

Wagner DW, Nisenbaum R, Heim C, et al. Psychometric properties of the CDC Symptom Inventory for the assessment of chronic fatigue syndrome. Popul Health Metrics 2005;3:8.

Wallman KE, Morton AR, Goodman C, et al. Exercise prescription for individuals with chronic fatigue syndrome. Med J Aust. 2005;183(3):142-143.

Chapter 31

Burckhardt CS, Mannerkorpi K, Hedenberg L, Bjelle A. A randomized controlled clinical trial of education and physical training for women with fibromyalgia. J Rheumatol. 1994;21:714-720.

Carville SF, Arendt-Nielsen L, Bliddal H, et al. EULAR evidence based recommendations for the management of fibromyalgia syndrome. Ann Rheum Dis. Online First. 2007 (cited 2007 October 3);3. Available from http://ard.bmj.com/cgi/content/abstract/ard.2007.071522v3. doi:10.1136/ard.2007.071522.

Dadabhoy D, Clauw DJ. Therapy insight: Fibromyalgia—different type of pain needing a different type of treatment. Nat Clin Pract Rheumatol. 2006;2(7):364-372.

Fisher NM. Osteoarthritis, rheumatoid arthritis, and fibromyalgia. In: Myers JN, Herbert WG, Humphrey WG, eds. ACSM's resources for clinical exercise physiology: Musculoskeletal, neuromuscular, neoplastic, immunologic, and hematologic conditions. Philadelphia: Lippincott Williams & Wilkins; 2002. p. 111-124.

Gowans SE, de Hueck A. Pool exercise for individuals with fibromyalgia. Curr Opin Rheumatol. 2007;19:168-173.

Häkkinen A, Häkkinen K, Hannonen P, Alen M. Strength training induced adaptations in neuromuscular function of premenopausal women with fibromyalgia: Comparison with healthy women. Ann Rheum Dis. 2001;60:21-26.

Jones KD, Burckhardt CS, Clark SR, Bennett RM, Potempa KM. A randomized controlled trial of muscle strengthening versus flexibility training in fibromyalgia. J Rheumatol. 2002;29:1041-1048.

Kingsley JD, Panton LB, Toole T, et al. The effects of a 12-week strength-training program on strength and functionality in women with fibromyalgia. Arch Phys Med Rehabil. 2005;86:1713-1721.

McCain GA, Bell DA, Mai FM, Halliday PD. A controlled study of the effects of a supervised cardiovascular fitness training program on the manifestations of primary fibromyalgia. Arthritis Rheum. 1988;31:1135-1141.

Mengshoel AM, Komnaes HB, Forre O. The effects of 20 weeks of physical fitness training in female patients with fibromyalgia. Clin Exp Rheumatol. 1992;10:345-349.

Meyer BB, Lemley KJ. Utilizing exercise to affect the symptomology of fibromyalgia: A pilot study. Med Sci Sports Exerc. 2000;32(10):1691-1697.

Nichols DS, Glenn TM. Effects of aerobic exercise on pain perception, affect, and level of disability in individuals with fibromyalgia. Physical Ther. 1994;74:327-332.

Nielens H, Booisset V, Masquelier E. Fitness and perceived exertion in patients with fibromyalgia syndrome. Clin J Pain. 2000;16:209-213.

Wigers SH, Stiles TC, Vogel PA. Effects of aerobic exercise versus stress management treatment in fibromyalgia. Scand J Rheumatol. 1996;25:77-86.

Wolfe F, Smythe HA, Yunus MB, et al. The American College of Rheumatology 1990 criteria for the classification of fibromyalgia. Arthritis Rheum. 1990;33:160-172.

Chapter 32

Beutler E, Waalen J. The definition of anemia: What is the lower limit of normal of the blood hemoglobin concentration? Blood. 2006;107(5):1747-1750.

Eichner ER. Sports medicine pearls and pitfalls: Anemia in athletes. Curr Sports Med Rep. 2007;6(1):2-3.

Gozal D, Thiriet P, Mbala E, et al. Effect of different modalities of exercise and recovery on exercise performance in subjects with sickle cell trait. Med Sci Sports Exerc. 1992;24(12):1325-1331.

Gregg SG, Willis WT, Brooks GA. Interactive effects of anemia and muscle oxidative capacity on exercise endurance. J Appl Physiol. 1989;67(2):765-770.

Jones SR, Binder RA, Donowho EM. Sudden death in sickle cell trait. New Engl J Med. 1970;282(6):323-325.

Koskolou MD, Roach RC, Calbet JA, Radegran G, Saltin B. Cardiovascular responses to dynamic exercise with acute anemia in humans. Am J Physiol. 1997;273(4 Pt 2):H1787-1793.

Krause JR, Stolc V. Serum ferritin and bone marrow biopsy iron stores, II: Correlation with low serum iron and Fe/TIBC ratio less than 15%. Am J Clin Pathol. 1980;74:461-464.

Lipschitz DA, Cook JD, Finch CA. A clinical evaluation of serum ferritin as an index of iron stores. N Engl J Med. 1974;290:1213-1216.

Mercer KW, Densmore JJ. Hematologic disorders in the athlete. Clin Sports Med. 2005;24(3):599-621.

Pollack A. FDA warning is issued on anemia drugs' overuse. New York Times. 2007 Mar 10.

Rimon E, Levy S, Sapir A, Gelzer G, Peled R, Ergas D, Sthoeger ZM. Diagnosis of iron deficiency anemia in the elderly by transferrin receptor–ferritin index. Arch Intern Med. 2002;162:445-449.

Singh AK, Szczech L, Tang KL, et al., CHOIR investigators. Correction of anemia with epoetin alfa in chronic kidney disease. N Engl J Med. 2006;355(20):2085-2098.

Sproule BJ, Mitchell JH, Miller WF. Cardiopulmonary physiological responses to heavy exercise in patients with anemia. J Clin Invest. 1960;39:378-388.

U.S. Food and Drug Administration. Information for healthcare professionals: Erythropoiesis stimulating agents (ESA) (cited 2008 Jan 8). Available from www.fda.gov/cder/drug/infopage/RHE/default.htm.

Chapter 33

Burke L, Parisotto R. Hematologic disorders. In: Myers JN, Herbert WG, Humphrey R, eds. ACSM's resources for clinical exercise physiology: Musculoskeletal, neuromuscular, neoplastic, immunologic, and hematologic conditions. Philadelphia: Lippincott Williams & Wilkins; 2002. p. 233-241.

Coppola L, Grassia A, Coppola A, Tondi G, Peluso G, Mordente S, Gombos G. Effects of a moderate-intensity aerobic program on blood viscosity, platelet aggregation and fibrinolytic balance in young and middle-aged sedentary subjects. Blood Coagul Fibrinol. 2004;15:31-37.

Hilberg T, Herbsleb M, Puta C, Gabriel HHW, Schramm W. Physical training increases isometric muscular strength and proprioceptive performance in haemophilic subjects. Haemophilia. 2003;9:86-93.

Kahn SR, Azoulay L, Hirsch A, Haber M, Strulovitch C, Shrier I. Acute effects of exercise in patients with previous deep venous thrombosis. Chest. 2003;123:399-405.

Lockard MM, Gopinathannair R, Paton CM, Phares DA, Hagberg JM. Exercise training-induced changes in coagulation factors in older adults. Med Sci Sports Exerc. 2007;39(4):587-592.

Mulder K, Cassis F, Seuser DRA, Naraya P, Dalzell R, Poulsen W. Risks and benefits of sports and fitness activities for people with haemophilia. Haemophilia. 2004;10(suppl 4):161-163.

Shrier I, Kahn SR. Effect of physical activity after recent deep venous thrombosis: A cohort study. Med Sci Sports Exerc. 2005;37(4):630-634.

Van Sralen KJ, Le Cessie S, Rosendaal FR, Doggen CJM. Regular sports activities decrease the risk of venous thrombosis. J Thromb Haemost. 2007;5:2186-2192.

Wang J-S. Exercise prescription and thrombogenesis. J Biomed Sci. 2006;13:753-761.

Wang J-S. Intense exercise increases shear-induced platelet aggregation in men through enhancement of von Willebrand factor binding, glycoprotein IIb/IIIa activation, and P-selectin expression on platelets. Eur J Appl Physiol. 2004;91:742-747.

Wang J-S, Liao C-H. Moderate-intensity exercise suppresses platelet activation and polymorphonuclear leukocyte interaction with surface-adherent platelets under shear flow in men. Thromb Haemost. 2004;91:587-594.

Weiss C, Egermann M, Bärtsch P. Exercise-induced activation of coagulation in subjects with activated protein C resistance. Blood Coagul Fibrinol. 2004;15:317-321.

Wittmeier K, Mulder K. Enhancing lifestyle for individuals with haemophilia through physical activity and exercise: Role of physiotherapy. Haemophilia. 2007;13(suppl 2):31-37.

Womack CJ, Nagelkirk PR, Coughlin AM. Exercise-induced changes in coagulation and fibrinolysis in healthy populations and patients with cardiovascular disease. Sports Med. 2003;3(11):795-807.

Chapter 34

Callahan LF, Mielenz T, Freuburger J, et al. A randomized controlled trial of the People With Arthritis Can Exercise Program: Symptoms, function, physical activity, and psychosocial outcomes. Arth Care Res. 2008;59(1):92-101.

Dagfinrud H, Hagen K. Physiotherapy interventions for ankylosing spondylitis. Cochrane Database Syst Rev. 2003;3.

De Carvalho MRP, Sasto EI, Tebexreni AS. Effects of supervised cardiovascular training program on exercise tolerance, aerobic capacity, and quality of life in patients with systemic lupus erythematosus. Arth Rheum (Arth Care Res). 2005;53(6):838-844.

De Jong Z, Munneke M, et al. Is a long-term high-intensity exercise program effective and safe in patients with rheumatoid arthritis? Results of a randomized controlled trial. Arth Rheum. 2003;48:2415-2424.

Feinglass J, Thompson JA, He XZ, et al. Effect of physical activity on functional status among older middle-age adults with arthritis. Arth Care Res. 2005;53(6):879-885.

Häkkinen A, Pakarinen A, Hannonen P, et al. Effects of prolonged combined strength and endurance training on physical fitness, body composition and serum hormones in women with rheumatoid arthritis and in healthy controls. Clin Exp Rheumatol. 2005;23:505-512.

Hurley MV, Walsh NE, Mitchell HL, et al. Clinical effectiveness of a rehabilitation program integrating exercise, self-management, and active coping strategies for chronic knee pain: A cluster randomized trial. Arth Rheum (Arth Care Res). 2007;57:1211-1219.

Mangione KK, McCully K, Gloviak A, et al. The effects of high-intensity and low-intensity cycle ergometry in older adults with knee osteoarthritis. J Gerontol Med Sci. 1999;54A:M184-M190.

Minor M, Stenstrom CH, Klepper SE, et al. Work group recommendations: 2002 Exercise and Physical Activity Conference, St. Louis, Missouri. Session V: Evidence of benefit of exercise and physical activity in arthritis. Arth Rheum (Arth Care Res). 2003;49:453-454.

Roddy E, Zhang W, Doherty M, et al. Evidence-based recommendations for the role of exercise in the management of osteoarthritis of the hip or knee—the MOVE consensus. Rheumatology. 2005;44:67-71.

Roos EM, Dahlberg L. Positive effects of moderate exercise on glycosaminoglycan content in knee cartilage. Arth Rheum. 2005;52:3507-3514.

Thorstensson CA, Roos EM, Petersson IF, Ekdahl E. Six-week high-intensity exercise program for middle-aged patients with knee osteoarthritis: Randomized controlled trial. BMC Musculoskel Dis. 2005;6:27.

Westby MA. Health professional's guide to exercise prescription for people with arthritis: A review of aerobic fitness activities. Arth Rheum (Arth Care Res). 2001;45(6):501-511.

Westby MD, Minor MA. Exercise and physical activity. In: Bartlett SJ, ed., Clinical care in the rheumatic diseases. 3rd ed. Atlanta: Association of Rheumatology Health Professionals; 2006. p. 211-219.

Chapter 35

Abenhaim L, Rossignol M, Valat JP, et al. The role of activity in the therapeutic management of back pain. Report of the International Paris Task Force on Back Pain. Spine. 2000;25(suppl 4):S1-33.

Dionne C, Dunn K, Croft PR, et al. A consensus approach toward the standardization of back pain definitions for use in prevalence studies. Spine. 2008 Jan 1;33(1)95-103.

Leggett S, Mooney V, Matheson L, Nelson B, Dreisinger T, Van Zytveld J, Vic L. Restorative exercise for clinical low back pain: A prospective two-center study with 1-year follow-up. Spine. 1999;24:889-898.

Malmivaara A, Hakkinen U, Aro T, et al. The treatment of acute low back pain: Bed-rest, exercises, or ordinary activity? N Engl J Med. 1995;332:351-355.

Protas EJ. Aerobic exercise in the rehabilitation of individuals with chronic low back pain: A review. Crit Rev Phys Rehabil Med. 1996;8:283-295.

Protas EJ. Physical activity and low back pain. In: Max M, ed. Pain 1999: An update review. Seattle: IASP Press; 1999. p. 145-152.

Simmonds MJ. Exercise and activity for persons with nonspecific back pain. In: Myers JN, Herbert WG, Humphrey R, eds. ACSM's resources for clinical exercise physiology: Musculoskeletal, neuromuscular, neoplastic, immunologic, and hematologic conditions. 3rd ed. Philadelphia: Lippincott Williams & Wilkins; 2002. p. 125-138.

Simmonds MJ. Measuring and managing pain and performance. Man Ther. 2006;11(3):175-179.

Smeets RJ, et al. Do patients with chronic low back pain have a lower level of aerobic fitness than healthy controls? Are pain, disability, fear of injury, working status, or level of leisure time activity associated with the difference in aerobic fitness level? Spine. 2006;31(1):90-97, discussion 98.

van Tulder M, Becker A, et al. European guidelines for the management of acute nonspecific low back pain in primary care. Eur Spine J. 2006;15 suppl 2:S169-191.

Wittink H, et al. Aerobic fitness testing in patients with chronic low back pain: Which test is best? Spine. 2000;25(13):1704-1710.

Wittink H, et al. The association of pain with aerobic fitness in patients with chronic low back pain. Arch Phys Med Rehabil. 2002;83(10):1467-1471.

Chapter 36

Bianchi ML, Orsini MR, Saraifoger S, et al. Quality of life in post-menopausal osteoporosis. Health Qual Life Outcomes. 2005;3:78.

Bonaiuti D, Shea B, Iovine R, et al. Exercises for preventing and treating osteoporosis in postmenopausal women. Cochrane Database Syst Rev. 2007;4.

Bonnick SL. The osteoporosis handbook. 3rd ed. Dallas: Taylor; 2000. p. 1-75.

Chen Z, Wang Z, Lohman T, et al. Dual-energy x-ray absorptiometry is a valid tool for assessing skeletal muscle mass in older women. J Nutr. 2007;137(12):2775-2780.

Cussler EC, Lohman TG, Going SB, et al. Weight lifted in strength training predicts bone change in postmenopausal women. Med Sci Sports Exerc. 2003;35(1):10-17.

FRAXTM WHO Fracture Risk Assessment Tool. World Health Organization Collaborating Centre for Metabolic Bone Diseases. University of Sheffield, UK: World Health Organization (cited 2008 Mar 4). Available from www.shef.ac.uk/FRAX/index.htm.

Kohrt WM, Bloomfield SA, Little KD, American College of Sports Medicine, et al. American College of Sports Medicine position stand: Physical activity and bone health. Med Sci Sports Exerc. 2004;36(11):1985-1996.

Lips P, van Schoor NM. Quality of life in patients with osteoporosis. Osteoporos Int. 2005;16(5):447-455.

Mauck KF, Clarke BL. Diagnosis, screening, prevention, and treatment of osteoporosis. Mayo Clin Proc. 2006;81(5):662-672.

Milliken LA, Going SB, Houtkooper LB, Flint-Wagner HG. Effects of exercise training on bone remodeling, insulin-like growth factors, and bone mineral density in postmenopausal women with and without hormone replacement therapy. Calcif Tissue Int. 2003;72(4):478-484.

NIH Consensus Development Panel on Osteoporosis Prevention, Diagnosis, and Therapy. Osteoporosis prevention, diagnosis, and therapy. JAMA. 2001;285:785-795.

Rikli RE. Reliability, validity, and methodological issues in assessing physical activity in older adults. [Comment]. Res Q Exerc Sport. 2000;71(2 suppl):S89-96.

Sambrook P, Cooper C. Osteoporosis. Lancet. 2006;367(9527): 2010-2018.

U.S. Department of Health and Human Services. Bone health and osteoporosis: A report of the surgeon general. Rockville, MD: U.S. Department of Health and Human Services, Office of the Surgeon General (cited 2008 Feb 20). Available from www. surgeongeneral.gov/library/bonehealth/content.html.

Van Schoor NM, Smit JH, Twisk JW, et al. Impact of vertebral deformities, osteoarthritis, and other chronic diseases on quality of life: A population-based study. Osteoporos Int. 2005;16(7):749-756.

Chapter 37

Lockette KF, Keyes AM. Conditioning with physical disabilities. Champaign, IL: Human Kinetics; 2000.

Pitetti KH, Manske RC. Amputation. In: Myers JN, Herbert WG, Humphrey R. ACSM's resources for clinical exercise physiology: Musculoskeletal, neuromuscular, neoplastic, immunologic, and hematologic conditions. Philadelphia: Lippincott Williams & Wilkins; 2002. p. 170-178.

Pitetti KH, Manske RC. Lower limb amputation. In: LeMura L, von Duvillard S. Clinical exercise physiology: Application and physiological principles. Baltimore: Lippincott Williams & Wilkins; 2003. p. 219-236.

Chapter 38

Bhambhani Y, Rowland G, Farag M. Effects of circuit training on body composition and peak cardiorespiratory responses in patients with moderate to severe traumatic brain injury. Arch Phys Med Rehabil. 2005;86(2):268-276.

Bhambhani Y, Rowland G, Farag M. Reliability of peak cardiorespiratory responses in patients with moderate to severe traumatic brain injury. Arch Phys Med Rehabil. 2003;84(11):1629-1636.

Browning R. Traumatic brain injury pharmacology guide. [Online]. 2000 Jan 23 (cited 2008 Mar 27). Available from http://tbi.unl.edu/savedTBI/drugs/guideforTBI. htm#Anti-Convulsants.

Dawodu ST. Traumatic brain injury: Definition, epidemiology, pathophysiology. [Online]. 2007 Jan 26 (accessed 2008 Mar 27). Available from www.emedicine.com/pmr/topic212. htm.

Driver S, O'Connor J, Lox C, Rees K. Evaluation of an aquatics programme on fitness parameters of individuals with a brain injury. Brain Inj. 2004;18(9):847-859.

Gaudet C, Wolcott GFR. Introduction to supporting individuals with acquired brain injury in developing a fitness program. [Online]. 2007 Mar 1 (cited 2008 Mar 27). Available from www.ncpad.org/disability/fact_sheet. php?sheet=111&view=all.

Gordon NF, Gulanick M, Costa F, et al. Physical activity and exercise recommendations for stroke survivors: An American Heart Association scientific statement from the Council on Clinical Cardiology, Subcommittee on Exercise, Cardiac Rehabilitation, and Prevention; the Council on Cardiovascular Nursing; the Council on Nutrition, Physical Activity, and Metabolism; and the Stroke Council. Circulation. 2004;109:2031-2041.

Gordon WA, Sliwinski M, Echo J, et al. The benefits of exercise in individuals with traumatic brain injury: A retrospective study. J Head Trauma Rehabil. 1998;134:58-67.

Gresham GE, Duncan PW, Adams HP, et al. Clinical practice guideline number 16: Post-stroke rehabilitation. Rockville, MD: U.S. Department of Health and Human Services; 1995. Public Health Service. Agency for Health Care Policy and Research. AHCPR pub. no. 95-0662.

Halar EM. Management of stroke risk factors during the process of rehabilitation: Secondary stroke prevention. Phys Med Rehabil Clin N Am. 1999;10(4):839-856.

Jankowski LW, Sullivan SJ. Aerobic and neuromuscular training: Effect on the capacity, efficiency, and fatigability of patients with traumatic brain injury. Arch Phys Med Rehabil. 1990;71:500-504.

LeBrasseur NK, Sayers SP, Ouellette MM, Fielding RA. Muscle impairments and behavioral factors mediate functional limitations and disability following stroke. Phys Ther. 2006;86:1342-1350.

Mead GE, Greig CA, Cunningham I, et al. Stroke: A randomized trial of exercise or relaxation. J Am Geriatr Soc. 2007;55:892-899.

Michael K, Macko RF. Ambulatory activity intensity profiles, fitness, and fatigue in chronic stroke. Stroke Rehabil. 2007;14(2):5-12.

Monga TN, Deforge DA, Williams J, Wolfe LA. Cardiovascular responses to acute exercise in patients with cerebrovascular accidents. Arch Phys Med Rehabil. 1988;69:937-940.

Mossberg KA, Ayala D, Baker T, et al. Aerobic capacity after traumatic brain injury: Comparison with a nondisabled cohort. Arch Phys Med Rehabil. 2007;88:315-320.

Mossberg KA, Greene BP. Reliability of graded exercise testing after traumatic brain injury: Submaximal and peak responses. Am J Phys Med Rehabil. 2005;84:492-500.

Myers J. Exercise testing. In: Woods SL, Sivarajan Froelicher ES, Motzer SU, Bridges EJ, eds. Cardiac nursing. 5th ed. Philadelphia: Lippincott Williams & Wilkins; 2004. p. 439-458.

National Center for Injury Prevention and Control. What is traumatic brain injury? [Online]. 2008 Jan 22 (accessed 2008 Mar 27). Available from www.cdc.gov/ncipc/tbi/ TBI.htm.

National Institute of Neurological Disorders and Stroke. NINDS post-stroke rehabilitation fact sheet. [Online]. 2008 (cited 2008 Mar 27). Available from www.ninds.nih.gov/disorders/stroke/poststrokerehab.htm.

O'Sullivan SB, Schmitz TJ. Physical rehabilitation assessment and treatment. 5th ed. Philadelphia: Davis; 2006.

Perna RB, Bordini EJ. Cognitive impairments in TBI: Pharmacological treatment considerations. TBI challenge! [Online]. 2001 (cited 2008 Mar 27);5(2). Available from www.biausa.org/word.files.to.pdf/good.pdfs/Cognitive%20impairment%20in%20tbi.pdf.\

Rimmer JH, Riley B, Creviston T, et al. Exercise training in a predominantly African-American group of stroke survivors. Med Sci Sports Exerc. 2000;32(12):1990-1996.

Chapter 39

American Spinal Injury Association. International standards for neurological classification of SCI revised 2002. www.asia-spinalinjury.org/publications/store.php.

Ehrman JK, Gordon PM, Visich PS, Keteyian SJ, eds. Spinal cord injury. In: Clinical exercise physiology. Champaign, IL: Human Kinetics; 2003. Chap. 27, p. 503-526.

Figoni SF, Kiratli BJ, Sasaki R. Spinal cord dysfunction. In: Myers JN, Herbert WG, Humphrey R, eds. ACSM's resources for clinical exercise physiology: Musculoskeletal, neuromuscular, neoplastic, immunologic, and hematologic conditions. Philadelphia: Lippincott Williams & Wilkins; 2002. p. 48-67.

Hicks AL, Martin KA, Ditor DS, et al. Long-term exercise training in persons with spinal cord injury: Effects on strength, arm ergometry performance and psychological well-being. Spinal Cord. 2003;41:34-43.

Jacobs PL, Nash MS. Exercise recommendations for individuals with spinal cord injury. Sports Med. 2004;34(11):727-751.

Lutkenhoff M, Oppenheimer SG, eds. SPINAbilities: A young person's guide to spina bifida. Bethesda, MD: Woodbine House; 1997.

Myers J, Lee M, Kiratli J. Cardiovascular disease in spinal cord injury: An overview of prevalence, risk, evaluation, and management. Am J Phys Med Rehabil. 2007;86(2):142-152.

Nash MS. Spinal cord injury. In: Frontera WF, Slovik DM, Dawson DM, eds. Exercise in rehabilitation medicine. 2nd ed. Champaign, IL: Human Kinetics; 2006. Chap. 13, p. 191-205.

Phillips WT, Kiratli BJ, Sarkarati M, et al. Effect of spinal cord injury on the heart and cardiovascular fitness. Curr Probl Cardiol. 1998 Nov 23;(11):641-716.

Valent L, Dallmeijer A, Houdijk H, et al. The effects of upper body exercise on the physical capacity of people with a spinal cord injury: A systematic review. Clin Rehabil. 2007;21(4):315-330.

Chapter 40

Aitkens SG, McCrory MA, Kilmer DD, Bernauer EM. Moderate resistance exercise program: Its effect in slowly progressive neuromuscular disease. Arch Phys Med Rehabil. 1993;74:711-715.

Bar-Or O. Pediatric sports medicine for the practitioner. New York: Springer-Verlag; 1983.

Bar-Or O, Reed SL. Rating of perceived exertion in adolescents with neuromuscular disease. In: Borg G, ed. Perception of exertion in physical work. Stockholm: Wenner-Gre; 1987. p. 137-148.

Brooke MH. A clinician's view of neuromuscular diseases. 2nd ed. Baltimore: Williams & Wilkins; 1986.

DeLateur BJ, Giaconi RM. Effect on maximal strength of submaximal exercise in Duchenne muscular dystrophy. Am J Phys Med. 1979;58:26-36.

Florence JM, Hagberg JM. Effect of training on the exercise responses of neuromuscular disease patients. Med Sci Sports Exerc. 1984;16:460-465.

Fowler WM Jr. Management of musculoskeletal complications in neuromuscular disease: Weakness and the role of exercise. Arch Phys Med Rehabil. 1988;2:489-507.

Gozal D, Thiriet P. Respiratory muscle training in neuromuscular disease: Long-term effects on strength and load perception. Med Sci Sports Exerc. 1999;31:1522-1527.

Kley R, Vorgerd M, Tarnopolsky M. Creatine for treating muscle disorders. Cochrane Database Syst Rev. 2007;CD004760.

Louis M, Lebacq J, Poortmans JR, et al. Beneficial effects of creatine supplementation in dystrophic patients. Muscle Nerve. 2003;27:604-610.

Mendell JR, Moxley RT, Griggs RC, et al. Randomized, double-blind six-month trial of prednisone in Duchenne's muscular dystrophy. N Engl J Med. 1989;320:1592-1597.

Milner-Brown HS, Miller RG. Muscle strengthening through high-resistance weight training in patients with neuromuscular disorders. Arch Phys Med Rehabil. 1988;69:14-19.

Scott OM, Hyde SA, Goddard C, et al. Effect of exercise in Duchenne muscular dystrophy. Physiotherapy. 1981;67:174-176.

Tarnopolsky M, Doherty TJ. Muscular dystrophy and other myopathies. In: Myers JN, Herbert WG, Humphrey R, eds. ACSM's resources for clinical exercise physiology: Musculoskeletal, neuromuscular, neoplastic, immunologic, and hematologic conditions. Philadelphia: Lippincott Williams & Wilkins; 2002. p. 78-88.

Tarnopolsky MA, Mahoney DJ, Vajsar J, et al. Creatine monohydrate enhances strength and body composition in Duchenne muscular dystrophy. Neurology. 2004;62:1771-1777.

Tarnopolsky M, Martin J. Creatine monohydrate increases strength in patients with neuromuscular disease. Neurology. 1999;52:854-857.

Tirosh E, Bar-Or O, Rosenbaum P. New muscle power test in neuromuscular disease: Feasibility and reliability. Am J Dis Child. 1990;144:1083-1087.

Tollback A, Eriksson S, Wredenberg A, et al. Effects of high resistance training in patients with myotonic dystrophy. Scand J Rehabil Med. 1999;31:9-16.

Walter MC, Lochmuller H, Reilich P, et al. Creatine monohydrate in muscular dystrophies: A double-blind, placebo-controlled clinical study. Neurology. 2000;54(9):1848-1850.

Chapter 41

Cantu R. Epilepsy and athletics. Clinics Sports Med. 1998;17(1):61-69.

Cordova F. Epilepsy and sport. Aust Fam Physician. 1993;22:558-562.

Dunn J. Other conditions requiring special consideration in physical education. In Grutz T, ed. Special physical education. 7th ed. Madison, WI: Brown & Benchmark; 1997. p. 305-308.

Ellerstein B, Eriksen HR, Hege R, Mostofsky DI, Ursin H. Exercise and epilepsy. In: Mostofsky DI, Loyning Y, eds. The neurobehavioral treatment of epilepsy. Hillsdale, NJ: Erlbaum; 1993. p. 107-122.

Gates J. Epilepsy and sports participation. Phys Sportsmed. 1993;19:98-104.

Gates J, Spiegel R. Epilepsy, sports and exercise. Sports Med. 1993;15(1):1-5.

Nakken KO. Physical exercise in epilepsy. In: Pfäfflin M, Fraser RT, Thorbecke R, Specht U, Wolf P, eds. Comprehensive care for people with epilepsy. Eastleigh: John Libbey; 2001. p. 137-145.

Nakken KO. Physical exercise in outpatients with epilepsy. Epilepsia. 1999;40(5):643-651.

Roth DL, Goode KT, Williams VL, Faught E. Physical exercise, stressful life experience, and depression in adults with epilepsy. Epilepsia. 1994;35:1248-1255.

Schmitt B, Thun-Hohenstein L, Vontobel H, Boltshauser E. Seizures induced by physical exercise: Report of two cases. Neuropediatrics. 1994;25:51-53.

van Linschoten R, Backx FJ, Mulder OG, Meinardi H. Epilepsy and sports. Sports Med. 1990;10:9-19.

Chapter 42

Mostert S, Kesselring J. Effects of a short-term exercise training program on aerobic fitness, fatigue, health perception and activity level of subjects with multiple sclerosis. Mult Scler. 2002;8:161-168.

Mulcare JA, Jackson K. Neuromuscular diseases and exercise. In: ACSM's resource manual for guidelines for exercise testing and prescription. Philadelphia: Lippincott Williams & Wilkins; 2006. p. 514-527.

Mulcare JA, Petajan JH. Multiple sclerosis. In: Myers JN, Herbert WG, Humphrey R, eds. ACSM's resources for clinical exercise physiology: Musculoskeletal, neuromuscular, neoplastic, immunologic, and hematologic conditions. Philadelphia: Lippincott Williams & Wilkins; 2002. p. 29-37.

O'Sullivan SB. Multiple sclerosis. In: O'Sullivan SB, Schmitz TJ, eds. Physical rehabilitation. 5th ed. Philadelphia: Davis; 2007. p. 777-818.

Petajan JH. Weakness. In: Burke JS, Johnson KP, eds. Multiple sclerosis: Diagnosis, medical management, and rehabilitation. New York: Demos; 2000.

Petajan JH, Gappmaier E, White AT, et al. Impact of aerobic training on fitness and quality of life in MS. Ann Neurol. 1996;34:432-441.

Ponichtera-Mulcare JA. Exercise and multiple sclerosis. Med Sci Sports Exerc. 1993;25:451-465.

Ponichtera-Mulcare JA, Mathews T, Barrett PJ, Glaser RM. Change in aerobic fitness of patients with multiple sclerosis during a 6-month training program. Sport Med Train Rehabil. 1997;7:265-272.

Ponichtera-Mulcare JA, Mathews T, Glaser RM, Gupta SC. Maximal aerobic exercise of individuals with multiple sclerosis using three modes of ergometry. Clin Kinesiol. 1995;49(1):4-12.

Schapiro RT. Symptom management in multiple sclerosis. New York: Demos; 1987.

Snook EM, Motl RW. Effect of Exercise Training on Walking Mobility in Multiple Sclerosis: A Meta-Analysis. Neurorehabil Neural Repair. 2009; 23:108-116.

White LJ, McCoy SC, Castellano V, et al. Resistance training improves strength and functional capacity in persons with multiple sclerosis. Mult Scler. 2004;10:668-674.

Chapter 43

Agre JC, Rodriquez AA. Neuromuscular function: Comparison of symptomatic and asymptomatic polio patients to control subjects. Arch Phys Med Rehabil. 1990;71:545-551.

Agre JC, Rodriquez AA, Franke TM. Strength, endurance, and work capacity after muscle strengthening exercise in postpolio subjects. Arch Phys Med Rehabil. 1997;78:681-687.

Birk TJ. Poliomyelitis and the post-polio syndrome: Exercise capacities and adaptations. Current research, future directions, and widespread applicability. Med Sci Sports Exerc. 1993;25:466-472.

Birk TJ, Pitetti KH. Postpolio and Guillain-Barré syndrome. In: Myers JN, Herbert WG, Humphrey R, eds. ACSM's resources for clinical exercise physiology: Musculoskeletal, neuromuscular, neoplastic, immunologic, and hematologic conditions. Philadelphia: Lippincott Williams & Wilkins; 2002. p. 68-77.

Chan KM, Amirjani N, Sumrain M, Clarke A, Strohschein FJ. Randomized controlled trial of strength training in post-polio patients. Muscle Nerve. 2003;27:332-338.

Dalakas MC, Bartfield H, Kurland LT. The post-polio syndrome: Advances in the pathogenesis and treatment. Ann NY Acad Sci. 1995;753:314-320.

Dean E, Ross J. Modified aerobic walking program: Effect on patients with post-polio syndrome symptoms. Arch Phys Med Rehabil. 1988;69:1033-1038.

Einarsson G. Muscle conditioning in late poliomyelitis. Arch Phys Med Rehabil. 1991;72:11-13.

Finch LE, Ventruini A, Mayo NE, Trojan DA. Effort-limited treadmill walk test-reliability and validity in subjects with postpolio syndrome. Am J Phys Med Rehabil. 2004;83:613-623.

Grimby G, Einarsson G, Medberg M, Aniansson A. Muscle adaptive changes in post-polio subjects. Scand J Rehabil Med. 1989;21:19-26.

Horemans HL, Johannes BJ, Beelen A, Stam HJ, Nollet F. Walking in postpoliomyelitis syndrome: The relationships between time-scored tests, walking in daily life and perceived mobility problems. J Rehabil Med. 2005;37:142-146.

Horemans HL, Nollet F, Beelen A, Drost G, et al. Pyridostigmine in postpolio syndrome: No decline in fatigue and limited functional performance. J Neurol Neurosurg Psychiatry. 2003;74:1655-1661.

Jones DR, Speier J, Canine J, Owen R, Stull GA. Cardiorespiratory responses to aerobic training by patients with postpoliomyelitis sequelae. JAMA. 1989;261:3255-3258.

Spector SA, Gordon PL, Feuerstein IM, Sivakumar K, Hurley BF, Dalakas MC. Strength gain without muscle injury after strength training in patients with postpolio muscular atrophy. Muscle Nerve. 1996;19:1282-1290.

Willen C, Cider A, Summerhagen KS. Physical performance in individuals with late effects of polio. Scand J Rehabil Med. 1999;31:244-249.

Chapter 44

Dal Bello-Haas VP, Florence J, Kloos AD, et al. A randomized controlled trial of resistance exercise in individuals with ALS. Neurology. 2007;68:2003-2007.

Dal Bello-Haas V, Florence JM, Krivickas LS. Therapeutic exercise for people with amyotrophic lateral sclerosis or motor neuron disease. Cochrane Database Syst Rev. 2008;2:CD005229. DOI:10.1002/14651858.CD005229.pub2.

Dal Bello-Haas V, Kloos AD, Mitsumoto H. Physical therapy for a patient through six stages of amyotrophic lateral sclerosis. Phys Ther. 1998;78:1312-1324.

Drory VE, Goltsman E, Reznik JG, et al. The value of muscle exercise in patients with amyotrophic lateral sclerosis. J Neurol Sci. 2001;191:133-137.

Kaspar BK, Frost LM, Christian L, et al. Synergy of insulin-like growth factor-1 and exercise in amyotrophic lateral sclerosis. Ann Neurol. 2005;57:649.

Kent-Braun JA, Miller RG. Central fatigue during isometric exercise in amyotrophic lateral sclerosis. Muscle Nerve. 2000;23:909-914.

Kirkinezos IG, Hernandez D, Bradley WG, et al. Regular exercise is beneficial to a mouse model of amyotrophic lateral sclerosis. Ann Neurol. 2003;53:804-807.

Krivickas LS. Exercise in neuromuscular disease. J Clin Neuromusc Dis. 2003;5:29-39.

Krivickas LS, Carter GT. Amyotrophic lateral sclerosis: Practical aspects of care. J Spinal Cord Med. 2002;25(4):274-276.

Krivickas LS, Dal Bello-Haas V, Danforth SE, Carter GT. Rehabilitation. In: Mitsumoto H, Przedborski S, Gordon P, eds. Amyotrophic lateral sclerosis. New York: Taylor & Francis; 2006. p. 691-720.

Krivickas LS, Yang JI, Kim SK, et al. Skeletal muscle fiber function and rate of disease progression in amyotrophic lateral sclerosis: Case series. Muscle Nerve. 2002;26:636-643.

Mahoney DJ, Rodriguez C, Devries M, et al. Effects of high-intensity endurance exercise training in the G93A mouse model of amyotrophic lateral sclerosis. Muscle Nerve. 2004;29:656-662.

Pinto AC, Alves M, Nogueira A, et al. Can amyotrophic lateral sclerosis patients with respiratory insufficiency exercise? J Neurol Sci. 1999;169:69-75.

Sanjak M, Paulson D, Sufit R, et al. Physiologic and metabolic response to progressive and prolonged exercise in amyotrophic lateral sclerosis. Neurology. 1987;37:1217-1220.

Sharma KR, Kent-Braun JA, Majumdar S, et al. Physiology of fatigue in amyotrophic lateral sclerosis. Neurology. 1995;45:733-740.

Veldink JH, Bar PR, Joosten EA, et al. Sexual differences in onset of disease and response to exercise in a transgenic model of ALS. Neuromusc Dis. 2003;13:737-743.

Chapter 45

Albright AL. Spasticity and movement disorders in cerebral palsy. J Child Neurol. 1996;11(suppl 1):S1-S4.

Allen J, Dodd K, Taylor N, McBurney H, Larkin H. Strength training can be enjoyable and beneficial for adults with cerebral palsy. Disabil Rehabil. 2004;26(19):1121-1128.

Bodensteiner JB. The management of cerebral palsy: Subjectivity and conundrum. J Child Neurol. 1996;11(2):75-76.

Bowen TR, Lennon N, Castagno P, et al. Variability of energy-consumption measures in children with cerebral palsy. J Pediatr Orthop. 1998;18:738-742.

Buckon CE, Thomas SS, Piatt JH, et al. Selective dorsal rhizotomy versus orthopedic surgery: A multidimensional assessment of outcome efficacy. Arch Phys Med Rehabil. 2004;85(3):457-465.

Campbell SK. Quantifying the effects of interventions for movement disorders resulting from cerebral palsy. J Child Neurol. 1996;11(suppl 1):S61-S70.

Carr LJ, Cosgrove AP, Gringras P, et al. Position paper on the use of botulinum toxin in cerebral palsy. Arch Dis Child. 1998;79:271-273.

Carroll KL, Leiser J, Paisley TS. Cerebral palsy: Physical activity and sport. Curr Sports Med Rep. 2006;5(6):319-322.

Chad KE, Bailey DA, McKay HA, et al. The effect of a weight-bearing physical activity program on bone mineral content and estimated volumetric density in children with spastic cerebral palsy. J Pediatr. 1999;135:115-117.

Damiano DL. Activity, activity, activity: Rethinking our physical therapy approach to cerebral palsy (III STEP Series). Phys Ther. 2006;86(11):1534-1537.

Damiano DL, Abel MF. Functional outcomes of strength training in spastic cerebral palsy. Arch Phys Med Rehabil. 1998;79:119-125.

Goldstein M. The treatment of cerebral palsy: What we know, what we don't know. J Pediatr. 2004;145:S45-S46.

Odding E, Roebroeck ME, Stam HJ. The epidemiology of cerebral palsy: Incidence, impairments and risk factors. Disabil Rehabil. 2006;28(4):183-191.

Suzuki N, Oshimi Y, Shinohara T, Kawasumi M, Mita M. Exercise intensity based on heart rate while walking in spastic cerebral palsy. Bull NYU Hosp Jt Dis. 2001;60(1):18-22.

Chapter 46

Cakit BD, Saracoglu M, Genc H, et al. The effects of incremental speed-dependent treadmill training on postural instability and fear of falling in Parkinson's disease. Clin Rehabil. 2007;21:698-705.

Crizzle AM, Newhouse IJ. Is physical exercise beneficial for persons with Parkinson's disease? Clin J Sport Med. 2006;16:422-425.

de Goede CJ, Keus SH, Kwakkel G, et al. The effects of physical therapy in Parkinson's disease: A research synthesis. Arch Phys Med Rehabil. 2001;82:509-515.

Dibble LE, Hale TF, Marucs RL, et al. High-intensity resistance training amplifies muscle hypertrophy and functional gains in persons with Parkinson's disease. Mov Disord. 2006;21:1444-1452.

Deane KH, Jones D, Ellis-Hill C, et al. A comparison of physiotherapy techniques for patients with Parkinson's disease. Cochrane Database Syst Rev. 2001;1:CD002815.

Deane KH, Jones D, Playford ED, et al. Physiotherapy for patients with Parkinson's disease: A comparison of techniques. Cochrane Database Syst Rev. 2001;3:CD002817.

Ellis T, de Goede J, Feldman RG, et al. Efficacy of a physical therapy program in patients with Parkinson's disease: A randomized controlled trial. Arch Phys Med Rehabil. 2005;86:626-632.

Falvo MJ, Schilling BK, Earhart GM. Parkinson's disease and resistive exercise: Rationale, review, and recommendations. Mov Disord. 2007 Sep 25. [e-pub ahead of print].

Garber CE, Friedman JH. Effects of fatigue on physical activity and function in patients with Parkinson's disease. Neurology. 2007;60:1119-1124.

Giladi N, Balash Y. The clinical approach to gait disturbances in Parkinson's disease; maintaining independent mobility. J Neural Transm (suppl). 2006;70:327-332.

Herman T, Giladi N, Gruendlinger L. Six weeks of intensive treadmill training improves gait and quality of life in patients with Parkinson's disease: A pilot study. Arch Phys Med Rehabil. 2007;88:1154-1158.

Jankovic J, Lang AE. Movement disorders: Diagnosis and assessment. In: Bradley WG, Daroff RB, Fenichel GM, Jankovic

J, eds. Neurology in clinical practice. 4th ed. Philadelphia: Butterworth-Heinemann (Elsevier); 2004. p. 293-322.

Miyai I, Fujimoto Y, Yamamoto H, et al. Long-term effect of body-weight supported treadmill training in Parkinson's disease: A randomized, controlled trial. Arch Phys Med Rehabil. 2002;83:1370-1373.

Protas EJ, Williams A, Qureshy H, et al. Gait and step training to reduce falls in Parkinson's disease. Neurorehabilitation. 2005;20:183-190.

Reuter I, Engelhardt M, Stecker K, et al. Therapeutic value of exercise training in Parkinson's disease. Med Sci Sports Exerc. 1999;31:1544-1549.

Robichaud JA, Corcos DM. Motor deficits, exercise, and Parkinson's disease. Quest. 2005;57:85-107.

Rodriques de Paula F, Teixeira-Salmela LF, Coelho de Morais Faria CD, et al. Impact of an exercise program on physical, emotional, and social aspects of quality of life of individuals with Parkinson's disease. Mov Disord. 2006;21:1073-1077.

Suteerawattananon M, Morris GS, Etnyre BR, et al. Effect of visual and auditory cues on individuals with Parkinson's disease. J Neurol Sci. 2004;219:63-69.

Wu SS, Frucht SJ. Treatment of Parkinson's disease: What's on the horizon? CNS Drugs. 2005;19:723-743.

Chapter 47

Balic MG, Mateos EC, Blasco CG, et al. Physical fitness levels of physically active and sedentary adults with Down syndrome. Adapt Phys Activ Q. 2000;17:310-321.

Bricout VA, Guinot M, Faure P, Flore P, Eberhard Y, Garnier P, Favre Juvin A. Are hormonal responses to exercise in young men with Down's syndrome related to reduced endurance performance? J Neuroendocrinol. 2008;20(5):558-565.

Cooper RA, Quartrano LA, Axelson PW, et al. Research on physical activity and health among people with disabilities: A consensus statement. J Rehabil Res Dev. 1999;36:142-153.

Dodd KJ, Shields N. A systematic review of the outcomes of cardiovascular exercise programs for people with Down syndrome. Arch Phys Med Rehabil. 2005;86:2051-2058.

Fernhall B. Mental retardation. In: LeMura LM, von Duvillard SP, eds. Clinical exercise physiology: Application and physiological principles. Lippincott Williams & Wilkins; 2004. p. 617-627.

Fernhall B, McCubbin JA, Pitetti KH. Prediction of maximal heart rate in individuals with mental retardation. Med Sci Sports Exerc. 2001;33(10):1655-1660.

Fernhall B, Pitetti KH, Rimmer JH, et al. Cardiorespiratory capacity of individuals with mental retardation including Down syndrome. Med Sci Sports Exerc. 1996;28(3):366-371.

Fernhall B, Pitetti KH, Vukovich MD, et al. Validation of cardiovascular fitness field tests in children with mental retardation. Am J Ment Retard. 1998;102:602-612.

Guerra M, Roman B, Geronimo C, Violan M, Cuadrado E, Fernhall B. Physical fitness level of sedentary and active individuals with Down syndrome. Adapt Phys Activ Q. 2000;17:310-321.

Jones MC, Walley RM, Leech A, et al. Using goal attainment scaling to evaluate a needs-led exercise programme for people with severe and profound intellectual disabilities. J Intellect Disabil. 2006;10(4):317-335.

Krebs PL. Intellectual disabilities. In: Winnick JP, ed. Adapted physical education and sport. 4th ed. Champaign, IL: Human Kinetics; 2005. p. 133-154.

Luckasson R, Borthwick-Duffy S, Buntinx WHE, et al. Mental retardation: Definition, classification and systems of supports. 10th ed. Washington, DC: American Association on Mental Retardation; 2002. p. 8-17, 145-168.

Millar AL, Fernhall B, Burkett LN. Effects of aerobic training in adolescents with Down syndrome. Med Sci Sports Exerc. 1993;25:270-274.

Ouellette-Kuntz H. Commentary: Comprehensive health assessments for adults with intellectual disabilities. Int J Epidemiol. 2007;36(1):147-148.

Pitetti KH, Boneh S. Cardiovascular fitness as related to leg strength in adults with mental retardation. Med Sci Sports Exerc. 1995;27:423-428.

Pitetti KH, Fernhall B. Comparing run performance of adolescents with mental retardation with and without Down syndrome. Adapt Phys Activ Q. 2004;21:219-228.

Pitetti KH, Fernhall B. Mental retardation. In: Skinner JS, ed. Exercise testing and exercise prescription for special cases. 3rd ed. Baltimore: Lippincott Williams & Wilkins; 2005. p. 392-403.

Pitetti KH, Tan D. Effects of a minimally supervised exercise program for mentally retarded adults. Med Sci Sports Exerc. 1991;23:594-601.

Pitetti KH, Yarmer DA. Lower body strength of children and adolescents with and without mild mental retardation: A comparison. Adapt Phys Activ Q. 2002;18, 68-81.

Rimmer JH, Heller T, Wang E, Valerio I. Improvements in physical fitness in adults with Down syndrome. Am J Ment Retard. 2004;109:165-174.

Rimmer JH, Kelly L. Effects of resistance training program on adults with mental retardation. Adapt Phys Activ Q. 1991;8:146-153.

Rintala P, McCubbin JA, Downs SB, et al. Cross-validation of the 1-mile walking test for men with mental retardation. Med Sci Sports Exerc. 1998;29:133-137.

Shields N, Taylor NF, Dodd KY. Effects of a community-based progressive resistance training program on muscle performance and physical function in adults with Down syndrome: A randomized controlled trial. Arch Phys Med Rehabil. 2008;89:1215-1220.

Sullivan WF, Heng J, Cameron D, et al. Consensus guidelines for primary health care of adults with developmental disabilities. Can Fam Physician. 2006;52(11):1410-1418.

Thompson JR, Hughes C, Schalock RL, et al. Integrating supports in assessment planning. Ment Retard. 2002;40(5):390-405.

Chapter 48

American Psychiatric Association. Diagnostic and statistical manual of mental disorders. 4th ed. Washington, DC: American Psychiatric Association; 2000.

Arkin S, Mahendra N. Discourse analysis of alzheimer's patients before and after intervention: Methodology. Aphasiology. 2001;15:533-569.

Bonner AP, Cousins SO. Exercise and Alzheimer's disease: Benefits and barriers. Activ Adapt Aging. 1996;20:21-34.

Bowlby C. Therapeutic activities with persons disabled by Alzheimer's disease and related disorders. Rockville, MD: Aspen; 1993.

Desai A. Diagnosis and treatment of Alzheimer's disease. Neurology. 2005;64:S34-36.

Hellen CR. Alzheimer's disease: Activity focused care. Boston: Butterworth-Heinemann; 1998.

National Center on Physical Activity and Disability. [Online]. Alzheimer's disease and exercise fact sheet. www.ncpad. org/disability/fact_sheet.php?sheet=138.

Nelson ME, et al. Physical activity and public health in older adults: Recommendations from the American College of Sports Medicine and the American Heart Association. Med Sci Sports Exerc. 2007;39:1435-1445.

Palleschi L, Vetta F, deGennaro E, et al. Effects of aerobic training on the cognitive performance of elderly patients with senile dementia of the Alzheimer type. Gerontol Geriatr. 1996;S5:47-50.

Petersen RC. Mayo Clinic guide to Alzheimer's disease. Rochester, MN: Mayo Clinic; 2006.

Richter RW. Alzheimer's disease: A physician's guide to practical management. Totowa, NJ: Humana Press; 2004.

Stewart KJ. Physical activity and aging. Ann NY Acad Sci. 2005;1055:193-206.

Teri LT, et al. Exercise plus behavioral management in patients with Alzheimer disease: A randomized controlled trial. JAMA. 2003;290:2015-2022.

Teri LT, McCurry SM, Buchner DM, et al. Exercise and activity level in Alzheimer's disease: A potential treatment focus. J Rehabil Res Dev. 1998;35:411-419.

Chapter 49

American Psychiatric Association. Diagnostic and statistical manual of mental disorders. 4th ed. Washington, DC: American Psychiatric Association; 1994.

Center for Mental Health Services and National Institute of Mental Health. Manderscheld RW, Sonnenschen MA, eds. Mental health, United States. Department of Health and Human Services pub. no. SMA 92-1942. Washington, DC: Superintendent of Documents; 1992.

Greist JH, Klein MH, Eschens RR, et al. Running as treatment for depression. Compr Psychiatry. 1979;20:41-54.

Hutchinson DS, Gagne C, Bowers A, et al. A framework for health promotion services for people with psychiatric disabilities. Psychiatr Rehabil J. 2006;29(4):241-250.

Hutchinson DS, Skrinar GS, Cross S. The role of improved physical fitness in rehabilitation and recovery. Psychiatr Rehabil J. 1999;22(4):355-359.

Martinsen EW, Medhus A, Sandvik L. Effects of aerobic exercise on depression: A controlled study. BMJ. 1985;291:109.

National Institute of Mental Health. When someone has schizophrenia. 2001. Accessed 2001 Jun 28 from www.mental-health-matters.com/articles/article.php?artID=212.

New Freedom Commission on Mental Health. Achieving the promise: Transforming mental health care in America. Final report. Department of Health and Human Services pub. no. SMA-03-3832. Rockville, MD; 2003.

Pelham TW, Campagna PD. Benefits of exercise in psychiatric rehabilitation of persons with schizophrenia. Can J Rehabil. 1991;5:159-168.

Plante TG, Rodin J. Physical fitness and enhanced psychological health. Curr Psychol: Res Rev. 1990;9:1-22.

Richardson C, Faulkner G, McDevitt J, et al. Integrating physical activity into mental health services for persons with serious mental illness. Psychiatr Serv. 2005;56:324-331.

Skrinar GS, Huxley NA, Hutchinson D. The role of a fitness intervention on people with serious psychiatric disabilities, Psychiatr Rehabil J. 2005;29(2):122-127.

U.S. Department of Health and Human Services. The surgeon general's call to action to improve the health and wellness of persons with disabilities. U.S. Department of Health and Human Services, Office of the Surgeon General; 2005.

Chapter 50

Buckworth J, Dishman RK. Anxiety. In: Exercise psychology. Champaign, IL: Human Kinetics; 2002. p. 115-130.

Buckworth J, Dishman RK. Stress. In: Exercise psychology. Champaign, IL: Human Kinetics; 2002. p. 75-89.

Burghardt PR, Fulk LJ, Hand GA, Wilson MA. The effect of chronic treadmill and wheel running behavior in rats. Brain Res. 2004;1019:84-96.

Carrasco GA, De Kar LDV. Neuroendocrine pharmacology of stress. Eur J Pharmacol. 2003;463:235-272.

Chaouloff F. Effects of acute physical exercise on central serotonergic systems. Med Sci Sports Exerc. 1997;29:58-62.

Dishman RK, Jackson EM. Exercise, fitness, and stress. Int J Sport Psychol. 2000;31:175-203.

Fulk LJ, Stock HS, Lynn A, et al. Chronic physical exercise reduces anxiety-like behavior in rats. Int J Sports Med. 2004;25:78-82.

Hand GA, Hewitt CB, Fulk LJ, et al. Differential release of corticotropin-releasing hormone (CRH) in the amygdala during different types of stressors. Brain Res. 2002;949:122-130.

Hand GA, Phillips KD, Wilson MA. Central regulation of stress reactivity and physical activity. In: Acevedo E, Ekkekakis P, eds. The psychobiology of exercise and sport. Champaign, IL: Human Kinetics; 2006. p. 189-201.

McEntee DJ, Halgin RP. Cognitive group therapy and aerobic exercise in the treatment of anxiety. J Coll Stu Psychother. 1999;13(3):37-56.

Chapter 51

Blanchfield BB, et al. The severely to profoundly hearing-impaired population in the United States: Prevalence estimates and demographics. J Am Acad Audiol. 2001;12:183-189.

Compton CL. Assistive technology for the enhancement of receptive communication. In: Alpiner JG, McCarthy PA, eds. Rehabilitation audiology: Children and adults. 3rd ed. Philadelphia: Lippincott Williams & Wilkins; 2000. p. 501-555.

Dair J, Ellis MK, Lieberman LJ. Prevalence of overweight among deaf children. Am Ann Deaf. 2006;151(3):318-326.

Dummer GM, Ellis MK. Physical fitness of deaf children with cochlear implants. Pediatr Exerc Sci. 2003;15(1):101-102.

Ellis MK, Darby LA. Effect of balance on the determination of peak oxygen consumption in hearing and non-hearing female athletes. Adapt Phys Activ Q. 1993;10:216-225.

Ellis MK, Lieberman LJ, Fittipauldi-Wert J, et al. Health-related fitness of deaf children: How do they measure up? Palaestra. 2005;21(3):20-25.

Ellis MK, Stewart DA. Revisiting the effects of balance and motor skill development in deaf children. Can Assoc Educ Deaf Hard Hearing J. 1997;23(2/3):125-134.

Goodman J, Hopper C. Hearing impaired children and youth: A review of psychomotor behavior. Adapt Phys Activ Q. 1994;9:214-236.

Longmuir PE, Bar-Or O. Factors influencing the physical activity levels of youths with physical and sensory disabilities. Adapt Phys Activ Q. 2000;17(1):40-53.

Loovis CF, Schall DG, Teter DL. The role of assistive devices in the rehabilitation of hearing impairment. Otolaryngol Clin North Am. 1997;30(5):803-847.

Rubenstein JT, Miller CA. How do cochlear prostheses work? Curr Opin Neurobiol. 1999;399-404.

Stewart D. Deaf sport: Impact of sports within the deaf community. Washington, DC: Gallaudet University; 1991.

Stewart DA, Dummer GM, Haubenstricker JL. Review of administration procedures used to assess the motor skills of deaf children and youth. Adapt Phys Activ Q. 1990;7(3):231-239.

Stewart DA, Ellis MK. Revisiting the role of physical education for deaf children. In: Moores DF, Martin DS, eds. Deaf learners: Developments in curriculum and instruction. Washington, DC: Gallaudet University Press; 2006. p. 75-92.

Stewart DA, Ellis MK. Sports and the deaf child. Am Ann Deaf. 2005;150(1):59-66.

Stewart DA, Kluwin T. Teaching deaf and hard of hearing students: Content, strategies, and curriculum. Boston: Allyn & Bacon; 2001.

Weil E, Wachterman M, McCarthy E, Davis RP, O'Day B, Iezzoni LI, Wee CC. Obesity among adults with disabling conditions. JAMA. 2002;288:1265-1268.

Winnick JP, Short FX. A comparison of the physical fitness of segregated and integrated hearing impaired adolescents. Clin Kinesiol. 1986;42(4):104-109.

Chapter 52

Buell C. Physical education and recreation for the visually handicapped. Rev. ed. Reston, VA: American Alliance for Health, Physical Education, Recreation and Dance; 1982.

Buell C. Physical education for blind children. 2nd ed. Springfield, IL: Charles C Thomas; 1984.

Craft DH, Lieberman L. Visual impairments and deafness. In: Winnick JP, ed. Adapted physical education and sport. 2nd ed. Champaign, IL: Human Kinetics; 1995. p. 143-166.

Dunn JM, Leitschuh CA. Special physical education. 8th ed. Dubuque, IA: Kendall/Hunt; 2006.

Leverenz LJ. The case of the skiing porcupines: The relationship of blind competitive skiers with their guides. Palaestra. 1986;2(2):16-19, 53.

Lieberman LL, Cowart JF. Games for people with sensory impairments. Champaign, IL: Human Kinetics; 1996.

Paciorek M, Jones J. Sports and recreation for the disabled. 2nd ed. Carmel, IN: Cooper; 1994.

Richards P. Popular activities and games for blind, visually impaired and disabled people. New York: American Foundation for the Blind Press; 1986.

Shapiro D. Athletic identity and perceived competence in children with visual impairments. Palaestra. 2003;19(4):6-7.

Sherrill C. Blindness and visual impairment. In: Adapted physical activity, recreation, and sport. 6th ed. New York: McGraw-Hill; 2004.

Winnick J. The performance of visually impaired youngsters in physical education activities: Implications for mainstreaming. Adapt Phys Activ Q. 1985;2(4):292-299.

Index

Note: The italicized *f* and *t* following page numbers refer to figures and tables, respectively.

About the ACSM

The **American College of Sports Medicine (ACSM)**, founded in 1954, is a professional membership society with more than 20,000 national, regional, and international members in more than 70 countries dedicated to improving health through science, education, and medicine. ACSM members work in a wide range of medical specialties, allied health professions, and scientific disciplines. Members are committed to the diagnosis, treatment, and prevention of sport-related injuries and the advancement of the science of exercise.

The ACSM promotes and integrates scientific research, education, and practical applications of sports medicine and exercise science to maintain and enhance physical performance, fitness, health, and quality of life.